Isolation and Identification of Bioactive Secondary Metabolites

Isolation and Identification of Bioactive Secondary Metabolites

Editors

Ana M. L. Seca
Antoaneta Trendafilova

MDPI • Basel • Beijing • Wuhan • Barcelona • Belgrade • Manchester • Tokyo • Cluj • Tianjin

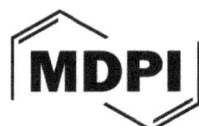

Editors
Ana M. L. Seca
cE3c/GBA, FCT—University
of Azores
Portugal

Antoaneta Trendafilova
Institute of Organic
Chemistry with Centre of
Phytochemistry, Bulgarian
Academy of Sciences
Bulgaria

Editorial Office
MDPI
St. Alban-Anlage 66
4052 Basel, Switzerland

This is a reprint of articles from the Special Issue published online in the open access journal *Foods* (ISSN 2304-8158) (available at: https://www.mdpi.com/journal/foods/special_issues/Bioactive_Secondary_Metabolites).

For citation purposes, cite each article independently as indicated on the article page online and as indicated below:

LastName, A.A.; LastName, B.B.; LastName, C.C. Article Title. *Journal Name* **Year**, *Volume Number*, Page Range.

ISBN 978-3-0365-3765-8 (Hbk)
ISBN 978-3-0365-3766-5 (PDF)

Cover image courtesy of Ana M. L. Seca

© 2022 by the authors. Articles in this book are Open Access and distributed under the Creative Commons Attribution (CC BY) license, which allows users to download, copy and build upon published articles, as long as the author and publisher are properly credited, which ensures maximum dissemination and a wider impact of our publications.

The book as a whole is distributed by MDPI under the terms and conditions of the Creative Commons license CC BY-NC-ND.

Contents

About the Editors ix

Ana M. L. Seca and Antoaneta Trendafilova
Secondary Metabolites in Edible Species: Looking beyond Nutritional Value
Reprinted from: *Foods* **2021**, *10*, 1131, doi:10.3390/foods10051131 1

Nayely Padilla-Montaño, Leandro de León Guerra and Laila Moujir
Antimicrobial Activity and Mode of Action of Celastrol, a Nortriterpen Quinone Isolated from Natural Sources
Reprinted from: *Foods* **2021**, *10*, 591, doi:10.3390/foods10030591 7

Silvie Rimpelová, Tomáš Zimmermann, Pavel B. Drašar, Bohumil Dolenský, Jiří Bejček, Eva Kmoníčková, Petra Cihlářová, Soňa Gurská, Lucie Kuklíková, Marián Hajdůch, Tomáš Ruml, Lubomír Opletal, Petr Džubák and Michal Jurášek
Steroid Glycosides Hyrcanoside and Deglucohyrcanoside: On Isolation, Structural Identification, and Anticancer Activity
Reprinted from: *Foods* **2021**, *10*, 136, doi:10.3390/foods10010136 25

Juan C. Ticona, Pablo Bilbao-Ramos, Ninoska Flores, M. Auxiliadora Dea-Ayuela, Francisco Bolás-Fernández, Ignacio A. Jiménez and Isabel L. Bazzocchi
(E)-Piplartine Isolated from *Piper pseudoarboreum*, a Lead Compound against *Leishmaniasis*
Reprinted from: *Foods* **2020**, *9*, 1250, doi:10.3390/foods9091250 45

Haichao Wen, Hui Cui, Hehe Tian, Xiaoxu Zhang, Liyan Ma, Charles Ramassamy and Jingming Li
Isolation of Neuroprotective Anthocyanins from Black Chokeberry (*Aronia melanocarpa*) against Amyloid-β-Induced Cognitive Impairment
Reprinted from: *Foods* **2021**, *10*, 63, doi:10.3390/foods10010063 57

Amani Taamalli, Anouar Feriani, Jesús Lozano-Sanchez, Lakhdar Ghazouani, Afoua El Mufti, Mohamed Salah Allagui, Antonio Segura-Carretero, Ridha Mhamdi and David Arráez-Roman
Potential Hepatoprotective Activity of Super Critical Carbon Dioxide Olive Leaf Extracts against CCl_4-Induced Liver Damage
Reprinted from: *Foods* **2020**, *9*, 804, doi:10.3390/foods9060804. 71

Stephanie Rodriguez, Mariano Walter Pertino, Chantal Arcos, Luana Reichert, Javier Echeverria, Mario Simirgiotis, Jorge Borquez, Alberto Cornejo, Carlos Areche and Beatriz Sepulveda
Isolation, Gastroprotective Effects and Untargeted Metabolomics Analysis of *Lycium Minutifolium* J. Remy (Solanaceae)
Reprinted from: *Foods* **2020**, *9*, 565, doi:10.3390/foods9050565. 89

Kawsar Hossen, Krishna Rany Das, Shun Okada, Arihiro Iwasaki, Kiyotake Suenaga and Hisashi Kato-Noguchi
Allelopathic Potential and Active Substances from *Wedelia Chinensis* (Osbeck)
Reprinted from: *Foods* **2020**, *9*, 1591, doi:10.3390/foods9111591 101

Virginia Hernández, M. Ángeles Botella, Pilar Hellín, Juana Cava, Jose Fenoll, Teresa Mestre, Vicente Martínez and Pilar Flores
Phenolic and Carotenoid Profile of Lamb's Lettuce and Improvement of the Bioactive Content by Preharvest Conditions
Reprinted from: *Foods* **2021**, *10*, 188, doi:10.3390/foods10010188 115

Zenon Węglarz, Olga Kosakowska, Jarosław. L. Przybył, Ewelina Pióro-Jabrucka and Katarzyna Bączek
The Quality of Greek Oregano (*O. vulgare* L. subsp. *hirtum* (Link) Ietswaart) and Common Oregano (*O. vulgare* L. subsp. *vulgare*) Cultivated in the Temperate Climate of Central Europe
Reprinted from: *Foods* **2020**, *9*, 1671, doi:10.3390/foods9111671 129

Janusz Malarz, Klaudia Michalska and Anna Stojakowska
Stem Lettuce and Its Metabolites: Does the Variety Make Any Difference?
Reprinted from: *Foods* **2021**, *10*, 59, doi:10.3390/foods10010059 143

Piret Saar-Reismaa, Katrin Kotkas, Viive Rosenberg, Maria Kulp, Maria Kuhtinskaja and Merike Vaher
Analysis of Total Phenols, Sugars, and Mineral Elements in Colored Tubers of *Solanum tuberosum* L.
Reprinted from: *Foods* **2020**, *9*, 1862, doi:10.3390/foods9121862 157

Hermenegildo R. Costa, Inês Simão, Helena Silva, Paulo Silveira, Artur M. S. Silva and Diana C. G. A. Pinto
Aglaomorpha quercifolia (L.) Hovenkamp & S. Linds a Wild Fern Used in Timorese Cuisine
Reprinted from: *Foods* **2021**, *10*, 87, doi:10.3390/foods10010087 169

Rosalba Leuci, Leonardo Brunetti, Viviana Poliseno, Antonio Laghezza, Fulvio Loiodice, Paolo Tortorella and Luca Piemontese
Natural Compounds for the Prevention and Treatment of Cardiovascular and Neurodegenerative Diseases
Reprinted from: *Foods* **2021**, *10*, 29, doi:10.3390/foods10010029 181

Lin-Lin Jiang, Xue Gong, Ming-Yue Ji, Cong-Cong Wang, Jian-Hua Wang and Min-Hui Li
Bioactive Compounds from Plant-Based Functional Foods: A Promising Choice for the Prevention and Management of Hyperuricemia
Reprinted from: *Foods* **2020**, *9*, 973, doi:10.3390/foods9080973 199

Antoaneta Trendafilova, Laila M. Moujir, Pedro M. C. Sousa and Ana M. L. Seca
Research Advances on Health Effects of Edible *Artemisia* Species and Some Sesquiterpene Lactones Constituents
Reprinted from: *Foods* **2021**, *10*, 65, doi:10.3390/foods10010065 223

About the Editors

Ana M. L. Seca has been an assistant professor at the University of Azores since 2000. She develops research in the Center for Ecology, Evolution and Environmental Changes—cE3c (ABG) as a full member, and in LAQV-REQUIMTE as a collaborator. She has a degree in Chemistry and an MSc in the Science and Technology of Paper and Forest Products, both obtained at the University of Aveiro, Portugal, where she also received her PhD in Chemistry in 2000. She has published 58 SCI papers and 8 book chapters. Her current research interests include the isolation and identification of secondary metabolites with potential pharmacological applications, and the synthesis of pharmaceutically relevant natural compound analogues.

Antoaneta Trendafilova is a professor from the Institute of Organic Chemistry with Centre of Phytochemistry, Bulgarian Academy of Sciences (IOCCP-BAS). She obtained her master's degree in Organic and Analytical Chemistry from the Faculty of Chemistry, Sofia University, and her PhD in Bioorganic Chemistry, Chemistry of Natural and Physiologically Active Compounds from IOCCP-BAS. She is the author of 100 research papers published across international journals. Her research interests include different aspects of natural product chemistry, such as the isolation, structural determination, and analysis of biologically active natural compounds and their chemotaxonomic significance.

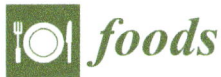

Editorial

Secondary Metabolites in Edible Species: Looking beyond Nutritional Value

Ana M. L. Seca [1,2,*] and Antoaneta Trendafilova [3,*]

1 cE3c—Centre for Ecology, Evolution and Environmental Changes/Azorean Biodiversity Group & Faculty of Sciences and Technology, University of Azores, Rua Mãe de Deus, 9500-321 Ponta Delgada, Portugal
2 LAQV-REQUIMTE, University of Aveiro, 3810-193 Aveiro, Portugal
3 Institute of Organic Chemistry with Centre of Phytochemistry, Bulgarian Academy of Sciences, Acad. G. Bonchev Str., bl. 9, 1113 Sofia, Bulgaria
* Correspondence: ana.ml.seca@uac.pt (A.M.L.S.); trendaf@orgchm.bas.bg (A.T.); Tel.: +351-296-650174 (A.M.L.S.); +359-296-06144 (A.T.)

Citation: Seca, A.M.L.; Trendafilova, A. Secondary Metabolites in Edible Species: Looking beyond Nutritional Value. *Foods* 2021, 10, 1131. https://doi.org/10.3390/foods10051131

Received: 10 May 2021
Accepted: 16 May 2021
Published: 19 May 2021

Publisher's Note: MDPI stays neutral with regard to jurisdictional claims in published maps and institutional affiliations.

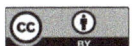

Copyright: © 2021 by the authors. Licensee MDPI, Basel, Switzerland. This article is an open access article distributed under the terms and conditions of the Creative Commons Attribution (CC BY) license (https://creativecommons.org/licenses/by/4.0/).

Secondary metabolites are organic molecules of low molecular weight, biosynthesized by any living being using a wide range of biosynthetic pathways, known as secondary metabolism. In evolutionary terms, secondary metabolism is seen as a set of specialized pathways that use a varied and specialized series of enzymes. Secondary metabolism aims to produce molecules with specific functions that promote the adaptability and survival of the species. However, secondary metabolites are not molecules essential to life, as are the lipids, carbohydrates and amino acids involved in basic life functions and produced by the primary metabolism. Terrestrial plants and algae, because they are sessile species, synthesize an admirable structural diversity of secondary metabolites.

Scientific research dedicated to the isolation and identification of secondary metabolites and the evaluation of their potential in different applications has already shown that these small molecules can be used in the promotion of human well-being, in the development of more sustainable agriculture and in the preservation of the environment.

Despite the knowledge already acquired, the consumer looks to the species used in cuisine, as a staple food, spice, or drinks, firstly based on its nutritional value (linked mainly to the primary metabolites present). The consumer is less focused on the different benefits related to the presence of secondary metabolites, such as the effect on the preservation and improvement of the organoleptic quality of the food, their medicinal and cosmetic effects, and as environmentally friendly herbicidal and pesticide agents.

Additionally, the research in this field is by no means complete. There are still many species, edible or not, whose profile in secondary metabolites is unknown and many other whose potential benefits to humanity have not yet been explored; and those in which some applications are already known, but the most relevant probably remains to be determined.

Thus, it remains pertinent to deepen the investigation on the isolation and identification of bioactive secondary metabolites, contributing so that the secondary metabolites present in a species are seen as an asset of that species, expanding the field of applications of the secondary metabolites and the species themselves, valuing them.

The special issue thematic "Isolation and Identification of Bioactive Secondary Metabolites" contributes to look at species beyond their nutritional value, giving them a wider and more efficient use, contributing to more sustainable management of natural resources.

This special issue brings together 12 original research papers which mainly demonstrate the value of several species, based on their secondary metabolites' composition, and based also in the effect of these metabolites on various applications.

Three of these research papers are dedicated to the identification and evaluation of secondary metabolites with potential pharmacological application.

Celastrol and pristimerin are two quinone-methide triterpenes isolated from species of Celastraceae family, which exhibit various biological activities such as cytotoxic, anti-obesity, and antidiabetic. In addition to the already known biological activities of these two natural compounds present in many species consumed in different world regions for their stimulating properties, Padilla-Montaño et al. [1] demonstrate for the first time the superior antibacterial effect of celastrol against *Bacillus subtilis*, when compared to pristimerin activity. Furthermore, they clarify the action mechanism of celastrol and its ability to act on multiple targets.

Rimpelová et al. [2] describe the cytotoxic effect of two cardiac glycosides, hyrcanoside and deglucohyrcanoside, isolated from seeds of *Coronilla varia* L. (this name is a synonym of *Securigera varia* (L.) Lassen) and reveal the high HEK 293T (transformed kidney cells) cell selectivity of deglucohyrcanoside, better than the well-known anticancer drug digitoxin.

Plants are a source of secondary metabolites that can act as antileishmanicidal agents. An example of this is the family of alkamides, characteristic constituents of *Piper* species that are widely used as culinary spices. (*E*)-Piplartine and (*E*)-demethoxypiplartine, two alkamides isolated from the leaves of *Piper pseudoarboreum* Yunck. exhibit higher potency against *Leishmania* spp. promastigotes and against *Leishmania amazonensis* amastigotes than the reference miltefosine. The activity of (*E*)-piplartine against cutaneous leishmaniasis is demonstrated in an in vivo model [3].

The beneficial health effects demonstrated by the pure secondary metabolites present in plants consumed in any region of the globe, promote these plants in addition to their possible nutritional value. Likewise, the health effects of semi-pure fractions from plant extracts chemically characterized may contribute to increase the value of these species.

The anthocyanins are a group of flavonoid derivatives which exhibit a broad range of bioactivities, such as antioxidant, antimicrobial and anti-inflammatory, and they can cross the blood-brain barrier acting on neurodegenerative targets. Wen et al. [4] present an optimized method for isolation of a rich-anthocyanins fraction from *Aronia melanocarpa* (Michx.) Elliott edible fruits, mainly constituted by four cyanidin 3-O-glycosides, and demonstrate, using an in vivo model, the neuroprotective effect of this fraction by improve spatial memory and protect against amyloid-β toxicity.

Compared with olive oil, the chemical composition and potential beneficial effects of olive leaves are still poorly investigated. Taamalli et al. [5] study the chemical composition of supercritical CO_2 extracts from fresh and dried olive leaves and their effect on hepatotoxicity caused by CCl_4 in a rat model. The authors identify and quantify 16 compounds (phenolic and terpenoid compounds) on the extracts being their composition significantly distinct. The in vivo study shows the hepatoprotective effect of both olive leaves extracts, due to significant improvement in hepatic fibrosis, biochemical parameters, and oxidative stress level after CCl_4-induced liver damage.

The edible infusion of bark from *Lycium minutifolium* J. Remy is used in Chilean traditional medicine to treat especially gastrointestinal disorders. This infusion and the ethyl acetate extract were studied by Rodriguez et al. [6] to identify the major secondary metabolites constituents (phenolic acids, flavonoids, coumarins, tropane and spermine alkaloids) and to obtain scientific data on the beneficial effect of these extracts, using an in vivo model and elucidating the action mechanism, to support its known gastroprotective properties. The edible infusion, at 100 mg/Kg, exhibit gastroprotective effect, on HCl/EtOH-induced gastric lesions in mice, higher than the ethyl acetate extract at same dose, and similar to the positive control at 30 mg/Kg.

Secondary metabolites biosynthesized by plant should not only be seen as potential pharmacological agents. Hossen et al. [7] demonstrate the allelopathic effect of *Wedelia chinensis* (Osbeck). Extracts of *Wedelia chinensis* exhibited high inhibitory activity against the root and shoot growth of cress, alfalfa, rapeseed, lettuce, foxtail fescue, Italian ryegrass, timothy, and barnyard grass and could be used for the biological control of weeds. Vanillic acid and gallic acid, isolated from the aqueous methanol extracts significantly arrested the growth of cress and Italian ryegrass seedlings. The concentrations of vanillic acid and gallic acid needed for 50% inhibition (I_{50} values) of the seedling growth of the cress and Italian ryegrass were 0.04–15.4 and 0.45–6.6 mM, respectively.

Several of the published articles on this special issue, in addition to identifying secondary metabolites, evaluate the variation of their content according to the cultivation conditions, between varieties and between different morphological parts of plant.

Hernández et al. [8] describe the phenolic, carotenoid and chlorophyll profile of lamb's lettuce (*Valerianella locusta* L. Laterr.), a vegetable used in various salads. LC/MS/MS analysis led to identification of 35 phenolic compounds including hydroxybenzoic and hydroxycinnamic acids, flavanols and flavanones. β-Carotene and lutein were the major carotenoids. It has also been found that different fertilization doses and salinity levels affected the concentrations of some compounds. The obtained results highlight the importance of these factors on the final metabolites contents of lamb's lettuce.

In another study, the differences between two subspecies: *Origanum vulgare* L. subsp. *hirtum* (Link) Ietsw. (Greek oregano) and *Origanum vulgare* L. subsp. *vulgare* (common oregano) growing in cultivation conditions within temperate climate of Central Europe were examined [9]. Greek oregano was distinguished by visibly higher number of glandular trichomes on the leaves and higher content of essential oil, total phenolic acids and rosmarinic acid in comparison to common oregano. Variation in the content of essential oil and rosmarinic acid in different stages of plant's development was also observed. The results of this study revealed that Greek oregano could be successfully adapted to different climatic conditions keeping essential oils with a chemical profile typical of Mediterranean cultivars.

In turn, Malarz et al. [10] study chemical constituents of the leaves from the old cultivar of asparagus lettuce (*Lactuca sativa* var. *angustana* cv. Grüner Stern) and compare them with those existing in other lettuce varieties, including wild lettuce. HPLC/DAD and ^{1}H NMR analysis of the methanolic extract of asparagus lettuce led to identification of five apocarotenoids, three sesquiterpene lactones, two lignans, five caffeic acid derivatives, and three flavonoids, some of which reported now for the first time in *L. sativa*. Stems, leaves and shoot tips of this variety were also examined to assess their phenolics and sesquiterpene lactone content, as well as DPPH scavenging activity. The results suggest that the leaves of the plant are the richest in antioxidant compounds. The investigated plant material, in terms of polyphenolic content and antioxidative activity, was similar to modern leafy cultivars of *L. sativa*.

Colored tubers of *Solanum tuberosum* L. are increasingly used in food, especially for their appealing colors. The contents of phenolic compounds and anthocyanins, well known for their antioxidant properties, as well as the content of sugars and minerals, were evaluated by Saar-Reismaa et al. [11] in the variety Blue Congo and its crossbreeds of Desiree and Granola and yellow-fleshed tubers. The results show that the content of antioxidant compounds varies among varieties and genotypes, being higher in purple-fleshed tubers than in yellow-fleshed ones. Moreover, the sugar content varies significantly between the studied specimens, with this content showing a positive correlation with the content of anthocyanins.

It is well-known that the profile of secondary metabolites varies depending on the morphological part of the plant. For species used in traditional medicine and gastronomy, it is imperative to know, in detail, the quantitative and qualitative composition of secondary metabolites in each morphological part. Only then will it be possible to take advantage of the potential of each part. Costa et al. [12] study the leaves and rhizome of *Aglaomorpha quercifolia* (L.) Hovenkamp & S. Linds (this name is currently considered synonymous with the Latin binominal name *Drynaria quercifolia* (L.) J.Sm.) used in Timor East in gastronomy and traditional medicine. The results show that the leaves are richest in fatty acids with high nutritional impact (ω6/ω3 ratio, atherogenicity index and thrombogenicity index), whereas the rhizome is richest in terpenes and steroids, some of them with proven medicinal properties.

This special issue also includes three literature review papers that emphasize the added value that the secondary metabolites, and the species they are isolated from, have in the development of new medicines to prevent/treat prevalent diseases.

Jiang et al. [13] present a comprehensive literature revision of the secondary metabolites present in plant-based functional foods that exhibit the ability to lower the level of uric acid, using in vitro and in vivo models. A detailed discussion concerning the targets and the action mechanism associated to their hypouricemic effect is presented.

Leuci et al. [14] review the most recent studies on the isolation and identification of secondary metabolites from plants and fungi, with impactful effects, in vitro and in vivo models, on targets related to the development of cardiovascular and neurodegenerative diseases.

The third review paper [15] focuses on edible species of the botanical genus *Artemisia*. The uses of these species in culinary and beverages and their nutritional value are reviewed, as well as some of their secondary metabolites belonging to the sesquiterpene lactone family. The pharmacological potential and possible adverse effects of these secondary metabolites and species are discussed based on results obtained in in vivo studies and clinical trials.

In conclusion, the fifteen articles published in this special edition reflect the latest research trends regarding the isolation, identification, and assessment of the beneficial effects of secondary metabolites, from edible or inedible species, contributing to these compounds and the plants of origin to be valued beyond the nutritional perspective.

Author Contributions: A.M.L.S. and A.T. conceived, designed, and wrote the editorial. Both authors have read and agreed to the published version of the manuscript.

Funding: This work was funded by FCT–Fundação para a Ciência e a Tecnologia, the European Union, QREN, FEDER, COMPETE, by funding the cE3c centre (UIDB/00329/2020) and the LAQV-REQUIMTE (UIDB/50006/2020) research units, and funded by the project EthnoHERBS (H2020-MSCA-RISE-2018, No. 823973). Thanks are due also to the University of Azores and Institute of Organic Chemistry with Centre of Phytochemistry, Bulgarian Academy of Sciences for their support.

Conflicts of Interest: The authors declare no conflict of interest.

References

1. Padilla-Montaño, N.; de León Guerra, L.; Moujir, L. Antimicrobial Activity and Mode of Action of Celastrol, a Nortriterpen Quinone Isolated from Natural Sources. *Foods* **2021**, *10*, 591. [CrossRef] [PubMed]
2. Rimpelová, S.; Zimmermann, T.; Drašar, P.B.; Dolenský, B.; Bejček, J.; Kmoníčková, E.; Cihlářová, P.; Gurská, S.; Kuklíková, L.; Hajdůch, M.; et al. Steroid Glycosides Hyrcanoside and Deglucohyrcanoside: On Isolation, Structural Identification, and Anticancer Activity. *Foods* **2021**, *10*, 136. [CrossRef] [PubMed]
3. Ticona, J.C.; Bilbao-Ramos, P.; Flores, N.; Dea-Ayuela, M.A.; Bolás-Fernández, F.; Jiménez, I.A.; Bazzocchi, I.L. (*E*)-Piplartine Isolated from *Piper pseudoarboreum*, a Lead Compound against Leishmaniasis. *Foods* **2020**, *9*, 1250. [CrossRef] [PubMed]
4. Wen, H.; Cui, H.; Tian, H.; Zhang, X.; Ma, L.; Ramassamy, C.; Li, J. Isolation of Neuroprotective Anthocyanins from Black Chokeberry (*Aronia melanocarpa*) against Amyloid-β-Induced Cognitive Impairment. *Foods* **2021**, *10*, 63. [CrossRef] [PubMed]
5. Taamalli, A.; Feriani, A.; Lozano-Sanchez, J.; Ghazouani, L.; El Mufti, A.; Allagui, M.S.; Segura-Carretero, A.; Mhamdi, R.; Arráez-Roman, D. Potential Hepatoprotective Activity of Super Critical Carbon Dioxide Olive Leaf Extracts against CCl4-Induced Liver Damage. *Foods* **2020**, *9*, 804. [CrossRef] [PubMed]
6. Rodriguez, S.; Pertino, M.W.; Arcos, C.; Reichert, L.; Echeverria, J.; Simirgiotis, M.; Borquez, J.; Cornejo, A.; Areche, C.; Sepulveda, B. Isolation, Gastroprotective Effects and Untargeted Metabolomics Analysis of *Lycium minutifolium* J. Remy (Solanaceae). *Foods* **2020**, *9*, 565. [CrossRef] [PubMed]
7. Hossen, K.; Das, K.R.; Okada, S.; Iwasaki, A.; Suenaga, K.; Kato-Noguchi, H. Allelopathic Potential and Active Substances from *Wedelia chinensis* (Osbeck). *Foods* **2020**, *9*, 1591. [CrossRef] [PubMed]
8. Hernández, V.; Botella, M.Á.; Hellín, P.; Cava, J.; Fenoll, J.; Mestre, T.; Martínez, V.; Flores, P. Phenolic and Carotenoid Profile of Lamb's Lettuce and Improvement of the Bioactive Content by Preharvest Conditions. *Foods* **2021**, *10*, 188. [CrossRef] [PubMed]
9. Węglarz, Z.; Kosakowska, O.; Przybył, J.L.; Pióro-Jabrucka, E.; Bączek, K. The Quality of Greek Oregano (*O. vulgare* L. subsp. *hirtum* (Link) Ietswaart) and Common Oregano (*O. vulgare* L. subsp. *vul-gare*) Cultivated in the Temperate Climate of Central Europe. *Foods* **2020**, *9*, 1671. [CrossRef]
10. Malarz, J.; Michalska, K.; Stojakowska, A. Stem Lettuce and Its Metabolites: Does the Variety Make Any Difference? *Foods* **2021**, *10*, 59. [CrossRef] [PubMed]
11. Saar-Reismaa, P.; Kotkas, K.; Rosenberg, V.; Kulp, M.; Kuhtinskaja, M.; Vaher, M. Analysis of Total Phenols, Sugars, and Mineral Elements in Colored Tubers of *Solanum tuberosum* L. *Foods* **2020**, *9*, 1862. [CrossRef] [PubMed]
12. Costa, H.R.; Simão, I.; Silva, H.; Silveira, P.; Silva, A.M.S.; Pinto, D.C.G.A. *Aglaomorpha quercifolia* (L.) Hovenkamp & S. Linds a Wild Fern Used in Timorese Cuisine. *Foods* **2021**, *10*, 87. [CrossRef]
13. Jiang, L.-L.; Gong, X.; Ji, M.-Y.; Wang, C.-C.; Wang, J.-H.; Li, M.-H. Bioactive Compounds from Plant-Based Functional Foods: A Promising Choice for the Prevention and Management of Hyperuricemia. *Foods* **2020**, *9*, 973. [CrossRef] [PubMed]

14. Leuci, R.; Brunetti, L.; Poliseno, V.; Laghezza, A.; Loiodice, F.; Tortorella, P.; Piemontese, L. Natural Compounds for the Prevention and Treatment of Cardiovascular and Neurodegenerative Diseases. *Foods* **2021**, *10*, 29. [CrossRef] [PubMed]
15. Trendafilova, A.; Moujir, L.M.; Sousa, P.M.C.; Seca, A.M.L. Research Advances on Health Effects of Edible *Artemisia* Species and Some Sesquiterpene Lactones Constituents. *Foods* **2021**, *10*, 65. [CrossRef] [PubMed]

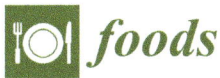

Article

Antimicrobial Activity and Mode of Action of Celastrol, a Nortriterpen Quinone Isolated from Natural Sources

Nayely Padilla-Montaño, Leandro de León Guerra and Laila Moujir *

Departamento de Bioquímica, Microbiología, Biología Celular y Genética, Facultad de Farmacia, Universidad de La Laguna, Avenida Astrofísico Fco Sánchez s/n, 382016 Tenerife, Spain; nayelypadilla@hotmail.com (N.P.-M.); lleongue@ull.edu.es (L.d.L.G.)
* Correspondence: lmoujir@ull.edu.es; Tel.: +34-922-318-513

Citation: Padilla-Montaño, N.; de León Guerra, L.; Moujir, L. Antimicrobial Activity and Mode of Action of Celastrol, a Nortriterpen Quinone Isolated from Natural Sources. *Foods* **2021**, *10*, 591. https://doi.org/10.3390/foods10030591

Academic Editors: Ana Maria Loureiro da Seca and Antoaneta Trendafilova

Received: 12 February 2021
Accepted: 5 March 2021
Published: 11 March 2021

Publisher's Note: MDPI stays neutral with regard to jurisdictional claims in published maps and institutional affiliations.

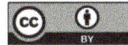

Copyright: © 2021 by the authors. Licensee MDPI, Basel, Switzerland. This article is an open access article distributed under the terms and conditions of the Creative Commons Attribution (CC BY) license (https://creativecommons.org/licenses/by/4.0/).

Abstract: Species of the Celastraceae family are traditionally consumed in different world regions for their stimulating properties. Celastrol, a triterpene methylene quinone isolated from plants of celastraceas, specifically activates satiety centers in the brain that play an important role in controlling body weight. In this work, the antimicrobial activity and mechanism of action of celastrol and a natural derivative, pristimerin, were investigated in *Bacillus subtilis*. Celastrol showed a higher antimicrobial activity compared with pristimerin, being active against Gram-positive bacteria with minimum inhibitory concentrations (MICs) that ranged between 0.16 and 2.5 µg/mL. Killing curves displayed a bactericidal effect that was dependent on the inoculum size. Monitoring of macromolecular synthesis in bacterial populations treated with these compounds revealed inhibition in the incorporation of all radiolabeled precursors, but not simultaneously. Celastrol at 3 µg/mL and pristimerin at 10 µg/mL affected DNA and RNA synthesis first, followed by protein synthesis, although the inhibitory action on the uptake of radiolabeled precursors was more dramatic with celastrol. This compound also caused cytoplasmic membrane disruption observed by potassium leakage and formation of mesosome-like structures. The inhibition of oxygen consumption of whole and disrupted cells after treatments with both quinones indicates damage in the cellular structure, suggesting the cytoplasmic membrane as a potential target. These findings indicate that celastrol could be considered as an interesting alternative to control outbreaks caused by spore-forming bacteria.

Keywords: celastrol; Celastraceae; antimicrobial activity; mechanism of action; *Bacillus subtilis*

1. Introduction

Historically, plants have provided a wide variety of active compounds, becoming a key element in the development of many cultures. The Celastraceae family, commonly known as the bittersweet family, comprises a group of plants distributed mainly in tropical and subtropical regions of the world including North Africa, South America, and East Asia. It has a long history in traditional medicine as a stimulant, diuretic, emmenagogue, anti-inflammatory, antibacterial, anti-cancer, and for the treatment of gastrointestinal disorders among others [1]. In the Canary Islands, East Africa, and the Arabian Peninsula, the leaves of members of this family are chewed to combat fatigue [1,2]. In our search for antimicrobial compounds from plants, we isolated celastrol and its methylated derivative, pristimerin, which are the first and the most frequently reported celastroloids. The term celastroloid refers to methylene quinone nor-triterpenes with a 24-nor-*D*: *A*-friedo-oleanane skeleton, which, later on, was extended to related phenolic nor-triterpenes [3] and their dimer and trimer congeners. The two natural pentacyclic triterpenoids celastrol and pristimerin are commonly found in the roots and bark of Celastraceae species. Both compounds show a wide range of pharmacological activities, including anti-cancer, anti-inflammatory, antioxidant, hepatoprotective, or immunomodulatory, among others [4–8]. The anti-cancer properties of celastrol, one of the most studied methylene quinones, have been attributed to apoptosis and autophagy induction, cell cycle arrest, and anti-metastatic and anti-angiogenic action [9,10]. Other works have evidenced the ability of celastrol in combating metabolic disorders such as obesity and type 2 diabetes [11]. Treatment with celastrol suppresses food intake, blocks reduction in energy consumption, and mediates weight loss by acting as a leptin sensitizer in mouse models [12,13].

In addition to these pharmacological activities, antimicrobial properties have also been demonstrated for these and other related triterpenoids such as tingenone, netzahualcoyone, or zeylasterone that exhibit inhibitory activity against Gram-positive bacteria [14–17]. Moreover, the anti-biofilm [18–20] and anti-fouling properties of celastrol and pristimerin have been reported on a wide variety of microorganisms [21], as well as anti-mycotic activity [22–27]. Besides, celastrol and its derivatives have also shown inhibitory activity against viruses producing hepatitis B and C [28,29], which makes them potentially useful compounds for the control of various diseases. This paper describes the antimicrobial activity and mechanism of action of celastrol and pristimerin using *Bacillus subtilis* as a model of spore-forming bacteria. Species of *Bacillus* have been associated with many food contaminations causing food-borne illness in humans [30], spoilage of processed food products [31,32], or certain pathologies such as pneumonia, bacteremia, and meningitis in immunosuppressed patients [33–35]. Regardless of variations in disease presentation, the etiologic agent is often the spore and the production of toxins that play a central role in the pathophysiology of the infection. Although it is generally accepted that the antimicrobial activity of terpenoid compounds involves damage on plasma membrane [36], little is known about how this affects other cellular processes essential to bacterial cell development. Thus, the action of these compounds on different metabolic pathways such as macromolecular synthesis, uptake of solutes and biosynthetic precursors, or the damage on membrane function was investigated.

2. Materials and Methods

2.1. Microorganisms

Strains used for determining antimicrobial activity included *Bacillus subtilis* ATCC 6051, *B. cereus* ATCC 21772, *B. megaterium* ATCC 25848, *B. pumilus* ATCC 7061, *Staphylococcus aureus* ATCC 6538, *S. epidermidis* ATCC 14990, *S. saprophyticus* ATCC 15305, *Enterococcus faecalis* CECT 795 (from Type Culture Spanish Collection), *Mycobacterium smegmatis* ATCC 19420, *Proteus mirabilis* CECT170, *Escherichia coli* ATCC 9637, *Pseudomonas aeruginosa* AK958 (from the University of British Columbia, Department of Microbiology collection), *Salmonella* spp. CECT 456, and *Candida albicans* CECT 1039.

Bacterial cultures were developed at 37 °C in nutrient broth (NB), except for *E. faecalis* and *M. smegmatis* that were grown in brain heart infusion broth (BHI), or *C. albicans* cultured in Sabouraud liquid medium. All media were purchased from Oxoid.

2.2. Quinones and Others Antibacterial Compounds

Celastrol and pristimerin were isolated, purified, and characterized from the roots of Celastraceae species as previously reported [37,38]. Pure compounds were dissolved in dimethyl sulfoxide (DMSO) before the evaluation. The reference antibacterial agents ciprofloxacin, rifampicin, tetracycline, penicillin, and clofoctol (Sigma-Aldrich, St. Louis, MO, USA) were used as controls according to the Clinical and Laboratory Standards Institute [39].

2.3. Determination of Minimum Inhibitory Concentration (MIC) and Minimum Bactericidal Concentration (MBC)

The antimicrobial activity was determined for each compound in triplicate by broth microdilution method (range 0.08–40 µg/mL) in 96-well microtiter plates, according to the M07-A9 approved standard of the Clinical and Laboratory Standards Institute (CLSI) [40]. Wells with the same proportions of DMSO were used as controls and never exceeded 1% (v/v). The starting concentration of microorganism ranged between 1 and 5×10^5 colony-forming units (CFU)/mL, and growth was monitored by measuring the increase in optical density at 550 nm (OD_{550}) with a microplate reader (Infinite M200, Tecan Group Ltd., Männedorf, Switzerland) and viable count in agar plates. The minimum inhibitory concentration (MIC) was defined as the lowest concentration of compound that completely inhibits growth of the organisms compared to the untreated cells. All wells with no visible growth were subcultured in duplicate by transferring (100 µL) to nutrient, BHI, or Sabouraud agar plates. After overnight incubation, colony counts were performed and the minimum bactericidal concentration (MBC) was defined as the lowest compound concentration that produces ≥99.9% killing of the initial inoculum.

2.4. Bacterial Killing Assays

Overnight liquid cultures of *B. subtilis* were diluted in Monod's flask containing 10 mL of NB medium, to give a working concentration ranging between 1 and 5×10^5 CFU/mL. Celastrol (3 µg/mL) or pristimerin (10 µg/mL) was added at time 0 (lag phase) or after 3 h of incubation (log-phase, $OD_{550} \approx 0.4$). These suspensions were incubated at 37 °C in a rotator shaker and growth was monitored by measuring the OD_{550} and CFU count on nutrient agar plates. Cultures with known antibiotics or without drugs were used as positive and negative controls, respectively. The assays were repeated at least three times.

2.5. Inoculum Effect

Overnight liquid cultures of *B. subtilis* were 10-fold serial diluted in NB medium to give different inoculum concentrations (10^3 to 10^7 CFU/mL). Celastrol (3 µg/mL) and pristimerin (10 µg/mL) were added and cultures were incubated at 37 °C in a rotatory shaker. Bacterial growth was monitored as described above. The assays were repeated at least three times.

2.6. Measurement of Radioactive Precursor Incorporation

Cultures of *B. subtilis* were diluted to obtain 10^6 CFU/mL in Davis–Mingioli medium [41] supplemented with glucose (1%), asparagine (0.1 g/L), and casamino acids (2 g/L) (pH 7). The cultures were grown at 37 °C under shaking for at least 3 h to obtain an optical density (OD_{550}) of 0.4. Volumes of 10 mL were transferred to prewarmed flasks containing celastrol (3 µg/mL) or pristimerin (10 µg/mL) and one of the precursors of DNA (1 µCi/mL [6-^{3}H] + 2 µg/mL unlabeled thymidine), RNA (1 µCi/mL [5-^{3}H] + 2 µg/mL unlabeled uridine), protein (5 µCi/mL [4,5-^{3}H] + 2 µg/mL unlabeled leucine), or cell wall peptidoglycan (0.1 µCi/mL N-Acetyl-D-[1-^{14}C] glucosamine). The samples were incubated at 37 °C under shaking. Volumes of 0.5 mL were collected and precipitated with 2 mL ice-cold 10% trichloroacetic acid (TCA) at different times. After 30 min of incubation in cold TCA, samples were filtered on glass microfiber filters grade GF/C (Whatman, Maidstone, UK)) and washed three times with 5 mL cold 10% TCA and once with 5 mL of 95% ethanol. The dried filters were placed in vials covered with a scintillation cocktail and counted in counter LKB Wallac Rackbeta (Perkin Elmer, Courtaboeuf, France). Macromolecular synthesis was measured by quantifying the incorporation of radiolabeled precursors (Amersham Biosciences Europe GmbH) into acid-insoluble material. Evaluations with DMSO added in the same proportion or a specific inhibitor of each biosynthetic pathway were included as negative and positive controls, respectively.

2.7. Measurement of Solutes Uptake

Solutes uptake was measured as total cell-associated counts after addition of quinones on cultures of *B. subtilis* growing exponentially ($OD_{550} \approx 0.2$). Growing cells containing half concentration of NB medium were transferred to prewarmed flasks containing celastrol (3 µg/mL) or pristimerin (10 µg/mL) and radiolabeled glucose (2 µCi/mL D-[1-^{14}C]-glucose) or the precursors of DNA, RNA, protein, and cell wall peptidoglycan (see concentrations in previous section). At different times (up to 30 min), 0.5 mL of samples was collected and filtered through Millipore filters of 0.45-µm pore size (Type HA, Millipore Corporation, Burlington, MA, USA). Filters were washed three times with 5 mL phosphate buffer, dried, and radioactivity was measured as above. Samples with clofoctol (5 µg/mL) or DMSO at the same concentration were included as positive and negative controls, respectively.

Furthermore, the effect of celastrol on the uptake and incorporation of radiolabeled precursors of DNA was also evaluated when the macromolecular synthesis was inhibited. *B. subtilis* cultures prepared as described above were treated for 30 min with the specific inhibitor ciprofloxacin (1.5 µg/mL) before the addition of labeled and unlabeled precursor. After 5 min, celastrol (3 µg/mL) or the same proportion of DMSO in control cultures was incorporated. At different times, precursor uptake and incorporation was measured as mentioned above. The assays were repeated at least three times.

2.8. Inhibition of DNA Gyrase

Inhibition of DNA gyrase was performed using the Gyrase Supercoiling kit 1 (#K001) (John Innes Enterprises Ltd., Norwich, UK) as described in the manufacturer's instructions. Two units of DNA gyrase were incubated with 0.5 µg relaxed plasmid pBR322 and 50 µg/mL of celastrol or pristimerin in a final volume of 30 µL. Ciprofloxacin at 25 and 50 µg/mL was used as positive control. The samples were incubated at 30 °C for 30 min and the products were visualized in 0.8% agarose gel containing 0.5 µg/mL ethidium bromide.

2.9. Integrity of Cell Membrane

Bacterial membrane damage was examined by determination of the release of material absorbing at 260/280 nm, detection of potassium (K^+) leakage, and the BacLight Live/Dead staining method (Invitrogen Molecular Probes, Eugene, OR, US). *B. subtilis* cultures in log-phase growth ($OD_{550} \approx 0.8$) were centrifuged at $15,000 \times g$ for 10 min at 4 °C and washed twice with saline buffer. The pellet was resuspended in the same buffer to obtain a bacterial concentration of $1–2 \times 10^8$ CFU/mL (or $1–2 \times 10^7$ CFU/mL for K^+ leakage experiments). Cell cultures were treated with celastrol (3 µg/mL) and incubated at 37 °C under shaking. Cultures with clofoctol (10 µg/mL) or DMSO at the same concentration were used as positive and negative controls, respectively. Samples were collected for quantification at different times over a 30-min period. Liberation of cytoplasmic materials was monitored by measuring the optical density (OD_{260} and OD_{280}) of the supernatant after removing cells by centrifugation (at $9500 \times g$ for 10 min, 4 °C) or after membrane filtration by means of an atomic absorption spectrophotometer (Model Thermo S-Series, Thermo Electron Corporation, Cambridge, UK) for K^+ release. The BacLight assay was analyzed after a 20-min dark-staining period following the manufacturer's instructions. The cells were visualized at $\times 1000$ magnification with an epifluorescence microscope (Leica DM4B, Leica Microsystems GmbH, Wetzlar, Germany) provided with a fluorescein–rhodamine dual filter.

2.10. Transmission Electron Microscopy

To further confirm the mode of action of celastrol on *B. subtilis*, transmission electron microscopy (TEM) analysis was performed. Suspensions of *B. subtilis* in log-phase growth (10^7 CFU/mL) were treated with celastrol (3 µg/mL) for 1 h at 37 °C and were harvested at $6500 \times g$ for 8 min at 4 °C. For comparative purposes, bacterial cells grown under the same conditions were also treated with pristimerin (10 µg/mL). Subsequently, bacteria were washed in fixative buffer, post-fixed in 1% osmium tetroxide in fixative buffer, and washed with distilled water. Sections (1 µm) were cut with a Reichert Ultracut ultramicrotome and stained with toluidine blue; ultra-thin sections were contrasted with uranyl acetate and lead. Preparations were observed under a Zeiss EM 912 transmission electron microscope. Images were captured with a Proscan Slow-scan CCD-Camera for TEM (Proscan, Scheuring, Germany) and Soft Imaging System software (version 5.2, Olympus Soft Imaging Solutions GmbH, Münster, Germany). Control experiments with the same proportion of DMSO were performed in parallel.

2.11. Oxygen Consumption

Suspensions of *B. subtilis* and *E. coli* in the log phase of growth ($OD_{550} \approx 0.8$) were centrifuged at 15,000× g for 10 min at 4 °C and washed twice with phosphate buffer 0.1 M (pH 7.0). Then, the pellet was suspended in the same buffer to obtain a bacterial concentration of 1–2 × 10^7 CFU/mL. Cells suspensions (2.7 mL) supplemented with 0.3 mL of 10% glucose were used to measure oxygen consumption at room temperature in a glass cell of Clark oxygen electrode equipped with a magnetic stirrer. Celastrol (at 3 µg/mL for *B. subtilis* and 20 µg/mL for *E. coli*) was added to the cell suspension, and the steady-state output of the oxygen electrode (after 4 min) was measured using a digital biological oxygen monitor (model YSI 5300, Yellow Springs, OH, USA). DMSO in the same proportion and sodium cyanate at 6.7 mM were used as negative and positive controls, respectively. Furthermore, disrupted cell preparations of *B. subtilis* and *E. coli* were used to determine the effect of celastrol on oxygen uptake using NADH (0.1 mM) as a substrate. Cultures grown in yeast extract and peptone (YP, 1% w/v) medium for 18 h at 37 °C under aeration were collected by centrifugation at 10,000× g for 10 min at 4 °C. Cells were washed twice in 0.1 M potassium phosphate buffer (pH 7.0), resuspended in the same buffer (5 mL of buffer per gram of cells), and sonicated (Labsonic M, Sartorius Stedim Biotech, Göttingen, Germany) for 15 min in 10-s bursts with 20-s stop intervals. Intact cells were removed by centrifugation at 4000× g for 10 min at 4 °C. The supernatant was centrifuged at 15,000× g for 10 min at 4 °C and the pellet was resuspended in the same buffer as before (5 mL). Aliquots (0.2 mL) of disrupted cells were incubated at room temperature in the same buffer (2.8 mL) containing NADH (0.1 mM).

2.12. Statistical Analysis

Three independent experiments were conducted for each evaluation and means and standard deviations (±SD) were calculated. Analysis of variance (one-way ANOVA) followed by Tukey's multiple comparison test ($p < 0.05$) to extract the specific differences between treatments were performed using R statistical software environment version 4.0.3 (R Foundation for Statistical Computing, Vienna, Austria).

3. Results and Discussion

3.1. Antimicrobial Activity

Table 1 shows the MICs and MBCs of celastrol and pristimerin against different microorganisms used in this study. Celastrol was active against all Gram-positive bacteria evaluated, with MIC values ranging between 0.16 (*B. subtilis*) and 2.5 µg/mL (*S. saprophyticus*). Compared to celastrol, pristimerin showed weaker activity on Gram-positive bacteria and no action on *S. aureus* and *M. smegmatis*. On the basis of these results, *B. subtilis* was selected to evaluate the mechanism of action of these quinones.

Table 1. Minimum inhibitory concentration (MIC) [1] and minimum bactericidal concentration (MBC) [1] of celastrol and pristimerin, expressed in µg/mL against different microorganisms [2].

Microorganisms	Celastrol		Pristimerin	
	MIC	MBC	MIC	MBC
Bacillus subtilis	0.156	2.5	1.25	10
B. cereus	0.625	2.5	10	>40
B. pumilus	0.625	2.5	2	10
B. megaterium	1.25	5	20	>40
Staphylococcus aureus	1.25	>40	>40	>40
S. epidermidis	0.312	15	1.25	>40
S. saprophyticus	2.5	10	10	10
Mycobacterium smegmatis	5	>40	>40	>40
Enterococcus faecalis	1.25	40	20	>40

[1] Values represent average obtained from a minimum of three experiments. [2] The quinone compounds were inactive against Gram-negative bacteria and the yeast assayed (MIC > 40 µg/mL).

Gram-negative bacteria and the yeast *C. albicans* were insensitive to the action of both compounds at the maximum concentration assayed (40 μg/mL). The inactivity of pristimerin against *S. aureus* was previously reported by our group [24], although in later works, da Cruz et al. [42] indicated MIC values of 25 μg/mL. The use of a bacterial strain of *S. aureus* less sensitive to the activity of the compound could explain this difference in the results. Gullo et al. [23] reported antimicrobial activity for pristimerin against *C. albicans* with an MIC of 250 μg/mL. In our evaluations, the maximum concentration tested was 40 μg/mL since higher concentrations of both compounds led to solubility problems.

These products differ in the functional group in ring E (Figure 1). As previously reported for other methylene quinones and phenolic nor-triterpenes compounds, replacement of the carboxylic group present in celastrol on C-29 by a methyl ester group reduces the antibacterial activity [14,43]. Celastrol has shown interesting pharmacological activities, although inconveniences related to poor water solubility, high toxicity, or poor stability have also been described [29,44]. Structural modifications in the triterpene quinones scaffolds could be of interest to obtain derivatives with improved antimicrobial activities and to overcome the pharmacokinetic limitations of these compounds.

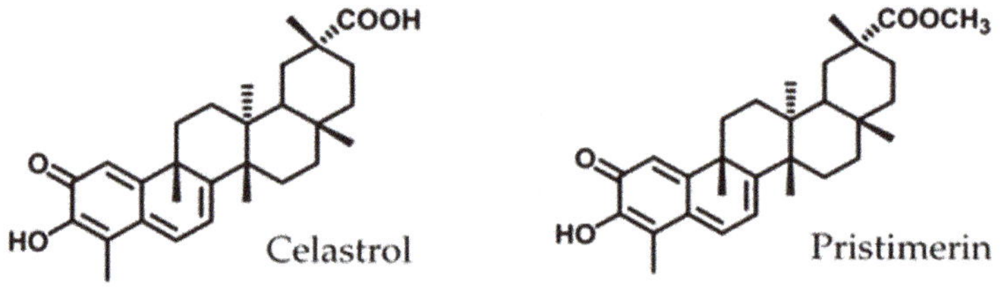

Figure 1. Structure of triterpenoid methylene quinones.

3.2. Effects of Methylene Quinones against B. subtilis

The time–kill curves of *B. subtilis* cultures showed a different behavior when celastrol and pristimerin were added at different growth stages (Figure 2). Addition of celastrol at 3 μg/mL in the lag phase (10^5 CFU/mL) had a bactericidal effect similar to ciprofloxacin with ≥ 3 Log_{10} in CFU reduction after 9 h of incubation (Figure 2A). Rifampicin and tetracycline also had a bactericidal behavior in the first hours of treatment, although the cultures recovered after 24 h of incubation. A bacteriostatic action and regrowth was observed with penicillin. Compared to celastrol, pristimerin at 10 μg/mL had a bacteriostatic effect, producing a minor reduction in the CFU counts (<3 Log_{10}). However, when pristimerin was incorporated in the log phase of growth (10^7 CFU/mL), a bactericidal action was observed, reducing the bacterial population 4.2 Log_{10} in 2 h of treatment, with up to 99.9% dead after 24 h of incubation (Figure 2B). In addition, the drop in optical density values (OD_{550}) revealed the bacteriolytic nature of this compound. Under these conditions of growth, celastrol had a bacteriostatic action, similar to that shown by ciprofloxacin, tetracycline, and rifampicin, with a clear regrowth of the culture after 24 h in the presence of rifampicin. Penicillin had a limited effect on the control of *B. subtilis* cells actively growing.

The action of the methylene quinones was also evaluated against different inoculum sizes of *B. subtilis* in lag-phase growth (Table 2). At the higher inoculum concentration (10^7 CFU/mL), celastrol showed a bacteriostatic activity during the exposition time and a lower reduction in CFU/mL compared to the log phase of growth (Figure 2B). A bacteriostatic effect was also observed at 10^6 and 10^5 CFU/mL and bactericide at 10^4 CFU/mL. Pristimerin showed a similar behavior to that obtained with celastrol. However, when this compound was added in the log phase of growth, a bacteriolytic effect was observed within 6 h of treatment (Figure 2B). These results indicate that both quinones show a stronger effect when *B. subtilis* is actively growing.

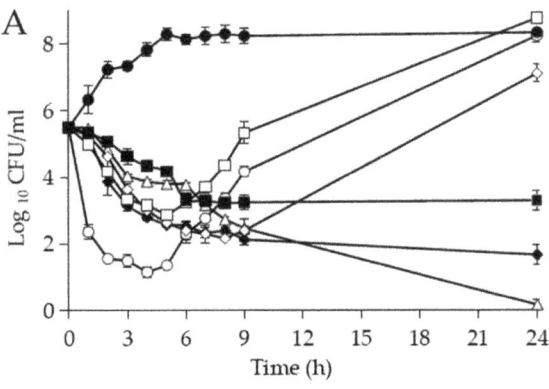

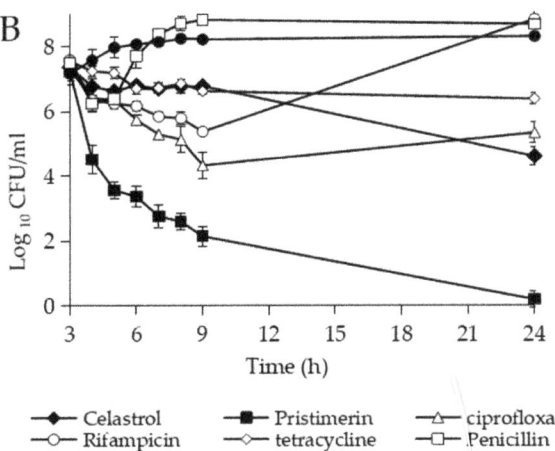

Figure 2. Time–kill curves of *B. subtilis* cultures expressed as Log_{10} of CFU counts after treatment with different antimicrobial substances (celastrol 3 μg/mL; pristimerin 10 μg/mL; ciprofloxacin 1.2 μg/mL; rifampicin 0.15 μg/mL; tetracycline 7.5 μg/mL; and penicillin 9 μg/mL) added in lag phase of growth (**A**) and log phase after three hours of preincubation (**B**). Cultures without drugs and with the maximum proportion of DMSO were used as controls. Error bars express SD with $n = 3$.

Table 2. Effect of celastrol at 3 μg/mL and pristimerin at 10 μg/mL on different inoculum sizes of *B. subtilis* at 3 and 6 h after treatment.

Triterpene	Dilution Factor	Mean Log_{10} CFU ± SD [1]		
		Initial Inoculum	Recovery at 3 h	Recovery at 6 h
Celastrol	10^7	7.58 ± 0.11	7.60 ± 0.15	7.58 ± 0.05
	10^6	6.41 ± 0.14	4.68 ± 0.27	4.08 ± 0.17
	10^5	5.54 ± 0.20	4.00 ± 0.21	3.15 ± 0.16
	10^4	4.67 ± 0.09	2.30 ± 0.25	1.27 ± 0.25
Pristimerin	10^7	7.58 ± 0.12	7.51 ± 0.07	7.47 ± 0.05
	10^6	6.35 ± 0.17	5.32 ± 0.20	4.71 ± 0.33
	10^5	5.32 ± 0.19	4.26 ± 0.16	3.27 ± 0.22
	10^4	4.75 ± 0.11	3.59 ± 0.12	1.56 ± 0.10

[1] Data are expressed as mean values ± standard deviations ($n = 3$).

3.3. Mechanism of Action

3.3.1. Effects of Macromolecular Synthesis and Initial Uptake of Solutes

Initially, the incorporation of radiolabeled precursors into DNA, RNA, protein, and cell wall synthesis was measured. After addition of celastrol and pristimerin, the incorporation of all precursors into the macromolecular synthesis was blocked, but not simultaneously (Figure 3). Celastrol at 3 µg/mL reduced by ≥70% the incorporation of [6-^{3}H] thymidine and [5-^{3}H] uridine within 5 and 10 min, respectively. The inhibitory effect of celastrol after 5 min was comparable to that observed with the specific inhibitor of the RNA synthesis, rifampicin. Pristimerin at 10 µg/mL needed at least 30 min to produce an inhibition of 57% and 47% of DNA and RNA synthesis, respectively (Figure 3A,B). Celastrol and pristimerin inhibited the incorporation of leucine into protein synthesis by >55% after 20 min, whereas tetracycline blocked this process (>70%) in 10 min. The incorporation of N-acetyl-D-[^{14}C] glucosamine into peptidoglycan decreased rapidly within 2 min after the addition of celastrol and pristimerin, with inhibition values of 58% and 70%, respectively. However, this effect was not constant over time and the incorporation of the precursor gradually increased after 5 min. Initially, the inhibitory effect produced by penicillin at 30 µg/mL on cell wall synthesis was slower (32% in 2 min) than with celastrol and pristimerin, but the incorporation of the precursor gradually increased this up to 85% in 30 min (Figure 3D). Clofoctol, a cytoplasmic membrane disruptor [45], had a variable effect on the incorporation of precursors but blocked all biosynthetic processes (>70% of inhibition) after 30 min of evaluation.

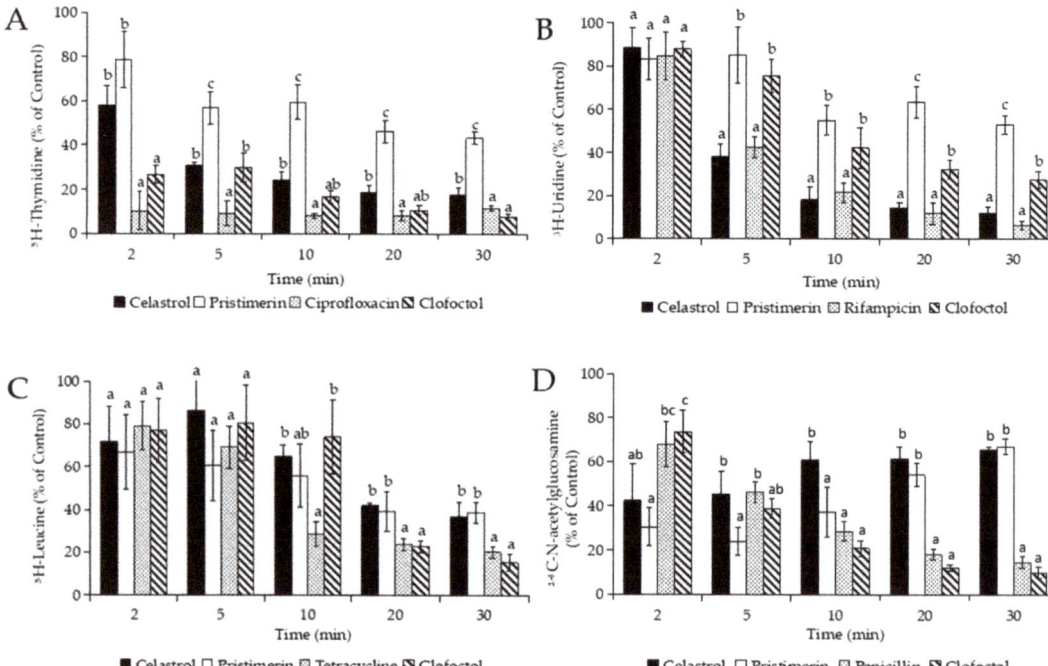

Figure 3. Incorporation of precursor in the synthesis of DNA (**A**), RNA (**B**), protein (**C**), and cell wall (**D**) of *B. subtilis* cultures in the presence of triterpene methylene quinones (celastrol 3 µg/mL; pristimerin 10 µg/mL), specific inhibitors of each pathway (ciprofloxacin 1.25 µg/mL; rifampicin 0.2 µg/mL; tetracycline 10 µg/mL; and penicillin 30 µg/mL), and clofoctol (5 µg/mL). Data are expressed as percentage (%) of precursors' incorporation compared to controls without drugs but with the maximum proportion of DMSO. Error bars express SD with *n* = 3. Different letters above bars mean significant differences between treated cultures (*p* < 0.05, one-way ANOVA; Tukey's test).

The inhibition of all processes of macromolecular synthesis is more compatible with an indirect effect on biosynthetic pathways rather than a specific action on specific targets [46,47]. Thus, the inhibition produced by celastrol and pristimerin on macromolecular synthesis could be related with damage on the cytoplasmic membrane, as it happens with clofoctol. For this reason, we firstly determined the effect of both compounds on the uptake of glucose by *B. subtilis*, measured as total cell-associated counts after cell isolation from free labeled precursors in the incubation medium. As shown in Figure 4, celastrol at 3 µg/mL drastically reduced (>70%) the uptake of D-[1-^{14}C]-glucose in only 2 min, whereas clofoctol needed at least 5 min to produce comparable reductions. Pristimerin weakly reduced the uptake of glucose and required up to 20 min to produce ≈50% inhibition.

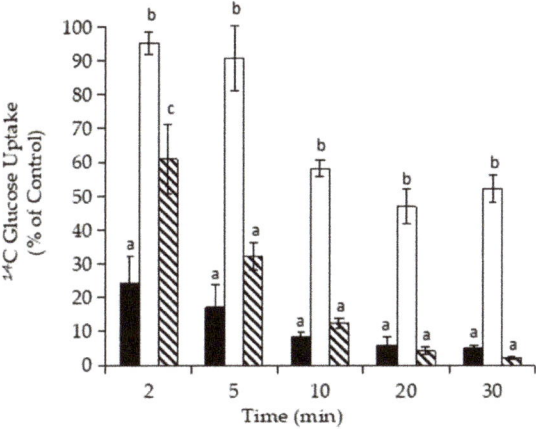

Figure 4. Glucose uptake assay on *B. subtilis* cultures after the addition of the quinones celastrol (3 µg/mL) and pristimerin (10 µg/mL). Clofoctol (5 µg/mL), a known inhibitor of macromolecule uptake, was added as a positive control. Data are expressed as percentage (%) of precursor incorporation compared to controls without drugs but with the maximum proportion of DMSO. Error bars express SD with n = 3. Different letters above bars mean significant differences between treated cultures (p < 0.05, one-way ANOVA; Tukey's test).

Based on these results, we decided to investigate whether the uptake of radiolabeled precursors would also be blocked in the presence of terpenoids, as was the case with glucose. The uptake of precursors (thymidine, uridine, leucine, and N-acetyl glucosamine) was determined in the presence of celastrol, the triterpenoid that showed the greatest inhibitory effect on glucose uptake and macromolecular synthesis. Figure 5 shows how the addition of celastrol at 3 µg/mL to *B. subtilis* cultures rapidly inhibited the uptake of [6-^{3}H] thymidine and [5-^{3}H] uridine by >50% between 2 and 5 min. The specific inhibitors of DNA and RNA synthesis, ciprofloxacin and rifampicin, did not affect the uptake of these precursors. The uptake of [4,5-^{3}H] leucine was inhibited by up to 43% after 20 min, while uptake of N-acetyl-D-[1-^{14}C] glucosamine was weakly affected and gradually increased during the experimentation time (Figure 5C,D). The addition of tetracycline blocked 75% the uptake of leucine in 10 min, whereas the transport of N-acetyl-D-[1-^{14}C] glucosamine into the cells was not affected in the presence of penicillin.

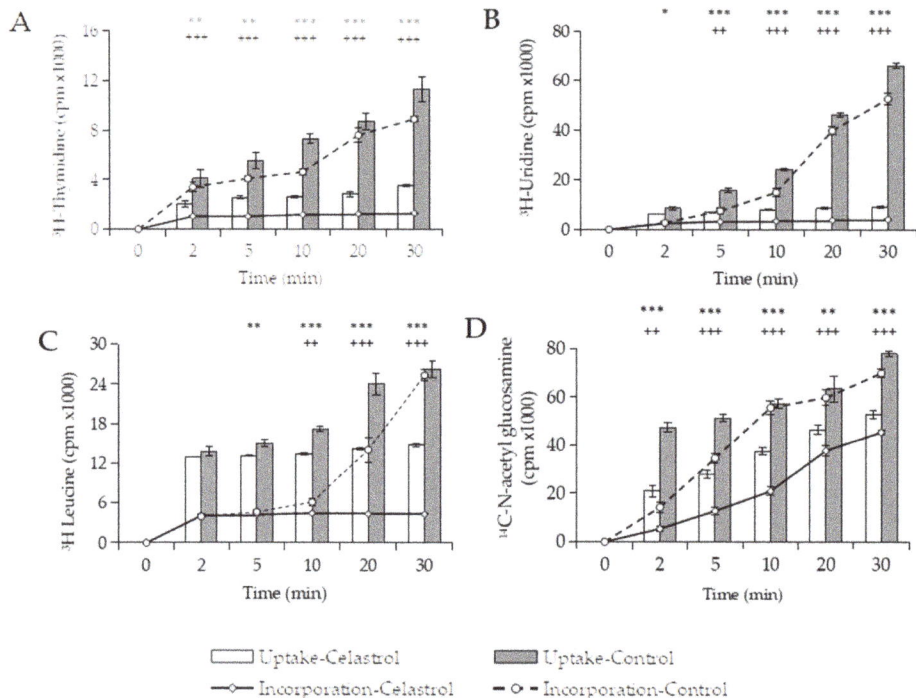

Figure 5. Incorporation (insoluble phase) and uptake (soluble phase) of DNA (**A**), RNA (**B**), protein (**C**), and cell wall (**D**) precursors on *B. subtilis* cultures in the presence of celastrol (3 µg/mL). Cultures in the same conditions but without celastrol and with the same proportion of DMSO were used as negative control. Error bars express SD with n = 3. Significant differences found in uptake (***: $p < 0.001$. **: $p < 0.01$. *: $p < 0.05$) or incorporation (+++: $p < 0.001$. ++: $p < 0.01$) compared with control (one-way ANOVA; Tukey's test).

Our results indicate that both uptake and incorporation processes in *B. subtilis* were affected by celastrol. Inhibition of macromolecular synthesis implies a low demand for biosynthetic precursors. Under these conditions, it would be reasonable to expect a slow-down in the uptake of precursors into the cell if both processes are coupled. In contrast, a primary blockage in precursor transport into the cells would also lead to inhibition of biosynthetic pathways due to low precursor availability. However, the uptake of precursors does not necessarily have to be linked to their incorporation in macromolecular synthesis. As Chou and Pogell [48] have previously suggested, if transport is inhibited and the process is not tightly coupled to macromolecular synthesis, the initial accumulation of precursors into the acid-soluble pool should be much more inhibited than their incorporation during macromolecular synthesis. In fact, these authors described how panamycin, an antibiotic that affects membrane-associated cellular functions, inhibits the uptake of uridine, while incorporation into biosynthetic processes is minimally affected. Thus, an ideal scenario would be one in which all of the precursors taken up by cells are in acid-soluble form to determine to what extent a blockage in molecular transport is a key process in the mechanism of action of the antibacterial agent [48].

Therefore, an experiment was conducted to investigate the effect of celastrol on the uptake of radiolabeled thymidine in *B. subtilis* when DNA synthesis was blocked by ciprofloxacin (1.25 µg/mL during 30 min). As seen in Figure 6, total radioactivity in control cells increased gradually throughout the incubation time. As expected, the incorporation of precursor slowed down when the biosynthetic process was specifically inhibited by ciprofloxacin. In this case, 5 min after the addition of the radiolabeled precursor, only ≈29%

of available thymidine was incorporated into macromolecular synthesis. By contrast, in the absence of ciprofloxacin, ≈74% of the precursor present in the cells was incorporated in the same time (Figure 5A). This observation suggests that uptake and incorporation are independent processes and that the precursors can accumulate in the cytoplasm in the absence of incorporation. The addition of celastrol at 3 µg/mL not only blocked the uptake of thymidine radiolabeled precursor in the treated cells but also produced a slight leakage of accumulated [6-^{3}H] thymidine from *B. subtilis*. This effect could be related to an action of celastrol on the integrity of the membrane, affecting its permeability and producing a release of the cytoplasmic content. Similar results have been observed on *S. aureus* cells treated with zeylasterone, another triterpenoid with antibacterial properties, for which an action on the cytoplasmic membrane has also been suggested [49]. Additionally, the arrest of uptake was accompanied by an immediate blockage of incorporation into macromolecular synthesis. The results obtained reinforce the idea that celastrol could first target the function of the cytoplasmic membrane by affecting the transport of solutes and other essential molecules into the cell.

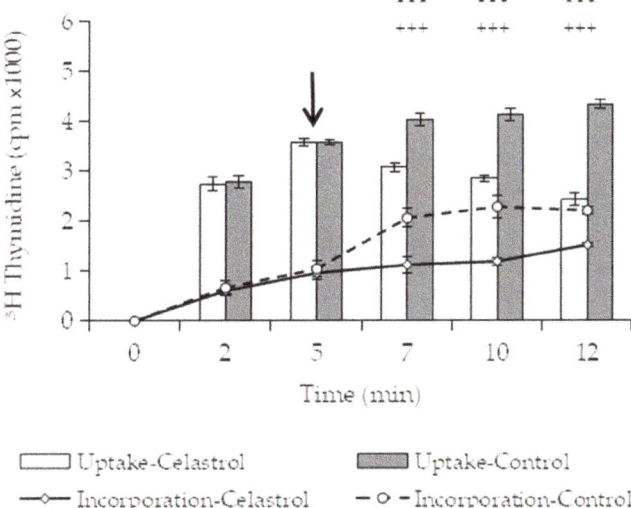

Figure 6. Incorporation (insoluble phase) and uptake (soluble phase) of radiolabeled ^{3}H-thymidine on *B. subtilis*. Bacterial culture were pretreated with ciprofloxacin (1.25 µg/mL), a specific inhibitors of DNA biosynthesis before the addition of the radiolabeled precursor (time 0). The triterpene celastrol (3 µg/mL), or the same proportion of DMSO used as control, was added at the time indicated by the arrow. Error bars express SD with n = 3. Significant differences found in uptake (***: $p < 0.001$) or incorporation (+++: $p < 0.001$) compared with control (one-way ANOVA; Tukey's test).

3.3.2. Effect of Celastrol on the Integrity and Functions of the Cytoplasmic Membrane

The cytoplasmic membrane is a delicate and metabolically active structure essential for the survival of microorganisms. It acts as a selective permeability barrier and prevents the loss of essential components of low molecular weight and nucleotide. Antibacterial agents targeting the cytoplasmic membrane affect its functions and cause a rapid release of low molecular weight compounds [50]. It has been described that the primary target site of the phenolic compounds in bacteria is the cytoplasmic membrane [51]. Damage to the cytoplasmic membrane impacts permeability barrier functions, which subsequently leads to a loss of structural integrity and a leakage of intracellular material. Thus, we also investigated the effect of celastrol on the cytoplasmic membrane of *B. subtilis* using (i) the BacLight test, (ii) detection of UV-absorbing material efflux, and (iii) determination of potassium leakage. Fluorescent dye and "LIVE/DEAD" BacLight Bacterial Viability Kits have the capability of monitoring the viability of bacteria as a function of the cell membrane integrity [52,53]. Surprisingly, microscopic observations after the BacLight assay showed that the cells treated with celastrol maintained membrane integrity like the untreated cells. In contrast, cultures treated with clofoctol showed red fluorescence, an observation indicating membrane damage (Supplementary Materials Figure S1). When UV-absorbing material from *B. subtilis* cultures was monitored, concentrations up to 20 µg/mL of celastrol did not alter the UV spectrum in comparison to the untreated cultures (Supplementary Materials Figure S2). Clofoctol used as a control clearly induced the release of UV-absorbing nucleotides in treated cells. Similar results were previously observed with netzahualcoyone, a terpenoid that interacts with the cytoplasmic membrane but also does not release materials that absorb at 260/280 nm [21]. We also determined the potassium released by *B. subtilis* cells as the first index of membrane damage [54]. Exposure to celastrol for 5 min induced intracellular potassium release compared with untreated cells, although the effect was significantly weaker than that observed with clofoctol (Figure 7). These data suggest that celastrol could act on biological membranes, altering their functions and modifying cell permeability.

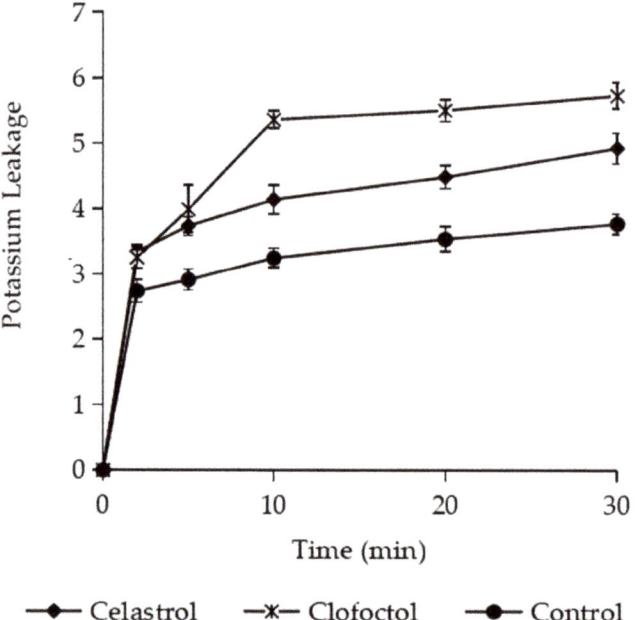

Figure 7. Potassium (K^+) leakage (µg/mL) from *Bacillus subtilis* cells exposed to celastrol (3 µg/mL). Cultures with clofoctol (5 µg/mL) or the maximum proportion of DMSO were used as positive and negative controls, respectively. Error bars express SD with $n = 3$.

3.3.3. Transmission Electron Microscopy

To determine whether celastrol induces noticeable cell membrane damage, transmission electron microscopy was performed on thin sections of *B. subtilis* treated with the terpenoid for 1 h. Compared to the untreated control, cells treated with celastrol exhibited abnormally long cells, variability in wall thickness, compact ribosomes underlying the plasma membrane, and mesosome-like structures arising from the septa (Figure 8).

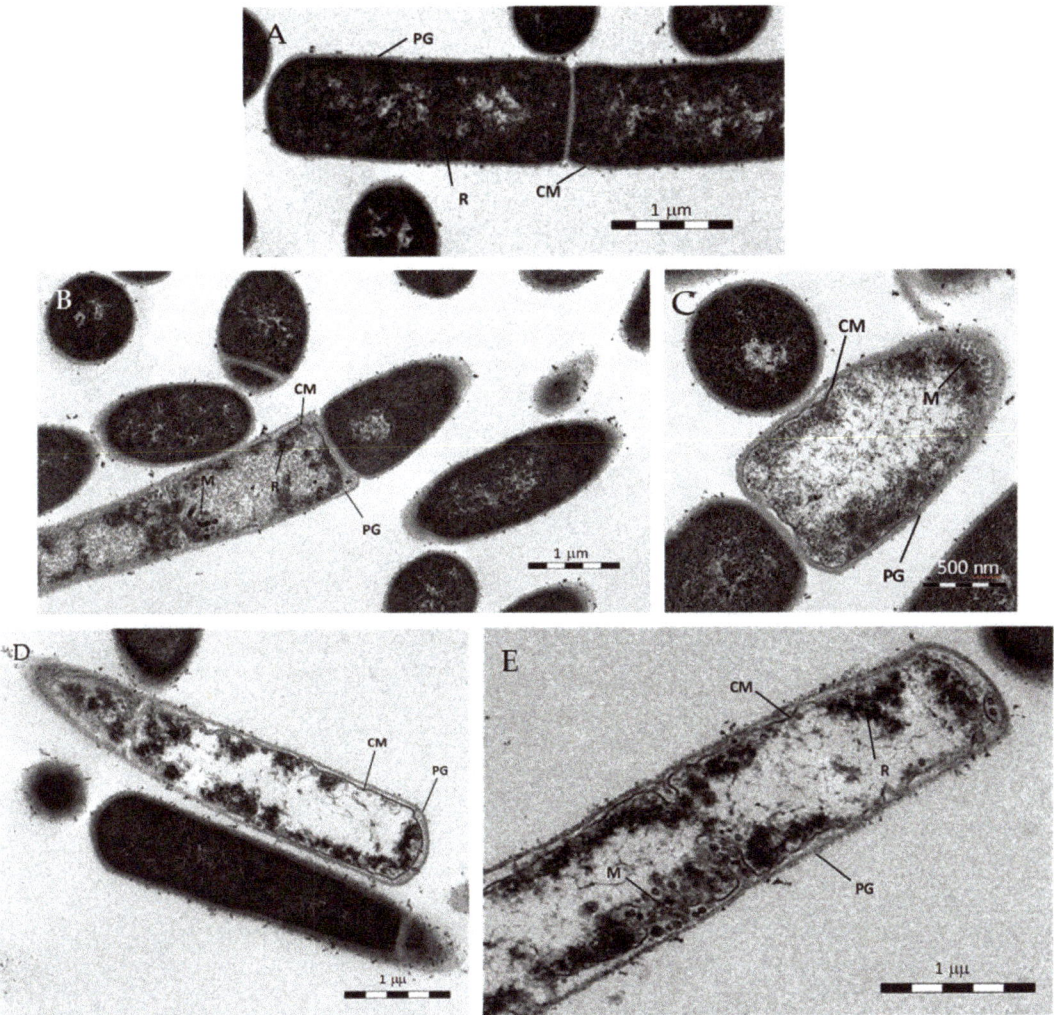

Figure 8. TEM of *B. subtilis* exposed for 1 h to celastrol at 3 µg/mL (**B,C**) or pristimerin at 10 µg/mL (**D,E**). Untreated cells (**A**). CM, cytoplasmic membrane; PG, peptidoglycan layer; R, ribosomes; M, mesosome-like structures.

Despite the multiple effects produced by celastrol, the technique did not allow the observation of visible damage to the cell membrane. For comparison purposes, *B. subtilis* treated with pristimerin at 10 µg/mL, which showed a bacteriolytic effect during killing curves assays, was also observed. As with celastrol, the cells were extremely long, spindle-shaped, with thin cell walls and slightly electrodense cytoplasm with ribosomes associated to the inner face of the membrane (Figure 8D,E). These observations resemble those obtained by da Cruz et al. [42] on cultures of *S. aureus* treated with pristimerin, where the cells presented a disrupted membrane, as well as a loss of cell integrity.

3.3.4. Effect of Celastrol on Cellular Respiration

Another fundamental function of the cytoplasmic membrane is cellular respiration. The respiratory chain plays an important role in the energetic metabolism of a cell, the maintenance of intracellular redox balance, or the protection against oxidative stress [55].

The membranes harbor the electron transport chain, a well-known system with oxygen as the final electron acceptor in aerobic respiration processes.

Thus, the effect of celastrol on oxygen consumption was also evaluated on cell cultures of *B. subtilis* and *E. coli*, as well as in acellular preparations of these bacteria obtained by cell disruption. Table 3 summarizes the results of the effect of celastrol on glucose-dependent oxygen uptake in intact cells of *B. subtilis* and *E. coli*. Both celastrol and NaCN produced an immediate inhibition of oxygen consumption in *B. subtilis*, reaching 60% at 8 min after their addition compared to the untreated control. As expected, celastrol barely affected the oxygen uptake in *E. coli*, as Gram-negative bacteria are insensitive to the terpene quinone.

Table 3. Mean values ± standard deviations of means (n = 3) of oxygen consumption rates (µL O_2/min) at different times in whole cells or membrane preparations of *B. subtilis* and *E. coli* without treatment or after treatments with celastrol at 3 µg/mL or sodium cyanide (NaCN) at 6.7 mM used as positive controls. The percentage (%) of inhibition in the oxygen consumption referring to the untreated cells (negative control) is shown in parentheses.

Bacteria	Time (min)	Oxygen Compsumption [1]					
		Whole Cells (Glucose 1%)			Membrane Fraction (NADH 0.1 mM)		
		Control	NaCN	Celastrol	Control	NaCN	Celastrol
B. subtilis	0	2.36 ± 0.10 [a]	2.30 ± 0.07 [a] (2.4%)	2.27 ± 0.12 [a] (3.9%)	0.54 ± 0.05 [a]	0.50 ± 0.06 [a] (6.9%)	0.52 ± 0.08 [a] (4.0%)
	2	3.69 ± 0.17 [a]	2.71 ± 0.05 [b] (26.5%)	2.74 ± 0.15 [b] (25.7%)	0.98 ± 0.11 [a]	0.66 ± 0.00 [b] (31.7%)	0.68 ± 0.01 [b] (30.6%)
	4	5.42 ± 0.46 [a]	2.77 ± 0.08 [b] (48.6%)	3.11 ± 0.04 [b] (42.4%)	1.27 ± 0.01 [a]	0.79 ± 0.00 [c] (37.7%)	0.82 ± 0.02 [b] (35.1%)
	6	7.09 ± 0.21 [a]	2.91 ± 0.03 [c] (58.9%)	3.30 ± 0.02 [b] (53.5%)	1.56 ± 0.05 [a]	0.89 ± 0.01 [b] (43.0%)	0.94 ± 0.03 [b] (39.4%)
	8	8.53 ± 0.14 [a]	2.97 ± 0.02 [c] (65.2%)	3.42 ± 0.04 [b] (59.8%)	1.80 ± 0.01 [a]	0.94 ± 0.00 [c] (47.9%)	1.01 ± 0.02 [b] (43.9%)
E. coli	0	2.16 ± 0.07 [a]	2.04 ± 0.06 [a,b] (5.5%)	2.00 ± 0.02 [b] (7.3%)	2.22 ± 0.07 [a]	2.10 ± 0.01 [a,b] (5.0%)	2.07 ± 0.05 [b] (6.5%)
	2	3.35 ± 0.14 [a]	2.16 ± 0.03 [c] (35.5%)	3.08 ± 0.08 [b] (7.9%)	3.07 ± 0.00 [a]	2.20 ± 0.05 [c] (28.2%)	2.41 ± 0.02 [b] (21.3%)
	4	4.34 ± 0.24 [a]	2.22 ± 0.03 [b] (48.8%)	3.95 ± 0.14 [a] (9.0%)	3.88 ± 0.01 [a]	2.30 ± 0.03 [c] (40.6%)	2.51 ± 0.01 [b] (35.3%)
	6	5.80 ± 0.32 [a]	2.32 ± 0.03 [c] (60.0%)	4.84 ± 0.10 [b] (16.6%)	4.74 ± 0.01 [a]	2.34 ± 0.02 [c] (50.6%)	2.61 ± 0.02 [b] (44.9%)
	8	6.79 ± 0.19 [a]	2.40 ± 0.05 [c] (64.6%)	5.53 ± 0.09 [b] (18.5%)	5.37 ± 0.00 [a]	2.40 ± 0.08 [c] (55.3%)	2.68 ± 0.01 [b] (50.0%)

[1] For each assessment, values with different superscript letters within each given time point indicate statistically significant differences (ANOVA, Tukey's multiple comparison test, $p < 0.05$).

The same evaluation was carried out on acellular preparations where the oxygen consumption was coupled to the oxidation of NADH. Unlike when whole cells were used, here, NADH oxidation only depended on the amount of dissolved oxygen and the function of the respiratory chain. In these conditions, the addition of celastrol and NaCN inhibited the oxygen consumption in *B. subtilis* and *E. coli* preparations. The different behavior shown by celastrol in intact and disrupted preparations of *E. coli* cells shows that the cell membranes of both Gram-positive and -negative bacteria are equally sensitive to its action. The outer membranes of Gram-negative bacteria act as a permeability barrier, holding celastrol physically distant from its target of action. These results indicate that celastrol has a direct effect on the electron transport chain, affecting the consumption of oxygen and, consequently, the oxidation of NADH associated with respiration processes. However, in the presence of celastrol, neither a spontaneous oxidation of NADH nor a reduction in NAD^+ was observed.

An additional experiment was carried out to verify previous results indicating an action of celastrol on the inhibition of enzymatic activity. Nagase et al. [56] reported that celastrol can inhibit topoisomerase II and trigger apoptosis in HL-60 cells. DNA gyrase is an important bacterial topoisomerase II that catalyzes ATP-dependent negative supercoiling of bacterial DNA. The essential role of gyrase is to maintain the topological constitution of DNA and, hence, the survival of bacteria [57]. Eukaryotic cells lack the enzyme, which has led to the development of specific antimicrobials targeting the gyrase functions [58]. Our results confirmed the effect of celastrol at 50 µg/mL on the gyrase activity of supercoiling plasmid pBR322, as did ciprofloxacin, used as a positive control (Supplementary Materials Figure S3). Interestingly, pristimerin has shown a weaker antibacterial action compared to celastrol and did not affect the enzymatic activity of gyrase. This mechanism of action has been suggested for other triterpenoid compounds showing activity against topoisomerases I and II [59]. Some models have been proposed for the mode of action of triterpenoids on topoisomerases, which can be either by binding to the enzyme at the DNA binding site or by binding to the ATP binding site, conformationally blocking DNA binding to the enzyme [60]. Thus, the effect on DNA supercoiling produced by celastrol could be related with an action on the gyrase rather than a direct DNA binding effect.

4. Conclusions

The antimicrobial action of celastrol and pristimerin, two natural triterpene methylene quinones, was evaluated, and the mechanism of action against the spore-forming bacteria *Bacillus subtilis* was also approached. Celastrol showed a higher antimicrobial effect compared with pristimerin, being active against Gram-positive bacteria. The results obtained in this study indicate that celastrol interacts with the cytoplasmic membrane of *B. subtilis*, preventing the transport of solutes into the cells and affecting basic membrane functions such as respiration processes. At the structural level, the membrane was not widely affected, suggesting a mechanism of action for celastrol other than a simple effect on structural components and subsequent membrane disruption. Furthermore, celastrol can also interact with enzymatic processes different from those exclusively located on the cytoplasmic membrane, as observed here for topoisomerase II. Although further investigations are required to elucidate a more precise mechanism of action, our results indicate that celastrol can act on multiple targets.

Supplementary Materials: The following are available online at https://www.mdpi.com/2304-8158/10/3/591/s1, Figure S1: Epifluorescence microscopy images of *B. subtilis* stained with propidium iodide and SYTO 9 after treatment with celastrol (3 µg/mL) for 30 and 60 min (A,B) or clofoctol (5 µg/mL) for 30 min (C). Control cells were treated with the maximum proportion of DMSO (D). Scale bars correspond to 10 µm. Figure S2: Release of 260 and 280 nm absorbing material from *B. subtilis* cells treated with celastrol at 3, 6, and 10 µg/mL and clofoctol at 5 µg/mL. Cells exposed to the maximum proportion of DMSO were used as control. Error bars express SD with $n = 3$. Figure S3: DNA supercoiling assays. Electrophoresis gel shows a control with a negatively supercoiled plasmid (line 1) with DMSO (line 2), and after its treatment with ciprofloxacin at 25 (line 3) and 50 µg/mL (line 4), celastrol at 50 µg/mL (line 5), and pristimerin at 50 µg/mL (line 6).

Author Contributions: Conceptualization, L.M. and L.d.L.G.; methodology, L.M. and L.d.L.G.; investigation, N.P.-M. and L.d.L.G.; data curation, L.M., N.P.-M. and L.d.L.G.; writing—original draft preparation, L.M. and L.d.L.G.; writing—review and editing, L.M. and L.d.L.G.; supervision, L.M. and L.d.L.G.; funding acquisition, L.M. All authors have read and agreed to the published version of the manuscript.

Funding: This study was supported by RTI2018-094356-B-C21 Spanish Ministerio de Economía, Industria y Competitividad (MINECO) and co-funded by the European Regional Development Fund (FEDER) projects.

Institutional Review Board Statement: Not applicable.

Informed Consent Statement: Not applicable.

Data Availability Statement: Not applicable.

Acknowledgments: Thanks are due to the Universidad de La Laguna and Servicio de Microscopia de la Universidad de Las Palmas de Gran Canaria.

Conflicts of Interest: The authors declare no conflict of interest.

References

1. González, A.G.; Bazzocchi, I.L.; Moujir, L.; Jiménez, I.A. Ethnobotanical uses of Celastraceae. Bioactive metabolites. In *Studies in Natural Products Chemistry: Bioactive Natural Products (Part D)*; Atta-ur, R., Ed.; Elsevier Science Publisher: Amsterdam, The Netherlands, 2000; Volume 23, pp. 649–738.
2. Simmons, M.P.; Cappa, J.J.; Archer, R.H.; Ford, A.J.; Eichstedt, D.; Clevinger, C.C. Phylogeny of the Celastreae (Celastraceae) and the relationships of *Catha edulis* (qat) inferred from morphological characters and nuclear and plastid genes. *Mol. Phylogenet. Evol.* **2008**, *48*, 745–757. [CrossRef] [PubMed]
3. Gunatilaka, A.A.L. Triterpenoid Quinonemethides and Related Compounds (celastroloids). In *Progress in the Chemistry of Organic Natural Products*; Herz, W., Kirby, G.W., Moore, R.E., Steglich, W., Tamm, C., Eds.; Springer: New York, NY, USA, 1996; Volume 67, pp. 1–123.
4. Bashir, A.Y.; Hozeifa, M.H.; Zhang, L.-Y.; Jiang, Z.-Z. Anticancer Potential and Molecular Targets of Pristimerin: A Mini-Review. *Curr. Cancer Drugs Targets* **2017**, *17*, 100–108. [CrossRef]
5. Hou, W.; Liu, B.; Xu, H. Celastrol: Progresses in structure-modifications, structure-activity relationships, pharmacology and toxicology. *Eur. J. Med. Chem.* **2020**, *189*, 112081. [CrossRef]
6. El-Agamy, D.S.; Shaaban, A.A.; Almaramhy, H.H.; Elkablawy, S.; Elkablawy, M.A. Pristimerin as a Novel Hepatoprotective Agent against Experimental Autoimmune Hepatitis. *Front. Pharmacol.* **2018**, *9*, 292. [CrossRef] [PubMed]
7. Venkatesha, S.H.; Moudgil, K.D. Celastrol and Its Role in Controlling Chronic Diseases. *Adv. Exp. Med. Biol.* **2016**, *928*, 267–289. [CrossRef]
8. Shi, J.; Li, J.; Xu, Z.; Chen, L.; Luo, R.; Zhang, C.; Gao, F.; Zhang, J.; Fu, C. Celastrol: A Review of Useful Strategies Overcoming its Limitation in Anticancer Application. *Front. Pharmacol.* **2020**, *11*, 558741. [CrossRef] [PubMed]
9. Cascão, R.; Fonseca, J.E.; Moita, L.F. Celastrol: A Spectrum of Treatment Opportunities in Chronic Diseases. *Front. Med.* **2017**, *4*, 69. [CrossRef]
10. Kashyap, D.; Sharma, A.; Tuli, H.S.; Sak, K.; Mukherjee, T.; Bishayee, A. Molecular targets of celastrol in cancer: Recent trends and advancements. *Crit. Rev. Oncol. Hematol.* **2018**, *128*, 70–81. [CrossRef]
11. Lan, G.; Zhang, J.; Ye, W.; Yang, F.; Li, A.; He, W.; Zhang, W.D. Celastrol as a tool for the study of the biological events of metabolic diseases. *Sci. China Chem.* **2019**, *62*, 409–416. [CrossRef]
12. Liu, J.; Lee, J.; Salazar Hernandez, M.A.; Mazitschek, R.; Ozcan, U. Treatment of Obesity with Celastrol. *Cell* **2015**, *161*, 999–1011. [CrossRef] [PubMed]
13. Pfuhlmann, K.; Schriever, S.C.; Baumann, P.; Kabra, D.G.; Harrison, L.; Mazibuko-Mbeje, S.E.; Contreras, R.E.; Kyriakou, E.; Simonds, S.E.; Tiganis, T.; et al. Celastrol-Induced Weight Loss Is Driven by Hypophagia and Independent From UCP1. *Diabetes* **2018**, *7*, 2456–2465. [CrossRef] [PubMed]
14. Moujir, L.; Gutiérrez-Navarro, A.M.; González, A.G.; Ravelo, A.G.; Luis, J.G. The relationship between structure and antimicrobial activity in quinones from the Celastraceae. *Biochem. Syst. Ecol.* **1990**, *18*, 25–28. [CrossRef]
15. Sotanaphun, U.; Lipipun, V.; Suttisri, R.; Bavovada, R. Antimicrobial activity and stability of tingenone derivatives. *Planta Med.* **1999**, *65*, 450–452. [CrossRef]
16. Moujir, L.; Gutiérrez-Navarro, A.M.; González, A.G.; Ravelo, A.G.; Luis, J.G. Mode of action of netzahualcoyone. *Antimicrob. Agents Chemother.* **1991**, *35*, 211–213. [CrossRef] [PubMed]
17. De León, L.; Moujir, L. Activity and mechanism of the action of zeylasterone against *B. subtilis*. *J. Appl. Microbiol.* **2007**, *104*, 1266–1274. [CrossRef] [PubMed]
18. Woo, S.-G.; Lee, A.-Y.; Lee, S.-M.; Lim, K.-H.; Ha, E.-J.; Eom, Y.-B. Activity of novel inhibitors of *Staphylococcus aureus* biofilms. *Folia Microbiol.* **2017**, *62*, 157–167. [CrossRef]
19. Ooi, N.; Eady, E.A.; Cove, J.H.; O'Neill, A.J. Redox-active compounds with a history of human use: Antistaphylococcal action and potential for repurposing as topical antibiofilm agents. *J. Antimicrob. Chemother.* **2015**, *70*, 479–488. [CrossRef] [PubMed]
20. Kim, H.-R.; Lee, D.; Eom, Y.-B. Anti-biofilm and Anti-Virulence Efficacy of Celastrol against *Stenotrophomonas maltophilia*. *Int. J. Med. Sci.* **2018**, *15*, 617–627. [CrossRef] [PubMed]
21. Pérez, M.; Sánchez, M.; Stupak, M.; García, M.; Rojo de Almeida, M.T.; Oberti, J.C.; Palermo, J.; Blustein, G. Antifouling Activity of Celastroids Isolated from *Maytenus* Species, Natural and Sustainable Alternatives for Marine Coatings. *Ind. Eng. Chem. Res.* **2014**, *53*, 7655–7659. [CrossRef]
22. Luo, D.Q.; Wang, H.; Tian, X.; Shao, H.J.; Liu, J.K. Antifungal properties of pristimerin and celastrol isolated from *Celastrus hypoleucus*. *Pest Manag. Sci.* **2005**, *61*, 85–90. [CrossRef]
23. Gullo, F.P.; Sardi, J.C.; Santos, V.A.; Sangalli-Leite, F.; Pitangui, N.S.; Rossi, S.A.; de Paula, E.; Silva, A.C.; Soares, L.A.; Silva, J.F.; et al. Antifungal activity of maytenin and pristimerin. *Evid. Based Complement. Alternat. Med.* **2012**, *2012*, 340787. [CrossRef]
24. Haque, E.; Irfan, S.; Kamil, M.; Sheikh, S.; Hasan, A.; Ahmad, A.; Lakshmi, V.; Nazir, A.; Mir, S.S. Terpenoids with antifungal activity trigger mitochondrial dysfunction in *Saccharomyces cerevisiae*. *Microbiology* **2016**, *85*, 436–443. [CrossRef]
25. Song, J.; Shang, N.; Baig, N.; Yao, J.; Shin, C.; Kim, B.K.; Li, Q.; Malwal, S.R.; Oldfield, E.; Feng, X.; et al. *Aspergillus flavus* squalene synthase as an antifungal target: Expression, activity, and inhibition. *Biochem. Biophys. Res. Commun.* **2019**, *512*, 517–523. [CrossRef]

26. Seo, W.-D.; Lee, D.-Y.; Park, K.H.; Kim, J.-H. Downregulation of fungal cytochrome c peroxidase expression by antifungal quinonemethide triterpenoids. *Appl. Biol. Chem.* **2016**, *59*, 281–284. [CrossRef]
27. Sun, Q.; Li, C.; Jing, L.; Peng, X.; Wang, Q.; Jiang, N.; Xu, Q.; Zhao, G. Celastrol ameliorates *Aspergillus fumigatus* keratitis via inhibiting LOX-1. *Int. Immunopharmacol.* **2019**, *70*, 101–109. [CrossRef] [PubMed]
28. Tseng, C.-K.; Hsu, S.-P.; Lin, C.-K.; Wu, Y.-H.; Lee, J.-C.; Young, K.-C. Celastrol inhibits hepatitis C virus replication by upregulating heme oxygenase-1 via the JNK MAPK/Nrf2 pathway in human hepatoma cells. *Antiviral. Res.* **2017**, *146*, 191–200. [CrossRef] [PubMed]
29. Zhang, H.; Lu, G. Synthesis of celastrol derivatives as potential non-nucleoside hepatitis B virus inhibitors. *Chem. Biol. Drug Des.* **2020**, *96*, 1380–1386. [CrossRef]
30. Kumar, T.D.K.; Murali, H.S.; Batra, H.V. Simultaneous detection of pathogenic *B. cereus, S. aureus* and *L. monocytogenes* by multiplex PCR. *Indian J. Microbiol.* **2009**, *49*, 283–289. [CrossRef]
31. Kubo, I.; Fujita, K.-I.; Nihei, K.-I.; Nihei, A. Antibacterial Activity of Akyl Gallates against *Bacillus subtilis*. *J. Agric. Food Chem.* **2004**, *52*, 1072–1076. [CrossRef]
32. Gopal, N.; Hill, C.; Ross, P.R.; Beresford, T.P.; Fenelon, M.A.; Cotter, P.D. The Prevalence and Control of *Bacillus* and Related Spore-Forming Bacteria in the Dairy Industry. *Front. Microbiol.* **2015**, *6*, 1418. [CrossRef]
33. Gaur, A.H.; Patrick, C.C.; McCullers, J.A.; Flynn, P.M.; Pearson, T.A.; Razzouk, B.I.; Thompson, S.J.; Shenep, J.L. *Bacillus cereus* Bacteremia and Meningitis in Immunocompromised Children. *Clin. Infect. Dis.* **2001**, *32*, 1456–1462. [CrossRef] [PubMed]
34. Dabscheck, G.; Silverman, L.; Ullrich, N.J. *Bacillus cereus* Cerebral Abscess during Induction Chemotherapy for Childhood Acute Leukemia. *J. Pediatr. Hematol. Oncol.* **2015**, *37*, 568–569. [CrossRef]
35. Hansford, J.R.; Phillips, M.; Cole, C.; Francis, J.; Blyth, C.; Gottardo, N.G. *Bacillus cereus* bacteremia and multiple brain abscesses during acute lymphoblastic leukemia induction therapy. *J. Pediatr. Hematol. Oncol.* **2014**, *36*, e197–e201. [CrossRef] [PubMed]
36. Cowan, M.M. Plant Products as Antimicrobial Agents. *Clin. Microbiol. Rev.* **1999**, *12*, 564–582. [CrossRef]
37. Nuñez, M.J.; Kennedy, M.L.; Jiménez, I.A.; Bazzocchi, I.L. Uragogin and blepharodin, unprecedented hetero-Diels-Alder adducts from Celastraceae species. *Tetrahedron* **2011**, *67*, 3030–3033. [CrossRef]
38. Taddeo, V.A.; Castillo, U.C.; Martínez, M.L.; Menjivar, J.; Jimenéz, I.A.; Nunez, M.J.; Bazzochi, I.L. Development and validation of an HPLC-PDA method for biologically active quinonemethide triterpenoids isolated from *Maytenus chiapensis*. *Medicines* **2019**, *6*, 36. [CrossRef]
39. Clinical and Laboratory Standards Institute (CLSI; formerly NCCLS); National Committee for Clinical Laboratory Standards. *Performance Standards for Antimicrobial Susceptibility Testing*; 16th Informational Supplement; CLSI Document M7-A7; Clinical and Laboratory Standards Institute: Wayne, PA, USA, 2006. Available online: https://clsi.org/ (accessed on 10 March 2021).
40. CLSI. *Methods for Dilution Antimicrobial Susceptibility Tests for Bacteria that Grow Aerobically; Approved Standard*, 9th ed.; CLSI Document M07-A9; Clinical and Laboratory Standards Institute: Wayne, PA, USA, 2012.
41. Davis, B.D.; Mignoli, E.S. Mutants of *Escherichia coli* requiring methionine or vitamin B_{12}. *J. Bacteriol.* **1950**, *60*, 17–28. [CrossRef]
42. Da Cruz Nizer, W.S.; Ferraz, A.C.; Moraes, T.F.S.; Lima, W.G.; Santos, J.P.; Duarte, L.P.; Ferreira, J.M.S.; de Brito Magalhães, C.L.; Vieira-Filho, S.A.; dos Santos PereiraAndrade, A.C.; et al. Pristimerin isolated from *Salacia crassifolia* (Mart. Ex. Schult.) G. Don. (Celastraceae) roots as a potential antibacterial agent against *Staphylococcus aureus*. *J. Ethnopharmacol.* **2021**, *266*, 113423. [CrossRef] [PubMed]
43. Moujir, L.; López, M.R.; Reyes, C.P.; Jiménez, I.A.; Bazzocchi, I.L. Structural requirements from antimicrobial activity of phenolic nor-triterpenes from Celastraceae species. *Appl. Sci.* **2019**, *9*, 2957. [CrossRef]
44. He, Q.-W.; Feng, J.-H.; Hu, X.-L.; Long, H.; Huang, X.-F.; Jiang, Z.Z.; Zhang, X.-Q.; Ye, W.-C.; Wang, H. Synthesis and Biological Evaluation of Celastrol Derivatives as Potential Immunosuppressive Agents. *J. Nat. Prod.* **2020**, *83*, 2578–2586. [CrossRef]
45. Yablonsly, F. Alteration of Membrane Permeability in *Bacillus subtilis* by Clofoctol. *J. Gen. Microbiol* **1983**, *129*, 1089–1195. [CrossRef]
46. Oliva, B.; Miller, K.; Caggiano, N.; O'neill, A.J.; Cuny, G.D.; Hoemarm, M.Z.; Hauske, J.R.; Chopra, I. Biological properties of novel antistaphylococcal quinoline-indole agents. *Antimicrob. Agents Chemother.* **2003**, *47*, 458–466. [CrossRef]
47. Wang, C.-M.; Jhan, Y.-L.; Tsai, S.-J.; Chou, C.-H. The Pleiotropic Antibacterial Mechanisms of Ursolic Acid against Methicillin-Resistant *Staphylococcus aureus* (MRSA). *Molecules* **2016**, *21*, 884. [CrossRef] [PubMed]
48. Chou, W.-G.; Pogell, B.M. Mode of Action of Pamamycin in *Staphylococcus aureus*. *Antimicrob. Agents Chemother.* **1981**, *20*, 443–454. [CrossRef] [PubMed]
49. De León, L.; López, M.R.; Moujir, L. Antibacterial properties of zeylasterone, a triterpenoid isolated from *Maytenus blepharodes*, against *Staphylococcus aureus*. *Microbiol. Res.* **2010**, *165*, 617–626. [CrossRef]
50. Epand, R.M.; Walker, C.; Epand, R.F.; Magarvey, N.A. Molecular mechanisms of membrane targeting antibiotics. *Biochim. Biophys. Acta* **2016**, *1858*, 980–987. [CrossRef]
51. Rempe, C.S.; Burris, K.P.; Lenaghan, S.C.; Stewart, C.N. The Potential of Systems Biology to Discover Antibacterial Mechanisms of Plant Phenolics. *Front. Microbiol.* **2017**, *8*, 422. [CrossRef] [PubMed]
52. Bunthof, C.J.; Van Schalkwijk, S.; Meijer, W.; Abee, T.; Hugenholtz, J. Fluorescent method for monitoring cheese starter permeabilization and lysis. *Appl. Environ. Microbiol.* **2001**, *67*, 4264–4271. [CrossRef]
53. Laflamme, C.; Lavigne, S.; Ho, J.; Duchaine, C. Assessment of bacterial endospore viability with fluorescent dyes. *J. Appl. Microbiol.* **2004**, *96*, 684–692. [CrossRef]

54. Lambert, P.A.; Hammond, S.M. Potassium fluxes, first indications of membrane damage in micro-organisms. *Biochem. Biophys. Res. Commun.* **1973**, *18*, 796–799. [CrossRef]
55. Kalnenieks, U.; Balodite, E.; Rutkis, R. Metabolic Engineering of Bacterial Respiration: High vs. Low P/O and the Case of *Zymomonas mobilis*. *Front. Bioeng. Biotechnol.* **2019**, *7*, 327. [CrossRef] [PubMed]
56. Nagase, M.; Oto, J.; Sugiyama, S.; Yube, K.; Takaishi, Y.; Sakato, N. Apoptosis Induction in HL-60 Cells and Inhibition of Topoisomerase II by Triterpene Celastrol. *Biosci. Biotechnol. Biochem.* **2003**, *67*, 1883–1887. [CrossRef]
57. Kolarič, A.; Anderluh, M.; Minovski, N. Two Decades of Successful SAR-Grounded Stories of the Novel Bacterial Topoisomerase Inhibitors (NBTIs). *J. Med. Chem.* **2020**, *63*, 5664–5674. [CrossRef] [PubMed]
58. D'Atanasio, N.; Capezzone de Joannon, A.; Di Sante, L.; Mangano, G.; Ombrato, R.; Vitiello, M.; Bartella, C.; Magarò, G.; Prati, F.; Milanese, C.; et al. Antibacterial activity of novel dual bacterial DNA type II topoisomerase inhibitors. *PLoS ONE* **2020**, *15*, e0228509. [CrossRef] [PubMed]
59. D'yakonov, V.A.; Dzhemileva, L.U.; Dzhemilev, U.M. Advances in the chemistry of natural and semisynthetic topoisomerase I/II inhibitors. In *Studied Natural Products Chemistry*; Atta-ur-Rahman, F., Ed.; Elsevier Science Publisher: Amsterdam, The Netherlands, 2017; Volume 54, pp. 21–86. [CrossRef]
60. Setzer, W.N. Non-Intercalative Triterpenoid Inhibitors of Topoisomerase II: A Molecular Docking Study. *Open Bioact. Compd. J.* **2008**, *1*, 13–17. [CrossRef]

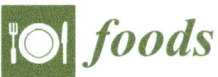

Article

Steroid Glycosides Hyrcanoside and Deglucohyrcanoside: On Isolation, Structural Identification, and Anticancer Activity

Silvie Rimpelová [1,†], Tomáš Zimmermann [2,†], Pavel B. Drašar [2], Bohumil Dolenský [3], Jiří Bejček [1], Eva Kmoníčková [4,5], Petra Cihlářová [2], Soňa Gurská [6], Lucie Kuklíková [1], Marián Hajdůch [6], Tomáš Ruml [1], Lubomír Opletal [7], Petr Džubák [6,*] and Michal Jurášek [2,*]

1. Department Biochemistry and Microbiology, University of Chemistry and Technology Prague, Technická 5, 166 28 Prague, Czech Republic; silvie.rimpelova@vscht.cz (S.R.); jiri.bejcek@vscht.cz (J.B.); lucie.kuklikova@vscht.cz (L.K.); tomas.ruml@vscht.cz (T.R.)
2. Department of Chemistry of Natural Compounds, University of Chemistry and Technology Prague, Technická 5, 166 28 Prague, Czech Republic; tomas.zimmermann@vscht.cz (T.Z.); pavel.drasar@vscht.cz (P.B.D.); Petra.Cihlarova@vscht.cz (P.C.)
3. Department of Analytical Chemistry, University of Chemistry and Technology Prague, Technická 5, 166 28 Prague, Czech Republic; bohumil.dolensky@vscht.cz
4. Department of Pharmacology and Toxicology, Faculty of Medicine in Pilsen, Charles University, Alej Svobody 76, 323 00 Pilsen, Czech Republic; eva.kmonickova@lfp.cuni.cz
5. Department of Pharmacology, Second Faculty of Medicine, Charles University, Plzeňská 311, 150 00 Prague, Czech Republic
6. Institute of Molecular and Translational Medicine, Faculty of Medicine and Dentistry, Palacký University and University Hospital in Olomouc, Hněvotínská 976/3, 779 00 Olomouc, Czech Republic; sona.gurska@upol.cz (S.G.); marian.hajduch@upol.cz (M.H.)
7. Department of Pharmaceutical Botany, Charles University, Akademika Heyrovského 1203, 500 05 Hradec Králové, Czech Republic; opletal@faf.cuni.cz
* Correspondence: petr.dzubak@upol.cz (P.D.); michal.jurasek@vscht.cz (M.J.)
† S.R. and T.Z. contributed equally to this work.

Abstract: Cardiac glycosides (CGs) represent a group of sundry compounds of natural origin. Most CGs are potent inhibitors of Na$^+$/K$^+$-ATPase, and some are routinely utilized in the treatment of various cardiac conditions. Biological activities of other lesser known CGs have not been fully explored yet. Interestingly, the anticancer potential of some CGs was revealed and thereby, some of these compounds are now being evaluated for drug repositioning. However, high systemic toxicity and low cancer cell selectivity of the clinically used CGs have severely limited their utilization in cancer treatment so far. Therefore, in this study, we have focused on two poorly described CGs: hyrcanoside and deglucohyrcanoside. We elaborated on their isolation, structural identification, and cytotoxicity evaluation in a panel of cancerous and noncancerous cell lines, and on their potential to induce cell cycle arrest in the G2/M phase. The activity of hyrcanoside and deglucohyrcanoside was compared to three other CGs: ouabain, digitoxin, and cymarin. Furthermore, by in silico modeling, interaction of these CGs with Na$^+$/K$^+$-ATPase was also studied. Hopefully, these compounds could serve not only as a research tool for Na$^+$/K$^+$-ATPase inhibition, but also as novel cancer therapeutics.

Keywords: cardiac glycosides; secondary plant metabolites; natural product isolation; hyrcanoside; deglucohyrcanoside; ouabain; cymarin; digitoxin; anticancer activity; Na$^+$/K$^+$-ATPase inhibitors

1. Introduction

Cancer is responsible for many people's deaths each year, and it represents the second most common cause of human death worldwide [1]. Even though this disease's incidence and mortality have declined over the past 20 years, there is still no reliable therapy for eradicating it. Recently, in addition to the traditional drug discovery approach, a novel strategy called drug repositioning has emerged. It lies in using the old for a novel purpose.

This approach is economically much more feasible and faster than the traditional approach of drug approval [2].

Interestingly, drug repositioning has also been used for some cardiac glycosides (CGs) as a potential remedy for cancer. Several undergoing clinical trials on CG administration for cancer in mono or combination therapy can be found in [3]. Moreover, also promising is the fact that a lower incidence in some types of cancer in patients on CG therapy (cardiac conditions) has been reported [4]. While another study claims the opposite [5], others stand somewhere in between [6,7]. However, what is quite certain and makes CGs a new hope for cancer treatment are clinical data showing that CGs, mainly digoxin, significantly prolong the survival of cancer patients otherwise treated with traditional chemotherapeutics. What is also beneficial is the fact that CGs at multiple levels affect the immune response and trigger immunogenic cell death, which significantly contributes to their anticancer activity [8].

CGs are secondary plant metabolites found mainly in *Digitalis purpurea* L. and *Digitalis lanata* Ehrh. (digitoxin, Dg; digoxin), *Strophanthus gratus* (ouabain, Ob), and *Nerium oleander* L. (oleandrin). Their biological effect is associated with the interaction with Na^+/K^+-ATPase (NKA), the integral membrane protein of animal cells maintaining the balance of sodium and potassium ions. The CG pharmacophore is the structure of $5\beta,14\beta$-androstane-$3\beta,14$-diol, which is substituted at the C-3 position by a saccharide moiety and the C-17 position by an unsaturated lactone [9]. According to the type of lactone, CGs are classified into cardenolides and bufadienolides; $5\beta,14\beta$-androstane-$3\beta,14$-diol may be substituted in some other positions [10]. Biological activity has been shown to decrease after saturation of the lactone double bond [11,12]. Furthermore, biological activity is also affected by the type and number of carbohydrate units at the C-3 position, and it increases with the decreasing number of carbohydrate units [13,14]. The only exception is aglycone, the biological activity of which is lower than that of its glycosylated variants [13,15].

As aforementioned, CGs, as a unique group of metabolites, have been extensively utilized for the treatment of various heart conditions, and recently, they were also explored as possible anticancer agents (reviewed in [16]). Based on the positive ionotropic effect they induce, they are introduced as drugs in the treatment of heart failure and cardiac arrhythmias. The ionotropic effect is associated with NKA inhibition, which leads to an increase in intracellular Na^+ concentration, resulting in an augmented influx of Ca^{2+} ions into the cell, followed by contraction of the heart muscle [17]. However, the interaction of CGs with NKA may not only be associated with disruption of Ca^{2+} homeostasis, as SERCA (Sarco-Endoplasmic Reticulum Calcium ATPase) inhibitors do [18]. It has also been found that at low (subclinical) concentrations of CGs, where there is little or no inhibition of NKA, this enzyme can serve as a receptor that activates non-receptor tyrosine kinases. This in turn leads to activation of mitogen-activated protein kinase (MAPK) and the triggering of the Ras/MAPK signaling pathway [19,20]. This further leads to stimulation or inhibition of cell proliferation, depending on the cell type: cancer cell proliferation is inhibited, while primary noncancerous cells are not [21–23].

Besides this, CGs are also potent activators of the immune system response by induction of immunogenic cell death, which is a tremendous advantage over some other currently used chemotherapeutics, such as cisplatin, which lacks this effect. The immunogenic cell death is achieved by calreticulin exposure to the cell surface and the secretion of ATP and high-mobility group box 1 protein [24].

One of the widely studied CGs in terms of cancer is digoxin, currently included in a clinical trial for cancer combination therapy, in which it is co-administered with cisplatin (ClinicalTrials.gov). Another interesting and, in cancer treatment, possibly potent CG is Dg. This cardenolide type of CG also binds and inhibits NKA [25], and was shown to be potent in inhibiting cancer cell proliferation and cell cycle arrest [26–28] already at low nanomolar concentrations. Such concentrations are commonly found in the blood plasma of patients treated with Dg due to heart failure [13–15].

However, both Dg and digoxin lack cancer cell selectivity, resulting in high systemic toxicity often encountered in patients on CG therapy. Based on this, the seeking of novel CGs with improved properties and enhanced performance has not yet been finished. Therefore, we report on two very interesting CGs: hyrcanoside (Hyr, Figure 1) and deglucohyrcanoside (deHyr, Figure 1), about which there has not yet been much information. Hyr is a secondary plant metabolite of *Coronilla varia* L. Regarding cytotoxicity, the only information available is on Hyr-containing alcoholic extracts inhibiting the growth of KB cell [29] and human lymphocytic leukemia (P-388) and nasopharynx carcinomas (9KB) [30]. From earlier reports, it is obvious that deglucohyrcanoside acts as digoxin, but its cytotoxicity is several times lower [31–33], which indicates the potential of this CG as a therapeutic used in cancer treatment.

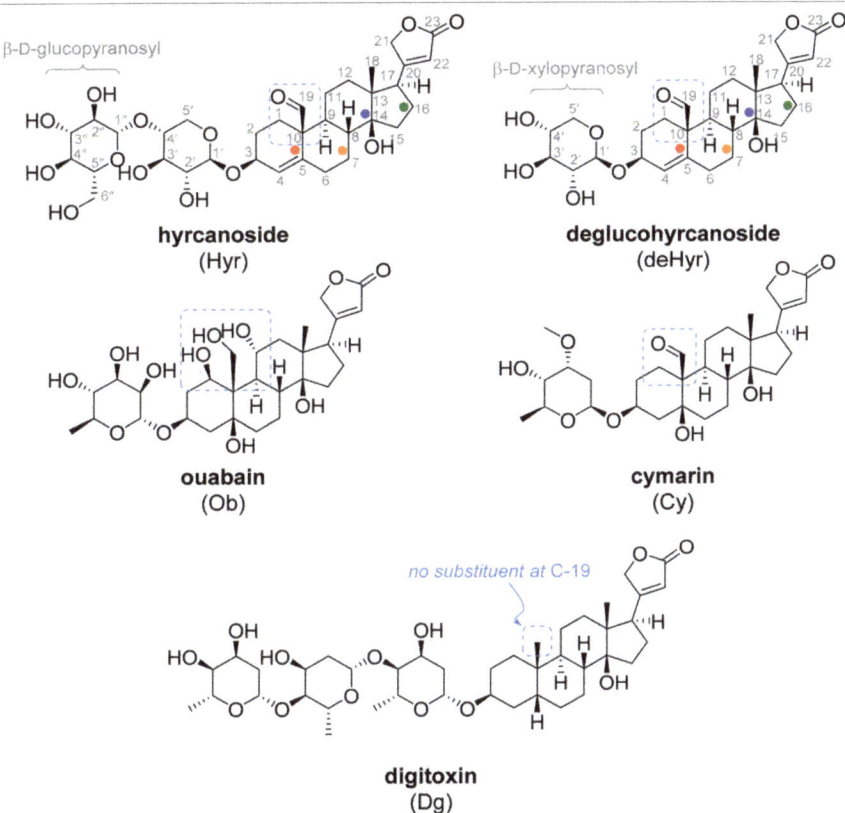

Figure 1. Structures of natural C-19-oxo cardiotonics and digitoxin. Carbon numbering of Hyr and deHyr is in grey. The ring designation of the steroid ring is highlighted by dots (i.e., the A ring is marked by a ● dot, B with ●, C with ●, and D with ● dot).

2. Materials and Methods

2.1. Materials

For thin-layer chromatography (TLC), aluminum silica gel sheets for detection in UV light (TLC Silica gel 60 F254, Merck, Prague, Czech Republic) were used. For TLC visualization, a diluted solution of H_2SO_4 in MeOH was used, and plates were heated. For column chromatography, 30–60 μm silica gel (ICN Biomedicals, Costa Mesa, CA, USA) was used. The NMR spectra were recorded by a 500 MHz instrument (JEOL, Tokyo, Japan) at 25 °C. The chemical shifts (δ) are presented in ppm, and the coupling constants (J) are presented in Hz. The ^{1}H and ^{13}C chemical shifts are referenced to tetramethylsilane using the solvent signals CHD$_2$SOCD$_3$ 2.50 ppm, CD$_3$SOCD$_3$ 39.52 ppm, CHD$_2$OD 3.31 ppm, and CD$_3$OD 49.00 ppm. For the signal assignments and obtaining of the coupling constants, combinations of the following standard NMR sequences were used: 1D and selective homodecoupled ^{1}H NMR spectra, ^{13}C NMR spectra with or without ^{1}H BB decoupling, 2D gCOSY, gTOCSY, dqf-COSY with 25% non-uniform sampling (NUS), 2D NOESY and ROESY (mix time 400 and 350 ms), 2D gHSQC and gHMBC (7 Hz) with adiabatic pulses and 25% NUS, 1D selective gNOESY1D and gROESY1D (various mix time), and gTOCSY1D (10, 15, 20, 40, 80, 160 ms). The content of Hyr and deHyr (dried extracts were dissolved in 50% MeOH) was verified using mass spectrometry, employing direct injection into the electrospray ionization source of QTRAP 6500+ (AB Sciex, Framingham, MA, USA) with a Turbo V Ion source. The mass spectrometer was operated in a positive scan mode with m/z ranging between 100 and 1000. The ion source settings were as follows: a temperature of 200 °C, a capillary voltage of 5500 V, curtain gas of 20 psi, nebulizer gas, and heater gas of 30 psi. The data were acquired and evaluated using Analyst 1.6.3 software (AB Sciex, Framingham, MA, USA). In further LC-MS analyses, the Quadrupole LC/MS (ESI ionization) with the Infinity III LC system (Agilent Technologies, Santa Clara, CA, USA) was used for LR-MS and HPLC analyses (C18 column: 100 mm, and UV detection).

2.2. Extraction of C. varia Seeds and Isolation of Compounds

Seeds of crown vetch (*Coronilla varia* L., Fabaceae, sometimes also *Securigera varia* (L.) Lassen, or *Coronilla pendula* Kit.) purchased from Agrostis Trávníky Ltd., Rousínov u Vyškova (CZ) were ground on an electric blade coffee grinder to a fine powder. Powdered seeds (500 g) were mixed with ethanol (500 mL) and kept at room temperature for seven days. Then, the mixture was filtered through frita, the filtrate was evaporated, re-dissolved in 200 mL of EtOH, and transferred onto a chromatography silicagel column (length of 24 cm, a diameter of 6 cm, 800 g of silica gel). Seed contents were eluted at first by ethanol and then by a gradient mixture of EtOH-H$_2$O (10:1→ 3:1, v/v), respectively. Thus, two fractions were obtained: ethanolic one (H1) and fractions eluted by the mixture of aqueous EtOH (H2). MS and TLC evaluations of fraction H1 showed that mainly daphnoretin, scopoletin, and umbelliferone (structures are shown in Figure S1) were present (after evaporation, a dry residue of 85 g) [29]. On the other hand, fraction H2 (we obtained a brown-red syrupy evaporate of 70 g) contained solely traces of the aforementioned three compounds plus (−)-epicatechin (Figure S1), deHyr, and some unidentified polar compounds [29]. As a major component, Hyr was identified. The content of both fractions was subjected to column chromatography.

Chromatographic purification of H1 (84 g) over a silica gel column (length of 24 cm, a diameter of 6 cm, 800 g of silica gel, using DCM-MeOH, 20:1→ 3:2, (v/v) as eluent) afforded mostly triacylglycerols, as expected, and some minor products. Only about 120 mg of crude Hyr was obtained. This was in accordance with the preliminary LC-MS spectra recorded for fraction H1, which showed only a negligible amount of compounds of interest. On the contrary, chromatographic purification of 69 g of the second major fraction H2 (length of 30 cm, a diameter of 4 cm, 600 g of silica gel, using DCM-MeOH, 10:1→ 3:2, v/v as an eluent) provided four fractions (f1–f4), and LC-MS confirmed the presence of both deHyr (in fraction 2) and Hyr (in fraction 4).

In addition, other known compounds contained in *C. varia* were detected by LC-MS in fraction f2, namely daphnoretin and umbelliferone in fraction f1 and (−)-epicatechin and scopoletin in f3 (structures are shown in Figure S1). DeHyr and Hyr fractions were further purified. Hyr fraction f4 of H2 was purified using a silica gel column (length of 30 cm, a diameter of 4 cm, 600 g of silicagel, using DCM-MeOH, 10:1→ 6:1, (v/v) as eluent) to provide fairly pure Hyr. Due to the fact that Hyr contains both hydrophilic disaccharide and lipophilic steroidal moiety, standard chromatographic purification was not efficient enough to provide pure Hyr (or deHyr). Thus, the final processing step was the crystallization of Hyr from the solution. Finally, the crude in absolute MeOH was dissolved, and the careful addition of Et$_2$O showed signs of crystals being formed. Crude Hyr was thus dissolved in MeOH (100 mL), then, Et$_2$O (50 mL) was slowly added and the solution left to stay at 4 °C overnight. The white solids formed were fritted and washed with ether. Hyr was obtained as white crystals (1.634 g, 2.40 mmol; 3.3%). Purified deHyr fraction H1 (length of 30 cm, a diameter of 4 cm, 600 g of silica gel, using DCM-MeOH, 10:1, v/v as an eluent) provided a notably lower amount of crude deHyr. This product was also crystallized by dissolving it in a mixture of MeOH (10 mL) and acetone (20 mL) with the subsequent addition of Et$_2$O (20 mL), then it was left overnight at 4 °C. This process provided deHyr as white crystals (96 mg, 0.19 mmol; 0.2%). MS analyses confirmed the corresponding molecular composition (Figures S6 and S7). The purity and identity of the isolated compounds were checked by LC analysis (Figures S8 and S9) and NMR (Section 3.1) spectroscopy, respectively.

2.3. In Silico Modeling

The Maestro program 2019-3 (Schrödinger, LLC, New York, NY, USA) was used for all structural modifications and subsequent molecular docking of the tested CGs into NKA. The CG structures were obtained from the ChemSpider database (www.chemspider.com). Using the LigPrep module, the missing hydrogen atoms were added to the ligands. Then, the ligands' structure was converted to 3D, and their energy was minimized using the OPLS3e force field. The structure of NKA with the code name 4RET (organism: *Sus scrofa*) was obtained from the ProteinDataBank database (www.rcsb.org). Non-protein moieties (aspartyl phosphate, cholesterol, sucrose, digoxin, Mg^{2+}, N-acetyl-D-glucosamine, phospholipids, and water) were removed from the NKA structure. This was followed by adding hydrogen atoms to the NKA structure. Then, the amino acids were assigned a protonation state corresponding to pH = 7 using the PROPKA function, and the energy of the molecule was minimized by the OPLS3e force field. Using the amino acids L-Thr$_{114}$, L-Asp$_{121}$, and L-Thr$_{797}$, a ligand-binding site was defined, which consisted of two cubes with an edge length of 15 and 35 Å (a small and large cube, respectively). The center of the molecule should not leave the smaller cube and the molecule as a whole should not leave the larger cube. Subsequently, a subset of a spherical pocket with a radius of 4 Å was defined using the constraints function, into which the C and D cycles of the steroid skeleton were fixed. The CG ligands were docked into NKA with an extra precision mode.

2.4. Cell Lines

If not indicated otherwise, the cell lines were purchased from the American Type Culture Collection (ATCC). The CCRF-CEM line is derived from T-cell childhood acute lymphoblastic leukemia, which shows the highest chemosensitivity in our tumor cell lines panel. K562 is the erythroid-myeloid precursor cell line derived from chronic myeloid leukemia carrying the *BCR-ABL* hybrid gene. A549, MCF-7, PC-3, 5637, U-2 OS, and MiaPaCa-2 are cells derived from lung, breast, prostate, bladder carcinoma, osteosarcoma, and pancreatic adenocarcinoma, respectively. HEK 293T are transformed human embryonic kidney cells, and L929 (Sigma, St. Louis, MS, USA) are transformed mouse fibroblasts. HCT116, cells from colorectal carcinoma, and their *p53* gene knock-out variant (HCT116p53-/-) were purchased from Horizon Discovery. This cell line is a model of human tumors bearing *p53* loss-of-function mutations or biallelic deletion of the *p53* gene, frequently associated with poor prognosis. The MRC-5 and BJ cells were used as noncancerous cells; more specifically, they are human fibroblasts from the lungs and foreskin, respectively. According to the supplier's recommendations, all cells were cultured at 37 °C in a 5% CO$_2$ atmosphere and 100% humidity. The culture media used were: DMEM, RPMI 1640, and MEM (according to a cell line); all were supplemented with 5 g L^{-1} glucose, 10% fetal calf serum, 2 mM glutamine, 100 U mL^{-1} penicillin, 100 µg mL^{-1} streptomycin, and NaHCO$_3$. Cells were passaged every two or three days using 0.25% trypsin plus 0.01% EDTA (ethylenediamine tetraacetic acid) in phosphate-buffered saline.

2.5. MTS Cytotoxic Assay

To evaluate compound cytotoxicity, cells were seeded in 384-well microtiter plates in a volume of 30 mL. The next day, aliquots of the tested derivatives were transferred with Echo550 acoustic liquid handler (Labcyte) to obtain dose response curves with dilution factor 4. The experiments were performed in technical duplicates and three or more biological replicates. After 72 h of incubation in a humidified incubator, 4 mL of the MTS/PMS stock solution were pipetted into each well. After another 1–4 h of incubation, the absorbance at 490 nm was measured using an EnVision Multilabel Plate Reader (PerkinElmer). IC_{50} values were calculated from the appropriate dose response curves in Dotmatics software using the following equation: IC_{50} = ($OD_{drug exposed well}$/mean $ODc_{ontrol\ wells}$) × 100% [34].

2.6. Mice and Peritoneal Primary Cells

Female mice of the inbred strain C57BL/6, eight to ten weeks old, were purchased from Charles River Deutschland (Sulzfeld, Germany). They were kept in transparent plastic cages in groups of ten. The animals were housed with food and water ad libitum, lighting was set on 6–18 h, and the temperature was set at 22 °C. All protocols were approved by the institutional ethics committee (MSMT15894/2013-310). Animals, killed by cervical dislocation, were intraperitoneally injected with 8 mL of sterile saline. Pooled peritoneal cells collected from mice were washed in sterile saline, re-suspended in the culture medium, and seeded into 96-well microplates in final 100-µL volumes (Costar, Cambridge, MA, USA). The final density of the cells was 0.25×10^6 per mL^{-1}. The cultures were maintained with or without compounds for 24 h at 37 °C with 5% CO_2 in a humidified Heraeus incubator in complete RPMI-1640 (Merck-Sigma, St. Louis, MS, USA), which contained 10% heat-inactivated fetal bovine serum, 2 mM of L-glutamine, 50 µg·mL^{-1} of gentamicin, and 5×10^{-5} M of 2-mercaptoethanol (all Merck-Sigma, St. Louis, MS, USA). Compounds (Ob, Cy (cymarin), Hyr, deHyr) were prepared as 100 mM stock solutions in dimethyl sulfoxide (DMSO) with cell culture grade. The next dilution continued immediately before the experiment with the culture medium. To eliminate the influence of DMSO, equal levels of DMSO were added to the experimental groups.

2.7. Viability of Mouse Primary Cells

The viability of mouse peritoneal cells was determined using a colorimetric assay based on the cleavage of the tetrazolium salt WST-1 by mitochondrial dehydrogenases in viable cells (Merck-Sigma, St. Louis, MS, USA). The cells were cultured as described above. After 24 h of culture, the WST-1 was added, and the cells were kept in the Heraeus incubator at 37 °C for an additional 3 h. Optical density at 450/690 nm was determined. The cytotoxicity of the tested CGs was expressed as a percentage. The test samples were related to control samples consisting of untreated cells and samples with 100% dead cells evoked by 1% Triton, according to the formula: ((exp. value − control value)/(Triton value − control value)) × 100. All control and experimental variants were run in quadruplicates. The data were analyzed using GraphPad Prism software 6.05 (GraphPad, San Diego, CA, USA). Values were expressed as the mean ± standard error of the mean (SEM).

2.8. Analysis of Cell Cycle Arrest and Cell Death

CCRF-CEM cells were seeded at a density of 1×10^6 cells per one mL in six-well plates (TPP) and treated the next day with CGs at concentrations corresponding to 1× or 5× the IC_{50} value. Together with the CG-treated cells, a vehicle-treated sample was harvested at the same time point. After 24 h, the cells were washed with cold phosphate-buffered saline, fixed dropwise in 70% ethanol, and stored overnight at −20 °C. The cells were then washed with hypotonic citrate buffer, treated with RNAse (50 µg mL^{-1}), and stained with propidium iodide. Flow cytometry using a 488 nm laser (FACS-Calibur, Becton Dickinson, NJ, USA) was used for measurement. The cell cycle was analyzed by the ModFitLT program (Verity), and apoptosis was measured in a logarithmic model expressing the percentage of particles with a lower propidium content than cells in the G0/G1 phase (<G1) of the cell cycle in the CellQuest program (Becton Dickinson). Half of the sample was used to label cells with pH3^{Ser10}-FITC antibody (Exbio) for subsequent flow cytometry analysis of mitotic cells [35].

2.9. BrDU Incorporation Analysis

The cells were cultured in the same way as the cell cycle analysis method. Just before harvesting, 5-bromo-2′-deoxyuridine (BrDU) of 10 µM concentration was added to the cells for pulse-labeling for 30 min. Then, the cells were fixed with −20 °C cold 70% ethanol and stored in a freezer for 16 h. Before antibody staining, the samples were incubated on ice for 30 min, washed once with phosphate-buffered saline (PBS), and re-suspended in 2 M of HCl for 30 min at room temperature to hydrolyze their DNA. After neutralization with 0.1 M of $Na_2B_4O_7$ (borax) solution, the cells were washed with PBS containing 0.5% Tween-20 and 1% BSA. This was followed by staining with the primary anti-BrDU antibody (Exbio) for 30 min at room temperature. Then, the cells were washed with PBS and stained with a secondary anti-mouse antibody conjugated to fluorescein isothiocyanate (Merck-Sigma, St. Louis, MS, USA) at room temperature in the dark. After another washing with PBS and incubation with propidium iodide (0.1 mg·mL^{-1}) and RNAse A (0.5 mg·mL^{-1}) for 1 h at room temperature in the dark, the cells were analyzed by flow cytometry using a 488 nm laser (FACSCalibur, Becton Dickinson, Franklin Lakes, NJ, USA) [35].

2.10. BrU Incorporation Analysis

The cells were cultured and processed as described above. Before harvesting, the cells were pulse-labeled with 1 mM of 5-bromouridine (BrU) for 30 min. The cells were then fixed in 1% buffered paraformaldehyde with 0.05% NP-40 at room temperature for 15 min, and then stored at 4 °C overnight. Before measurement, they were washed with 1% glycine in PBS, washed again with PBS, and stained with primary anti-BrdU antibody cross-reactive to BrU (Exbio) for 30 min at room temperature in the dark. From this point on, the experiment was performed exactly as in the method described above [35].

3. Results and Discussion

3.1. Isolation and Identification of Hyr and deHyr

Isolation of the desired substances from the plant seeds consisted of several steps (Figure 2). First, it was necessary to grind the seeds and extract them. This procedure is described in detail in Section 2.1. Two extraction solvent systems were used: EtOH and aqueous EtOH, providing two extracts designated as H1 and H2, respectively. According to MS and TLC analyses, the desired substances (Hyr and deHyr) were mainly present in the H2 fraction. This was followed by purification of the extracts by chromatographic separation on silica gel. Separation of the components from extract H2 yielded pure Hyr (3.3%) and a very small amount of deHyr (0.0002%). Hembree et al. [30] described the isolation of Hyr and deHyr from 14.8 kg of powdered seeds with the yield of semi-pure Hyr of 2.57 g (0.00017%) and 70 mg (0.000005%) of deHyr. We hypothesize that the low yield of deHyr can be explained by its absence in the plant material, and the trace amount is formed during the processing. Taken together, our procedure has improved the yield of pure Hyr and deHyr by ca. 20,000 and 40 times, respectively.

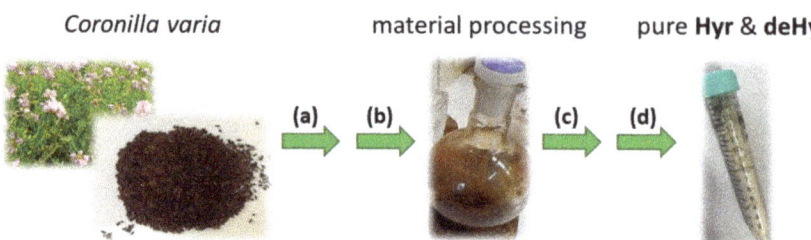

(a) seed grinding and extraction
(b) rough chromatographic separation
(c) further chromatographic purifications
(d) Hyr and deHyr crystallization

Figure 2. Diagram presenting the process leading to the isolation of Hyr and deHyr from the seeds of *Coronilla varia*.

A thorough literature search has revealed that the name hyrcanoside has also been used for other chemical structures. Two different compounds were named hyrcanoside (Figure S2). A cardenolide, (3β)-3-[(4-O-β-D-glucopyranosyl-β-D-xylopyranosyl)oxy]-14-hydroxy-19-oxocarda-4,20(22)-dienolide (Hyr) (CAS Registry No. 15001-93-1; Figure 2 and Figure S2—compound Hyr), mostly named hyrcanoside (*Coronilla*) [30,31], which is the substance isolated from *Coronilla varia* (or from *C. varia* Prilipko, a synonym of *Securigera cretica* (L.) Lassen, *Securigera securidaca* (L.) Degen et Dörfler, and some other plants) [36], and a phenolglycoside that was isolated from *Dorema hyrcanum* Koso-Pol. or *Dorema glabrum* Fisch. & C.A. Mey., 1-[2-[(6-O-α-D-glucopyranosyl-β-D-glucopyranosyl)oxy]-6-hydroxy-4-methoxyphenyl]ethanone (CAS Registry No. 60197-59-3; Figure S2—compound s1) [37,38]. Hereby, we suggest naming this compound hyrcanoside (*Dorema*).

To make things even more complicated, Abubakirov [39] lists the structure of Hyr (Figure 1 and Figure S2) named as securidaside, and declares it identical with steroidal hyrcanoside. However, Zatula et al., in a series of earlier research articles [40–42], presents securidaside as C4(5) saturated, 5α,11β-hydroxy derivative s2 (CAS Registry No. 18309-58-5; for structure, see Figure S2). Zatula et al. in 1969 corrected [43] the structure to be identical with Hyr, from which it was cited by Abubakirov [39].

We also attempted to confirm the molecular structures of Hyr and deHyr by ^{1}H and ^{13}C NMR spectra (Table S1). Unfortunately, our values of the ^{13}C chemical shifts were not in full accordance with the ones recorded in DMSO-d_6 [30], nor in CD$_3$OD [44] (Hyr is named as securigenin glycoside s3; see Figures S4 and S5). Thus, we performed the signal assignment of all ^{13}C and ^{1}H signals of both Hyr and deHyr in both solvents. By the combination of 2D HSQC, HMBC, NOESY, TOCSY, and dqf-COSY spectra, followed by the series of the selective 1D TOCSY, NOESY, ROESY, and homodecoupled ^{1}H spectra, we were able to assign all of the signals, including stereo positions (Table S1). We concluded that our assignments and characteristics of Hyr are fully consistent with its known crystal structure and molecular models [44]. Comparison of ^{1}H and ^{13}C chemical shifts of Hyr in CD$_3$OD revealed that the chemical shifts of C3′ and H3′ signals are interchanged with C5″ and H5″, respectively [44]. After this correction, the ^{13}C chemical shifts differed from −0.15 to 0.03 ppm, and ^{1}H chemical shifts differed from −0.01 to −0.08 ppm; thus, we concluded that our Hyr isolated from *C. varia* and the securigenin glycoside s3 (= Hyr, Figure S3; the designation is different for data comparison) [44] isolated from *S. securidaca* are identical compounds. In contrast, the values of ^{13}C chemical shifts of Hyr differed more significantly in DMSO-d_6 [30]. Even when the obvious interchange of the signals for C4 and C22 were corrected, there were still several deviations (1–11 ppm), which cannot be removed by an interchange. Since the compound was isolated from the same herb and its structure was confirmed by comparison with the synthetic standard, we concluded that the ^{13}C chemical shifts are confused in [30].

3.2. In Silico Modeling

Since CGs are well-known to be NKA inhibitors, we strived to determine whether Hyr and deHyr share the same fate. Using molecular docking, which is a method for studying protein-ligand complex interactions, we performed an in silico study of these CGs and NKA. The data were compared with Ob, Dg, and Cy. The structures of all five examined NKA ligands consisted of a steroid skeleton, which is substituted by a lactone and a saccharide moiety at the C-17 and C-3 position, respectively. Hyr and deHyr were docked into the NKA binding site, which is located in the transmembrane domain of the NKA α-subunit between the helices one to six. This binding site is divided into a polar (L-Gln$_{111}$, L-Glu$_{117}$, L-Asp$_{121}$, L-Asn$_{122}$, and L-Thr$_{797}$) and nonpolar part (L-Ile$_{315}$, L-Phe$_{316}$, L-Gly$_{319}$, L-Phe$_{783}$, L-Phe$_{786}$, and L-Leu$_{793}$) [45]. In Figures 3 and 4, the far and near views of the CGs docked into NKA are shown in the lowest binding energy mode (Table 1). From Table 1, based on the binding energies, it is clear that the NKA-Ob and NKA-Hyr complexes were the most and the least stable ones, respectively, from the docked ligands.

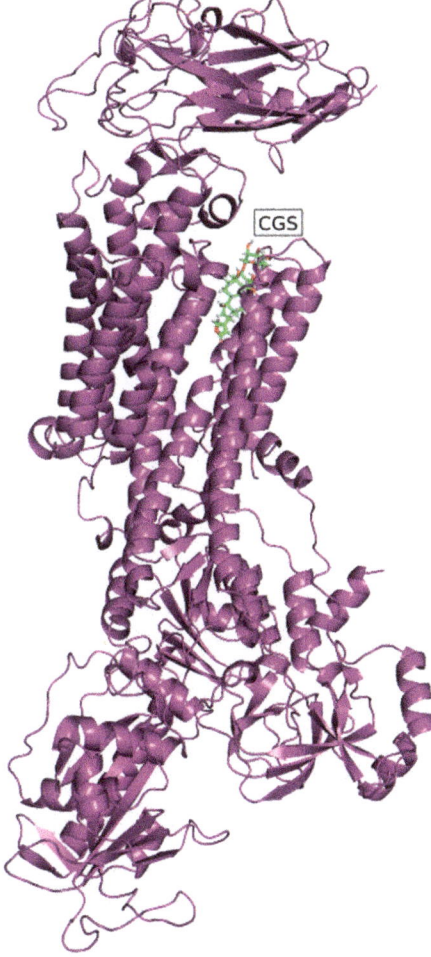

Figure 3. Far view of ouabain (green) docked into Na$^+$/K$^+$-ATPase (purple) with the lowest binding energy. Images were taken using PyMOL 2.3.3 (Schrödinger, LLC, New York, NY, USA).

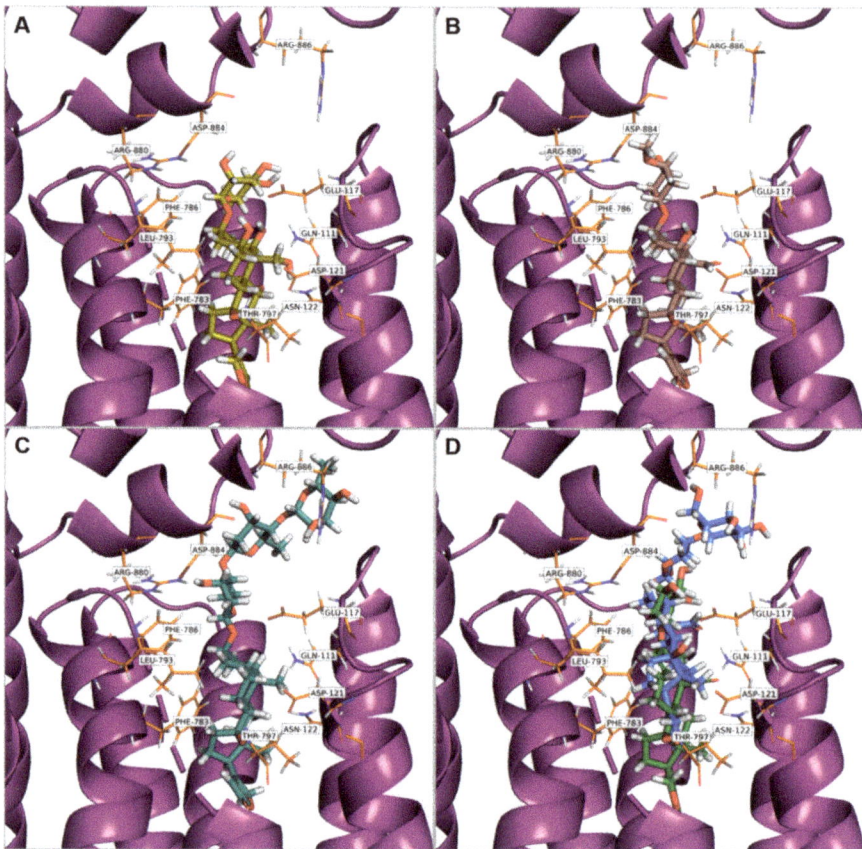

Figure 4. Near view of cardiac glycosides (stick representations) docked into Na$^+$/K$^+$-ATPase (purple, image representations; orange, individual residues, stick representations) with the lowest binding energy mode. The cardiac glycoside binding site in the Na$^+$/K$^+$-ATPase is indicated. (**A**) Ouabain, (**B**) cymarin, (**C**) digitoxin, (**D**) hyrcanoside (in blue) and deglucohyrcanoside (in green). The images were taken using PyMOL 2.3.3 (Schrödinger, LLC, New York, NY, USA).

Table 1. Binding energies of cardiac glycosides docked into Na$^+$/K$^+$-ATPase.

Ligand *	Binding Energies (kcal·mol^{-1})
Ob	−9.85
deHyr	−8.48
Dg	−7.47
Cy	−6.42
Hyr	−5.85

* Ob = ouabain; deHyr = deglucohyrcanoside; Dg = digitoxin; Cy = Cymarin; Hyr = Hyrcanoside.

The NKA-Ob complex, which served as a reference, contained a hydrogen bridge between the conserved β-hydroxyl group at the C-14 position and L-Thr$_{797}$, and between the hydroxyl group at the C-1 and C-19 positions with L-Gln$_{111}$ and C-11 and C-5 with L-Asn$_{122}$ and L-Glu$_{117}$, respectively. Thus, Ob was docked into NKA as expected, i.e., with its polar surface facing the polar amino acids. Similarly, the nonpolar surface of Ob was oriented towards the nonpolar part of the NKA cavity.

Another CG docked into NKA, the second reference ligand Dg, interacted like Ob with L-Thr$_{797}$ via the β-hydroxyl group at the C-14. Unlike Ob, Dg contains only one of the aforementioned β-hydroxyl groups at the C-14, but even so, the orientation of its steroid skeleton was identical to that of Ob, underlining the importance of nonpolar interactions (especially with L-Phe$_{783}$ and L-Leu$_{793}$) for CG binding to NKA.

Similarly, the other CG ligands were docked to the binding site of NKA with the same steroid skeleton orientation as Ob and Dg; β-Hydroxyl groups at the C-14 position interacting with L-Thr$_{797}$ were also present in the NKA-deHyr and NKA-Cy complexes. In the case of Cy, interactions of the carbonyl group at the C-19 and β-hydroxyl group at the C-5 with L-Gln$_{111}$ and L-Glu$_{117}$, respectively, were also found. The interaction of the conserved β-hydroxyl group of C-14 with L-Thr$_{797}$ was also present in the NKA-deHyr complex. However, it was not present in the NKA-Hyr complex; on the contrary, this hydroxyl group interacted with L-Glu$_{117}$, which lies closer to the NKA cavity surface. The absence of Hyr interaction with L-Thr$_{797}$ of NKA was because Hyr did not penetrate deep enough into the CG binding site of NKA as the other evaluated ligands. This is probably caused by the presence of β-D-glucopyranosyl as a second saccharide unit (with the first being β-D-xylopyranosyl in the case of both Hyr and deHyr, as is illustrated in Figure 1) at the C-3 position of Hyr. Hyr interactions with the key amino acid residues (L-Glu$_{115}$, L-Glu$_{116}$, and L-Arg$_{886}$) of NKA were detected only from the β-D-glucopyranosyl unit, not from the β-D-xylopyranosyl, as it was in the case of deHyr interaction with L-Glu$_{116}$ and L-Glu$_{117}$.

For other glycosylated ligands (Ob, Dg, Cy), the saccharide moiety also contributed to their binding to NKA. Ob and Cy interacted with L-Arg$_{880}$ and L-Glu$_{312}$ by α-L-rhamnopyranosyl present in Ob and β-D-cymaropyranosyl present in Cy. In the case of Dg, there was an interaction of the first β-D-digitoxopyranose with L-Arg$_{880}$ and L-Asp$_{884}$ of NKA and the third β-D-digitoxopyranose with L-Arg$_{886}$.

To summarize, all ligands (Ob, Dg, deHyr, Hyr, and Cy) that docked into the NKA binding site differed in the type of glycosylation at the C-3 position, as well as in the number of hydroxyl and carbonyl groups present at the steroid skeleton. As is evident from our findings, the number of these groups is important for the strength of the bond with NKA. Ob, which contains the most hydroxyl groups in its structure and is, therefore, able to form the most hydrogen bridges with NKA, was docked with the lowest binding energy (Table 1). The importance of these interactions, especially with L-Gln$_{111}$ and L-Asn$_{122}$, is documented by the crystal structure of NKA with Ob in [45], and in several mutagenesis studies in which a significant reduction in CG affinity to NKA was observed due to their substitution.

Dg, deHyr, and Cy have also docked as Ob to the CG binding site in NKA with the same orientation of the steroid skeleton as Ob in the aforementioned NKA crystal structure [45]. The same orientation of the steroid skeleton was also observed in the crystal structure of NKA with digoxin [46] and strebloside, which is a structural analog of Cy [47]. However, deHyr and Cy showed higher binding energies compared to Ob caused by a lower number of interactions with NKA, which is due to the lower number of substituents on the steroid skeleton. For the same reason, the reference ligand Dg also had higher binding energy compared to Ob. As for Hyr, it was also docked with the same steroid skeleton orientation as Ob and Dg, however, its binding energy was higher not only compared to these ligands, but also compared to other glycosylated ligands, including deHyr, which contains only one saccharide unit in its structure. Precisely due to the presence of two saccharide units, Hyr did not dock as deeply into the NKA binding cavity as did the other tested ligands. It has been reported that the number of carbohydrate units affects the strength of the NKA–CG interaction [48], and, for this reason, there was an increase in binding energy for Hyr compared to deHyr. However, this argument does not apply to Dg, which contains trisaccharide in its structure, meaning that the size of the binding energy is determined by a combination of both factors, i.e., the appropriate type of substituents on the steroid skeleton and the degree of glycosylation. Overall, Hyr was docked with higher binding energy due to both the different number of substituents on the steroid skeleton and the different degrees of glycosylation compared to other glycosylated ligands.

3.3. Anticancer Potential of the Evaluated Steroid Glycosides

CGs as well-established therapeutics for the treatment of cardiac insufficiencies and arrhythmias have lately been subjected to drug repurposing, since it has been reported that they also exhibit great anticancer potential. Often, however, high systemic toxicity was also described. However, this phenomenon could be circumvented by higher cancer cell selectivity and/or a partial decrease in the overall toxicity. Therefore, as a next step, we evaluated the cytotoxicity and cancer cell selectivity of the CGs, Hyr, and deHyr (compared with Ob, Cy, and Dg), isolated from *C. varia* in a panel of human cancer cell lines. The activity was compared with toxicity results from noncancerous primary human cells, as well as mouse cells, which should be, in general, less sensitive to CGs due to different NKA isoforms.

The cytotoxicities of the CGs after 72 h of incubation were expressed as the half-maximal inhibitory concentrations (IC_{50}), which are summarized in Table 2. The results showed marked differences in *in vitro* toxicity between the CGs both in potency and selectivity. For all compounds, we detected a concentration-dependent cytotoxicity profile in all evaluated cell lines. From the results, it is obvious that Hyr and deHyr, even though they exhibited lower cytotoxicities to cancerous cell lines than that of well-described CGs Ob and Dg, manifested a good selectivity for cancer cells when compared to noncancerous cells. As for Hyr, the most pronounced selectivity (compared against MRC-5 cells) was observed for human cancer cells from lung (A549), pancreas (MiaPaCa-2), breast (MCF-7), and transformed kidney cells (HEK 293T). Fairly good selectivity was also detected for human leukemic cells, cells from colorectal carcinoma regardless of *p53* deletion, and cells from bladder carcinoma. Concerning deHyr, it exhibited the highest cancer cell selectivity (compared to BJ cells) for A549 cells, which was followed by good selectivity for leukemic, pancreatic, breast, prostate, and colorectal (with and without *p53* deletion) cancer cells. Dg and Cy shared almost identical selectivity (compared to BJ cells) to cancer cells derived from lung and colon carcinoma, as well as to leukemic cells (Ob mainly to A549 cells).

As expected, cytotoxicity of the tested CGs was significantly affected by the type of attached saccharide at the C-3 position of the steroid skeleton. Based on the data gained in this study, we concluded that the derivatives with one attached carbohydrate moiety exhibited the highest cytotoxicity compared to derivatives glycosylated to a higher extent, which is in agreement with what is known for the sugar vs. cytotoxicity relationship for CGs in general [13]. However, interestingly, the least toxic CG, Hyr, contains two saccharide moieties. It exhibited even lower toxicity than Dg, which contains trisaccharide. This contradiction might be explained by the molecular docking into NKA, in which the presence of the third carbohydrate unit stabilized Dg in the NKA cavity to a greater extent than in the case of Hyr.

Table 2. Summary of cytotoxic activities (IC$_{50}$, nM) of the examined cardiac glycosides: ouabain (Ob), cymarin (Cy), digitoxin (Dg), hyrcanoside (Hyr), and deglucohyrcanoside (deHyr) after 72 h of incubation with cancerous and noncancerous human and mouse cells.

Compound Cell Line	Ob	Cy	Dg	Hyr	deHyr
			IC$_{50}$ [nM] [a]		
CCRF-CEM	32 ± 5.8	14 ± 2.1	20 ± 3.5	660 ± 38	110 ± 21
K562	57 ± 6.2	25 ± 4.5	19 ± 2.2	800 ± 52	130 ± 21
A549	22 ± 0.94	15 ± 1.8	19 ± 2.0	550 ± 38	90 ± 14
HCT116	30 ± 3.6	21 ± 2.5	20 ± 1.5	670 ± 37	140 ± 16
HCT116p53-/-	28 ± 7.6	19 ± 3.8	27 ± 9.6	730 ± 98	130 ± 23
MiaPaCa-2	49 ± 2.01	44 ± 8.6	79 ± 2.8	491 ± 23	120 ± 5.2
MCF-7	52 ± 5.6	29 ± 8.1	78 ± 1.1	566 ± 29	119 ± 6.4
U-2 OS	59 ± 1.1	43 ± 1.8	45 ± 2.1	1104 ± 59	165 ± 11
5637	110 ± 11	89 ± 5.5	58 ± 1.6	1511 ± 51	398 ± 46
PC-3	49 ± 1.4	26 ± 2.9	69 ± 2.2	756 ± 29	122 ± 4.7
HEK 293T	35 ± 1.2	3.02 ± 1.4	69 ± 2.1	383 ± 8.9	38 ± 0.97
MRC-5	39 ± 1.6	26 ± 2.4	78 ± 1.9	302 ± 43	77 ± 12
BJ	54 ± 9.9	54 ± 10	47 ± 12	1450 ± 250	230 ± 35
L929	>10,000	>10,000	>10,000	>10,000	>10,000

[a] Cytotoxic activity was determined by MTS assay following 72 h of incubation. The values represent the mean of IC$_{50}$ from three independent experiments. The tested cell lines: CCRF-CEM (childhood T-cell acute lymphoblastic leukemia), K562 (chronic myeloid leukemia), A549 (lung adenocarcinoma), HCT116 (colorectal carcinoma), HCT116p53-/- (HCT116 with deleted *p53* gene), MiaPaCa-2 (adenocarcinoma of pancreas), MCF-7 (breast carcinoma), U-2 OS (osteosarcoma), 5637 (bladder carcinoma), PC-3 (prostate carcinoma), and HEK 293T (transformed kidney cells). Noncancerous human cells: MRC-5 (lung fibroblasts) and BJ (fibroblasts from foreskin). L929, mouse transformed fibroblasts. The colors in the first slope represent the types of the cells: orange—human cancerous or transformed cell lines, blue—human primary noncancerous cells, green—mouse cells.

Besides the number of saccharide moieties, the distribution of substituents on the steroid skeleton of CGs also significantly affected their overall cytotoxicity. As aforementioned in the docking part of this study, the binding site for CGs is divided in terms of amino acid distribution into a polar and nonpolar part, which means that the presence of polar substituents on the steroid skeleton affects the level of NKA inhibition to a greater extent. Of the monoglycosylated CGs in this study, the highest cytotoxicity was exhibited by Cy, which, like deHyr, contains a carbonyl group at the C-19, but also contains a β-hydroxyl group at the C-5 position. In contrast, Ob contains β-hydroxyl group at the C-1, α-OH at C-10, and C-19 positions, but it lacks the β-OH at the C-5. Thus, it seems that the β-hydroxyl group of the C-5 might contribute to the overall cytotoxicity. However, as evidenced by Levrier et al., the cytotoxicity is also significantly affected by the carbonyl group at the C-19; when a hydroxyl group at the C-19 is substituted for a carbonyl moiety, the cytotoxicity of the resulting derivative increases approximately 150-fold [49]. The carbonyl group is also present in Cy, which was the most cytotoxic from the CGs in this study. Therefore, based on our data, we conclude that the cytotoxicity of the five CGs evaluated was mainly influenced by the carbonyl group at the C-19, the β-hydroxyl group at the C-5, and the decreasing number of carbohydrate units.

The trend of the dose response curves for the evaluated CGs was somewhat similar for all examined human cell lines. Nonetheless, the situation substantially differed for mouse fibroblasts (L929; see Table 2), for which none of the CGs exhibited any signs of cytotoxicity up to the highest tested concentration (10 μM), which is probably caused by increased resistance of the mouse α-subunit of NKA to CGs [50]. Amino acid substitutions Q111R and N122D are present in the murine α-subunit of NKA [51] and, therefore, mouse cells can tolerate up to at least 1000 times higher concentrations of CGs than corresponding human cells [52].

3.4. Steroid Glycoside Toxicity to Mouse Macrophages

Even though it is known that CGs trigger immunogenic cell death and that they stimulate the immune response, not much is known about their effect on primary macrophages.

For the first time, we bring data on the effect of Ob, Hyr, deHyr, and Cy on these cells: primary macrophages, the innate immune cells. For this task, the cells were isolated directly from mice, and cell viability after 24-h CG treatment was determined by WST-1. The results are summarized in Figure 5. It is obvious that the viability of mouse macrophages was reduced in the presence of all tested compounds in comparison to untreated control cells, but, for some, only marginally. The viability of mouse macrophages treated with Ob decreased only by 10–20% (compared to the control) quite independently on the used concentration (1 nm–100 μM), while cytotoxicity of Cy and Hyr was more pronounced—about 60% of the control. The most cytotoxic to mouse macrophages was deHyr, which reduced their viability to 50% of the control. Surprisingly, a dose-dependent decrease in cell viability was not found for any of the compounds, despite a wide range of tested concentrations: 0.001–100.0 μM.

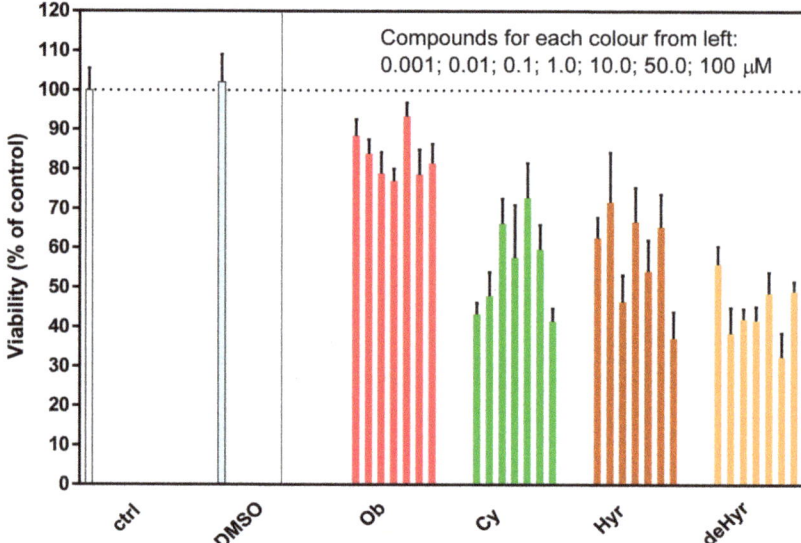

Figure 5. Viability of mouse peritoneal cells. Isolated cells were cultured for 24 h. Individual compounds, i.e., ouabain (Ob), cymarin (Cy), hyrcanoside (Hyr), and deglucohyrcanoside (deHyr), were applied at concentrations of 0.001, 0.01, 0.1, 1.0, 10.0, 50.0, and 100 μM. The effect of DMSO was also analyzed; its concentration corresponded to 50 μM concentration of compounds. WST-1 assay was used for viability evaluation. The results are expressed as the percent of untreated controls (ctrl) ± SEM (standard error of the mean) of n = 8 values from two independent experiments.

To summarize, in our in vitro conditions, the most cytotoxic was deHyr; Cy and Hyr made a position between deHyr and Ob. Cytotoxicity of Ob was previously studied in neuronal-like SH-SY5Y cells after 24 and 48 h, for which Ob reduced their viability by 40 and 10%, respectively [53]. Distinct effects of Ob on the survival of human and rat vascular smooth muscle cells, endothelial cells, and astrocytes were confirmed by Akimova et al. [54]. Unlike human cells, their rodents counterparts perfectly survived in the presence of high concentrations of Ob (3–3000 μM), despite the complete inhibition of the NKA and inversion of the $[Na^+]_I/[K^+]_i$ ratio. These dramatic differences in Ob effects on rat and mouse cells are driven by variations of rodent α1 NKA isoform. This difference could also explain the non-existing dose-dependent curve in mouse macrophages.

It is generally accepted that CGs, such as clinically used digoxin, are cytotoxic. This is a rational reason to employ such compounds in anticancer therapy instead of the regulation of cardiac function. It seems that some cancer cell lines (especially the ones derived from lung and colon carcinoma) are more sensitive to cardenolides consisting of a lactone ring with five carbons than noncancerous cells. Recent data also document that another lesser known cardenolide derivative, nerigoside, was more cytotoxic in two colorectal cancer cell lines HT29 and SW620 when compared to normal human epithelial cell line NCM460 (determined by a similar in vitro viability assay, as in our study) [55]. Our pilot results showed that the cytotoxic effect of the tested CGs on mouse macrophages was not fully devastating, but the results significantly differed from mouse fibroblasts, for which no toxicity was detected up to 10 μM concentration, while for mouse macrophages, only Ob did not exhibit significant cytotoxicity (up to 100 μM concentration), which corresponds to the known fact that mouse cells are generally insensitive or less sensitive to CGs than human cells based on the expression of different NKA isoforms. Contrary to L929, in mouse macrophages, Cy reached IC_{50} already at the lowest tested concentration of 1 nM, deHyr ca. at 10 nM, and Hyr at ca. 100 nM concentration. The reason for this difference between the two types of mouse cells remains elusive.

3.5. Cell Cycle and Cell Death Analysis

Next, we wanted to find out whether Hyr and deHyr can arrest the cell cycle of cancer cells, as has been previously reported for Dg and Ob, which were evaluated in cancer cells of various origin. For a more detailed description of the biological activity of the studied derivatives, we performed cell cycle analysis of the most sensitive CCRF-CEM cells after 24 h of CG treatment (Table 3).

Table 3. Effect of cytotoxic compounds on cell cycle, apoptosis, and DNA/RNA synthesis in CCRF-CEM lymphoblasts (% of positive cells). Flow cytometry analysis was used to quantify cell cycle distribution and the percentage of apoptotic cells. The sum of the percentages for G0/G1, S, and G2/M is equal to 100%. [a] Phospho-Histone3 (Ser10); [b] BrDU, 5-bromo-2-deoxyuridine; [c] BrU, 5-bromouridine.

Compound *	< G1	G0/G1	S	G2/M	M [a]	BrDU [b]	BrU [c]
Control	2.74	43.36	33.86	22.34	1.69	33.10	34.51
Ob 1 × IC_{50}	20.68	40.42	25.78	33.80	1.73	40.53	39.77
Ob 5 × IC_{50}	33.31	33.94	40.80	25.27	0.63	19.29	6.56
Cy 1 × IC_{50}	2.89	35.78	39.87	24.35	1.43	32.34	35.63
Cy 5 × IC_{50}	7.01	40.34	31.17	28.49	1.08	21.37	27.52
Dg 1 × IC_{50}	7.56	33.21	36.28	30.51	1.97	35.91	42.99
Dg 5 × IC_{50}	10.35	33.71	22.26	44.03	1.28	23.52	3.88
Hyr 1 × IC_{50}	2.82	38.48	35.22	26.30	1.41	30.58	28.80
Hyr 5 × IC_{50}	5.82	42.13	23.01	34.86	0.95	23.58	3.82
deHyr 1 × IC_{50}	22.02	44.90	17.60	37.50	1.44	37.40	38.91
deHyr 5 × IC_{50}	27.43	39.12	34.53	26.34	1.56	6.08	12.17

* Ob = ouabain; deHyr = deglucohyrcanoside; Dg = digitoxin; Cy = Cymarin; Hyr = Hyrcanoside.

After 24-h incubation with 1× IC_{50} of CGs, CCRF-CEM cells were still viable. The percentage of the sub G0/1 population was only slightly increased compared to the untreated control, while treatment with 5× IC_{50} caused a typical increase in the cell number present in the sub G0/G1 phase, together with augmented DNA fragmentation. All five evaluated CGs induced an increase in the G2/M phase population. The decrease in cells in the S and G0/G1 populations was caused by the proportional accumulation of cells in the G2/M phase. We did not observe positivity for pH3^{Ser10}, and negativity indicated G2 arrest. Such a finding is consistent with a recently reported study showing ATR-CHK2-CDC25C-mediated G2/M cell cycle arrest after Dg treatment [56].

BrDU is incorporated into newly synthesized DNA, and BrDU pulse labeling is therefore commonly used as a proliferation marker. Low BrDU incorporation into the DNA of treated cells with all compounds at 5× IC_{50} reflected inhibition of DNA synthesis, indicating irreversible apoptotic changes. The percentage of BrU positive cells incorporating 5-bromouridine is proportional to the transcriptional activity of CCRF-CEM cells.

These values significantly decreased upon treatment with $5\times$ IC$_{50}$ of CGs, but not with $1\times$ IC$_{50}$.

Previously, the ability to arrest the cell cycle of cancer cells in the G2/M phase has been already described for Ob, oleandrin, digoxin, Dg, and its synthetic analog monoD [26,57–59]. In this study, the same effect was observed for all tested CGs, although in some, there was an increase in the G2/M phase already at $1\times$ IC$_{50}$, and in others only at $5\times$ IC$_{50}$. For substances in which the G2/M phase increased at $1\times$ IC$_{50}$, on the contrary, it decreased at $5\times$ IC$_{50}$, which means that each substance had its concentration optimum, above which G2/M decreased again. The same trend was observed by Elbaz et al. [26]. Lower incorporation of BrDU and BrU at $5\times$ IC$_{50}$ concentrations indicated that DNA and RNA synthesis decreased at these concentrations, although in some cases the number of S-phase cells may be higher, even though nucleic acid synthesis is no longer present and thus, the incorporation of BrDU and BrU decreases.

4. Conclusions

In this work, we describe a procedure for the isolation of two CGs, Hyr and de-Hyr, by aqueous EtOH extraction from seeds, with an overall yield of 3.3% and 0.0002%, respectively. This was an improvement by several times of magnitude than what has been reported so far. Both CGs, Hyr and deHyr, were assessed for their anticancer activity, which was compared to other well-known CGs Ob, Dg, and Cy. From the results, it is clear that Ob and deHyr outperformed the other CGs, which correlates with the docking study into NKA. The highest anticancer (based on the cancer cell selectivity) potential of all CGs was found against cells derived from lung and colorectal carcinoma. Moreover, all evaluated CGs arrested the cell cycle of CRF-CEM in the G2/M phase. Thus, even though further elaboration in deciphering detailed mechanisms of Hyr and deHyr and other CG anticancer activity is needed, the first results already indicate that these CGs could have a potential for a therapeutic application in cancer treatment. From the number of publications on CGs as anticancer drugs, it is obvious that they have come into the foreground as candidates of anticancer therapy with new mechanisms of actions than the standardly used chemotherapeutics, such as antimitotics [60] or cisplatin, and that their induction of the immune system response brings another added value in the treatment. We assume that our results can contribute to further development of drugs based on NKA interaction, and maybe additional molecular targets with selective cytotoxicity for cancer cells.

Supplementary Materials: The following are available online at https://www.mdpi.com/2304-8158/10/1/136/s1; Figure S1: Other known components of *C. varia*; Figure S2: Structures related to naming mismatch; Figure S3: Structures of so-called "securigenin glycosides"; Figure S4: The ^{1}H and ^{13}C chemical shifts of deHyr in CD$_3$OD and CD$_3$SOCD$_3$; Figure S5: The ^{1}H and ^{13}C chemical shifts of Hyr in CD$_3$OD and CD$_3$SOCD$_3$; Figures S6 and S7: MS spectrum of Hyr and deHyr, respectively; Figures S8 and S9: HPLC chromatograms of Hyr and deHyr, respectively; Table S1: ^{1}H and ^{13}C NMR characteristics of Hyr (securigenin s3), deHyr and related securigenins s4 and s5.

Author Contributions: S.R., T.Z., M.J., P.B.D., P.D., B.D., M.H., T.R., L.O., and E.K. conceived and designed the experiments; T.Z., S.R., B.D., M.J., J.B., E.K., P.C., L.K., S.G. and P.D. performed the experiments; T.Z., M.J., P.B.D., S.R., E.K., and B.D. analyzed the data; S.R., M.J., J.B., and P.D. wrote the article. All authors have read and agreed to the published version of the manuscript.

Funding: This work was supported by an internal grant from the budget for the implementation of the activities of the Institutional Plan of the UCT Prague in 2020, the grant of Specific university research A1_FPBT_2020_001, A2_FPBT_2020_015, grant No. A1_FPBT_2020_004, the grant of the Czech Ministry of Education, Youth and Sports (CZ-OPENSCREEN—LM2018130 and EATRIS-CZ—LM2018133), OPPC CZ.2.16/3.1.00/24503, NPU I LO1601, the internal grant of Palacký University (IGA_LF_2020_019) and Czech Science Foundation 14-04329S.

Institutional Review Board Statement: The study was conducted according to the guidelines of the Declaration of Helsinki. All protocols were approved by the institutional ethics committee (No. MSMT15894/2013-310).

Informed Consent Statement: Not applicable for studies not involving humans.

Conflicts of Interest: The authors declare no conflict of interest.

References

1. WHO. Available online: https://www.who.int/news-room/fact-sheets/detail/cancer (accessed on 7 December 2020).
2. Xue, H.; Li, J.; Xie, H.; Wang, Y. Review of drug repositioning approaches and resources. *Int. J. Biol. Sci.* **2018**, *14*, 1232–1244. [CrossRef] [PubMed]
3. Clinical Trials. Available online: ClinicalTrials.gov (accessed on 7 December 2020).
4. Platz, E.A.; Yegnasubramanian, S.; Liu, J.O.; Chong, C.R.; Shim, J.S.; Kenfield, S.A.; Stampfer, M.J.; Willett, W.C.; Giovannucci, E.; Nelson, W.G. A novel two-stage, transdisciplinary study identifies digoxin as a possible drug for prostate cancer treatment. *Cancer Discov.* **2011**, *1*, 68–77. [CrossRef] [PubMed]
5. Osman, M.H.; Farrag, E.; Selim, M.; Osman, M.S.; Hasanine, A.; Selim, A. Cardiac glycosides use and the risk and mortality of cancer; systematic review and meta-analysis of observational studies. *PLoS ONE* **2017**, *12*, e0178611. [CrossRef] [PubMed]
6. Couraud, S.; Azoulay, L.; Dell'Aniello, S.; Suissa, S. Cardiac glycosides use and the risk of lung cancer: A nested case–control study. *BMC Cancer* **2014**, *14*, 573. [CrossRef]
7. Karasneh, R.A.; Murray, L.J.; Cardwell, C.R. Cardiac glycosides and breast cancer risk: A systematic review and meta-analysis of observational studies. *Int. J. Cancer* **2017**, *140*, 1035–1041. [CrossRef]
8. Kepp, O.; Menger, L.; Vacchelli, E.; Adjemian, S.; Martins, I.; Ma, Y.; Sukkurwala, A.Q.; Michaud, M.; Galluzzi, L.; Zitvogel, L.; et al. Anticancer activity of cardiac glycosides. At the frontier between cell-autonomous and immunological effects. *Oncoimmunology* **2012**, *1*, 1640–1642. [CrossRef]
9. Schönfeld, W.; Weiland, J.; Lindig, C.; Masnyk, M.; Kabat, M.M.; Kurek, A.; Wicha, J.; Repke, K.R.H. The lead structure in cardiac glycosides is 5β,14β-androstane-3β,14-diol. *Naunyn Schmiedebergs Arch. Pharmacol.* **1985**, *329*, 414–426. [CrossRef]
10. Morsy, N. References. In *Aromatic and Medicinal Plants—Back to Nature*; El-Shemy, H., Ed.; IntechOpen: London, UK, 2017; pp. 29–45. ISBN 978-953-51-7348-9.
11. Manunta, P.; Hamilton, B.P.; Hamlyn, J.M. Structure-activity relationships for the hypertensinogenic activity of ouabain. *Hypertension* **2001**, *37*, 472–477. [CrossRef]
12. Magpusao, A.N.; Omolloh, G.; Johnson, J.; Gascón, J.; Peczuh, M.W.; Fenteany, G. Cardiac glycoside activities link Na$^+$/K$^+$ ATPase ion-transport to breast cancer cell migration via correlative SAR. *ACS Chem. Biol.* **2015**, *10*, 561–569. [CrossRef]
13. Wang, H.Y.; Xin, W.; Zhou, M.; Stueckle, T.A.; Rojanasakul, Y.; O'Doherty, G.A. Stereochemical survey of digitoxin monosaccharides: New anticancer analogues with enhanced apoptotic activity and growth inhibitory effect on human non-small cell lung cancer cell. *ACS Med. Chem. Lett.* **2011**, *2*, 73–78. [CrossRef]
14. Iyer, A.K.V.; Zhou, M.; Azad, N.; Elbaz, H.; Wang, L.; Rogalsky, D.K.; Rojanasakul, Y.; O'Doherty, G.A.; Langenhan, J.M. A direct comparison of the anticancer activities of digitoxin MeON-neoglycosides and O-glycosides. *ACS Med. Chem. Lett.* **2010**, *1*, 326–330. [CrossRef] [PubMed]
15. López-Lázaro, M.; Pastor, N.; Azrak, S.S.; Ayuso, M.J.; Austin, C.A.; Cortés, F. Digitoxin inhibits the growth of cancer cell lines at concentrations commonly found in cardiac patients. *J. Nat. Prod.* **2005**, *68*, 1642–1645. [CrossRef] [PubMed]
16. Ayogu, J.I.; Odoh, A.S. Prospects and therapeutic applications of cardiac glycosides in cancer remediation. *ACS Comb. Sci.* **2020**, *22*, 543–553. [CrossRef] [PubMed]
17. Reuter, H.; Henderson, S.A.; Han, T.; Ross, R.S.; Goldhaber, J.I.; Philipson, K.D. The Na$^+$-Ca^{2+} exchanger is essential for the action of cardiac glycosides. *Circ. Res.* **2002**, *90*, 305–308. [CrossRef] [PubMed]
18. Peterková, L.; Kmoníčková, E.; Ruml, T.; Rimpelová, S. Sarco/endoplasmic reticulum calcium ATPase inhibitors: Beyond anticancer perspective. *J. Med. Chem.* **2020**, *63*, 1937–1963. [CrossRef] [PubMed]
19. Haas, M.; Askari, A.; Xie, Z. Involvement of Src and epidermal growth factor receptor in the signal-transducing function of Na$^+$/K$^+$-ATPase. *J. Biol. Chem.* **2000**, *275*, 27832–27837. [CrossRef]
20. Haas, M.; Wang, H.; Tian, J.; Xie, Z. Src-mediated inter-receptor cross-talk between the Na$^+$/K$^+$-ATPase and the epidermal growth factor receptor relays the signal from ouabain to mitogen-activated protein kinases. *J. Biol. Chem.* **2002**, *277*, 18694–18702. [CrossRef]
21. Danen, E.H.J.; Sonneveld, P.; Sonnenberg, A.; Yamada, K.M. Dual stimulation of Ras/mitogen-activated protein kinase and Rhoa by cell adhesion to fibronectin supports growth factor–stimulated cell cycle progression. *J. Cell Biol.* **2000**, *151*, 1413–1422. [CrossRef]
22. Prassas, I.; Karagiannis, G.S.; Batruch, I.; Dimitromanolakis, A.; Datti, A.; Diamandis, E.P. Digitoxin-induced cytotoxicity in cancer cells is mediated through distinct kinase and interferon signaling networks. *Mol. Cancer Ther.* **2011**, *10*, 2083–2093. [CrossRef]
23. McConkey, D.J.; Lin, Y.; Nutt, L.K.; Ozel, H.Z.; Newman, R.A. Cardiac glycosides stimulate Ca^{2+} increases and apoptosis in androgen-independent, metastatic human prostate adenocarcinoma cells. *Cancer Res.* **2000**, *60*, 3807–3812.
24. Menger, L.; Vacchelli, E.; Adjemian, S.; Martins, I.; Ma, Y.; Shen, S.; Yamazaki, T.; Sukkurwala, A.Q.; Michaud, M.; Mignot, G.; et al. Cardiac glycosides exert anticancer effects by inducing immunogenic cell death. *Sci. Transl. Med.* **2012**, *4*, 143–199. [CrossRef] [PubMed]
25. Katz, A.; Lifshitz, Y.; Bab-Dinitz, E.; Kapri-Pardes, E.; Goldshleger, R.; Tal, D.M.; Karlish, S.J.D. Selectivity of digitalis glycosides for isoforms of human Na,K-ATPase. *J. Biol. Chem.* **2010**, *285*, 19582–19592. [CrossRef] [PubMed]

26. Elbaz, H.A.; Stueckle, T.A.; Wang, H.Y.L.; O'Doherty, G.A.; Lowry, D.T.; Sargent, L.M.; Wang, L.; Dinu, C.Z.; Rojanasakul, Y. Digitoxin and a synthetic monosaccharide analog inhibit cell viability in lung cancer cells. *Toxicol. Appl. Pharmacol.* **2012**, *258*, 51–60. [CrossRef] [PubMed]
27. Xu, Y.; Li, J.; Chen, B.; Zhou, M.; Zeng, Y.; Zhang, Q.; Guo, Y.; Chen, J.; Ouyang, J. Cardiac glycosides inhibit proliferation and induce apoptosis of human hematological malignant cells. *Int. J. Clin. Exp. Pathol.* **2016**, *9*, 9268–9275.
28. Zhang, Y.Z.; Chen, X.; Fan, X.X.; He, J.X.; Huang, J.; Xiao, D.K.; Zhou, Y.L.; Zheng, S.Y.; Xu, J.H.; Yao, X.J.; et al. Compound library screening identified cardiac glycoside digitoxin as an effective growth inhibitor of gefitinib-resistant non-small cell lung cancer via downregulation of alpha-tubulin and inhibition of microtubule formation. *Molecules* **2016**, *21*, 374. [CrossRef]
29. Williams, L.M.; Cassady, J.M. Potential antitumor agents: A cytotoxic cardenolide from *Coronilla varia* L. *J. Pharm. Sci.* **1976**, *65*, 912–914. [CrossRef]
30. Hembree, J.A.; Chang, C.J.; McLaughlin, L.J.; Peck, G.; Cassady, J.M. Potential antitumor agents: A cytotoxic cardenolide from *Coronilla varia*. *J. Nat. Prod.* **1979**, *42*, 293–298. [CrossRef]
31. Slavík, J.; Zácková, P.; Michlová, J.; Opletal, L.; Sovová, M. Phytotherapeutic aspects of diseases of the circulatory system. III. Cardiotonic and cardiotoxic effects of hyrcanoside and deglucohyrcanoside isolated from *Coronilla varia* L. *Ceska Slov. Farm.* **1994**, *43*, 298–302.
32. Zácková, P.; Sovová, M.; Horáková, M.; Opletalová, V. Study of *Coronilla varia* L. III. Pharmacological evaluation of its effects on heart function. *Ceskoslovenska Farm.* **1982**, *31*, 242–246.
33. Gersl, V. Effects of *Coronilla varia* Linné extract and lanatoside C in rabbits with experimental acute heart overloading in vivo. *Sb. Ved. Pr. Lek. Fak. Karlov. Univerzity Hradci Kral. Suppl.* **1980**, *23*, 445–457.
34. Jurášek, M.; Džubák, P.; Rimpelová, S.; Sedlák, D.; Konečný, P.; Frydrych, I.; Gurská, S.; Hajdúch, M.; Bogdanová, K.; Kolář, M.; et al. Trilobolide-steroid hybrids: Synthesis, cytotoxic and antimycobacterial activity. *Steroids* **2017**, *117*, 97–104. [CrossRef] [PubMed]
35. Řehulka, J.; Vychodilová, K.; Krejčí, P.; Gurská, S.; Hradil, P.; Hajdúch, M.; Džubák, P.; Hlaváč, J. Fluorinated derivatives of 2-phenyl-3-hydroxy-4(1*H*)-quinolinone as tubulin polymerization inhibitors. *Eur. J. Med. Chem.* **2020**, *192*, 112176. [CrossRef] [PubMed]
36. Bagirov, R.B.; Komissarenko, N.F. New cardenolides from seeds of *Coronilla hyrcana*. *Khimiya Prir. Soedin.* **1966**, *2*, 251–257.
37. Nurmukhamedova, M.R.; Nikonov, G.K. Glycosides from *Dorema hyrcanum*. *Khimiya Prir. Soedin.* **1976**, *3*, 101–102.
38. Khushbaktova, Z.A.; Mukhtasimova, R.; Syrov, V.N.; Sultanov, M.B. O farmakologicheskikh svoistvach novogo fenolglykozida—girkanozida [Pharmacological properties of a new phenolglycoside—hyrcanoside]. *Dokl. Akad. Nauk.* **1983**, *39*, 54–55.
39. Abubakirov, N.K. The chemistry of cardiac glycosides in the Soviet union. *Khimiya Prir. Soedin.* **1971**, *7*, 553–571. [CrossRef]
40. Zatula, V.V.; Maksyutina, N.P.; Kolesnikov, D.G. Cardenolides of *Securigera securidaca*. *Khimiya Prir. Soedin.* **1965**, *1*, 153–156.
41. Zatula, V.V.; Chernobrovaya, N.V.; Kolesnikov, D.G. A chemical study of the structure of securigenin and its bioside securidaside. *Khimiya Prir. Soedin.* **1966**, *2*, 438–439. [CrossRef]
42. Zatula, V.V. Kil'kisne vyznachennia sekurydazydu v nasinni sekuryhery mechovydnoi [Quantitative determination of securidazide in seeds of *Securigera securidaca*]. *Farmatsevtychnyi Zhurnal (Kiev)* **1968**, *23*, 85–88.
43. Zatula, V.V.; Kovalev, I.P.; Kolesnikov, D.G. The structure of securigenin and securigenol. *Khimiya Prir. Soedin.* **1969**, *5*, 127–128. [CrossRef]
44. Tofighi, Z.; Moradi-Afrapoli, F.; Ebrahimi, S.N.; Goodarzi, S.; Hadjiakhoondi, A.; Neuburger, M.; Hamburger, M.; Abdollahi, M.; Yassa, N. Securigenin glycosides as hypoglycemic principles of *Securigera securidaca* seeds. *J. Nat. Med.* **2017**, *71*, 272–280. [CrossRef] [PubMed]
45. Laursen, M.; Yatimea, L.; Nissena, P.; Fedosova, N.U. Crystal structure of the high-affinity Na$^+$,K$^+$-ATPase–ouabain complex with Mg^{2+} bound in the cation binding site 1. *Proc. Natl. Acad. Sci. USA* **2013**, *110*, 10958–10963. [CrossRef] [PubMed]
46. Laursen, M.; Gregersena, J.L.; Yatimea, L.; Nissena, P.; Fedosova, N.U. Structures and characterization of digoxin- and bufalin-bound Na$^+$,K$^+$-ATPase compared with the ouabain-bound complex. *Proc. Natl. Acad. Sci. USA* **2015**, *112*, 1755–1760. [CrossRef] [PubMed]
47. Chen, W.L.; Ren, Y.; Ren, J.; Erxleben, C.; Johnson, M.E.; Gentile, S.; Kinghorn, A.D.; Swanson, S.M.; Burdette, J.E. (+)-Strebloside-induced cytotoxicity in ovarian cancer cells is mediated through cardiac glycoside signaling networks. *J. Nat. Prod.* **2017**, *80*, 659–669. [CrossRef] [PubMed]
48. Paula, S.; Tabet, M.R.; Ball, W.J. Interactions between cardiac glycosides and sodium/potassium-ATPase: Three-dimensional structure-activity relationship models for ligand binding to the E2-Pi form of the enzyme versus activity inhibition. *Biochemistry* **2005**, *44*, 498–510. [CrossRef] [PubMed]
49. Levrier, C.; Kiremire, B.; Guéritte, F.; Litaudon, M. Toxicarioside M, a new cytotoxic 10β-hydroxy-19-nor-cardenolide from *Antiaris toxicaria*. *Fitoterapia* **2012**, *83*, 660–664. [CrossRef] [PubMed]
50. Perne, A.; Muellner, M.K.; Steinrueck, M.; Craig-Mueller, N.; Mayerhofer, J.; Schwarzinger, I.; Sloane, M.; Uras, I.Z.; Hoermann, G.; Nijman, S.M.B.; et al. Cardiac glycosides induce cell death in human cells by inhibiting general protein synthesis. *PLoS ONE* **2009**, *4*, e8292. [CrossRef]
51. Price, E.M.; Lingrel, J.B. Structure-function relationships in the Na,K-ATPase alpha subunit: Site-directed mutagenesis of glutamine-111 to arginine and asparagine-122 to aspartic acid generates a ouabain-resistant enzyme. *Biochemistry* **1988**, *27*, 8400–8408. [CrossRef]

52. Calderon-Montano, J.M.; Burgos-Moron, E.; Lopez-Lazaro, M. The in vivo antitumor activity of cardiac glycosides in mice xenografted with human cancer cells is probably an experimental artifact. *Oncogene* **2014**, *33*, 2947–2948. [CrossRef]
53. Zhang, X.J.; Mei, W.L.; Tan, G.H.; Wang, C.C.; Zhou, S.L.; Huang, F.R.; Chen, B.; Dai, H.F.; Huang, F.Y. Strophalloside induces apoptosis of SGC-7901 cells through the mitochondrion-dependent caspase-3 pathway. *Molecules* **2015**, *20*, 5714–5728. [CrossRef]
54. Akimova, O.A.; Tverskoi, A.M.; Smolyaninova, L.V.; Mongin, A.A.; Lopina, O.D.; La, J.; Dulin, N.O.; Orlov, S.N. Critical role of the α1-Na(+), K(+)-ATPase subunit in insensitivity of rodent cells to cytotoxic action of ouabain. *Apoptosis* **2015**, *20*, 1200–1210. [CrossRef] [PubMed]
55. Wen, S.Y.; Chen, Y.Y.; Deng, C.M.; Zhang, C.Q.; Jiang, M.M. Nerigoside suppresses colorectal cancer cell growth and metastatic potential through inhibition of ERK/GSK3β/β-catenin signaling pathway. *Phytomedicine* **2019**, *57*, 352–363. [CrossRef] [PubMed]
56. Lei, Y.; Gan, H.; Huang, Y.; Chen, Y.; Chen, L.; Shan, A.; Zhao, H.; Wu, M.; Li, X.; Ma, Q.; et al. Digitoxin inhibits proliferation of multidrug-resistant HepG2 cells through G2/M cell cycle arrest and apoptosis. *Oncol. Lett.* **2020**, *20*, 71. [CrossRef] [PubMed]
57. Hiyoshi, H.; Abdelhady, S.; Segerström, L.; Sveinbjörnsson, B.; Nuriya, M.; Lundgren, T.K.; Desfrere, L.; Miyakawa, A.; Yasui, M.; Kogner, P.; et al. Quiescence and γH2AX in neuroblastoma are regulated by ouabain/Na,K-ATPase. *Br. J. Cancer* **2012**, *106*, 1807–1815. [CrossRef]
58. Newman, R.A.; Kondo, Y.; Yokoyama, T.; Dixon, S.; Cartwright, C.; Chan, D.; Johansen, M.; Yang, P. Autophagic cell death of human pancreatic tumor cells mediated by oleandrin, a lipid-soluble cardiac glycoside. *Integr. Cancer Ther.* **2007**, *6*, 354–364. [CrossRef]
59. Wang, T.; Xu, P.; Wang, F.; Zhou, D.; Wang, R.; Meng, L.; Wang, X.; Zhou, M.; Chen, B.; Ouyang, J. Effects of digoxin on cell cycle, apoptosis and NF-κB pathway in Burkitt's lymphoma cells and animal model. *Leuk. Lymphoma* **2017**, *58*, 1673–1685. [CrossRef]
60. Škubník, J.; Jurášek, M.; Ruml, T.; Rimpelová, S. Mitotic poisons in research and medicine. *Molecules* **2020**, *25*, 4632. [CrossRef]

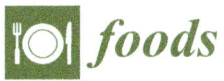 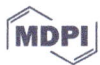

Article

(E)-Piplartine Isolated from *Piper pseudoarboreum*, a Lead Compound against *Leishmaniasis*

Juan C. Ticona [1,2,†], Pablo Bilbao-Ramos [3,4,†], Ninoska Flores [2], M. Auxiliadora Dea-Ayuela [3,5], Francisco Bolás-Fernández [3], Ignacio A. Jiménez [1,*] and Isabel L. Bazzocchi [1,*]

1. Instituto Universitario de Bio-Orgánica Antonio González and Departamento de Química Orgánica, Universidad de La Laguna, Avenida Francisco Sánchez 2, 38206 La Laguna, Tenerife, Spain; biojuancarlos@hotmail.com
2. Instituto de Investigaciones Fármaco Bioquímicas, Facultad de Ciencias Farmacéuticas y Bioquímicas, Universidad Mayor de San Andrés, Avenida Saavedra 2224, Miraflores, La Paz, Bolivia; eflores5umsa@gmail.com
3. Departamento de Parasitología, Facultad de Farmacia, Universidad Complutense de Madrid, Plaza Ramón y Cajal s/n, 28040 Madrid, Spain; pablobil15@yahoo.com (P.B.-R.); mda_3000@yahoo.es (M.A.D.-A.); francisb@ucm.es (F.B.-F.)
4. Laboratorio de Parasitología y Entomología, Instituto Nacional de Laboratorios de Salud (INLASA), Pasaje Rafael Zubieta 1889, Zona Miraflores, La Paz, Bolivia
5. Departamento de Farmacia, Universidad CEU-Cardenal Herrera, Avenida Seminario s/n, 46113 Moncada, Valencia, Spain
* Correspondence: ignadiaz@ull.edu.es (I.A.J.); ilopez@ull.edu.es (I.L.B.); Tel.: +34-922-318594 (I.A.J. & I.L.B.)
† Both authors contribute equally to this paper.

Received: 30 July 2020; Accepted: 3 September 2020; Published: 7 September 2020

Abstract: The current therapies of leishmaniasis, the second most widespread neglected tropical disease, have limited effectiveness and toxic side effects. In this regard, natural products play an important role in overcoming the current need for new leishmanicidal agents. The present study reports a bioassay-guided fractionation of the ethanolic extract of leaves of *Piper pseudoarboreum* against four species of *Leishmania* spp. promastigote forms, which afforded six known alkamides (1–6). Their structures were established on the basis of spectroscopic and spectrometric analysis. Compounds **2** and **3** were identified as the most promising ones, displaying higher potency against *Leishmania* spp. promastigotes (IC_{50} values ranging from 1.6 to 3.8 µM) and amastigotes of *L. amazonensis* (IC_{50} values ranging from 8.2 to 9.1 µM) than the reference drug, miltefosine. The efficacy of (E)-piplartine (**3**) against *L. amazonensis* infection in an in vivo model for cutaneous leishmaniasis was evidenced by a significant reduction of the lesion size footpad and spleen parasite burden, similar to those of glucantime used as the reference drug. This study reinforces the therapeutic potential of (E)-piplartine as a promising lead compound against neglected infectious diseases caused by *Leishmania* parasites.

Keywords: *Piper pseudoarboreum*; bioassay-guided fractionation; leishmanicidal activity; alkamides; (E)-piplartine

---

1. Introduction

Leishmaniases are neglected tropical diseases caused by the infection with *Leishmania* parasites, and are transmitted by the bite of a sand fly belonging to the genera *Lutzomyia* and *Phlebotomus*. Leishmaniases are endemic in large areas of the tropics, subtropics, and the Mediterranean basin, and are among the major neglected tropical diseases causing morbidity worldwide. Recently, it has broken out of its traditional boundaries and has been reported in new geographic locations with atypical disease manifestations involving novel parasite variants. Cutaneous leishmaniasis (CL) is endemic in more than 70 countries, with an estimated annual incidence of 1.5–2 million new cases, and clinical manifestations ranging from small skin nodules to massive destruction of the mucous tissues. CL is mainly caused by *Leishmania major* in the Old World and by *L. amazonensis* and *L. braziliensis* in the New World, specifically in Brazil [1]. In spite of the high prevalence, and advances in the chemotherapy for leishmaniasis, the current available drugs, including pentavalent antimonials, amphotericin B, miltefosine, paromomycin, and pentamidine are compromised by the emergence of resistance, variable sensitivity between species, adverse side effects, requirements for long courses of administration, and high cost [2]. These drawbacks and the absence of vaccines underline the urgent need for searching alternative treatments with acceptable efficacy and safety profile.

Natural products are an important source of leishmanicidal drugs owing to their accessibility, structural diversity, low cost, and possible rapid biodegradation [3–5]. In South America, where resorting to medicinal plants represents a primary health care measure of the native population, several species of *Piper* genus are widely used as a remedy to relieve the symptoms of leishmaniasis disease. Thus, the leaves of *Piper aduncum*, *P. loretoanum*, and *P. hispidum* are used as poultices for healing wounds and to treat the symptoms of CL [6,7]. In addition, *Piper* species are used as culinary spices, and as a food preservative to control food spoilage and pathogenic microorganisms. In particular, *P. nigrum* (black pepper) is worldwide popular as a flavoring for food [8]. Phytochemical investigations of *Piper* species have reported numerous metabolites with ecological and medicinal properties, including amides, pyrones, lignanes, terpenes, and flavonoids [8]. Alkamides, also named piperamides, are characteristic bioactive constituents in *Piper* species [9]. In particular, (*E*)-piplartine, also called piperlongumine, is the major natural alkaloid from *P. longum* and *P. tuberculatum*, and in vitro and in vivo studies have demonstrated its promising pharmacological properties such as antioxidant, anxiolytic, anti-atherosclerosis, antidiabetic, and antiparasitic against neglected tropical diseases [10]. Moreover, (*E*)-piplartine is reported to kill a large variety of cancer cells while remaining nontoxic to normal cells, highlighting its therapeutic potential [11,12].

In previous investigations, we reported the isolation of an unprecedented chlorine-containing piperamide along with several known compounds and their antileihmanicidal activity from *Piper pseudoarboreum* [13]. In continuous research toward the discovery of natural occurring leihmanicidal agents, we report herein on the isolation and structure elucidation of six known alkamides from the leaves of *P. pseudoarboreum* Yunker through a bioassay-guided fractionation carried out against four promastigote strains of *Leishmania*. Compounds **2** and **3** were further evaluated on intracellular amastigotes of *L. amazonensis* and *L. infantum*. (*E*)-piplartine (**3**) was selected to be assayed in an in vivo model for cutaneous leishmaniasis.

2. Materials and Methods

2.1. General Experimental Procedures

The structure of the isolated compounds were elucidated using spectrometric and spectroscopic methods, and comparison with data previously reported. The Nuclear Magnetic Resonance (NMR) experiments were recorded on Bruker Avance 400 and 500 spectrometers (Bruker Co. Billerica, MA, USA); chemical shifts were referred to the residual solvent signal (CDCl$_3$: δ_H 7.26, δ_C 77.36) (acetone d_6: δ_H 2.09, δ_C 30.60 and 205.87), using trimethylsilane (TMS) as internal standard. Electron Impact Mass Spectrometry (EIMS) and High Resolution Electron Impact Mass Spectrometry (HREIMS) were recorded on a Micromass Autospec spectrometer (Micromass, Manchester, UK). Silica gel 60 (15–40 mm) and silica gel 60 F254 for column chromatography and Thin Layer Chromatography (TLC), respectively, were purchased from Panreac (Barcelona, Spain). Sephadex LH-20 was obtained from Pharmacia Biotech (Pharmacia, Uppsala, Sweden). Centrifugal planar chromatography was carried out in a Chromatotron instrument (model 7924T, Harrison Research Inc., Palo Alto, CA, USA) on manually coated silica gel 60 GF$_{254}$ (Merck, Darmstadt, Germany) using 4-mm plates. The spots were visualized by UV light and heating silica gel plates sprayed with H$_2$O-H$_2$SO$_4$-AcOH (1:4:20).

2.2. Chemicals and Reagents

All solvents used were of analytical grade and purchased from Panreac (Barcelona, Spain). (*E*)-Piplartine, Scheneider's insect medium, RPMI-1640, fetal bovine serum (FBS), 4-(2-hydroxyethyl)-1-piperazineethanesulfonic acid (HEPES), resazurin sodium salt, and sodium dodecyl sulphate (Sigma-Aldrich, St Louis, MO, USA), L-glutamine (Avantor Performance Material Inc., PA, USA), trypsin (Merck, Darmstadt, Germany), penicillin Penilevel® 100.000 U.I. (ERN laboratories, Barcelona, Spain), streptomycin sulphate (Reig Jofré laboratories, Barcelona, Spain), and Glucantime® (Merial Laboratories, Barcelona, Spain).

2.3. Plant Material

Leaves of *Piper pseudoarboreum* Yunck. were collected in November 2009 at Iquitos, Maynas Province, Department of Loreto, Perú. The plant material was identified by the botanist Juan Celedonio Ruiz Macedo, and a voucher specimen (AMZ 11114) was deposited at the Amazonense Herbarium of the Universidad Nacional de la Amazonia Peruana, Iquitos, Perú.

2.4. Extraction, Bioassay-Guided Fractionation and Isolation

The dried leaves of *P. pseudoarboreum* (200.3 g) were powdered and extracted in a Soxhlet apparatus with 5 L of 96% ethanol. The solvent was evaporated to give 42.9 g (21.4%) of extract. The ethanolic extract (EtOH) was partitioned into dichlorometane (DCM), ethyl acetate (EtOAc), and water (H_2O). After removing the organic solvents under reduced pressure, the DCM (9.2 g, 4.6%) and EtOAc (1.2 g, 0.6%) fractions were obtained, whereas the aqueous-soluble extract was lyophilized providing the H_2O fraction (8.9 g, 4.5%). The most active organic fraction (DCM, 9.2 g) was chromatographed over silica gel column eluting with mixtures of hexanes-EtOAc (10:0 to 0:10, 1 L each one) to obtain seven sub-fractions (F1–F7). The most active fraction, F6 (1.5 g), was subjected to column chromatography over Sephadex LH-20 by isocratic elution (MeOH-$CHCl_3$, 1:1) to afford fifteen sub-fractions, which were combined based on their TLC profiles (F6A to F6F). Preliminary nuclear magnetic resonance (NMR) studies revealed that sub-fraction F6B was rich in aromatic alkamides, and were further investigated. Thus, F6B (448.1 mg) was chromatographed by centrifugal planar chromatography on 4-mm silica gel plates, using mixtures of hexanes-EtOAc (60:40 to 50:40) as eluent to give eleven sub-fractions (F6B1 to F6B11). Sub-fraction F6B2 (21.5 mg) was further purified on silica gel by preparative TLC (3 × development, hexanes-2-propanol, 8:2) to give compounds **1** (1.7 mg) and **5** (1.4 mg). Purification of sub-fraction F6B4 (18.3 mg) by preparative TLC (2 × development, CH_2Cl_2-Et_2O, 95:5) yielded compounds **3** (11.4 mg) and **4** (2.2 mg), whereas sub-fraction F6B7 (23.8 mg) gave compounds **2** (19.8 mg) and **6** (0.9 mg) after purification by preparative TLC (2 × development, hexanes-2-propanol, 8:2). The compounds were identified by NMR spectroscopy and comparison with data reported in the literature.

2.5. Biological Studies

2.5.1. Parasites

Autochthonous isolates of *Leishmania infantum* (MCAN/ES/92/BCN83) were obtained from an asymptomatic dog from the Priorat region (Catalunya, Spain), and kindly provided by Prof. Montserrat Portús (University of Barcelona). *L. braziliensis* (2903), *L. amazonensis* (MHOM/Br/79/Maria) and *L. guyanensis* (141/93) were kindly given by Prof. Alfredo Toraño (Instituto de Salud Carlos III, Madrid).

2.5.2. Cells

J774 murine macrophages were grown and maintained in RPMI-1640 medium supplemented with 10% heat-inactivated FBS, penicillin G (100 U/mL), and streptomycin (100 μg/mL) at 37 °C and 5% CO_2 air atmosphere.

2.5.3. Animals

Male BALB/c mice of 20–25 g body weigh were purchased from Harlan Interfauna Ibérica (Barcelona, Spain). All rodents were housed in plastic cages in a 12 h dark–light cycle under controlled temperature (25 °C) and humidity (70%) conditions. During the study, animals had unrestricted access to food and water.

2.5.4. In Vitro Promastigotes Susceptibility Assay

In vitro antileishmanial assay was performed using a method described elsewhere [14]. Briefly, promastigotes were grown in vitro in a Schneider's insect medium supplemented with 20% heat-inactivated FBS, penicillin (100 U/mL) and streptomycin (100 µg/mL) at 26 °C in 25 mL in tissue culture flasks, and were cultured in 96-well plastic plates (2.5×10^5 parasites/well). Compounds dissolved in dimethylsulfoxide 1% (DMSO) at the suitable concentration to be tested in serial dilutions (a first screening using 100 µg/mL, and then 100, 50, 25, 12.5, 6.25, 3.12, 1.56 and 0.78 µg/mL) to get a final volume of 200 µL were added to each well. After an incubation of 48 h at 26 °C, 20 µL of 2.5 mM resazurin solution was added. Plates were then analyzed by fluorescence emission (535_{ex}–590_{em} nm) using a fluorometer Infinite 200 (Tecan i-Control, Tecan Group Ltd, Männedorf, Switzerland). All tests were carried out in triplicate, and miltefosine was used as the reference drug. The antileishmanial activity of each compound was estimated by calculating the GI% (percentage of growth inhibition) and then the IC_{50} value (concentration of the compound that produced a 50% reduction in parasites).

2.5.5. Cytotoxicity Assay

The cytotoxicity assay of the tested compounds was performed according to a previously described method [14]. Briefly, J774 macrophages (5×10^4 cells/well) were placed in 96-well flat-bottom plates with 100 µL of RPMI-1640 medium, and allowed to attach at 37 °C and 5% CO_2 for 2 h. Afterwards, 100 µL of RPMI-1640 medium containing the test compound in varying concentrations (100, 50, 25, 12.5, 6.25, 3.12, 1.56, and 0.78 µg/mL) were added to the cells and incubated for another 48 h. Growth controls and signal-to-noise were included. Following the aforementioned incubation time, 20 µL of 2.5 mM resazurin solution in PBS was added, and the plates were placed again in the incubator for another 3 h to evaluate cell viability. The ability of cells to reduce resazurin was determined by fluorometry as in the promastigote assay. Each concentration was assayed in triplicate. Cytotoxicity was expressed as the 50% reduction of cell viability of treated culture cells with respect to untreated culture (CC_{50}).

2.5.6. In Vitro Amastigote Assay

The effectiveness against intracellular amastigotes was evaluated using a fluorometric method described elsewhere [15]. Briefly, macrophages (5×10^4 cells) and stationary *Leishmania* promastigotes in a ratio of 1:10 (macrophage/parasite) were seeded in each well of a microtiter plate, suspended in 200 µL of culture medium and incubated at 33 °C and 5% CO_2 for 24 h. After this incubation time, the temperature was increased up to 37 °C for another 24 h. Cells were washed with medium several times in order to remove free non-infective promastigotes, and the supernatant was replaced by 200 µL/well of culture medium containing two-fold serial dilutions of the test compounds (ranging from 5 to 0.038 µg/mL) and the reference drug (ranging from 50 to 0.38 µg/mL). The culture medium was removed carefully to be replaced by 200 µL/well of the lysis solution (RPMI-1640 with 0.048% HEPES and 0.006% sodium dodecyl sulfate (SDS)) and incubated at room temperature for 20 min. Thereafter, the plates were centrifuged at $3500\times g$ for 5 min and the lysis solution was replaced by 200 µL/well of Schneider's insect medium. The culture plates were incubated at 26 °C for another 3 days for the transformation of viable promastigotes into amastigotes. Afterwards, 20 µL/well of 2.5 mM resazurin was added and incubated for 3 h. Plates were analyzed by fluorescence emission, and IC$_{50}$ was determined as described above. All tests were carried out in triplicate. Miltefosine was used as reference drug and was evaluated at the same conditions.

2.5.7. In Vivo Experiments

BALB/c mice were infected subcutaneously at the left hand-foot with 1×10^7 promastigotes of *L. amazonensis* on day 0. Right hind paw was used as a negative control (no infection). Thirty five days after infection, chronic cutaneous leishmaniasis was developed, and animals were randomly divided into three groups ($n = 8$/group): animals treated with (*E*)-piplartine received in the foot lesions (intralesion) doses of 25 mg/kg/day for 4 days in a 15 µL volume of phosphate saline dilution/propylene glycol (9:1), a group treated with glucantime receiving 25 mg/kg/day for 4 days by intraperitoneal route, and the control group. The measurement of cutaneous lesion was monitored at 0, 35, 50, and 100 days post-infection, using a Vernier calliper to measure footpad size. The number of viable *L. amazonensis* parasites in the spleen of the different groups of mice was estimated using the limiting dilution assay method at the end of the experiment (day 100 post-infection) [16]. Mice were sacrificed, and the spleen were aseptically removed, weighed, and homogenized in Schneider's medium supplemented with 10% FBS. Briefly, serial dilutions were prepared and distributed to 96-well microtiter plates under sterile conditions, and incubated at 26 °C. On day 7 post-incubation, wells were analyzed using an inverted microscope. The number of parasites per milligram of tissue was determined based on the tissue weight and the parasite load from the culture dilutions [17].

2.5.8. Ethical Consideration

All animals were handled according to the European Union legislation Directive 2010/63/EU and Spanish law Real Decreto 53/2013 on the protection of animals used for scientific purposes. The experimental protocols involving the use of animals were approved by the local ethical committee of the University Complutense of Madrid (CEXAN170415) http://147.96.70.122/Web/Actas/CEXAN170415.pdf.

2.5.9. Statistical Analysis

For in vitro assays, the antileishmanial activity (IC$_{50}$) and cytotoxic activity (CC$_{50}$) of compounds were analyzed by Probit test, using SPSS v20.0 software. All results were expressed as means ± standard error of the mean (S.E.M). For in vivo assays, results were analyzed by Shapiro-Wilk's normality test, and then by one-way ANOVA with Tukey's HSD post-hoc test. Significant differences were considered at p-value < 0.05, using SPSS v20.0 and Microsoft Excel 2010 software.

3. Results and Discussion

The ethanolic extract of the leaves of *P. pseudoarboreum* was evaluated against promastigote forms of *L. amazonensis*, *L. braziliensis*, *L. guyanensis*, and *L. infantum*. The active EtOH crude extract was further fractionated by liquid–liquid partition to obtain DCM, EtOAc, and H$_2$O fractions, which were assayed for their in vitro activity against the four *Leishmania* strains.

The DCM fraction showed an improved profile compared to the crude extract, displaying IC$_{50}$ values ranging from 14.7 to 19.1 µg/mL for the four *Leishmania* strains assayed, whereas the EtOAc and H$_2$O fractions showed to be inactive (IC$_{50}$ > 50 µg/mL). Thus, DCM fraction was further fractionated to yield seven sub-fractions. Sub-fractions F1–F4 showed to be inactive (IC$_{50}$ > 100 µM), whereas sub-fraction F5 showed some degree of activity on the four *Leishmania* strains (IC$_{50}$ 15.7–20.8 µg/mL) and F7 exhibited only slight potency on *L. amazonensis* and *L. braziliensis*. Moreover, the most active sub-fraction F6 exhibited higher potency than miltefosine, used as the reference drug (IC$_{50}$ ranging from 2.2 to 3.4 µM vs. 17.7 to 30.7 µM), although showed a slightly low selectivity index taking J774 macrophages as reference mammalian cells (CC$_{50}$ values ranging from 1.9 to 3.0 vs. 4.4 to 7.7) (Table 1).

Table 1. Leishmanicidal activity on promastigotes forms and cytotoxic activity on macrophages of the extract, fractions, sub-fractions, and isolated compounds [a] from *P. pseudoarboreum*.

Sample	L. amazonensis		L. braziliensis		L. guyanensis		L. infantum		J774
	IC_{50}[b] ± SD	SI[d]	IC_{50}[b] ± SD	SI[d]	IC_{50}[b] ± SD	SI[d]	IC_{50}[b] ± SD	SI[d]	CC_{50}[c] ± SD
EtOH	31.4 ± 2.5	1.8	21.3 ± 1.0	2.6	41.3 ± 1.4	1.3	32.3 ± 1.4	1.7	55.0 ± 4.1
DCM	17.7 ± 0.3	1.9	14.7 ± 0.8	2.3	19.1 ± 0.2	1.8	18.4 ± 0.3	1.9	34.1 ± 3.4
F5	18.5 ± 0.1	1.2	15.7 ± 2.8	1.4	20.8 ± 0.8	1.1	20.3 ± 0.3	1.1	22.6 ± 2.2
F6	2.5 ± 0.0	2.6	2.2 ± 0.1	3.0	3.4 ± 0.2	1.9	3.0 ± 0.1	2.2	6.5 ± 1.3
F7	40.0 ± 1.1	0.8	46.7 ± 5.1	0.7	-	-	-	-	30.8 ± 2.8
1	28.0 ± 1.0	0.8	28.7 ± 1.0	0.8	24.6 ± 0.0	0.9	27.7 ± 1.7	0.8	23.2 ± 3.1
2	1.7 ± 0.3	6.6	1.7 ± 0.0	6.6	2.1 ± 0.0	5.5	3.8 ± 0.3	3.0	11.5 ± 0.7
3	2.2 ± 0.0	4.7	1.6 ± 0.3	6.6	2.2 ± 0.3	4.7	2.2 ± 1.6	4.7	10.4 ± 0.9
4	3.5 ± 0.0	3.6	2.5 ± 0.0	5.0	3.8 ± 0.0	3.3	5.4 ± 0.3	2.4	12.6 ± 3.8
5	-	-	-	-	88.0 ± 2.4	0.6	-	-	52.2 ± 23.0
M [e]	30.7 ± 0.9	4.4	17.7 ± 0.4	7.7	19.4 ± 1.2	7.0	17.7 ± 1.8	7.7	135.9 ± 10.3

[a] Fractions and compounds not included in the table were inactive ($IC_{50} > 50$ µg/mL and $IC_{50} > 100$ µM, respectively). [b] IC_{50}: concentration able to inhibit 50% of parasites. The IC_{50} values of the ethanol extract (EtOH) and dichloromethane (DCM) and F5–F7 fractions are expressed as µg/mL ± standard deviation. The IC_{50} values of the compounds are expressed as µM ± standard deviation. [c] CC_{50} concentration able to inhibit 50% of murine macrophages. [d] SI: selectivity index (CC_{50}/IC_{50}). [e] M: miltefosine was used as a positive control.

Therefore, sub-fraction F6 was submitted to multiple chromatographic steps on silica gel and Sephadex LH-20 affording the known alkamides 1–6 (Figure 1). Their chemical structures were elucidated on the basis of their spectroscopic data (Supplementary Materials Figures S1–S6) and comparison with data reported in the literature. Thus, the isolated metabolites were identified as sintenpyridone (1) [18], (E)-demethoxypiplartine (2) [19], (E)-piplartine (also known as piperlongumine, 3) [19], (Z)-piplartine (4) [20], 3,4-epoxy-8,9-dihydropiplartine (5) [21], and 10,11-dihydropiperine (6) [20].

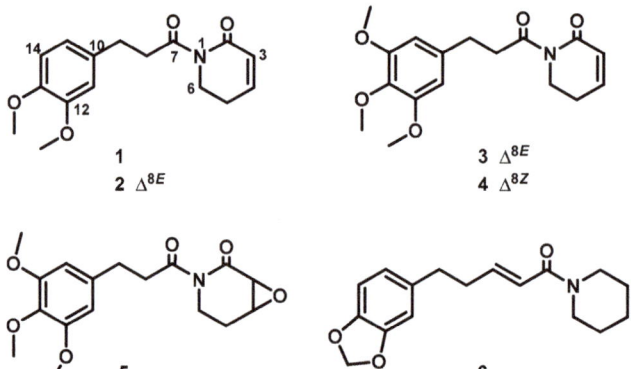

Figure 1. Chemical structures of piperamides (1–6) isolated from *Piper pseudoarboreum*.

Alkamides 1–6 were tested by in vitro assays against the four strains of *Leishmania* promastigotes. The results indicated that alkamides 2 and 3 were 4.7 to 18-fold more potent (IC_{50} ranging from 1.6 to 3.8 µM) than miltefosine (IC_{50} ranging from 17.7 to 30.7 µM), and exhibited a selectivity index ranging from 3.0 to 6.6 for all *Leishmania* strains tested (Table 1). Recently, Araújo-Vilges and co-workers reported that (E)-piplartine was able to reduce the growth of *L. amazonensis* promastigotes (MHOM/BR/pH8) in a dose-dependent pattern, exhibiting an IC_{50} value of 179.0 µg/mL [22]. On the other hand, Capello et al. [23] reported that no antileishmanial activity on macrophages infected with *L. (L.) amazonensis* was found for (E)-piplartine at 50 µg/mL. We assume that such differences in potency depend to a great extent on the infecting *Leishmania* strain used in the assay and cell culture procedures.

Regarding the influence of the substitution pattern in the alkamide scaffold on the leishmanicidal activity, it seems that α,β-unsaturated carbonyl groups in both, the acyl chain and the lactam ring are critical functionalities for the activity (**2, 3,** and **4** vs. **1, 5,** and **6**). Moreover, isomerization of the unsaturated acyl chain leads to slight changes in the activity (**3** vs. **4**). No straightforward conclusion can be drawn from the type of functional group on the aromatic ring.

Based on the in vitro results on promastigote forms, alkamides **2** and **3** were selected to be evaluated on intracellular amastigotes of *L. amazonensis* and *L. infantum*. The results revealed that compounds **2** and **3** exhibited some degree of activity, showing two-fold higher potency on *L. amazonesis* (IC_{50} 9.1 and 8.2 µM, respectively) than on *L. infantum* (IC_{50} 17.1 and 16.1 µM, respectively). Moreover, both compounds exhibited higher activity than miltefosine on both assayed *Leishmania* strains. Furthermore, these compounds were 5- to 6-fold more potent than miltefosine on *L. amazonensis* (Table 2).

Table 2. Leishmanicidal activity on amastigote forms of alkamides 2 and 3.

Compounds	*L. amazonesis*		*L. infantum*	
	IC_{50} [a] ± SD	SI [b]	IC_{50} ± SD	SI [b]
2	9.1 ± 0.2	1.3	17.1 ± 0.1	0.7
3	8.2 ± 0.1	1.3	16.1 ± 0.1	0.7
M [c]	49.3 ± 0.2	2.8	23.6 ± 0.4	5.8

[a] IC_{50}: concentrations able to inhibit 50% of the parasites, and values are expressed as µM ± standard deviation (SD). [b] SI: selectivity index (CC_{50} of murine macrophages/IC_{50}). [c] M: Miltefosine was used as a positive control.

Taking into consideration its potency and efficacy on *Leishmania* promastigote and amastigote forms, and although a poor selectivity index, (*E*)-piplartine was selected for in vivo assays to investigate its potential as a lead compound targeting CL since previous toxicological studies indicate a good safety profile in murine models [10]. Previous works report the in vitro evaluation of (*E*)-piplartine against *Leishmania* spp. promastigotes [22,24] and *L. amazonensis* intracellular amastigote forms [25] as well as an in vivo study against *L. donovani* in a hamster model of visceral leishmaniasis [24]. However, to our knowledge, in vivo studies on CL have not been reported.

The in vivo assay in BALB/c mice infected with *L. amazonensis* for CL was performed by treatment of three randomly separated mice groups (8 mice per group). Thirty five days after infection, the treated mice group with (*E*)-piplartine received in the foot lesions (intralesion) a dose of 25 mg/kg/day for 4 days, whereas the treated group with glucantime received by intraperitoneal route 25 mg/kg/day for 4 days. The lesion size footpad was measured four times before infection and treatment, after treatment and at the end of the experiment (days 0, 35, 50, and 100) (Figures 2 and 3). The individual lesion size was calculated from two measurements (differences between the left and the right footpad).

Moreover, with the aim to establish the visceralization of the chronic infection disease, all mice were sacrificed at the end of the experiment to determine parasite burden in spleen by culture on microtiter plates. This in vivo assay indicated that from the day of infection to the day before treatment with (*E*)-piplartine, the progress of the lesion size was similar in the three mice groups (day 35), whereas after the end of treatment (day 50), the mean progress of lesions within groups treated with (*E*)-piplartine and glucantime were reduced by around 35% with respect to the untreated group. At the end of the experiment, both treated groups showed more than 40% reduction in the lesion size and 55% in spleen parasite burden compared to untreated mice group. The intralesion (*E*)-piplartine treatment efficacy was comparable to the intraperitoneal glucantime treatment, with *p*-values of 0.800 and 0.832 for the lesion size and spleen parasite burden, respectively, and significantly higher than the untreated control group, with *p*-values of 0.045 and 0.027, respectively (Table 3).

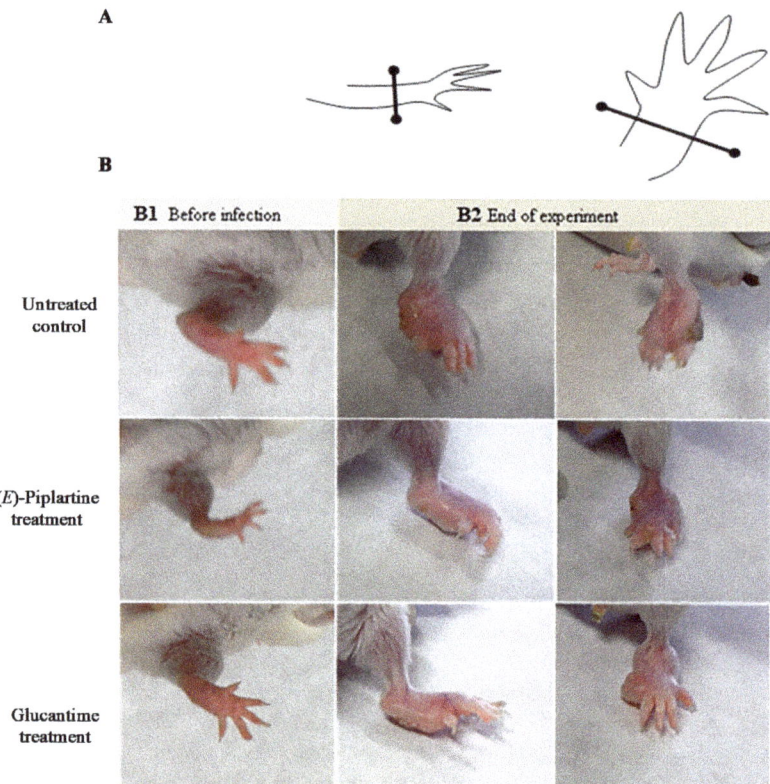

Figure 2. Effect of the treatment with (*E*)-piplartine on chronic cutaneous leishmaniasis in BALB/c mice. (**A**) Graphic representation of footpad measurement: thickness (**left**) and width (**right**). Lesion size is expressed as the difference in size between the infected and contralateral non-infected footpads. (**B**) Representative images of a mouse infected with *Leishmania amazonensis*, at day 0 (**B1**) and at the end of experiment (**B2**).

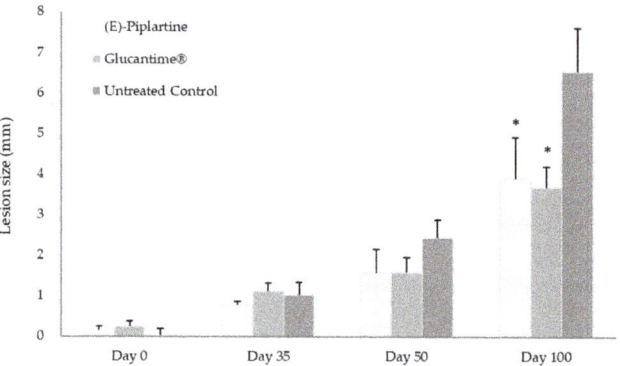

Figure 3. Effectiveness of (*E*)-piplartine in the treatment of chronic cutaneous leishmaniasis. Lesion size was measured four times (day 0, day 35, day 50, and day 100) and expressed as a mean of the group in mm. At end of the experiment, lesion size of (*E*)-piplartine vs. glucantime treated mice groups did not show statistically significant differences with p-value > 0.800; untreated control group vs. (*E*)-piplartine and glucantime showed significant differences with p-value < 0.000 *.

Table 3. Efficacy of (E)-piplartine in the control of the visceralization in chronic Cutaneous Leishmaniasis.

Mice Groups	Spleen Parasite Burden [a]		
	Number and Percentage	SEM [b] and Percentage	p-Value with Untreated Control
Untreated control	277.17 (100%)	±43.3 (15.6%)	-
(E)-Piplartine treated	122.6 (44.2%)	±40.3 (14.5%)	0.045
Glucantime® treated	111.6 (40.3%)	±46.8 (16.9%)	0.027

[a] Number of parasites per gram in spleen measured on day 100 of infection. [b] SEM: Standard error of the mean.

Thus, the results indicated that (E)-piplartine was effective in the in vivo assay (Figures 2 and 3, and Table 3) as evidenced by a significant reduction in the lesion size footpad after infection, and in the spleen parasite burden at the end of the experiment (day 100 post-infection). These findings, together with previous safety [22,25] and pharmacokinetic studies [10,26], provide additional experimental evidence of the potential of (E)-piplartine as a promising leishmanicidal lead compound.

In this study, the intralesional route for (E)-piplartine was chosen in order to develop a prospective formulation for topical administration. This administration route is an attractive alternative for CL, offering significant advantages over systemic therapy with: fewer adverse side effects, easy administration, and low costs [27]. This later point is relevant as in regions with limited resources there are no dispensaries or qualified personnel for intramuscular or intravenous drug administration [28]. In addition, topical formulations can penetrate over the skin to diminish disease progression at the beginning of the infection [29].

Although the mechanism of action of (E)-piplartine has not been established on *Leishmania* parasites, previous studies performed on cancer cell lines [12,30,31] have demonstrated that this alkamide is able to inhibit the proliferative process by activation of mitochondrial apoptosis pathways and induction of reactive oxygen species. Considering these studies, the effect of (E)-piplartine on *Leishmania* parasites could also be related to the activation of apoptotic events. Moreover, further studies should be undertaken in order to determine the leishmanicidal mechanism of action of this promising lead compound.

4. Conclusions

The results reported herein reinforce the efficacy of (E)-piplartine against neglected tropical diseases caused by *Leishmania* spp., and deserve future investigations for further lead optimization with desired drug-likeness properties for the treatment of leishmaniasis. Furthermore, (E)-piplartine is a natural alkamide occurring in several species in the widely distributed *Piper* genus, and therefore, the in vivo studies results support and may validate the traditional uses of some *Piper* species by the indigenous people to treat the symptoms of cutaneous leishmaniasis.

Supplementary Materials: The following are available online at http://www.mdpi.com/2304-8158/9/9/1250/s1, Figures S1–S6: ^{1}H and ^{13}C NMR spectra of compounds **1–6**.

Author Contributions: Conceptualization, I.A.J. and F.B.-F.; methodology, I.A.J., M.A.D.-A., and J.C.T.; investigation, J.C.T. and P.B.-R.; data curation, M.A.D.-A. and N.F.; writing—the original draft preparation; N.F. and I.A.J.; writing—reviewed and editing, I.L.B.; funding acquisition, I.L.B. and F.B.-F. All authors have read and agreed to the published version of the manuscript.

Funding: This research was funded by RTI2018-094356-B-C21 Spanish MINECO project, cofunded by the European Regional Development Fund (FEDER) and PCI-Iberoamerica A/030160/10 and AP/039767/11 projects from Spanish MAEC-AECID. J.C.T. and P.B.-R. are grateful to Spanish MAEC-AECID for their fellowships.

Acknowledgments: The authors would like to thank the botanist Juan Celedonio Ruiz Macedo, Amazonense Herbarium of the Universidad Nacional de la Amazonia Peruana, Iquitos, Perú, for the identification of the plant material.

Conflicts of Interest: The authors declare no conflict of interest.

References

1. World Health Organization, Update March 2019. Available online: http://www.who.int/news-room/fact-sheets/detail/leishmaniasis (accessed on 8 April 2020).
2. Passero, L.F.D.; Cruz, L.A.; Santos-Gomes, G.; Rodrigues, E.; Laurenti, M.D.; Lago, J.H.G. Conventional versus natural alternative treatments for Leishmaniasis: A Review. *Curr. Top. Med. Chem.* **2018**, *18*, 1275–1286. [CrossRef]
3. Bekhit, A.A.; El-Agroudy, E.; Helmy, A.; Ibrahim, T.M.; Shavandi, A.; Bekhit, A.E.A. Leishmania treatment and prevention: Natural and synthesized drugs. *Eur. J. Med. Chem.* **2018**, *60*, 229–244. [CrossRef] [PubMed]
4. Hussian, H.; Al-Harrasi, A.; Al-Rawahi, A.; Green, I.R.; Gibbons, S. Fruitful decade for antileishmanial compounds from 2002 to late 2011. *Chem. Rev.* **2014**, *114*, 10369–10428. [CrossRef] [PubMed]
5. Newman, D.J.; Cragg, G.M. Natural products as sources of new drugs over the nearly four decades from 01/1981 to 09/2019. *J. Nat. Prod.* **2020**, *83*, 770–803. [CrossRef] [PubMed]
6. Braga, F.G.; Bouzada, M.L.; Fabri, R.L.; de O Matos, M.; Moreira, F.O.; Scio, E.; Coimbra, E.S. Antileishmanial and antifungal activity of plants used in traditional medicine in Brazil. *J. Ethnopharmacol.* **2007**, *111*, 396–402. [CrossRef] [PubMed]
7. Odonne, G.; Bourdy, G.; Castillo, D.; Estevez, Y.; Lancha-Tangoa, A.; Alban-Castillo, J.; Deharo, E.; Rojas, R.; Stien, D.; Sauvain, M. Ta'ta', Huayani: Perception of leishmaniasis and evaluation of medicinal plants used by the Chayahuita in Peru. Part II. *J. Ethnopharmacol.* **2009**, *126*, 149–158. [CrossRef] [PubMed]
8. Salehi, B.; Zakaria, Z.A.; Gyawali, R.; Ibrahim, S.A.; Rajkovic, J.; Shinwari, Z.K.; Khan, T.; Sharifi-Rad, J.; Ozleyen, A.; Turkdonmez, E.; et al. Piper species: A comprehensive review on their phytochemistry, biological activities and applications. *Molecules* **2019**, *24*, 1364. [CrossRef]
9. Rios, M.Y.; Olivo, H.F. Natural and synthetic alkamides: Applications in pain therapy. *Studies Nat. Prod. Chem.* **2014**, *43*, 79–121.
10. Bezerra, D.P.; Pessoa, C.; de Moraes, M.O.; Saker-Neto, N.; Silveira, E.R.; Costa-Lotufo, L.V. Overview of the therapeutic potential of piplartine (piperlongumine). *Eur. J. Pharm. Sci.* **2013**, *48*, 453–463. [CrossRef]
11. Adams, D.J.; Dai, M.; Pellegrino, G.; Wagner, B.K.; Stern, A.M.; Shamji, A.F.; Schreiber, S.L. Synthesis, cellular evaluation, and mechanism of action of piperlongumine analogs. *Proc. Natl. Acad. Sci. USA* **2012**, *109*, 15115–15120. [CrossRef]
12. Li, L.; Zhao, Y.; Cao, R.; Li, L.; Cai, G.; Li, J.; Qi, X.; Chen, S.; Zhang, Z. Activity-based protein profiling reveals GSTO1 as the covalent target of piperlongumine and a promising target for combination therapy for cancer. *Chem. Commun.* **2019**, *55*, 4407–4410. [CrossRef] [PubMed]
13. Flores, N.; Ticona, J.C.; Bilbao-Ramos, P.; Dea-Ayuela, M.A.; Ruiz-Macedo, J.C.; Bazzocchi, I.L.; Bolás-Fernández, F.; Jiménez, I.A. An unprecedented chlorine-containing piperamide from *Piper pseudoarboreum* as potential leishmanicidal agent. *Fitoterapia* **2019**, *134*, 340–345. [CrossRef]
14. Galiana-Rosello, C.; Bilbao-Ramos, P.; Dea-Ayuela, M.A.; Rolón, M.; Vega, C.; Bolás-Fernández, F.; García-España, E.; Alfonso, J.; Coronel, C.; González-Rosende, M.E. In vivo and in vitro anti-leishmanial and trypanocidal studies of new N-benzene- and N-naphthalenesulfonamide derivatives. *J. Med. Chem.* **2013**, *56*, 8984–8998. [CrossRef] [PubMed]
15. Bilbao-Ramos, P.; Sifontes-Rodríguez, S.; Dea-Ayuela, M.A.; Bolás-Fernández, F. A fluorometric method for evaluation of pharmacological activity against intracellular *Leishmania* amastigotes. *J. Microbiol. Methods* **2012**, *89*, 8–11. [CrossRef] [PubMed]
16. Titus, R.G.; Marchand, M.; Boon, T.; Louis, J.A. A limiting dilution assay for quantifying *Leishmania major* in tissues of infected mice. *Parasite Immunol.* **1985**, *7*, 545–555. [CrossRef] [PubMed]
17. Rodrigues, R.F.; Charret, K.S.; Campos, M.C.; Amaral, V.; Echevarria, A.; dos Reis, C.; Canto-Cavalheiro, M.M.; Leon, L.L. The in vivo activity of 1,3,4-thiadiazolium-2-aminide compounds in the treatment of cutaneous and visceral leishmaniasis. *J. Antimicrob. Chemother.* **2012**, *67*, 182–190. [CrossRef]
18. Chen, J.J.; Huang, Y.C.; Chen, Y.C.; Huang, Y.T.; Wang, S.W.; Peng, C.Y.; Teng, C.M.; Chen, I.S. Cytotoxic amides from *Piper sintenense*. *Planta Med.* **2002**, *68*, 980–985. [CrossRef]
19. Duh, C.Y.; Wu, Y.C.; Wang, S.K. Cytotoxic pyridone alkaloids from *Piper aborescens*. *Phytochemistry* **1990**, *29*, 2689–2691. [CrossRef]
20. Navickiene, H.M.D.; Alécio, A.C.; Kato, M.J.; Bolzani, V.D.; Young, M.C.; Cavalheiro, A.J.; Furlan, M. Antifungal amides from *Piper hispidum* and *Piper tuberculatum*. *Phytochemistry* **2000**, *55*, 621–626. [CrossRef]

21. Seeram, N.P.; Lewis, P.A.; Jacobs, H.; McLean, S.; Reynolds, W.F.; Tay, L.L.; Yu, M. 3,4-Epoxy-8,9-dihydropiplartine. A new imide from *Piper verrucosum*. *J. Nat. Prod.* **1996**, *59*, 436–437. [CrossRef]
22. Araújo-Vilges, K.M.; Oliveira, S.V.; Couto, S.C.P.; Fokoue, H.H.; Romero, G.A.S.; Kato, M.J.; Romeiro, L.A.S.; Leite, J.R.S.A.; Kuckelhaus, S.A.S. Effect of piplartine and cinnamides on *Leishmania amazonensis*, *Plasmodium falciparum* and on peritoneal cells of Swiss mice. *Pharm. Biol.* **2017**, *55*, 1601–1607. [CrossRef] [PubMed]
23. Capello, T.M.; Martins, E.G.A.; Farias, C.F.; Figueiredo, C.R.; Matsuo, A.L.; Passero, L.F.; Oliveira-Silva, D.; Sartorelli, P.; Lago, J.H.G. Chemical composition and in vitro cytotoxic and antileishmanial activities of extract and essential oil from leaves of *Piper cernuum*. *Nat. Prod. Commun.* **2015**, *10*, 285–288. [CrossRef] [PubMed]
24. Bodiwala, H.S.; Singh, G.; Singh, R.; Dey, C.S.; Sharma, S.S.; Bhutani, K.K.; Singh, I.P. Antileishmanial amides and lignans from *Piper cubeba* and *Piper retrofractum*. *J. Nat. Med.* **2007**, *61*, 418–421. [CrossRef]
25. Moreira, F.L.; Riul, T.B.; Moreira, M.L.; Pilon, A.C.; Dias-Baruffi, M.; Araújo, M.S.S.; Lopes, N.P.; de Oliveira, A.R.M. Leishmanicidal effects of piperlongumine (piplartine) and its putative metabolites. *Planta Med.* **2018**, *84*, 1141–1148. [CrossRef]
26. Moreira, F.L.; Habenschus, M.D.; Barth, T.; Marques, L.M.; Pilon, A.C.; da Silva Bolzani, V.; Vessecchi, R.; Lopes, N.P.; de Oliveira, A.R. Metabolic profile and safety of piperlongumine. *Sci. Rep.* **2016**, *6*, 33646. [CrossRef]
27. Carneiro, G.; Aguiar, M.G.; Fernandes, A.P.; Ferreira, L.A. Drug delivery systems for the topical treatment of cutaneous leishmaniasis. *Expert Opin. Drug Deliv.* **2012**, *9*, 1083–1097. [CrossRef]
28. WHO. Leishmania. Treatment. Available online: https://www.who.int/health-topics/leishmaniasis#tab=tab_3 (accessed on 8 April 2020).
29. Bilbao-Ramos, P.; Serrano, D.R.; Ruiz Saldaña, H.K.; Torrado, J.J.; Bolás-Fernández, F.; Dea-Ayuela, M.A. Evaluating the potential of ursolic acid as bioproduct for cutaneous and visceral leishmaniasis. *Molecules* **2020**, *25*, 1394. [CrossRef]
30. Liu, Z.; Shi, Z.; Lin, J.; Zhao, S.; Hao, M.; Xu, J.; Li, Y.; Zhao, Q.; Tao, L.; Diao, A. Piperlongumine-induced nuclear translocation of the FOXO3A transcription factor triggers BIM-mediated apoptosis in cancer cells. *Biochem. Pharmacol.* **2019**, *163*, 101–110. [CrossRef]
31. Rawat, L.; Hegde, H.; Hoti, S.; Nayak, V. Piperlongumine induces ROS mediated cell death and synergizes paclitaxel in human intestinal cancer cells. *Biomed. Pharmacother.* **2020**, *128*, 110243. [CrossRef]

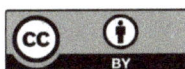

© 2020 by the authors. Licensee MDPI, Basel, Switzerland. This article is an open access article distributed under the terms and conditions of the Creative Commons Attribution (CC BY) license (http://creativecommons.org/licenses/by/4.0/).

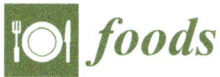

Article

Isolation of Neuroprotective Anthocyanins from Black Chokeberry (*Aronia melanocarpa*) against Amyloid-β-Induced Cognitive Impairment

Haichao Wen [1,2], Hui Cui [1,2], Hehe Tian [1,2], Xiaoxu Zhang [2], Liyan Ma [2,3], Charles Ramassamy [4] and Jingming Li [1,2,*]

1. Center for Viticulture and Enology, College of Food Science and Nutritional Engineering, China Agricultural University, Beijing 100083, China; wenhc@cau.edu.cn (H.W.); cuihuidaisy@163.com (H.C.); tianhehe@cau.edu.cn (H.T.)
2. College of Food Science and Nutritional Engineering, China Agricultural University, Beijing 100083, China; zxxjoypeace@foxmail.com (X.Z.); lyma1203@cau.edu.cn (L.M.)
3. Supervision, Inspection & Testing Center for Agricultural Products Quality, Ministry of Agriculture, Beijing 100083, China
4. Institut National de la Recherche Scientifique-Institut Armand Frappier, Laval, QC H7V 1B7, Canada; Ramassamy@iaf.inrs.ca
* Correspondence: lijingming@cau.edu.cn; Tel.: +86-010-62737039; Fax: +86-010-62738658

Abstract: Black chokeberry (*Aronia melanocarpa*) fruits are rich in anthocyanins, which are vital secondary metabolites that possess antioxidative properties. The aim of this study was to isolate and purify the anthocyanins from black chokeberry by simulated moving bed (SMB) chromatography, and to investigate the neuroprotective effect of SMB purified anthocyanin against Aβ-induced memory damage in rats. The parameters of the SMB process were studied and optimized. Anthocyanin extracts were identified by HPLC and UPLC-QTOF-MS, and antioxidant abilities were evaluated. The Aβ-induced animal model was established by intracerebral ventricle injection in rat brain. Through the SMB purification, anthocyanins were purified to 85%; cyanidin 3-*O*-galactoside and cyanidin 3-*O*-arabinoside were identified as the main anthocyanins by UPLC-QTOF-MS. The SMB purified anthocyanins exhibited higher DPPH and ABTS free radical scavenging abilities than the crude anthocyanins extract. Furthermore, rats receiving SMB purified anthocyanins treatment (50 mg/kg) showed improved spatial memory in a Morris water maze test, as well as protection of the cells in the hippocampus against Aβ toxicity. These results demonstrate that anthocyanins could serve as antioxidant and neuroprotective agents, with potential in the treatment of Alzheimer's disease.

Keywords: black chokeberry; anthocyanin; simulated moving bed; antioxidant activity; neuroprotection; Alzheimer's disease

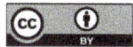

1. Introduction

Black chokeberry (*Aronia melanocarpa*) is used as an ornamental plant and as a food and colorant. It is rich in the secondary metabolites such as anthocyanins and flavonoids which play vital roles in protecting against oxidative stress and biotic stress [1]. The main anthocyanins in the black chokeberry are cyanidin 3-*O*-galactoside, cyanidin 3-*O*-arabinoside, cyanidin 3-*O*-glucoside, and cyanidin 3-*O*-xyloside. These compounds exhibit many bioactivities such as antioxidant, antiproliferative, antimicrobial, anti-inflammation, and modulate hepatic lipid metabolism activities [1–4]. Meanwhile, anthocyanins have been shown to prevent and remedy diseases such as cardiovascular disease, liver failure, obesity, and diabetes [5]. Moreover, anthocyanins can cross the blood-brain barrier (BBB) and delay aging-related degenerative diseases [6–8]. However, the stability of anthocyanins is influenced by many factors such as structure, the presence of solvents, pH, temperature, oxygen, and enzymes and other concomitant substances; as such it is still impossible to isolate and purify monomeric anthocyanin from complex natural compounds [9].

Neurodegenerative disorders are becoming more and more prevalent, leading to living and economic burdens on the family members of affected individuals. Alzheimer's disease (AD), one of the most common causes of dementia, is associated with many risk factors including alcohol use, smoking, hypertension, exposure to metals, and oxidative stress [10]. A hallmark of AD is the accumulation of insoluble forms of amyloid-β (Aβ) in the plaques in extracellular spaces and in the walls of blood vessels [10]. Although the pathogenesis of AD is not fully understood, a great deal of research has supported the hypothesis that reactive oxygen species (ROS) impair antioxidant defense systems and induce neuron apoptosis [11]. Many secondary metabolites, like phenolic compounds from Ginkgo biloba, green tea, curcumin, grape, and blueberry, have been reported to protect neuronal cells against oxidative stress in in vivo and in vitro models [12–16].

Simulated moving bed (SMB) chromatography is a continuous countercurrent process which has been used in the separation stage for the large-scale production of compounds such as glucose and fructose [17] and chiral drugs. SMB chromatography is characterized by the separation of a few grams of thermally unstable compounds [18] and chiral drugs, which differ little in terms of their physicochemical properties [19]. Compared to semipreparative liquid chromatography, SMB requires less adsorbent and solvent, and target compounds may be derived with low loss [17,20]. Although SMB is suitable for the isolation of unstable secondary metabolites like phenolic compounds, further studies on its use are necessary. To the best of our knowledge, this study is the first to isolate and purify anthocyanins by SMB chromatography and study both their protective effects against oxidative stress and their neuroprotective ability against Aβ-induced damage in rats.

The specific aims of this study are to develop a new, highly-efficient method to isolate and purify the anthocyanins from black chokeberry, and to investigate the antioxidant activity of the SMB purified anthocyanin extract. An Aβ-induced damage animal model was used to test the effects of SMB-purified anthocyanins on spatial learning and memory ability, as well as nerve cell viability in vivo.

2. Materials and Methods

2.1. Chemicals

Cyanidin 3-O-glucoside standard (99%) was purchased from Sichuan Weikeqi Biological Technology CO., LTD (Chengdu, Sichuan, China) and Cyanidin 3-O-galactoside (Cyn-3-gal, 95%) was obtained from HaoChen Ecological Agriculture Development CO., LTD (Shanghai, China). The $Aβ_{1-40}$ peptides were purchased from Beijing Biosynthesis Biotechnology CO., LTD (Beijing, China). 1,1-diphenyl-2-picrylhydrazyl (DPPH) and 2,2′-azino-bis(3-ethylbenzothiazoline-6-sulfonic acid) diammonium salt (ABTS), 6-hydroxy-2,5,7,8-tetramethylchroman-2-carboxylic acid (Trolox) were purchased from TCI (Shanghai) Development CO., LTD (Shanghai, China). All other organic solvents were of analytical grade.

2.2. Plants Material

Black chokeberry fruits were harvested at the full maturity stage in September 2017 from black chokeberry demonstration planting base in Wafangdian City (39°49′21″ N, 121°54′32″ E, Dalian, Liaoning, China). Fruits were transported at 4 °C and stored at −40 °C for a maximum of 6 months.

2.3. Extraction of Anthocyanins

The black chokeberry fruits were crushed and homogenized using a stainless steel blender, and then extracted twice with 65% ethanol in a 1:8 (w/v) ratio with 1% acetic acid in an ultrasonic wave bath for 10 min. Then, the supernatants were collected after centrifugation at 6485× g (10,000 rpm in an Anke GL-20G-II centrifuge, Shanghai Anke company, Ltd., Shanghai, China) at 25 °C for 15 min. The supernatants were evaporated until approximately a 90% volume was achieved, and then loaded onto a column (2.6 × 60 cm) containing 100 g of the Amberlite® XAD-7HP macroporous resin (Sigma Aldrich Co., St. Louis, MO, USA). The column was washed with deionized water, and then eluted with 1% acetic acid in 35% ethanol at a flow rate of 1 mL/min. Then, the crude extract solutions were evaporated, lyophilized, and stored at −40 °C.

2.4. Purification of Anthocyanins by SMB

Simulated moving bed chromatography (HYSMB6-500) was provided by Beijing Xiang Yue Huang Yu Technology Development Co., Ltd. (Beijing, China). The mathematical principle model is based on a rigorous mathematical first-principles model and the accurate dynamic models of multicolumn continuous chromatographic processes [18]. The anthocyanin extract solutions were homogenized by ultrasound and dissolved in 25% ethanol with 1% acetic acid at a concentration of 50 g/L through a 0.45 μm membrane to form the raw material solution used as the first SMB feed. In this SMB system (Figure 1), a four-zone working model was set up including an eluting zone (zone I), a refining (zone II) and an adsorbing zone (zone III), and a washing zone (zone IV) with two columns per zone. The SMB was equipped with eight columns (10 mm × 150 mm) with C18 (30 μm) filler configured as 2/2/2/2. The fluid was 25% ethanol with 1% acetic acid. Pump F and D pumped into the feeding and desorbent for eluting, and pump E and R pumped out the extract and raffinate. Q_E, Q_R, Q_D, and Q_F are the flow rates of extract, raffinate, desorbent and feed, respectively. The SMB purified anthocyanin extract (SMB ACN) solutions were dried under vacuum in a rotary evaporator and lyophilized into powder, and then stored at −40 °C. HPLC-PDA was used to monitor of the extract and raffinate during the SMB process, and the purity was calculated by the area of the corresponding anthocyanin peak to the total peak area at 278 nm.

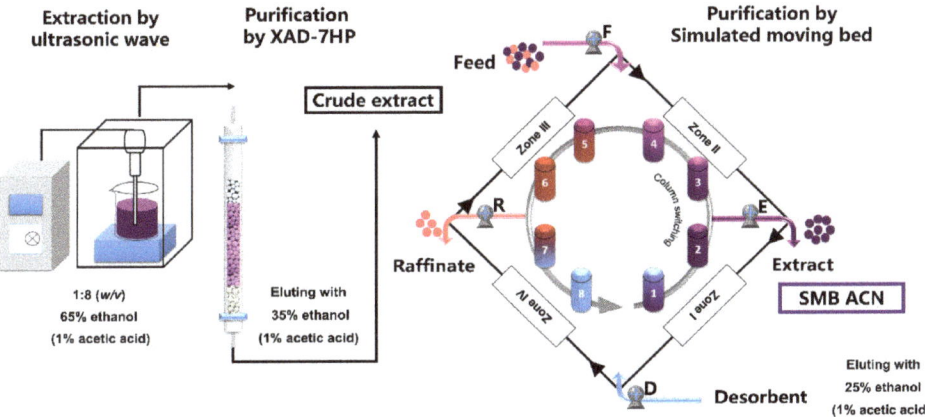

Figure 1. Schematic illustration of the isolation and purification of anthocyanins from black chokeberry fruits. The anthocyanins were isolated by an ultrasonic extraction method and the crude extract was prepared by XAD-7HP macroporous resins as the feed of simulated moving bed chromatography (SMB). The separation zones of SMB were zones II and III, and the solid phase was regenerated in zones I and IV with two columns per zone. The liquid phase (black) consisted of feed and desorbent for inlets, and extract and raffinate for outlets by pump E and pump R. The liquid phase was continuously fed the crude extract by pump F and eluted with ethanol by pump D. Then, SMB ACN was collected from the extract. The columns switched counter-clockwise (gray) at the switching time intervals.

2.5. HPLC-PDA and UPLC-QTOF-MS Analysis

The anthocyanins extract powders were dissolved in water with 10% acetic acid and 1% phosphoric acid. Then, all samples were centrifuged at 9339× g (12,000 rpm) at 4 °C for 10 min, and the supernatants were used for HPLC-PDA and UPLC-QTOF-MS analysis.

The HPLC system consisted of a pump (LC-20 AT) and a photodiode array (PDA) detector (SPD-10A) (Shimadzu Corp., Tokyo, Japan). The analytical column was the Intertsil ODS-SP C18 column (4.6 × 250 mm, 5 µm, GL Sciences Inc., Tokyo, Japan). Mobile phase A was 10% acetic acid and 1% phosphoric acid in water, and mobile phase B was 100% acetonitrile. Elution was performed at a flow rate of 1.0 mL/min, and the solvent gradient was as follows: 0–8 min, 10% B; 8–12 min, B from 10% to 40%; 12–15 min, 40% B; 15–25 min, from 40% to 10% B. The injection volume was 20 µL and the column was thermostated at 25 °C. The analysis wavelengths were 278 nm for monitoring the SMB process and 520 nm for quantifying the anthocyanins [21]. The UV-VIS spectra were scanned from 220 to 800 nm. Cyanidin 3-*O*-galactoside were quantified using cyanidin 3-*O*-galactoside ($y = 18{,}674x + 11{,}660$, $R^2 = 0.9994$) and cyanidin 3-*O*-glucoside, cyanidin 3-*O*-arabinoside and cyanidin 3-*O*-xyloside were quantified using cyanidin 3-*O*-glucoside ($y = 25{,}228x + 10{,}850$, $R^2 = 0.9990$). The purity was determined by the area normalization method of these four anthocyanins on HPLC-PDA at 278 nm. The anthocyanin contents were determined by comparing retention times and absorption spectra, and further confirmed by UPLC-QTOF-MS.

A Waters ACQUITY UPLC system coupled with a Xevo G2QTOF mass spectrometer (Waters Corporation, Milford, MA, USA) was used for anthocyanins confirmation as previously described [22]. The separation of anthocyanins was conducted on a HSS T3 column (2.1 mm × 100 mm, 1.8 µm). The mobile phase was (A) water + 0.2% formic acid and (B) acetonitrile + 0.2% formic acid: 0 to 1 min, 5% B; 1 to 2 min, 5% to 40% B; 4 to 8 min, 95% B; 8.1 to 10 min, 5% B. The injection volume was 2 µL and the flow rate was 0.3 mL/min. The ESI parameters were set as follows: negative mode, capillary voltage 2.2 kV, sampling cone voltage 30 V, extraction cone voltage 4 V, source temperature 100 °C, desolvation gas (nitrogen) temperature 400 °C, cone gas flow rate 20 L/h, desolvation gas (nitrogen) flow rate 800 L/h, collision energies 6 eV and mass range from 50 to 1200 Da. The anthocyanin structure was determined according to its fragmentation pattern of deprotonated and product ions.

2.6. DPPH Free Radical Scavenging Assay

The ROS scavenging capacity was determined by the DPPH free radical scavenging assay as previously reported [23]. The assay was performed in a 96-well plate using serial dilutions of 5 µL aliquots of each Cyn-3-gal (14 to 449 mg/L), anthocyanins crude extract (2.5 to 80.0 mg/L) and SMB ACN (0.03 to 1.0 g/L). DPPH solution (200 µL, 0.06 mM) was added to each well, and the plate was incubated at room temperature in the dark for 30 min. The absorbance was determined at 520 nm using a Thermo Multiskan MK3 Automated Microplate Reader (Thermo Fisher Scientific, Waltham, MA, USA). The EC_{50} value was calculated using a calibration curve of Trolox (25 to 250 mg/L) by SPSS.

2.7. ABTS Free Radical Scavenging Assay

The ABTS•+ scavenging capacity assay was determined as previously described with some modifications [24]. The ABTS•+ solution was produced by reacting aqueous ABTS solution (7 mM) with potassium persulfate (2.45 mM). Diluted ABTS•+ solution with an absorbance of 0.70 ± 0.02 at 734 nm was employed in the analysis. The reactions were performed by adding 4 mL of ABTS•+ solution and 0.4 mL of each Cyn-3-gal (14 to 449 mg/L), anthocyanins crude extract (2.5 to 40.0 g/L) and SMB ACN (0.03 to 1.0 g/L). After 6 min of incubation at room temperature, absorbance values were measured on a spectrophotometer at 734 nm. The EC_{50} value of ABTS•+ scavenging capacity was calculated using a Trolox calibration curve (25 to 250 mg/L).

2.8. Experimental Animals

Thirty-six Sprague-Dawley (SD) rats (male, weighing 250 ± 20 g, specific pathogen-free) were purchased by Beijing HFK Bioscience Co. Ltd. (Beijing, China). The rats were kept at the animal facility with free access to standard chow and water at 22 ± 2 °C, the relative humidity of 45 ± 15% and 12 h light/dark cycle. All animals had adapted for one week before experiments. SD rats were randomly divided into 3 groups ($n = 12$) of sham, Aβ, Aβ + SMB ACN. The group of Aβ and Aβ + SMB ACN were treated by intracerebral ventricle injection of Aβ$_{1-40}$, and then Aβ + SMB ACN group were administered by intragastric administration with anthocyanins (50 mg/kg anthocyanins 85%) for one month. The experiment was approved by the Animal Ethical and Welfare Committee (No. IRM-DWLL-2017095).

2.9. Preparation of Aβ-Induced Damage Rat Model

The Aβ$_{1-40}$ oligomers were prepared according to a previously reported method [25]. Briefly, Aβ$_{1-40}$ peptide was prepared as a stock solution at a concentration of 1 mg/mL in sterile sodium chorionic solution, followed by aggregation via incubation at 37 °C for 4 days.

Rats were anesthetized with 10% chloral hydrate (0.3 mL/100 g i.p.) and the head was symmetrically held in the stereotaxic apparatus (ZS-FD, ZS Dichuang, Beijing, China). The scalp skin was clean shaved and the skull was exposed. One hole was drilled on the skull at coordinates of −0.8 mm posterior to the bregma and 1.4 mm lateral according to the atlas of Paxinos and Watson [26,27]. The needle was injected 4 mm deep into the ventricle with a speed of 1 μL/min for 5 μL and left in place for 5 min after the injection of Aβ$_{1-40}$. The sham rats were injected with 0.9% saline. The surgical wound was sutured and the animals were returned to their cages with free access to food and water, and allowed to recover for 1 day [28].

2.10. Morris Water Maze

After one month of intragastric administration with anthocyanins, the Morris water maze (MWM) test was performed as previously described [29]. The circular pool was 150 cm in diameter and 60 cm in depth with an invisible platform (12 cm in diameter and 25 cm in depth). The water in the pool was mixed with black ink. During the experiment, the temperature of the water remained within 22 to 24 °C, and all landmarks around the maze remained the same. The MWM included spatial learning and acquisition trials (hidden platform trials) and a spatial probe trial. Before the spatial acquisition trials, each rat was put into the water to adapt for 2 min and the platform was visible, located in the middle of the first quadrant for one day. Then, water was added to the pool with the platform 1 cm below the water surface. During the hidden platform trials, each rat was placed into the water from one of the start positions, facing the wall. The spatial acquisition trials were conducted over four days, with four trials per day. If the animal reached the platform, the timer was stopped. If the animal failed to find the platform within 90 s, the animal was placed on the platform for 15 s to help it learn the platform's location. The spatial probe test was on day 5, and then the platform was removed. The rats were released from the third quadrant (180° from the original platform position) and the time spent crossing the target quadrant and the number of times the region in which the platform was previously located was crossed were recorded over a 90 s period. After testing, the rats were dried with a towel to keep them warm. The animals were recorded with a video camera, and the data were analyzed using ANY-maze behavioral tracking software (Stoelting Co., Wood Dale, IL, USA)

2.11. Nissl Staining

For Nissl staining of the brain, the rats were euthanized by intraperitoneal injection of 0.3% chloral hydrate, and were transcardially perfused with 100 mL of saline (0.9% w/v NaCl). Then, the brains were removed and put in the 15 mL of 4% paraformaldehyde.

Serial coronal hippocampal sections with a thickness of 25 µm were cut using a cryostat (Leica Microsystems, Wetzlar, Germany). The sections were washed twice for 5 min in 0.01 M PBS and incubated in 1% toluidine blue staining solution for 5–10 min at room temperature. Then, the sections were rinsed in distilled water, soaked in 95% ethanol for 30 min, and dehydrated in 100% ethanol. After dehydration, brains were placed in xylene and cover slipped using resin medium. The neurons were quantified using image software (Image J 1.45 s), with three sections from three rats for each group.

2.12. Statistical Analysis

The data are presented as mean ± SD in triplicate from at least using GraphPad Prism 7.0 software (GraphPad Software, San Diego, CA, USA). $p < 0.05$ was considered statistically significant by LSD test. The results were analyzed by ANOVA and the EC_{50} value was calculated using the Probit Analysis by SPSS 20.0 software (IBM, Armonk, NY, USA).

3. Results

3.1. Isolation and Purification of Black Chokeberry Anthocyanins by SMB

Anthocyanins from black chokeberry were extracted and preliminarily purified by the XAD-7HP macroporous resin column. Four-section SMB was employed to separate the anthocyanins crude extract. After approximately 20 switching times, a cyclic steady state was reached. As shown in Table 1, the optimal parameters of flow rate were Q_F = 0.42 mL/min, Q_E = 1.5 mL/min, Q_R = 6.5 mL/min, and Q_D = 4.5 mL/min. The HPLC-PDA chromatograms of feed, raffinate and extract by running H are presented in Figure 2A–C. Anthocyanins and impurities are separated in column 3 to 6 (Figure 1). The purity of the SMB ACN was estimated to be 68% to 85%. These results in run A, B and G indicated that a switching time of 141 s maximally purified the anthocyanins. At a certain switching time, the slight decrease of flow rate in the feed, extract and raffinate zone increased the purity comparing run B to C, E to G and D to H. These results confirmed that the performance of SMB was mainly associated with the switching time and flow rate of feed, extract and raffinate [30].

Table 1. Operation parameters and separation performance of the SMB.

Run	Flow Rates (mL/min)				Switch Time ts (s)	Purity (%)
	Q_E	Q_R	Q_D	Q_F		
A	1.5	6.5	4.5	0.45	135	68.7
B	1.5	6.5	4.5	0.45	140	78.2
C	1.5	6.5	4.5	0.40	140	73.1
D	1.5	8.0	4.5	0.42	141	71.4
E	3.5	6.5	4.5	0.45	141	70.3
F	1.5	6.0	4.5	0.42	141	77.5
G	1.5	6.5	4.5	0.45	141	78.3
H	1.5	6.5	4.5	0.42	141	85.1

In order to analyze the anthocyanins crude extract and SMB CAN, HPLC-PDA was used to quantify and UPLC-QTOF-MS to identify the anthocyanins. An HPLC chromatogram of the crude extract showed four peaks (Figure 3A). The λ_{max} value of UV-VIS spectra was 516 nm for cyanidin. The SMB ACN mainly showed two peaks by HPLC-PDA (Figure 3B) which were identified by UPLC-QTOF-MS (Figure 3C,D). Peak 1 of cyanidin 3-O-galactoside (m/z 449.1089/287.0560) appeared as a principal peak, and peak 2 was identified as a cyanidin 3-O-arabinoside by detection of the respective parent and product ion pairs (m/z 419.0975/287.0557). The four compounds of crude extract were cyanidin 3-O-galactoside (72.9% of total anthocyanins), cyanidin 3-O-glucoside (2.7%), cyanidin 3-O-arabinoside (21.0%), and cyanidin 3-O-xyloside (3.4%) (Table 2), which is in accordance with the Oszmianski's results [31]. The mass of total anthocyanins in the crude extract was

2.29 ± 0.19 g/100 g of dry extract, and the mass of total anthocyanins in the SMB ACN was 61.02 ± 6.46 g/100 g of the fraction rich in dry anthocyanins.

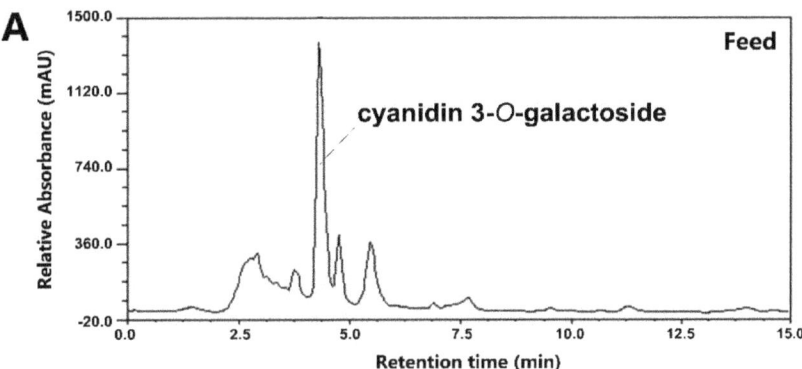

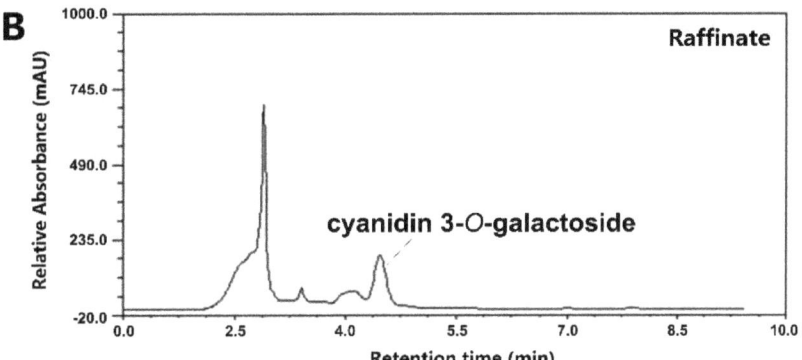

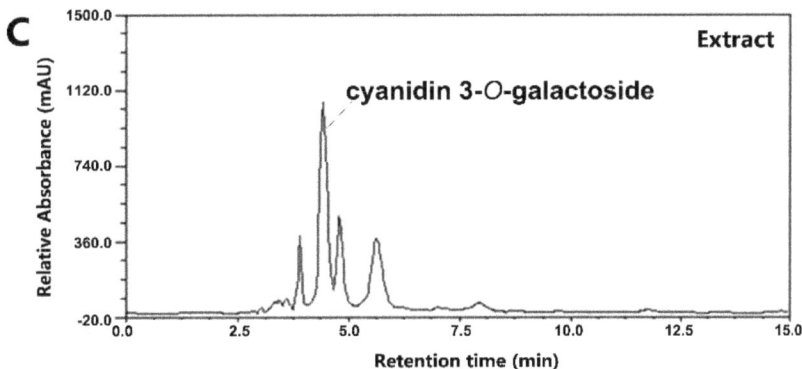

Figure 2. HPLC-PDA chromatogram of the feed (**A**), the raffinate (**B**), and the extract (**C**) during the SMB process monitored at 278 nm.

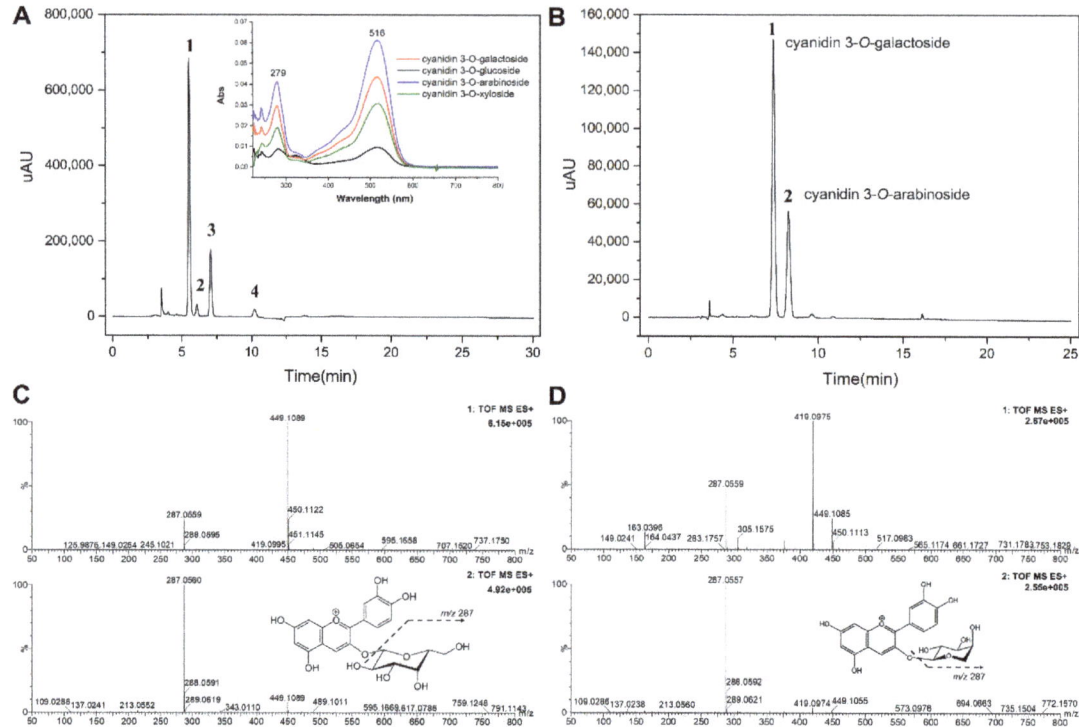

Figure 3. (**A**) HPLC-PDA chromatogram and UV-VIS scanning spectra of the black chokeberry anthocyanins crude extract at 520 nm and peak identities (1: cyanidin 3-O-galactoside; 2: cyanidin 3-O-glucoside; 3: cyanidin 3-O-arabinoside; 4: cyanidin 3-O-xyloside); (**B**) HPLC-PDA chromatogram of the SMB ACN at 520 nm and peak identities (1: cyanidin 3-O-galactoside; 2: cyanidin 3-O-arabinoside); The UPLC-QTOF-MS mass spectra and structure of cyanidin 3-O-galactoside (**C**) and cyanidin 3-O-arabinoside (**D**) of the SMB ACN peak 1 and peak 2.

Table 2. HPLC quantification and UPLC-QTOF-MS identification of anthocyanins in Black chokeberry crude extract and SMB ACN.

Peak	RT HPLC (min)	Compound	Molecular Formula	ESI(+)MS/MS2 (m/z)	Crude Extract (mg/100 g FW)	SMB ACN (mg/g DW)
1	4.809	cyanidin 3-O-galactoside	$C_{21}H_{21}O_{11}$	449.1089([M]+) 287.0560([M-gal]+)	500.4 ± 38.7	449.1 ± 30.8
2	5.169	cyanidin 3-O-glucoside	$C_{21}H_{21}O_{11}$	449.1088([M]+) 287.0558([M-glu]+)	18.6 ± 1.8	ND
3	5.923	cyanidin 3-O-arabinoside	$C_{20}H_{19}O_{10}$	419.0975([M]+) 287.0557([M-arab]+)	144.2 ± 14.0	161.2 ± 33.8
4	8.219	cyanidin 3-O-xyloside	$C_{20}H_{19}O_{10}$	419.0975([M]+) 287.0556([M-xyl]+)	23.4 ± 1.8	ND

Data presented in fresh fruit weight (FW) and dried extract weight (DW). ND: not detected.

The SMB continuously purified the anthocyanins, and efficiently enriched the two main anthocyanins and eliminated the impurity. A similar observation was made by Wang, who reported the use of a two-step simulated moving bed chromatographic process to purify the EGCG from tea polyphenol [32]. It was suggested that the SMB was a highly efficient way to separate and purify the secondary metabolites from a natural extract. Due to the instability of secondary metabolites like anthocyanins and the complexity of the plant phenols, the extraction process of monomer was extremely difficult. Therefore, these results indicated that SMB may be a feasible and effective strategy to isolate and purify the anthocyanins from black chokeberry.

3.2. The Free Radical Scavenging Abilities of Black Chokeberry Anthocyanin Extracts

To evaluate the SMB purification process, we tested the DPPH and ABTS free radical scavenging abilities of the black chokeberry anthocyanins crude extract and the SMB purified anthocyanin extract. As shown in Figure 4, the EC_{50} values of anthocyanins crude extract were significantly higher than Trolox, Cyn-3-gal and SMB ACN of the free radical scavenging abilities ($p < 0.001$). The DPPH• and ABTS•+ scavenging of crude extract (54.18 ± 19.59 g/L and 4.21 ± 1.50 g/L) were 65- and 30-fold more than SMB ACN (0.83 ± 0.20 g/L and 0.14 ± 0.06 g/L). The lower EC_{50} of SMB ACN indicated a higher antioxidant activity. Moreover, the ABTS radical scavenging ability of SMB ACN was similar to Cyn-3-gal and Trolox ($p > 0.05$). These results suggest that the SMB process increased the free radical scavenging ability of the anthocyanin extract.

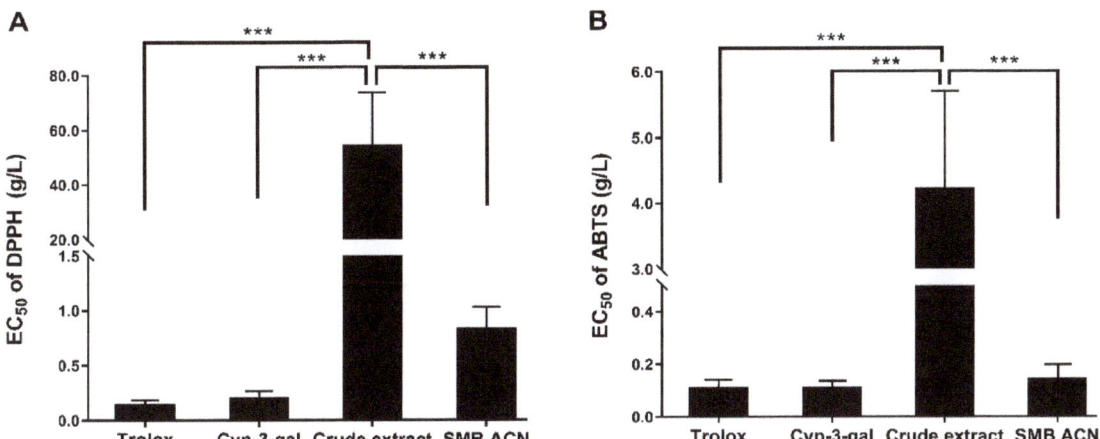

Figure 4. (**A**) DPPH free radical scavenging activity of Trolox, cyanidin 3-O-galactoside (Cyn-3-gal), anthocyanins crude extract and SMB ACN; (**B**) ABTS free radical scavenging activity of Trolox, Cyn-3-gal, anthocyanins crude extract and SMB ACN. Date represent mean ± SD (n = 6) were expressed by the EC_{50} inhibition of the free radical scavenging and the *** $p < 0.001$ by LSD test of one-way ANOVA.

The results showed that the ABTS free radical scavenging abilities of anthocyanins extracts were higher than those of DPPH; notably, cyanidin 3-O-galactoside had a high free radical scavenging ability due to its hydroxyl group. It may be that the anthocyanin extracts neutralized the DPPH free radicals mainly by hydrogen atom transfer and the ABTS•+ by a fast, non-selective electron transferring process. Therefore, the application of the SMB chromatography purified and enriched the anthocyanins and improved the antioxidant ability than crude extract. Deneva et al. found that anthocyanins were the second biggest contributor to antioxidant activity after the proanthocyanidins among black chokeberry polyphenols [3]. Moreover, cyanidin-3-O-glucoside could regulate cellular antioxidant defense induced by $A\beta_{1-40}$ in SH-SY5Y cells through the Nrf2 signaling pathway [33]. The purified anthocyanins may scavenge the free radicals and inhibit the $A\beta_{1-40}$ neurotoxicity. Therefore, the next section of this study is concerned with SMB ACN, investigating its neuroprotective activity against amyloid-β induced in rats.

3.3. The Protection of Anthocyanins on Memory Impairment in Aβ-Induced Toxicity Rats

The Morris water maze (MWM) is a method to assess spatial learning and memory in rats. The escape latency time of all groups had a decreasing tendency over four days

(Figure 5A). The results showed that the SMB ACN treatment group presented a less steep learning curve between days 1 and 2, which might indicate that anthocyanins had increased the short-term memory. The sham group showed a more stable spatial learning rate than the Aβ+SMB ACN group. In the probe trial, the time spent in the targeted quadrant of the sham group was shorter compared to the Aβ group impaired by Aβ$_{1-40}$, which indicated that the Aβ group showed lower long-tern learning and memory ability (Figure 5B). The rats given the anthocyanins extract achieved more platform crossings in comparison with the Aβ-induced group, and showed a nonsignificant difference with the sham group (Figure 5C). The results indicated that anthocyanin group had a significantly higher spatial learning ability than the Aβ-induced group ($p < 0.05$). Interestingly, the sham group achieved higher scores than the Aβ group, although this was not significant, and may have been due to intervariability among the rats. As shown in Figure 5D, the Aβ + SMB ACN group allayed behavioral deficits compared to the Aβ group regarding the swim path. The behavioral test results showed that the purified anthocyanins extract alleviated the damage induced by amyloid-β to spatial learning and memory.

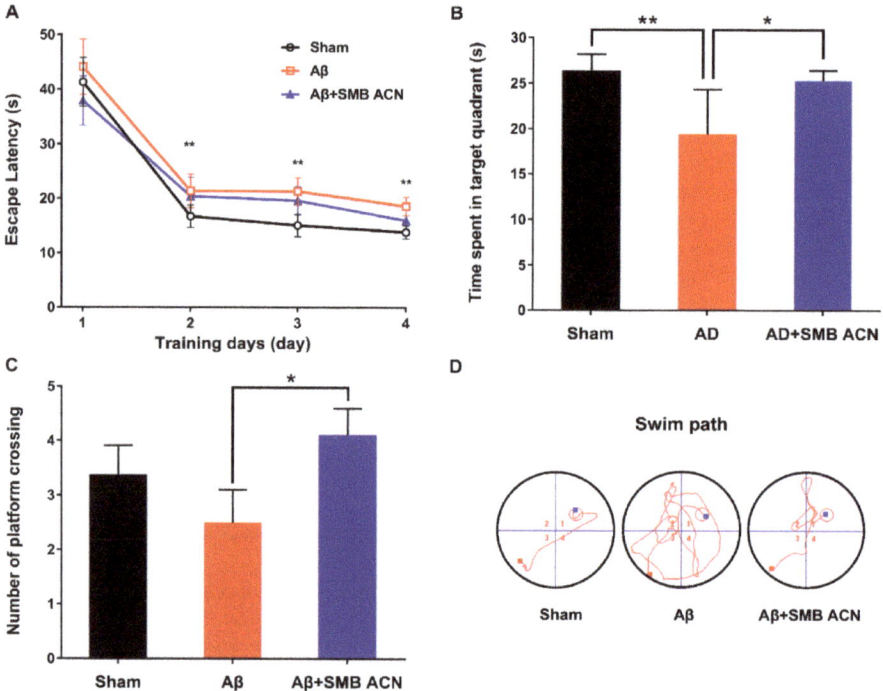

Figure 5. SMB ACN treatment alleviated Aβ induced spatial learning deficits. (**A**) The escape latency during the spatial acquisition trials of Sham, Aβ and Aβ + SMB ACN group; (**B**) The time spent in the target quadrant of the spatial probe test; (**C**) The number of platform crossing of the spatial probe test; (**D**) The swim path of the spatial acquisition trial. The results were expressed by mean ± SD ($n = 12$) and the * $p < 0.05$, ** $p < 0.01$ by LSD test of one-way ANOVA.

Previous reports have shown that anthocyanin galactosides are better maintained in the intestines compared to glucosides, while arabinosides or xylosides showed negligible losses [34]. Notably, cyanidin 3-O-galactoside and cyanidin 3-O-arabinoside crossed the blood-brain barrier into the cortex and hippocampus [16]. Moreover, the neuroprotective ability of black chokeberry has been reported; additionally, anthocyanins have been associated with antiaging [7]. Anthocyanins were shown to regulate the cell cycle and senescence by regulating the expression of the DNA damage signaling pathway and antioxidant enzymes in neuronal cells [7,11]. Our results support the hypothesis that the administration of SMB ACN ameliorates learning and memory impairment by Aβ-induced severe behavioral dysfunction.

3.4. The Neuroprotective Effect of SMB Anthocyanins Extract in Rat Brain

To further elucidate the neuroprotective effect of anthocyanins, we examined the hippocampus. The Nissl staining stains the nuclei of all cells, as well as clumps of material surrounding the nuclei of neurons. Neuronal loss in the brain, especially in the CA1 region of the hippocampus [35] and basal forebrain, is one of the most important pathological hallmarks of Alzheimer's disease [36]. The pyramidal cells in the CA1 and CA3 regions of the hippocampus in the brain modulates memory and emotions [37].

The results showed that the survival of neuron cells in the CA1 and CA3 of the sham group was greater than in the $A\beta_{1-40}$ treated group ($p < 0.05$) (Figure 6). The neurons in the Aβ group were disorganized and deformed with deep stain nuclei due to the neurotoxicity of Aβ. The results of the sham group indicated that the injection into the ventricle of the brain did not damage the hippocampus region. The neurons and kernel in the visual field of the Aβ + SMB ACN group were clearer and more intact than the Aβ group, and the numbers of pyramidal cells in the CA1 and CA3 were significantly increased ($p < 0.05$). The neurons in the $A\beta_{1-40}$ treated group were damaged with extensive degenerative changes including sparse cell arrangements, swollen cell bodies, loss of integrity, shrunken cytoplasm and oval or triangular nucleus [38,39]. These results confirmed that $A\beta_{1-40}$ can induce cellular loss and disorganization of the pyramidal cells, and indicated that the treatment of anthocyanins can reverse these changes to alleviate the loss of memory.

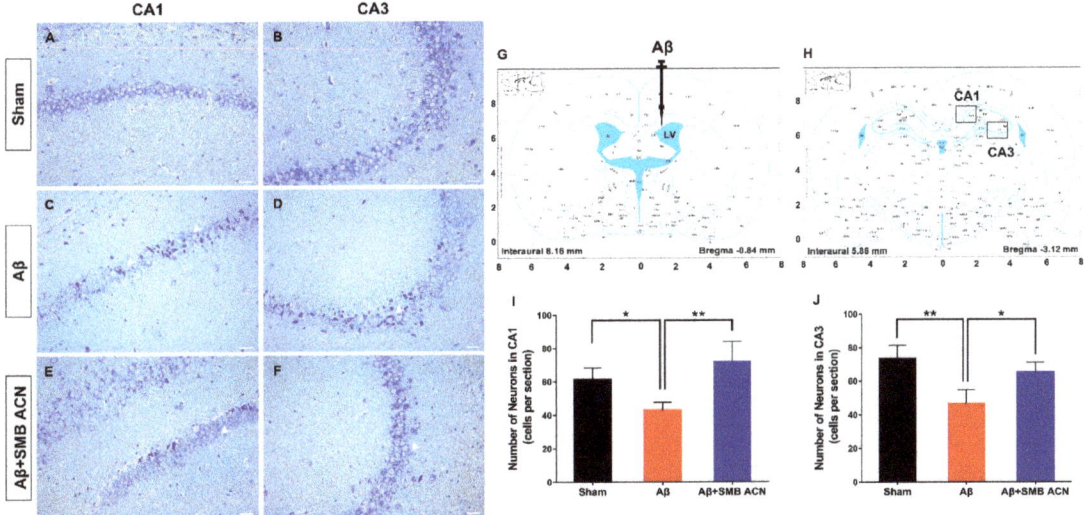

Figure 6. Representative images of Nissl staining in the CA1 and CA3 regions of the hippocampus of sham group (**A,B**), Aβ group (**C,D**), and Aβ + SMB ACN group (**E,F**). (**G**) The site of intracerebral ventricle injection in rat brain (Black) and the sites of the section in CA1 and CA3 region of the hippocampus (**H**). The number indicated the surviving neurons in CA1 (**I**) and CA3 (**J**), * $p < 0.05$ and ** $p < 0.01$. Stained sections of each group were viewed at 200× magnification. Scale bar = 100 μm.

This research shows that purified anthocyanins by SMB exhibit excellent antioxidative activity against oxidative stress and prevent amyloid-β induced neurotoxicity in the brain. However, we still need to investigate the mechanism of antioxidative ability in vivo and the bioavailability of anthocyanins and their metabolites to determine the efficacy of such a treatment. The cell signaling pathway of anthocyanins regulating the cellular antioxidant system and alleviating the Aβ neurotoxicity still needs to be examined. We used UPLC-QTOF-MS to analyze a black chokeberry anthocyanins crude extract and found many secondary metabolites, such as polyphenols, that have antioxidant activities. In a future study, the neuroprotective ability of black chokeberry may found to be associated with the ability of these secondary metabolite compounds to protect neuronal cells against oxidative stress.

4. Conclusions

In this study, the anthocyanins from black chokeberry (*Aronia melanocarpa*) were isolated and purified by XAD-7HP macroporous resin and SMB chromatography, yielding a purity of 85%. The main purified anthocyanins (cyanidin 3-*O*-galactoside and cyanidin 3-*O*-arabinoside) had a strong antioxidant ability and ameliorated learning and memory impairment among Aβ-induced neurotoxicity rats. Taken together, these results demonstrate that simulated moving bed chromatography could be a feasible and effective strategy to separate highly bioactive anthocyanins from black chokeberry. The present study was an attempt to establish a method to isolate secondary metabolites from natural plants to exploit their neuroprotective abilities.

Author Contributions: Conceptualization, L.M. and J.L.; methodology, H.W., H.C., and H.T.; software, H.W. and X.Z.; validation, X.Z. and C.R.; investigation, H.W., H.C., and H.T.; data curation, L.M. and J.L.; writing—original draft preparation, H.W. and X.Z.; writing—review and editing, H.W., H.C., C.R. and J.L.; visualization, H.W.; supervision, L.M. and J.L.; project administration, J.L. All authors have read and agreed to the published version of the manuscript.

Funding: This work was funded by the National Natural Science Foundation of China, grant number 31571840.

Institutional Review Board Statement: The study was approved and conducted according to the Animal Ethical and Welfare Committee (Approval No. IRM-DWLL-2017095).

Informed Consent Statement: Not applicable.

Data Availability Statement: The data are not publicly available because the research is still ongoing.

Conflicts of Interest: The authors declare no conflict of interest.

References

1. Kim, B.; Ku, C.S.; Pham, T.X.; Park, Y.; Martin, D.A.; Xie, L.; Taheri, R.; Lee, J.; Bolling, B.W. Aronia melanocarpa (chokeberry) polyphenol-rich extract improves antioxidant function and reduces total plasma cholesterol in apolipoprotein E knockout mice. *Nutr. Res.* **2013**, *33*, 406–413. [CrossRef] [PubMed]
2. Stanisavljević, N.; Samardžić, J.; Janković, T.; Šavikin, K.; Mojsin, M.; Topalović, V.; Stevanović, M. Antioxidant and antiproliferative activity of chokeberry juice phenolics during in vitro simulated digestion in the presence of food matrix. *Food Chem.* **2015**, *175*, 516–522. [CrossRef] [PubMed]
3. Denev, P.; Číž, M.; Kratchanova, M.; Blazheva, D. Black chokeberry (*Aronia melanocarpa*) polyphenols reveal different antioxidant, antimicrobial and neutrophil-modulating activities. *Food Chem.* **2019**, *284*, 108–117. [CrossRef] [PubMed]
4. Bhaswant, M.; Shafie, S.R.; Mathai, M.L.; Mouatt, P.; Brown, L. Anthocyanins in chokeberry and purple maize attenuate diet-induced metabolic syndrome in rats. *Nutrition* **2017**, *41*, 24–31. [CrossRef] [PubMed]
5. Thilavech, T.; Adisakwattana, S. Cyanidin-3-rutinoside acts as a natural inhibitor of intestinal lipid digestion and absorption. *BMC Complement. Altern. Med.* **2019**, *19*, 1–10. [CrossRef] [PubMed]
6. Amin, F.U.; Shah, S.A.; Badshah, H.; Khan, M.; Kim, M.O. Anthocyanins encapsulated by PLGA@PEG nanoparticles potentially improved its free radical scavenging capabilities via p38/JNK pathway against Aβ1-42-induced oxidative stress. *J. Nanobiotechnol.* **2017**, *15*, 12. [CrossRef]
7. Wei, J.; Zhang, G.; Zhang, X.; Xu, D.; Gao, J.; Fan, J.; Zhou, Z. Anthocyanins from Black Chokeberry (*Aroniamelanocarpa* Elliot) Delayed Aging-Related Degenerative Changes of Brain. *J. Agric. Food Chem.* **2017**, *65*, 5973–5984. [CrossRef]
8. Faria, A.; Meireles, M.; Fernandes, I.; Santos-Buelga, C.; Gonzalez-Manzano, S.; Dueñas, M.; Freitas, V.; Mateus, N.; Calhau, C. Flavonoid metabolites transport across a human BBB model. *Food Chem.* **2014**, *149*, 190–196. [CrossRef]
9. Klisurova, D.; Petrova, I.; Ognyanov, M.; Georgiev, Y.; Kratchanova, M.; Denev, P. Co-pigmentation of black chokeberry (*Aronia melanocarpa*) anthocyanins with phenolic co-pigments and herbal extracts. *Food Chem.* **2019**, *279*, 162–170. [CrossRef]
10. Masters, C.L.; Bateman, R.; Blennow, K.; Rowe, C.C.; Sperling, R.A.; Cummings, J.L. Alzheimers disease. *Nat. Rev. Dis. Primers* **2015**, *1*, 15056. [CrossRef]

11. Pacheco, S.M.; Soares, M.S.P.; Gutierres, J.M.; Gerzson, M.F.B.; Carvalho, F.B.; Azambuja, J.H.; Schetinger, M.R.C.; Stefanello, F.M.; Spanevello, R.M. Anthocyanins as a potential pharmacological agent to manage memory deficit, oxidative stress and alterations in ion pump activity induced by experimental sporadic dementia of Alzheimers type. *J. Nutr. Biochem.* **2018**, *56*, 193–204. [CrossRef] [PubMed]
12. Liu, X.; Hao, W.; Qin, Y.; Decker, Y.; Wang, X.; Burkart, M.; Schoetz, K.; Menger, M.D.; Fassbender, K.; Liu, Y. Long-term treatment with Ginkgo biloba extract EGb 761 improves symptoms and pathology in a transgenic mouse model of Alzheimer's disease. *Brain Behav. Immun.* **2015**, *46*, 121–131. [CrossRef] [PubMed]
13. Schimidt, H.L.; Garcia, A.; Martins, A.; Mello-Carpes, P.B.; Carpes, F.P. Green tea supplementation produces better neuroprotective effects than red and black tea in Alzheimer-like rat model. *Food Res. Int.* **2017**, *100*, 442–448. [CrossRef] [PubMed]
14. Ghosh, S.; Banerjee, S.; Sil, P.C. The beneficial role of curcumin on inflammation, diabetes and neurodegenerative disease: A recent update. *Food Chem. Toxicol.* **2015**, *83*, 111–124. [CrossRef]
15. Wen, H.; Fu, Z.; Wei, Y.; Zhang, X.; Ma, L.; Gu, L.; Li, J. Antioxidant Activity and Neuroprotective Activity of Stilbenoids in Rat Primary Cortex Neurons via the PI3K/Akt Signalling Pathway. *Molecules* **2018**, *23*, 2328. [CrossRef]
16. Andres-Lacueva, C.; Shukitt-Hale, B.; Galli, R.L.; Jauregui, O.; Lamuela-Raventos, R.M.; Joseph, J.A. Anthocyanins in aged blueberry-fed rats are found centrally and may enhance memory. *Nutr. Neurosci.* **2005**, *8*, 111–120. [CrossRef]
17. Hong, S.B.; Choi, J.H.; Chang, Y.K.; Mun, S. Production of high-purity fucose from the seaweed of Undaria pinnatifida through acid-hydrolysis and simulated-moving bed purification. *Sep. Purif. Technol.* **2019**, *213*, 133–141. [CrossRef]
18. Toumi, A.; Engell, S.; Diehl, M.; Bock, H.G.; Schlöder, J. Efficient optimization of simulated moving bed processes. *Chem. Eng. Process.* **2007**, *46*, 1067–1084. [CrossRef]
19. Strube, J.; Jupke, A.; Epping, A.; Schmidt-Traub, H.; Schulte, M.; Devant, R. Design, optimization, and operation of SMB chromatography in the production of enantiomerically pure pharmaceuticals. *Chirality* **1999**, *11*, 440–450. [CrossRef]
20. Wang, E.; Yin, Y.; Xu, C.; Liu, J. Isolation of high-purity anthocyanin mixtures and monomers from blueberries using combined chromatographic techniques. *J. Chromatogr. A* **2014**, *1327*, 39–48. [CrossRef]
21. Wojdyło, A.; Nowicka, P. Anticholinergic effects of Actinidia arguta fruits and their polyphenol content determined by liquid chromatography-photodiode array detector-quadrupole/time of flight-mass spectrometry (LC-MS-PDA-Q/TOF). *Food Chem.* **2019**, *271*, 216–223. [CrossRef]
22. Yang, J.; Wen, H.; Zhang, L.; Zhang, X.; Fu, Z.; Li, J. The influence of ripening stage and region on the chemical compounds in mulberry fruits (Morus atropurpurea Roxb.) based on UPLC-QTOF-MS. *Food Res. Int.* **2017**, *100*, 159–165. [CrossRef]
23. Mensor, L.L.; Menezes, F.S.; Leitão, G.G.; Reis, A.S.; Santos, T.C.; Coube, C.S.; Leitão, S.G. Screening of Brazilian plant extracts for antioxidant activity by the use of DPPH free radical method. *Phytother. Res.* **2001**, *15*, 127–130. [CrossRef]
24. Re, R.; Pellegrini, N.; Proteggente, A.; Pannala, A.; Yang, M.; Rice-Evans, C. Antioxidant activity applying an improved ABTS radical cation decolorization assay. *Free Radical Bio. Med.* **1999**, *26*, 1231–1237. [CrossRef]
25. Wen, M.; Ding, L.; Zhang, L.; Zhou, M.; Xu, J.; Wang, J.; Wang, Y.; Xue, C. DHA-PC and DHA-PS improved Aβ1–40 induced cognitive deficiency uncoupled with an increase in brain DHA in rats. *J. Funct. Foods* **2016**, *22*, 417–430. [CrossRef]
26. Paxinos, G.; Watson, C. *The Rat Brain in Stereotaxic Coordinates*, 6th ed.; Elsevier Academic Press: New York, NY, USA, 2006.
27. Wen, M.; Xu, J.; Ding, L.; Zhang, L.; Du, L.; Wang, J.; Wang, Y.; Xue, C. Eicosapentaenoic acid-enriched phospholipids improve Aβ1–40-induced cognitive deficiency in a rat model of Alzheimer's disease. *J. Funct. Foods* **2016**, *24*, 537–548. [CrossRef]
28. Sohanaki, H.; Baluchnejadmojarad, T.; Nikbakht, F.; Roghani, M. Pelargonidin improves memory deficit in amyloid β25-35 rat model of Alzheimer's disease by inhibition of glial activation, cholinesterase, and oxidative stress. *Biomed. Pharmacother.* **2016**, *83*, 85–91. [CrossRef]
29. Chen, L.; Huang, J.; Yang, L.; Zeng, X.-A.; Zhang, Y.; Wang, X.; Chen, M.; Li, X.; Zhang, Y.; Zhang, M. Sleep deprivation accelerates the progression of alzheimer's disease by influencing Aβ-related metabolism. *Neurosci. Lett.* **2017**, *650*, 146–152. [CrossRef]
30. Lü, Y.-B.; Su, B.-G.; Yang, Y.-W.; Ren, Q.-L.; Wu, P.-D. Simulated moving bed separation of tocopherol homologues: Simulation and experiments. *J. Zhejiang Univ. Sci. A* **2009**, *10*, 758–766. [CrossRef]
31. Oszmianski, J.; Sapis, J.C. Anthocyanins in fruits of *Aronia melanocarpa* (chokeberry). *J. Food Sci.* **1988**, *53*, 1241–1242. [CrossRef]
32. Wang, S.; Liang, Y.; Zheng, S. Separation of epigallocatechin gallate from tea polyphenol by simulated moving bed chromatography. *J. Chromatogr. A* **2012**, *1265*, 46–51. [CrossRef] [PubMed]
33. Meng, L.; Li, B.; Li, D.; Wang, Y.; Lin, Y.; Meng, X.; Sun, X.; Liu, N. Cyanidin-3-*O*-glucoside attenuates amyloid-beta (Aβ1-40)-induced oxidative stress and apoptosis in SH-SY5Y cells through a Nrf2 mechanism. *J. Funct. Foods* **2017**, *38*, 474–485. [CrossRef]
34. He, J.; Magnuson, B.A.; Giusti, M.M. Analysis of anthocyanins in rat intestinal contents–impact of anthocyanin chemical structure on fecal excretion. *J. Agric. Food Chem.* **2005**, *53*, 2859–2866. [CrossRef] [PubMed]
35. Miguel-Hidalgo, J.J.; Cacabelos, R. β-Amyloid (1–40)-induced neurodegeneration in the rat hippocampal neurons of the CA1 subfield. *Acta Neuropathol.* **1998**, *95*, 455–465. [CrossRef]
36. Miguel-Hidalgo, J.J.; Alvarez, X.A.; Cacabelos, R.; Quack, G. Neuroprotection by memantine against neurodegeneration induced by β-amyloid (1–40). *Brain Res.* **2002**, *958*, 210–221. [CrossRef]
37. Sarbishegi, M.; Heidari, Z.; Mahmoudzadeh-Sagheb, H.; Valizadeh, M.; Doostkami, M. Neuroprotective effects of Withania coagulans root extract on CA1 hippocampus following cerebral ischemia in rats. *Avicenna J. Phytomed.* **2016**, *6*, 399–409.

38. Sun, X.; Xu, H.; Meng, X.; Qi, J.; Cui, Y.; Li, Y.; Zhang, H.; Xu, L. Potential use of hyperoxygenated solution as a treatment strategy for carbon monoxide poisoning. *PLoS ONE* **2013**, *8*, e81779. [CrossRef]
39. Kim, M.J.; Rehman, S.U.; Amin, F.U.; Kim, M.O. Enhanced neuroprotection of anthocyanin-loaded PEG-gold nanoparticles against Aβ1-42-induced neuroinflammation and neurodegeneration via the NF-KB/JNK/GSK3β signaling pathway. *Nanomed. NBM* **2017**, *13*, 2533–2544. [CrossRef]

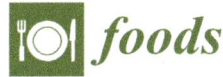 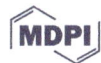

Article

Potential Hepatoprotective Activity of Super Critical Carbon Dioxide Olive Leaf Extracts against CCl$_4$-Induced Liver Damage

Amani Taamalli [1,2], Anouar Feriani [3], Jesús Lozano-Sanchez [4,5,*], Lakhdar Ghazouani [3], Afoua El Mufti [3], Mohamed Salah Allagui [6], Antonio Segura-Carretero [4,5], Ridha Mhamdi [2] and David Arráez-Roman [4,5]

- [1] Department of Chemistry, College of Sciences, University of Hafr Al Batin, P.O. Box 1803, Hafr Al Batin 39524, Saudi Arabia; ataamalli@uhb.edu.sa
- [2] Laboratoire de Biotechnologie de l'Olivier, Centre de Biotechnologie de Borj-Cedria, B.P.901, Hammam-Lif 2050, Tunisia; ridha.mhamdi@cbbc.rnrt.tn
- [3] Research Unit of Macromolecular Biochemistry and Genetics, Faculty of Sciences of Gafsa, Gafsa 2112, Tunisia; ferianianwer@yahoo.fr (A.F.); ghazouani2005@yahoo.fr (L.G.); mufti.afoua-90@hotmail.com (A.E.M.)
- [4] Research and Development Functional Food Centre (CIDAF), Health Science Technological Park, Avenida del Conocimiento 37, Edificio BioRegión, 18016 Granada, Spain; ansegura@ugr.es (A.S.-C.); darraez@ugr.es (D.A.-R.)
- [5] Department of Analytical Chemistry, Faculty of Sciences, University of Granada, 18071 Granada, Spain
- [6] Laboratory of Animal Ecophysiology, Faculty of Sciences of Sfax, Sfax 3018, Tunisia; amsallagui@yahoo.fr
- * Correspondence: jesusls@ugr.es

Received: 21 May 2020; Accepted: 16 June 2020; Published: 18 June 2020

Abstract: Virgin olive oil has demonstrated its effective activity against oxidative stress. However, data on the bioactive effect of olive leaves or their major constituents on the liver are scarce. The present research work was conducted to evaluate the hepatoprotective effects of supercritical carbon dioxide (SC-CO$_2$) extracts from fresh and dried olive leaves on hepatotoxicity caused by carbon tetrachloride (CCl$_4$) in rat models. For this purpose, healthy albino rats of 180–250 g weight were used. The assessment of biochemical markers was carried out on blood and liver tissue. Then, a histopathological study was carried out on liver tissue. The obtained results showed that fresh and dried olive leaf extracts ameliorate the perturbed biochemical parameters caused by CCl$_4$ treatment. Furthermore, the results registered for the histopathological study are in accordance with the biochemical parameters and the protective capacity of SC-CO$_2$ extracts against DNA damage, indicating that olive leaf extracts helped to improve liver fibrosis caused by CCl$_4$ treatment.

Keywords: olive leaves; supercritical fluid extraction; antioxidants

1. Introduction

Oxidative stress constitutes a disturbance characterized by an imbalance between the generation of free radicals and antioxidant defenses [1]. The reactive oxygen (ROS e.g., O2$^-$, OH, ROO) and nitrogen species (RNS, e.g., NO, ONOO$^-$) are generated in a variety of intracellular processes and their overproduction produces cell damage in lipids, proteins and DNA [2].

The liver is the largest organ in the vertebrate body and the site for intense metabolism [3]. It is involved in several vital functions and it has a great capacity to detoxify toxic substances and synthesize useful principles. Therefore damage to the liver inflicted by hepatotoxic substances is of grave consequences [4]. The hepatotoxin CCl$_4$ has been used as a model component causing cellular necrosis in the liver. It induces hepatotoxicity in rats, rabbits and humans [5] and mediates its hepatotoxicity after biotransformation by hepatic microsomal cytochrome 450 (CYT 450) to generate trichloromethyl free radicals which launch attacks on membrane proteins, thiols and lipids. This leads to the peroxidation of the lipid membrane which results in necrotic cell death [6]. To prevent such disease, both enzymatic and non-enzymatic mechanisms are present in the cell [7]. The body protects itself from oxygen free radical toxicity by enzymatic antioxidant mechanisms (e.g., glutathione peroxidase, GSH; glutathione reductase, GR; superoxide dismutase, SOD; and catalase, CAT) and by non-enzymatic antioxidants (e.g., vitamins, uric acid, albumin, bilirubin, and many others) [8].

Liver pathologies constitute a serious global health issue despite recent therapeutic advances. Nevertheless, some plants have been used for liver disorders and showed to be therapeutically useful agents [5]. Diverse plant extracts were assessed for their hepatoprotective effect against different experimentally induced liver toxicities [9–15].

From the large diversity of the plant components, special importance has been assigned to their polyphenols, which have shown their capacity to counteract oxidative stress through various mechanisms [16]. An interesting approach used to obtain such compounds is to source them from food industry residues, which are in general disposed of or used to produce animal feed [17]. The olive tree (*Olea europaea*, L.), amongst the oldest known cultivated trees in the world and mentioned in the Holy Qur'ân and Ahadith [18], has been known for its long history of medicinal and nutritional values. Historically, olive leaves were used as a folk remedy for combating fevers and other diseases, such as malaria. Numerous researchers showed the important role of this plant in improving cardiovascular risk factors [19], cancer [20] and other diseases. A recent publication reviewed the relevant role of phenolic compounds present in *Olea europaea*, L. products and by-products in human health [21], while another review focused on the potential protective effect of secoiridoids from *Olea europaea* L. in cancer, cardiovascular, neurodegenerative, aging-related, and immune-inflammatory diseases [20].

Olive leaves constitute a huge abundant residue resulting from olive tree pruning and olive oil processing. It has been estimated that olive pruning produces 25 kg of olive leaves and twigs per tree annually. In addition these by-products present, only about 10% of olives actually arrive at the mills [22]. All of this makes olive leaves a very interesting, cheap source with potentially useful bioactive components such as secoiridoids, triterpenes, lignans, and flavonoids [23]. Oleuropein and hydroxytyrosol, as major compounds of olive leaves, have been reported to exert numerous pharmacological properties, including anticancer, antidiabetic, and anti-inflammatory activities [14]. Recently, the hepatoprotective activity of olive leaves against damage induced by CCl_4 [24,25], cadmium [26,27], paracetamol [28], thioacetamide [29], ethanol [5], fluoxetine [30] and deltamethrin [31] has receieved increasing interest in animal experiemts. However, available data about the hepatoprotective effect of olive leaf extracts or their major constituents are still scarce. Hence, there is not enough literature about the hepatoprotective effect of olive leaves against CCl_4 induced damage. The existing published articles focused on methanolic or butanolic extracts of dried olive leaves obtained by Soxhlet apparatus [24] and ethanolic extract from dried olive leaves standardized to 16–24% of oleuropein [25]. As far we know, this is the first study on the hepatoprotective effect of Tunisian olive leaves on CCl_4-induced toxicity.

Nowadays, supercritical fluid extraction (SFE), an environmentally friendly and selective technique, has become one of the most popular green extraction techniques [32] used mainly in large-scale industrial applications. This technique has several advantages such as high efficacy, rapidity, non-toxicity, the absence of thermal degradation resulting a very high quality extracts, and the possible direct coupling to analytical instrumental technique [33] with a particular green interest due to the use of supercritical fluids such as CO_2 instead organic solvents [34]. It has been increasingly used in recent years around the world for the processing of nutraceuticals as a "natural" alternative to traditional solvent-extraction processes [35]. It has acquired some relevance for the extraction of polyphenols from plant sources [36]. No previous literature reported the evaluation of olive leaf supercritical fluid extract for its hepatoprotective activity. In our present work, we used fresh and dried leaves from which extracts were obtained using a green advanced extraction technology.

Taking into account all these aspects, this study aimed to assess and compare the hepatoprotective capacity of supercritical carbon dioxide (SC-CO_2) extracts of fresh and dried olive leaves in CCl_4-induced toxicity in rat models. For this purpose, serum biochemical parameters alanine aminotransferase (ALT), aspartate aminotransferase (AST), alcaline phosphatase (ALP and lactate dehydrogenase (LDH)), liver tissue parameters malondialdehyde (MDA), protein carbonyls (PC), total superoxide dismutase (SOD), catalase (CAT) and glutathione peroxydase (GPX) in addition to histopathological and DNA damage assays were evaluated. As far as we know, this is the first evaluation of the hepatoprotective activity of (SC-CO_2) extracts from fresh and dried olive leaves acquired via green technology. Moreover, no available literature evaluated the effect of olive leaf extracts containing phenolic compounds and triterpenoid on induced hepatotoxicity in rats.

2. Materials and Methods

2.1. Plant Material, Supercritical CO_2 Extraction and Chemical Characterization

Olive leaves from the El Hor olive variety cultivated in Kairouan (center of Tunisia) were collected in January 2018 (voucher code OE00182). The cultivar was identified by Pr. Mokhtar Zarrouk. Dried leaves were kept under shade at 25 °C and fresh leaves were ground using an Ultra Centrifugal Mill ZM 200 (RetschGmbH, Haan, Germany). Extraction of phytochemicals was carried out according to a previously reported method [37]. Briefly, 10 g of ground leaves were homogenized with sea sand in a ratio 1:1.5 (m/m), loaded onto the extraction vessel, packed with glass wool and pressurized until working conditions. Extractions were carried out at 150 bar and 40 °C using a mixture of CO_2 and ethanol (6.6%) as the extraction solvent which passed through the extraction cell for one hour at 23 g/min. The obtained extract was finally collected and the solvent was evaporated under vacuum at 38 °C. The extraction yields were 9.3% and 16.7% for fresh and dried leaves, respectively.

Olive leaf extracts were analyzed for their phenolic and triterpenoids composition by high performance liquid chromatography coupled to electrospray ionization and time of flight mass spectrometry (HPLC-ESI-TOF/MS). To achieve this goal, SFE extracts were reconstituted in an extraction co-solvent up to a concentration of 5000 mg/L and filtered through a 0.2 µm polytetrafluoroethylene (PTFE) syringe filter prior to further analysis. Qualitative and quantitative determination of both phenolic compounds and terpenoids were carried out according to the previously reported method [38]. Quantitation was carried out using available commercial standards of six phenolics and two terpenoids: hydroxytyrosol, vanillin, luteolin, ferulic acid, (+)-pinoresinol, oleuropein, oleanolic, and maslinic acids. These standards were purchased from Sigma–Aldrich (St. Louis, MO, USA), Arbo Nova (Turku, Finland), and Extrasynthèse (Lyon, France). The stock solutions containing these analytes were prepared by dissolving the appropriate amount in methanol or methanol/water (50/50, v/v) at a concentration level of 1 mg/L. All calibration curves showed good linearity over the range of study with a minimum value of $R^2 = 0.994$.

2.2. Experimental Animals and Toxicity Test

Healthy adult male albino rats weighing 180–250 g were used. The animals were provided from Pasteur institute and housed in a plastic cage under controlled temperature (24 ± 2 °C), 12 h light/dark cycle and 55 ± 5% relative humidity. The animals were guarded in the laboratory (Faculty of Sciences, Gafsa, Tunisia) for seven days before experiences with free access to standard laboratory food (SNA –Sfax) and water ad libitum. Animals were treated in accordance with guidelines and according to the Medical Ethics Committee for the Care and Use of Laboratory Animals of the Pasteur Institute of Tunis, Tunisia (approval number: FST/LNFP/Pro 152012).

The toxicity of SC-CO_2 extracts of fresh leaves and dried leaves mixed with corn oil was tested by gavage administration of four doses at 5, 10, 20 and 30 mg/kg body weight (b.w.). Animals ($n = 6$ in each group) were carefully controlled for progress of any toxicological symptoms at 30 min and then 4, 12, 24 and 48 h.

2.3. Animals and Experimental Design of the CCl$_4$-Induced Hepatotoxicity

To test the potential hepatoprotective effects of olive leaf extracts, experiments were conducted in six groups according to the following administration (Scheme 1): group I—negative control with administration of vehicle only (corn oil); group II—administration of carbon tetrachloride (CCl$_4$) in corn oil 50 µL/kg [39]; group III—daily administration of fresh leaf extracts dissolved in corn oil (FLE, 30 mg/kg); group IV—daily administration of dried leaf extracts dissolved in corn oil (DLE, 30 mg/kg); group V—administration of FLE (30 mg/kg) and simultaneous treatment with CCl$_4$ (50 µL/kg) +; group VI—administration of DLE (30 mg/kg) and simultaneous treatment with CCl$_4$ (50 µL/kg).

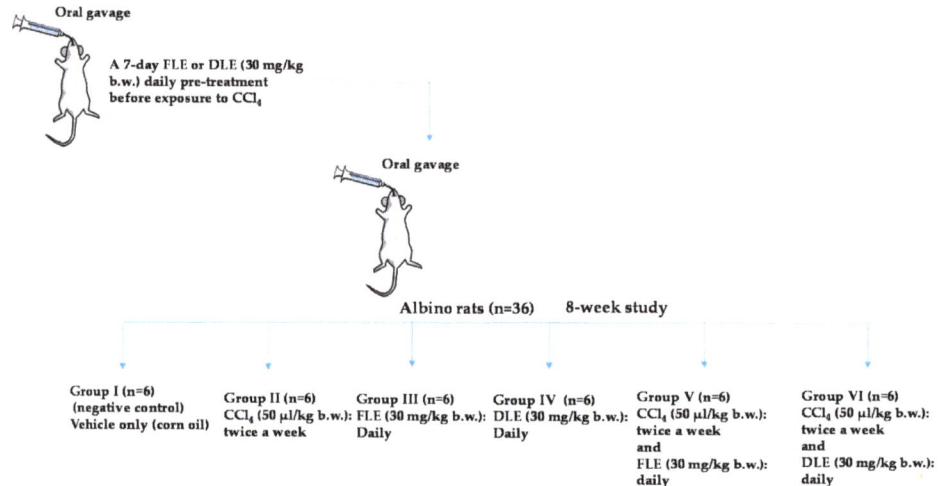

Scheme 1. Graphical scheme summarizing the experimental design, n: number of rats.

The CCl$_4$ was administered by gastric gavage twice per week (on every Tuesday and Thursday) over eight weeks. A daily pretreatment with FLE or DLE was realized 7 days before CCl$_4$ exposure and then daily throughout the research work by gastric gavage. The rats were sacrificed at the end of eight weeks and 24 h after the last dose of the hepatotoxin.

2.4. Analysis of Liver-Damage Serum Markers

Blood samples were obtained by cardiac puncture. After coagulation, the samples were centrifuged at 3000× g for 10 min and serum was stored at −20 °C for further analysis. Levels of alanine aminotransferase, aspartate aminotransferase, alcaline phosphatase and lactate dehydrogenase were determined by spectrophotometric assays according to the commercially available diagnostic kits (Biomaghreb, Ariana, Tunisia).

2.5. Biological Determination of Liver Tissue

2.5.1. Preparation of Tissue Extracts

The liver tissues were homogenized into 2 mL of ice-cold lyses buffer (pH = 7.4) using a grinder (homogenizer ultra-turrax). Then, the homogenate was centrifuged (12,000 rpm, 4 °C) for 15 min. The obtained supernatant was frozen at −20 °C to determine the oxidative stress biomarkers: malondialdehyde (MDA), protein carbonyls (PC), SOD, CAT and GPX.

2.5.2. Measurement of Lipid Peroxidation and Protein Oxidation in Hepatic Tissue

The lipid peroxidation was estimated in control and treated rats by the quantification of thiobarbituric acid-reactive substances (TBARS) using the method described previously [24]. Briefly, the solution containing 100 µL of liver tissue extract and 100 µL of trichloroacetic acid (TCA, 5%) was centrifuged at 4000× g for 10 min. Then, in a boiling water bath, 100 µL of the supernatant was incubated with 200 µL of thiobarbituric acid reagent (TBA, 0.67%) for 15 min. The absorbance was read at 530 nm, the degree of lipid peroxidation was measured as thiobarbituric acid reactive substances (TBARS) and the result was expressed as nmol of MDA equivalents per gram of tissue (nmol MDA equivalents/g tissue).

The protein carbonyl (PC) level was determined using the method described in the literature [40]. In this method, the carbonyl group of proteins was measured in the resulting pellets by reaction with 2,4-dinitrophenylhydrazine to form protein hydrazone which was measured spectrophotometrically at 370 nm.

2.5.3. Determination of Enzymatic Antioxidants Activities

Total SOD activity, expressed as units per milligram of protein, was determined by measuring the inhibition of pyrogallol activity [41]. One unit (U) corresponded to the enzyme activity necessary to inhibit the oxidation of half of the pyrogallol.

Catalase activity was determined in tissue supernatants using hydrogen peroxide (H_2O_2) as substrate according to the literature [42]. H_2O_2 degradation was accompanied by a decrease in absorbance and it was confirmed by measuring the absorbance at 240 nm for 1 min, and the enzyme activity was expressed as mmol H_2O_2 consumed per minute per milligram of protein.

Glutathione peroxidase activity was assayed by the subsequent oxidation of NADPH at 340 nm, using the method described by Flohé and Günzler [43], and the results were expressed as nmol of GSH oxidized per minute per milligram of protein.

Finally, protein concentration in liver homogenates was measured by the Bradford technique ((BCA) Protein Assay Kit, Pierce Biotechnology Inc., Rockford, USA) with bovine serum albumin (BSA) as standard.

2.6. Histopathological Study

The liver samples of the rats were fixed in 10% buffered formalin. After fixation, the tissues were dehydrated in a graded series of alcohol, cleared in xylene, embedded in paraffin, and cut into 5 µm thick slices. These serial tissue sections were stained with hematoxylin and eosin (HE) for routine histological examination. Sirius Red and Masson's trichrome staining were used to visualize the collagen deposit in hepatic tissue, which was coloured blue using Masson's trichrome and red by Sirius Red staining. The specimens were observed and photographed through a light microscope (Olympus CX31, Hamburg, Germany).

2.7. DNA Fragmentation Assay

Genomic DNA in the liver tissue of control and treated rats was isolated by phenol–chloroform DNA extraction method. The separation of intact and fragmented DNA fractions was visualized in an agarose gel by ethidium bromide staining, following the protocol described in the literature [44].

2.8. Statistical Analysis

Statistical analysis was performed using GraphPad Prism 4.02 (GraphPad Software, San Diego, CA, USA). One-way analysis of variance (ANOVA) together with Tukey test were applied to observe significant differences between the tested treatments at a significance level ($p < 0.05$).

3. Results

3.1. Identification of Phenolic and Triterpenoid Composition in SC-CO_2 Olive Leaf Extracts

In Table 1 are summarized the different compounds detected in both FLE and DLE. The analysis of the extract composition permitted the chemical characterization of 16 compounds. Quantitative results showed in this table include the amount of each identified compound in the administered dose to evaluate the hepatoprotective effects.

Table 1. Identified and quantified phytochemicals in the SC-CO_2 olive leaf extracts.

m/z [M − H]⁻	Molecular Formula	Compound	FLE	DLE	Classification
389.1089	$C_{16}H_{22}O_{11}$	Secologanoside	-	0.15 ± 0.2	Phenolic compound
153.0557	$C_8H_{10}O_3$	Hydroxytyrosol	-	19 ± 1	Phenolic compound
403.1246	$C_{17}H_{24}O_{11}$	Elenolic acid glucoside isomer 1	-	0.05 ± 0.01	Phenolic compound
151.0401	$C_8H_8O_3$	Vanillin	3 ± 0.3	13.0 ± 0.4	Phenolic compound
403.1246	$C_{17}H_{24}O_{11}$	Elenolic acid glucoside isomer 2	-	0.70 ± 0.01	Phenolic compound
193.0506	$C_{10}H_{10}O_4$	Ferulic acid	-	0.40 ± 0.01	Phenolic compound
539.177	$C_{25}H_{32}O_{13}$	Oleuropein isomer 1	-	42 ± 1	Phenolic compound
539.177	$C_{25}H_{32}O_{13}$	Oleuropein isomer 2	-	1.10 ± 0.01	Phenolic compound
417.1555	$C_{22}H_{26}O_8$	Syringaresinol	2.4 ± 0.1	-	Phenolic compound
357.1344	$C_{20}H_{22}O_6$	Pinoresinol	1.1 ± 0.3	0.8 ± 0.2	Phenolic compound
415.1398	$C_{22}H_{24}O_8$	Acetoxypinoresinol	37 ± 1	1 ± 0.1	Phenolic compound
299.0561	$C_{16}H_{12}O_6$	Diosmetin	2 ± 0.2	0.040 ± 0.002	Phenolic compound
471.348	$C_{30}H_{48}O_4$	Maslinic acid	935 ± 7	-	Triterpenoid
455.3531	$C_{30}H_{48}O_3$	Oleanolic acid	1902 ± 8	867 ± 6	Triterpenoid
455.3531	$C_{30}H_{48}O_3$	Ursolic acid	1539 ± 11	1479 ± 7	Triterpenoid
401.1453	$C_{18}H_{26}O_{10}$	Benzyl alcohol pentose	-	0.05 ± 0.00	Other polar compound

Value = X ± SD (μg of compound per 30 mg of extract), not detected (-).

A clear qualitative and quantitative difference was observed between fresh and dried leaves. In fresh leaves only vanillin, lignans (pinoresinol and acetoxypinoresinol), diosmetin and triterpenoids (maslinic, ursolic and oleanolic acids) were detected. This could be related to the impact of drying on the quality and the composition of olive leaf extract. Regarding the administered dose, acetoxypinoresinol was the major phenolic compound and constituted 37 μg in FLE, whereas in DLE, oleuropein formed the major phenolic compound (42 μg) followed by hydroxytyrosol (19 μg). Regarding triterpenoids, ursolic acid was the major compound in both extracts, being higher in fresh olive leaf extract.

3.2. Biochemical Measurements

3.2.1. Effect on Plasma Biochemical Markers

Table 2 summarizes the impact of the hepatotoxin and olive leaf extract administration on liver function tests. Compared to the control group, the ALT, AST, ALP and LDH activities in serum of rats treated with CCl_4 increased significantly ($p < 0.001$) after eight weeks reaching 336, 417, 231 and 261 U/L, respectively, indicating acute hepatocellular damage (Table 2). Nevertheless, the oral administration of olive leaf extracts (dose of 30 mg/kg b.w.) during intoxication showed a significant decrease in AST, ALT, ALP and LDH activities compared to CCl_4 only-treated rats.

Table 2. Effect of CCl_4, FLE and DLE administration on hepatic biochemical markers.

	AST (U/L)	ALT (U/L)	ALP (U/L)	LDH (U/L)
Control	355 ± 8	285 ± 4	161 ± 5	205 ± 5
CCl_4	417± 4 ***	336 ± 9 ***	231.9± 0.8 ***	261 ± 5 ***
FLE	371 ± 4	276 ± 2	171 ± 4	199 ± 8
CCl_4 + FLE	402 ± 3 [+]	308 ± 9 [++]	207 ± 2 [++]	240 ± 5 [++]
DLE	354 ± 5	281 ± 6	158 ± 9	207 ± 7
CCl_4 + DLE	389 ± 4 [+++]	316 ± 3 [+]	211 ± 3 [+]	242 ± 4 [+]

AST: aspartate aminotransferase; ALT: alanine aminotransferase; ALP: alkaline, phosphatase and LDH: lactate dehydrogenase. Values are expressed as mean ± SD of six rats in each group. CCl_4 group versus control group: ** $p < 0.01$; *** $p < 0.001$. CCl_4 + FLE or CCl_4 + DLE group versus CCl_4 group: [+] $p < 0.05$; [++] $p < 0.01$; [+++] $p < 0.001$.

The observed decrease was more pronounced in terms of AST activity when DLE was administered (389 U/L, $p < 0.001$) during CCl_4 toxicity. Contrastingly, FLE administration in intoxicated rats caused a slightly more important decrease than with DLE administration in terms of ALT, ALP and LDH activities (Table 1).

3.2.2. Lipid Peroxidation and Protein Carbonyls

The effect on lipid peroxidation and protein carbonyls contents are summarized in Table 3. For CCl_4-intoxicated rats, the TBARS level increased significantly (4.6 nmol MDA equivalents/g tissue) when compared with the control group (1.13 nmol MDA equivalents/g of tissue). Nevertheless, treatment with olive leaf extracts significantly reduced the lipid peroxidation level in CCl_4-treated rats to 2.9 nmol MDA equivalents/g tissue in the case of FLE + CCl_4 and 2.7 nmol MDA equivalents/g of tissue in the case of DLE + CCl_4.

Likewise, protein carbonyl amounts significantly increased (*** $p < 0.001$) further CCl_4 intoxication (2.7 nmol/mg protein) in comparison to the control group (1 nmol/mg protein). However, FLE pretreatment of intoxicated rats showed a more pronounced effect than DLE pretreatment when compared to intoxicated rats (1.6 nmol/mg protein) with values of 1.0, 2.7 and 2.03 nmol/mg protein for control, CCl_4 and DLE+ CCl_4 treatment, respectively.

A significant increase (** $p < 0.01$) was registered in terms of SOD, CAT and GPx activities among those in the CCl_4-treated group (141 U/mg protein, 136 µmol of H_2O_2 destroyed/min per mg protein and 100 nmol of NADPH oxidized/min per mg protein, respectively) when compared to the control group (89 U/mg protein, 109 µmol of H_2O_2 destroyed/min per mg protein and 83 nmol of NADPH oxidized/min per mg protein, respectively). In contrast, SOD, CAT and GPx activities significantly decreased ($p < 0.05$) in intoxicated rats pretreated with DLE or FLE when compared to the rats who received only CCl_4 (Table 3).

Table 3. Effect of CCl$_4$, FLE and DLE on liver oxidative stress.

	TBARS (nmol MDA Equivalents/g Tissue)	PC (nmol/mg Protein)	SOD (U/mg Protein)	CAT (μmol of H$_2$O$_2$ Destroyed/min per mg Protein)	GPx (nmol of NADPH Oxidized/min per mg Protein)
Control	1.13 ± 0.2	1.0 ± 0.1	89 ± 3	109 ± 8	83 ± 3
CCl$_4$	4.6 ± 0.3 ***	2.7 ± 0.3 ***	141 ± 9 ***	136 ± 6 **	100 ± 4 **
FLE	1.4 ± 0.4	0.9 ± 0.2	78 ± 4	98 ± 4	73 ± 4
CCl$_4$ + FLE	2.9 ± 0.7 $^+$	1.6 ± 0.1 $^{+++}$	125 ± 3 $^+$	119 ± 4 $^+$	81 ± 1 $^{++}$
DLE	1.0 ± 0.7	1.1 ± 0.2	87 ± 2	98 ± 9	74 ± 7
CCl$_4$ + DLE	2.7 ± 0.4 $^{++}$	2.03 ± 0.05 $^{++}$	123 ± 5 $^{++}$	120 ± 1 $^+$	87 ± 5 $^+$

Values are expressed as mean ± SD of six rats in each group. CCl$_4$ group versus control group: ** $p < 0.01$; *** $p < 0.001$. CCl$_4$ + FLE or CCl$_4$ + DLE group versus CCl$_4$ group: $^+$ $p < 0.05$; $^{++}$ $p < 0.01$; $^{+++}$ $p < 0.001$.

3.2.3. Evaluation of Enzymatic Antioxidant Activities

Table 3 also shows the effects of olive leaf extracts on the antioxidant enzymes. It is noteworthy to say that CCl_4 caused a significant increase in SOD, CAT and GPx activities (141 U/mg protein, 136 µmol of H_2O_2 destroyed/min per mg protein and 100 nmol of NADPH oxidized/min per mg protein, for SOD, CAT and GPx, respectively) when compared to the control group (89 U/mg protein, 109 U/mg protein and 83 U/mg protein, for SOD, CAT and GPx, respectively). Contrastingly, olive leaf extract administration caused a significant decrease in the activity of such enzymes when compared to CCl_4-treated animals, resulting in levels close to those of the control group, especially for GPx activity (81 and 87 nmol of NADPH oxidized/min per mg protein, respectively, in comparison to the control rats with 83 nmol of NADPH oxidized/min per mg protein).

3.3. Histopathological Examinations

3.3.1. Hematoxylin and Eosin (HE) Staining

(HE) staining of hepatic tissues of control and all treated rats are demonstrated in Figure 1. As it can be observed, the figure shows the hepatoprotective effect of FLE and DLE after CCl_4 hepatotoxin administration.

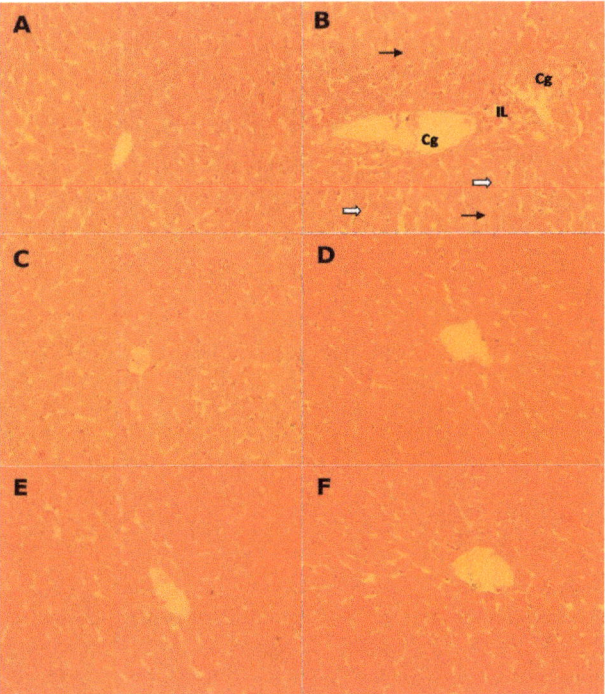

Figure 1. Pathological histology analysis in rat liver tissues after HE staining (magnification: 200×): (**A**) controls, (**B**) CCl_4-treated (CCl_4); (**C**) FLE-treated (FLE), and (**D**) CCl_4-treated co-treated with FLE (CCl_4 + FLE). (**E**) DLE-treated (DLE), and (**F**) CCl_4-treated cotreated with DLE (CCl_4 + DLE). Each microphotograph shows a section of an individual liver. Extensive focal necrosis (⇨), a moderate Kupffer cell hyperplasia (→), congestion and dilatation of the central vein (Cg) and leukocyte infiltration (LI).

The control rats' hepatic sections revealed a normal form of hepatic cells; polyhedral hepatocytes and sinusoids boundaries exhibited a single layer of fenestrated endothelial and Kupffer cells (Figure 1A). FLE and DLE alone had no significant effects on liver histology (Figure 1C,E) whilst hepatoxin administration resulted in cells injury (Figure 1B). This was marked by extensive focal necrosis, a moderate Kupffer cell hyperplasia, congestion and dilatation of the central vein, and leukocyte infiltration. Finally, following the administration of CCl_4 + FLE or CCl_4 + DLE, focal neutrophils were infiltrated in some space and a number of centrilobular veins were congested (Figure 1D,F).

3.3.2. Sirius Red and Masson's Trichrome Staining

Sirius Red and Masson's trichrome staining of hepatic cells are shown in Figures 2 and 3.

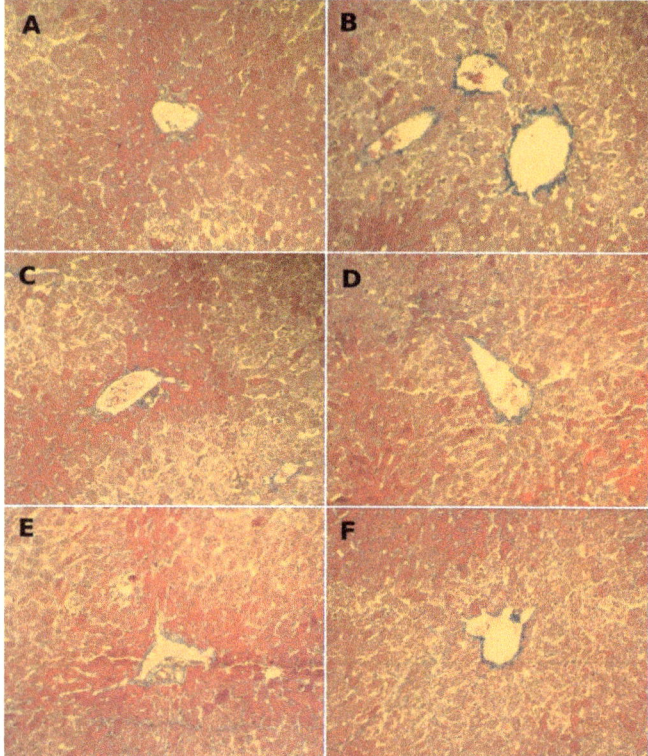

Figure 2. Effect of FLE and DLE on hepatic connective tissue fibrosis caused by CCl_4 treatment: assessment by Masson's trichrome stain (G × 200). (**A**) Control, (**B**) CCl_4-treated, blue-stained zone indicates increasing fibrosis. (**C**) FLE-treated (30 mg/kg), and (**D**) co-treated with CCl_4 and FLE (30 mg/kg); (**E**) DLE-treated (30 mg/kg) showing normal structure and (**F**) co-treated with CCl_4 and DLE (30 mg/kg) showing results close to the control.

Microscopic observations of the hepatic tissues of control group (Figure 2A) and those of groups pretreated with FLE and DLE (Figures 2 and 3C,E) show a normal distribution of collagen fibers between the portal spaces and the centrilobular vein manifested by a low red and blue color. After treatment with CCl_4 (Figures 2 and 3B), fibrous collagen bridges (shown by the intense red and blue stains) were formed between portal spaces and the centrilobular, marking hepatic fibrosis.

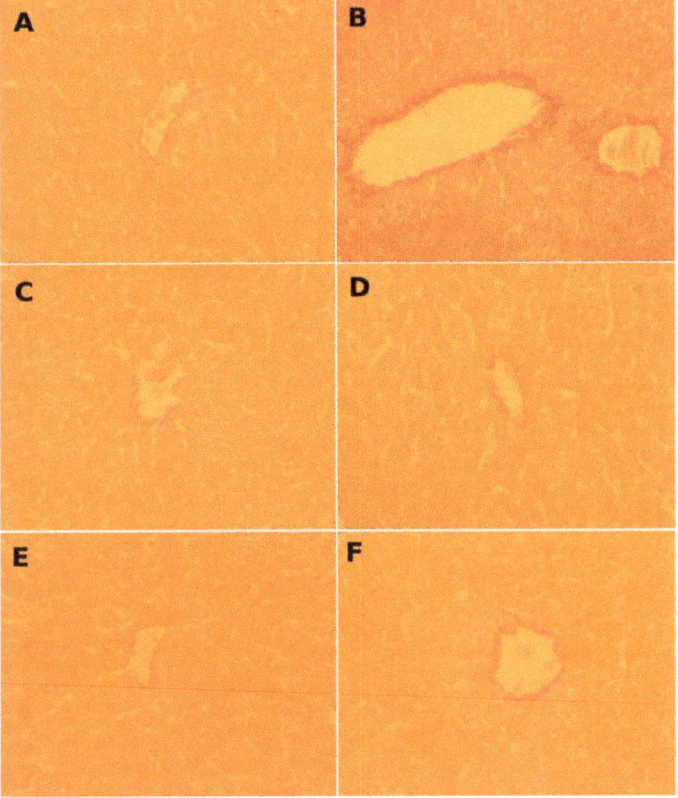

Figure 3. Micrograph showing the effect of FLE and DLE on hepatic fibrosis caused by CCl_4. Assessment by Sirius red stain (G × 200). (**A**) Control, (**B**) CCl_4-treated, showing intensified red stain. (**C**) FLE-treated (30 mg/kg), and (**D**) co-treated with CCl_4 and FLE (30 mg/kg). (**E**) DLE-treated (30 mg/kg) showing normal collagen deposition and (**F**) co-treated with CCl_4 and DLE (30 mg/kg).

Concerning the association with FLE and DLE, the study revealed that these extracts exerted a protective effect against CCl_4-induced hepatic fibrotic scarring, observed through the decreasing red and blue staining when compared to that of control (Figures 2 and 3D,F).

3.4. Effects of Olive Leaf Extracts on the DNA Fragmentation

As shown in Figure 4, the DNA extracted from the hepatic sections has changed qualitatively. The control group DNA (lane 1) and that of FLE or DLE-treated groups (lanes 3 and 4) showed an intact band. However, we observed that DNA degraded after treatment with the CCl_4 (lane 2 and lane 6), marked by an obvious smearing and laddering which indicates apoptosis. In the FLE + CCl_4 and DLE+ CCl_4 rats (lane 5 and lane 7), the olive leaf extract addition shows its effect on preventing DNA damage and provides results close to those of the control rats, as observed in Figure 4.

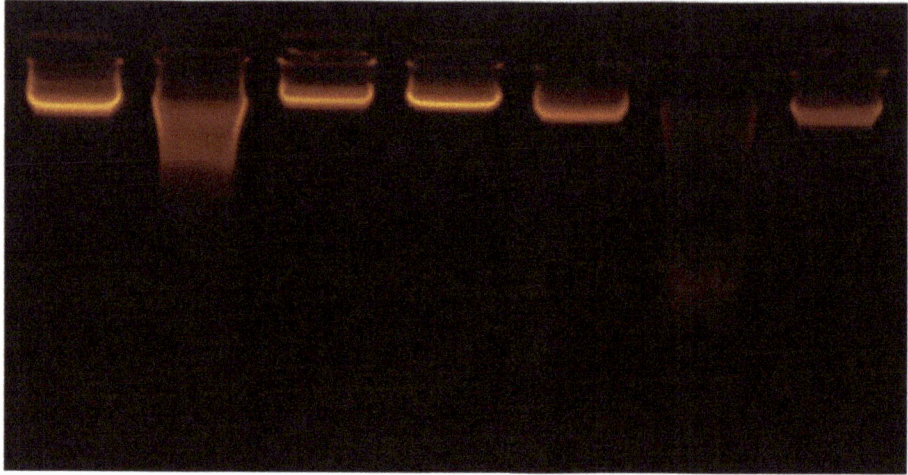

Figure 4. Agarose gel electrophoresis of DNA fragmentation. Lane 1: control hepatic tissue DNA; lane 2 and lane 6: CCl_4 intoxicated liver DNA, lane 3 and lane 4: FLE- or DLE-treated liver DNA; lane 5 and lane 7: FLE + CCl_4- or DLE + CCl_4- treated liver DNA.

4. Discussion

Despite recent therapeutic advances, many liver diseases remain relentlessly progressive because specific therapies to target the underlying etiologies of the liver diseases are not available. Therefore, the demand for liver transplantation is likely to increase unless more effective therapeutic and anti-fibrotic agents are developed [45].

In this research work, healthy adult male albino rats were used as an experimental model for the evaluation of olive leaf extracts on induced hepatotoxicity. Among the known hepatotoxic agents, CCl_4 is the best model of oxidative stress-induced liver damage and is commonly used to assay the hepatoprotective capacity of drugs [46].

The obtained results revealed that the oral gavage of SC-CO_2 olive leaf extracts effectively attenuated the CCl_4-induced hepatic damage and fibrotic scarring in rats. The hepatotoxin-caused injury was marked through the antioxidant enzyme markers' determination in the study of hepatic tissues and DNA. The results obtained in our current study are in accordance with those reported in previous works related to the impact of CCl_4 on the liver [39,46–51].

CCl_4 is reported to produce free radicals, which affect the cellular permeability of hepatocytes, subsequently leading to elevated levels of serum biochemical parameters such as ALT, AST and ALP [51]. This marks a damaged structural and functional integrity of the liver cell membranes, since these cytosolic enzymes are only released into circulation after hepatic cellular damage. An increase in ALT enzyme activity is almost always due to hepatocellular damage and is usually accompanied by an increase in AST and ALP. Oral administration of both fresh and dried olive leaf extracts produced a significant decrease in serum ALT, AST and ALP levels in CCl_4-induced rats, pointing to their hepatoprotective effect. The reduced concentrations of these markers as a result of olive leaf extract administration observed during the present study might be due to the presence of bioactive compounds such as phenolic and triterpenoid compounds; although, there is a difference observed between fresh and dried leaf extracts (Table 1). As in the present study, previous research works on olive leaf extracts showed that CCl_4 caused significant elevation of ALT, AST, ALP activities, while pretreatment with olive leaf extracts significantly suppresses the increase in their levels [24,25]. It has been reported that effective hepatoprotective agents must suppress the increase in ALT activity and bring it closer to a normal level in order to induce liver-healing. This would suggest that agents that can lower ALP levels may be useful in hepatoprotection [9].

The fluidity of the biological membrane as well as some enzyme activities can be affected by lipid peroxidation [36]. In our research work, we observed how treatment with FLE and DLE extracts significantly reduced lipid peroxidation level in CCl_4 treated rats, which suggests that the lipid-oxidation inhibition was exerted by the $SC-CO_2$ olive leaf extracts. The generated toxic radicals could be masked through the antioxidants present in the extracts. Amongst the reactive species marker of oxidative stress in cells, we find the highly reactive compound MDA [6]. An increase in MDA levels in tissue sections as a result of CCl_4 treatment signifies that lipid oxidation has increased, which subsequently causes tissue injury and the intrinsic cell system failure to eliminate exogenous hepatotoxin agents. In our study, the treatment with $SC-CO_2$ olive leaf extracts showed a significant reduction in lipid peroxidation levels in CCl_4-treated rats, demonstrating the capacity of the extracts to reduce such severe alterations. The same behavior was observed for the elevated level of protein carbonyl groups considered as an indicator of protein oxidation. Our results are in agreement with those reported in the literature. In fact, when investigating the protective activity of dried olive leaf extract on CCl_4-induced liver damage in rats, the researchers reported that the concentration of MDA significantly increased in rats administered CCl_4 when compared to the control group [25]. A similar observation for increasing MDA levels was reported in another study [24] after which a significant decrease was registered in pretreated rats with (methanolic or butanolic) olive leaf extracts in comparison to CCl_4-treated rats. Moreover, ethanolic olive leaf extract produced a significant decrease in lipid peroxidation levels in the liver of rats with fluoxetine-induced hepatotoxicity [30].

GPx is an enzyme with peroxidase activity which assures the protection from oxidative damage [9]. GPx catalyzes the reduction in H_2O_2 or organic peroxide to water or alcohol [52]. Other important antioxidant enzymes are SOD and CAT. SOD is a key enzyme with the ability to convert superoxide radicals into hydrogen peroxide and molecular oxygen, while CAT enhances the conversion of H_2O_2 to water and molecular oxygen.

In this study, high activities of GPx, SOD and CAT were observed following CCl_4 intoxication. Similar observation for SOD was reported in another research on the hepatoprotective effect of extracts of *Cnestis ferruginea* against CCl_4-induced toxicity [46]. High antioxidant enzyme activities of tissues and organs do not mean efficient protective potential against oxidative stress caused by CCl_4 intoxication. It was found that antioxidant enzyme mRNA expression and enzyme activity were induced by the exposure of hepatocytes to hydrogen peroxide for 24 h [53]. Thus, the increase in CAT, SOD, and GPx activities observed in the liver are probably partly due to the elevated hydrogen peroxide content generated during the metabolism of CCl_4 in the body, which lead to up-regulation of gene expression of antioxidant enzyme mRNA and consequently induced an increase in their activities in the liver tissue [54]. The elevated catalase and GPX activities in liver tissue may indicate a large increase in hydrogen peroxide; however, we cannot state to what degree the process of hydrogen peroxide removal is effective [55].

Additionally, the pretreatment of CCl_4-intoxicated rats with FLE or DLE showed a marked decrease in the activities of antioxidant enzymes compared to the CCl_4-only group. The protective effect of the extracts in CCl_4-treated rats is manifested by their capacity to maintain the redox balance marked by the levels of antioxidant enzymes that changed to a figure close to that registered for the control group [9].

Histopathological studies also support the biochemical analysis. The liver histology was improved after co-treatment with $SC-CO_2$ extracts in comparison to the CCl_4 only-treated group, suggesting the hepatoprotective capacity of tested extracts against tissue fibrosis. Olive leaves exerted a significant protective effect against CCl_4-induced liver damage as marked by the improvement of serum oxidative stress biomarkers and the histology of tissue sections.

The results also showed that CCl_4 administration could induce hepatic fibrosis detected by Sirius Red and Masson's Trichrome staining, as manifested by excessive collagen deposition in the hepatic tissue. These findings were in line with other studies showing that CCl_4 is able to induce liver fibrosis [56]. The fibrosis status could be related to the activation of hepatic stellate cells (HSCs) as a result of elevated levels of a variety of inflammatory cytokines induced by CCl_4 intoxication, as reported in previous studies [57].

Administering FLE or DLE along with CCl_4 significantly reduced liver fibrosis. These data support the efficacy of FLE or DLE in reducing the hepatocellular toxic effects of CCl_4 and in suppressing the activation and proliferation of HSCs. This positive effect could be due to inflammation reduction. These findings are in line with recent studies that indicate that herbal bioactive molecules are effective against fibrosis in hepatic tissues [58,59].

Despite that significant effect observed for both DLE and FLE extracts, the different composition of tested extracts highlights the importance of phenolic compounds from different classes and triterpenoids as bioactive compounds. Concerning chemical differences related to phenolic compounds, it has to be taken into account that the DLE extract was characterized by the presence of high quantities of hydroxytyrosol and oleuropein isomer. Evaluating the hepatoprotective effect of oleuropein purified from olive leaves, it was found that its administration during ethanol-induced toxicity in rats improves the antioxidant defense system and reduces the levels of lipid peroxides [5]. In another study, oleuropein- and hydroxytyrosol-rich olive leaf extracts revealed hepatoprotective effects against high-fat diet-induced metabolic disorders in rats [14]. With regard to triterpenoids, maslinic acid was only detected and quantified in the FLE extract. Nevertheless, the hepatoprotective effects of triterpenoids present in SC-CO2 olive leaf extracts have not been reported previously.

Since active phenolics and triterpenoids may have not only additive but also synergic effects on hepatoprotection, future investigations are warranted to develop purified triterpenoid extracts and determine correlations between the olive leaf isolated compounds and the hepatoprotective activity parameters.

5. Conclusions

The findings of the present study revealed the capacity of olive leaf extracts obtained by supercritical CO_2 extraction in repairing injuries caused by CCl_4-induced hepatotoxicity in a rat model. The obtained results show that fresh and dried olive leaf extracts are able to ameliorate the perturbed biochemical parameters caused by CCl_4 treatment. Moreover, SC-CO_2 olive leaf extract administration resulted in a reduction in elevated levels of liver lipid peroxidation, and a reduction in protein carbonyls due to CCl_4 administration was observed. Serum biochemical markers affirmed the capacity of SC-CO_2 extracts to protect DNA, and histopathological studies confirmed the capacity of olive leaf extracts to improve liver fibrosis caused by CCl_4 treatment. Therefore, olive leaf contributes to health benefits and it is a potential source of powerful antioxidant compounds. In conclusion, the current research indicates that SC-CO_2 extracts from olive leaves have an in vivo protective effect against CCl_4-induced injury in rats' livers. Such a biological study is extremely important to highlight the usefulness of olive tree leaves among plants stated as having hepatoprotective activities. Olive leaves, precious by-products from which we have recovered bioactive compounds by green extraction technology, can be reused for agronomic, food, nutraceutical, and pharmaceutical applications.

Author Contributions: Conceptualization, A.T., A.F. and J.L.-S.; methodology, A.F. and A.T.; software, A.F., A.E.M.; A.T.; validation, D.A.-R., M.S.A. and L.G.; investigation, A.T.; A.F., A.E.M.; data curation, A.T.; A.F.; writing—original draft preparation, A.T.; writing—review and editing, A.F. and J.L.-S.; visualization, D.A.-R.; supervision, R.M. and D.A.-R.; project administration, R.M., A.S.-C. and J.L-S. All authors have read and agreed to the published version of the manuscript.

Funding: This study was supported by the Tunisian Ministry of Higher Education and Scientific Research (LR15CBBC05), the Spanish Ministry of Economy and Competitiveness (MINECO) (project AGL2015-67995-C3-2) and Junta de Andalucia, Andalucian Government, Spain (B-AGR-466-UGR18).

Acknowledgments: The authors would like to thank Rached Raddadi, Hafedh Trabelsi, and Jihen Jeffel, technicians at Anatomopathology Laboory, Gafsa, Tunisia, for their assistance in histological studies.

Conflicts of Interest: The authors declare no conflict of interest.

References

1. Karthikeyan, J. Enzymatic and non-enzymatic antioxidants in selected Piper species. *Indian J. Exp. Biol.* **2003**, *41*, 135–140.
2. Pereira Rodrigues, O. *Characterization of Phenolic Constituents of Medicinal Plants and Evaluation of Pharmacological Activities: Focus in Antioxidant and Anti-Inflammatory Properties*; University of Salamanca-Faculty of Pharmacy: Salamanca, Spain, 2013.
3. Krishna, M.G.; Pallavi, E.; Ravi, K.B.; Ramesh, M.; Venkatesh, S. Hepatoprotective activity of Ficus carica Linn. leaf extract against carbon tetrachloride-induced hepatotoxicity in rats. *Daru* **2007**, *15*, 162–166.
4. Nandakishor, S.D. Effect of Microbially Synthesized Eicosapentaenoic Acid on Carbon Tetrachloride Induced Hepatotoxicity. *J. Dev. Drugs* **2014**, *4*, 2–5. [CrossRef]
5. Alirezaei, M.; Dezfoulian, O.; Kheradmand, A.; Neamati, S.; Khonsari, A.; Pirzadeh, A. Hepatoprotective effects of purified oleuropein from olive leaf extract against ethanol-induced damages in the rat. *Iran. J. Vet. Res.* **2012**, *13*, 218–226.
6. Brent, J.A.; Rumack, B.H. Role of free radicals in toxic hepatic injury I. Free radical biochemistry. *Clin. Toxicol.* **1993**, *31*, 139–171. [CrossRef]
7. Mccord, J.M. Human disease, free radicals, and the oxidant/antioxidant balance. *Clin. Biochem.* **1993**, *26*, 351–357. [CrossRef]
8. Koruk, M.; Taysi, S.; Savas, M.C.; Yilmaz, O.; Akcay, F.; Karakok, M. Oxidative stress and enzymatic antioxidant status in patients with nonalcoholic steatohepatitis. *Ann. Clin. Lab. Sci.* **2004**, *34*, 57–62.
9. Alqasoumi, S.I.; Abdel-Kader, M.S. Screening of some traditionally used plants for their hepatoprotective effect. In *Phytochemicals as Nutraceuticals—Global Approaches to Their Role in Nutrition and Health*; Venketeshwer, R., Ed.; InTechOpen: London, UK, 2012; pp. 255–278. ISBN 978-953-51-0203-8.
10. Bagali, R.S.; Jalalpure, S.S.; Patil, S.S. In-vitro Antioxidant and In-Vivo Hepatoprotective Activity of Ethenolic Extract of Tectona grandis Bark Against CCl4 Induced Liver Injury in Rats. *Pharmacogn J.* **2020**, *12*, 598–602. [CrossRef]
11. Kingsley, U.I. Ameliorative effect of hydroalcoholic extracts of Nigella sativa seed against CCl4-induced acute liver injury in rats. *J. Drug Deliv. Ther.* **2020**, *10*, 164–169.
12. Vani, M.; Rahaman, S.A.; Rani, A.P. Hepatoprotective studies of floral extracts of Gomphrena serrata L. and piperic acid on CCl 4 induced hepatotoxicity. *Indian J. Nat. Prod. Resour.* **2019**, *10*, 238–251.
13. Rashmi, K.; Shenoy, K.B. Hepatoprotective studies of aqueous leaf and root extracts of Barringtonia acutangula (L.) Gaertn. against ethanol induced hepatic stress in rats. *Indian J. Tradit. Knowl.* **2020**, *19*, 152–157.
14. Fki, I.; Sayadi, S.; Mahmoudi, A.; Daoued, I.; Marrekchi, R.; Ghorbel, H. Comparative Study on Beneficial Effects of Hydroxytyrosol- and Oleuropein-Rich Olive Leaf Extracts on High-Fat Diet-Induced Lipid Metabolism Disturbance and Liver Injury in Rats. *Biomed Res. Int.* **2020**, *2020*, 1–15. [CrossRef] [PubMed]
15. Feriani, A.; Tir, M.; María, A.; Caravaca, G.; Contreras, M.; Taamalli, A.; Segura-Carretero, A.; Ghazouani, L.; Mufti, A.; Tlili, N.; et al. Zygophyllum album leaves extract prevented hepatic fibrosis in rats, by reducing liver injury and suppressing oxidative stress, inflammation, apoptosis and the TGF-β1/Smads signaling pathways. Exploring of bioactive compounds using HPLC–DAD–ES. *Inflammopharmacology* **2020**. [CrossRef] [PubMed]
16. Pereira, O.; Macias, R.; JPerez, M.; JGMarin, J.; Cardoso, S. Protective effects of phenolic constituents from Cytisus multiflorus, Lamium album L. and Thymus citriodorus on liver cells. *J. Funct. Foods* **2013**, *5*, 1170–1179. [CrossRef]
17. Herrero, M.; Temirzoda, T.N.; Segura-Carretero, A.; Quirantes, R.; Plaza, M.; Ibañez, E. New possibilities for the valorization of olive oil by-products. *J. Chromatogr. A* **2011**, *1218*, 7511–7520. [CrossRef]

18. El-seedi, H.R.; Khalifa, S.A.M.; Yosri, N.; Khatib, A.; Chen, L.; Saeed, A.; Efferth, T.; Verpoorte, R. Plants mentioned in the Islamic Scriptures (Holy Qur'ân and Ahadith): Traditional uses and medicinal importance in contemporary times. *J. Ethnopharmacol.* **2019**, *243*, 112007. [CrossRef]
19. Schwingshackl, L.; Krause, M.; Schmucker, C.; Hoffmann, G.; Rücker, G.; Meerpohl, J.J. Impact of different types of olive oil on cardiovascular risk factors: A systematic review and network meta-analysis. *Nutr. Metab. Cardiovasc. Dis.* **2019**, *29*, 1030–1039. [CrossRef]
20. Castejón, M.L.; Montoya, T.; Alarcón-de-la-Lastra, C.; Sánchez-Hidalgo, M. Potential Protective Role Exerted by Secoiridoids from *Olea europaea* L. in Cancer, Cardiovascular, Neurodegenerative, Aging-Related, and Immunoinflammatory Diseases. *Antioxidants* **2020**, *9*, 149. [CrossRef]
21. Romani, A.; Ieri, F.; Urciuoli, S.; Noce, A.; Marrone, G.; Nediani, C.; Bernini, R. Health Effects of Phenolic Compounds Found in Extra-Virgin Olive Oil, By-Products, and Leaf of *Olea europaea* L. *Nutrients* **2019**, *11*, 1776. [CrossRef]
22. Talhaoui, N.; Trabelsi, N.; Taamalli, A.; Verardo, V.; Gómez-Caravaca, A.M.; Fernández-Gutiérrez, A.; Arraez-Roman, D. Olea europaea as Potential Source of Bioactive Compounds for Diseases Prevention. In *Studies in Natural Products Chemistry*; Atta-ur-Rahman, Ed.; Elsevier: Amsterdam, The Netherlands, 2018; Volume 57, pp. 389–411. ISBN 9780444640574.
23. Taamalli, A.; Arráez Román, D.; Gómez Caravaca, A.M.; Zarrouk, M.; Segura Carretero, A. Geographical Characterization of Tunisian Olive Tree Leaves (cv. Chemlali) Using HPLC-ESI-TOF and IT/MS Fingerprinting with Hierarchical Cluster Analysis. *J. Anal. Methods Chem.* **2018**, *2018*, 1–10. [CrossRef]
24. Soliman, S.S.; Soliman, M.A.E. Protective Activities of Some Extracts from Olea europaea Leaves towards CCl$_4$-Induced Hepatotoxicity in Rats. *Chem. Res. J.* **2019**, *4*, 62–75.
25. Vidičević, S.; Jelena, T.; Stanojević, Ž.; Isaković, A.; Mitić, D.; Ristić, D.; Dekanski, D. Standardized Olea europaea L. leaf extract exhibits protective activity in carbon tetrachloride-induced acute liver injury in rats: The insight into potential mechanisms. *Arch. Physiol. Biochem.* **2019**, 1–9. [CrossRef]
26. Jemai, H.; Mahmoudi, A.; Feryeni, A.; Fki, I.; Bouallagui, Z.; Choura, S.; Chamkha, M.; Sayadi, S. Hepatoprotective Effect of Oleuropein-Rich Extract from Olive Leaves against Cadmium-Induced Toxicity in Mice. *Biomed Res. Int.* **2020**, *2020*, 1–9. [CrossRef] [PubMed]
27. Al-basher, G.I. Anti-fibrogentic and hepatoprotective potential of methanolic olive extract on cadmium induced toxicity in rats. *Life Sci. J.* **2018**, *15*, 1–11. [CrossRef]
28. Taha, M.E.S.; Kamal, A.M.; Ibrahim, D.R. Possible protective effect of olive leaves extract on paracetamol induced hepatotoxicity in male albino rats. *Biosci. J.* **2020**, *36*, 245–255. [CrossRef]
29. Al-Attar, A.M.; Alrobai, A.A.; Almalki, D.A. Effect of Olea oleaster and Juniperus procera leaves extracts on thioacetamide induced hepatic cirrhosis in male albino mice. *Saudi J. Biol. Sci.* **2016**, *23*, 363–371. [CrossRef]
30. Elgebaly, H.A.; Mosa, N.M.; Allach, M.; El-massry, K.F.; El-Ghorab, A.H.; Al Hroob, A.M.; Mahmoud, A.M. Olive oil and leaf extract prevent fluoxetine-induced hepatotoxicity by attenuating oxidative stress, inflammation and apoptosis. *Biomed. Pharmacother.* **2018**, *98*, 446–453. [CrossRef]
31. Maalej, A.; Mahmoudi, A.; Bouallagui, Z.; Fki, I.; Marrekchi, R.; Sayadi, S. Olive phenolic compounds attenuate deltamethrin-induced liver and kidney toxicity through regulating oxidative stress, inflammation and apoptosis. *Food Chem. Toxicol.* **2017**, *106*, 455–465. [CrossRef]
32. Nastic, N.; Borras-Linares, I.; Lozano-Sánchez, J.; Švarc-Gajić, J.; Segura-carretero, A. Comparative assessment of phytochemical profiles of comfrey (*Symphytum officinale* L.) root extracts Obtained by Different Extraction Techniques. *Molecules* **2020**, *25*, 837. [CrossRef]
33. Sánchez-Camargo, A.D.; Parada-Alonso, F.; Ibáñez, E.; Cifuentes, A. Recent applications of on-line supercritical fluid extraction coupled to advanced analytical techniques for compounds extraction and identification. *J. Sep. Sci.* **2018**, 1–42. [CrossRef]
34. Armenta, S.; Garrigues, S.; Esteve-turrillas, F.A.; De la Guardia, M. Green extraction techniques in green analytical chemistry. *Trends Anal. Chem.* **2019**, *116*, 248–253. [CrossRef]
35. Temelli, F.; Guculu-Ustundag, O. Supercritical technologies for further processing of edible oils. In *Bailey's Industrial Oil and Fat Products*; Shahidi, F., Ed.; John Wiley & Sons, Inc.: Hoboken, NJ, USA, 2005; pp. 397–432.
36. Carrasco-Pancorbo, A.; Cerretani, L.; Bendini, A.; Segura-Carretero, A.; Gallina-Toschi, T.; Fernández-Gutiérrez, A. Analytical determination of polyphenols in olive oils. *J. Sep. Sci.* **2005**, *28*, 837–858. [CrossRef] [PubMed]

37. Taamalli, A.; Arráez-Román, D.; Barrajón-Catalán, E.; Ruiz-Torres, V.; Pérez-Sánchez, A.; Herrero, M.; Ibañez, E.; Micol, V.; Zarrouk, M.; Segura-Carretero, A.; et al. Use of advanced techniques for the extraction of phenolic compounds from Tunisian olive leaves: Phenolic composition and cytotoxicity against human breast cancer cells. *Food Chem. Toxicol.* **2012**, *50*, 1817–1825. [CrossRef]
38. Taamalli, A.; Lozano, J.; Jebabli, H.; Trabelsi, N.; Abaza, L.; Segura-Carretero, A.; Cho, J.Y.; Arraez-Roman, D. Monitoring the bioactive compounds status in Olea europaea according to collecting period and drying conditions. *Energies* **2019**, *12*, 947. [CrossRef]
39. Tipoe, G.L.; Leung, T.M.; Liong, E.C.; Lau, T.Y.H.; Fung, M.L.; Nanji, A.A. Epigallocatechin-3-gallate (EGCG) reduces liver inflammation, oxidative stress and fibrosis in carbon tetrachloride (CCl4)-induced liver injury in mice. *Toxicology* **2010**, *273*, 45–52. [CrossRef] [PubMed]
40. Levine, R.L.; Garland, D.; Oliver, C.N.; Amici, A.; Climent, I.; Lenz, A.G.; Ahn, B.W.; Shaltiel, S.; Stadtman, E.R. Determination of carbonyl content in oxidatively modified proteins. In *Methods in Enzymology*; Elsevier: Hoboken, NJ, USA, 1990; pp. 464–478.
41. Marklund, S.; Marklund, G. Involvement of the superoxide anion radical in the autoxidation of pyrogallol and a convenient assay for superoxide dismutase. *Eur. J. Biochem.* **1974**, *47*, 469–474. [CrossRef]
42. Aebi, H. Catalase in vitro. In *Methods in Enzymology*; Packer, L., Ed.; Elsevier: New York, NY, USA, 1984; pp. 121–126.
43. Flohé, L.; Günzler, W. Assays of glutathione peroxidase. In *Methods in Enzymology*; Packer, L., Ed.; Elsevier: New York, NY, USA, 1984; pp. 114–121.
44. Kanno, S.-I.; Shouji, A.; Hirata, R.; Asou, K.; Ishikawa, M. Effects of naringin on cytosine arabinoside (Ara-C)-induced cytotoxicity and apoptosis in P388 cells. *Life Sci.* **2004**, *75*, 353–365. [CrossRef] [PubMed]
45. Al-Attar, A.M.; Shawush, N.A. Influence of olive and rosemary leaves extracts on chemically induced liver cirrhosis in male rats. *Saudi J. Biol. Sci.* **2015**, *22*, 157–163. [CrossRef]
46. Rahmat, A.; Dar, F.; Choudhary, I. Protection of CCl 4 -induced liver and kidney damage by phenolic compounds in leaf extracts of Cnestis ferruginea (de Candolle). *Pharmacognosy Res.* **2014**, *6*, 19–28. [CrossRef]
47. Szende, B.; Timár, F.; Hargitai, B. Olive oil decreases liver damage in rats caused by carbon tetrachloride (CCl4). *Exp. Toxicol. Pathol.* **1994**, *46*, 355–359. [CrossRef]
48. Dineshkumar, G.; Rajakumar, R.; Mani, P.; Johnbastin, T.M.M. Hepatoprotective activity of leaves extract of eichhornia crassipes against CCl4 induced hepatotoxicity albino rats. *Int. J. Pure Appl. Zool.* **2013**, *1*, 209–212.
49. Tlili, N.; Feriani, A.; Allagui, M.S.; Saadoui, E.; Khaldi, A.; Nasri, N. Effects of Rhus tripartitum fruit extract on CCl4-induced hepatotoxicity and cisplatin-induced nephrotoxicity in rats. *Can. J. Physiol. Pharmacol.* **2015**, *94*, 1–28. [CrossRef] [PubMed]
50. Essawy, A.E.; Abdel-Moneim, A.M.; Khayyat, L.I.; Elzergy, A.A. Nigella sativa seeds protect against hepatotoxicity and dyslipidemia induced by carbon tetrachloride in mice. *J. Appl. Pharm. Sci.* **2012**, *2*, 021–025. [CrossRef]
51. Kumar, P.V.; Sivaraj, A.; Elumalai, E.K.; Kumar, B.S. Carbon tetrachloride-induced hepatotoxicity in rats—Protective role of aqueous leaf extracts of Coccinia grandis. *Int. J. Pharm. Tech. Res.* **2009**, *1*, 1612–1615.
52. Castro, L.; Freeman, B.A. Reactive oxygen species in human health and disease. *Nutrition* **2001**, *17*, 163–165. [CrossRef]
53. Rohrdanz, E.; Kahl, R. Alterations of antioxidant enzyme expression in response to hydrogen peroxide. *Free Radic. Biol. Med.* **1998**, *24*, 27–38. [CrossRef]
54. Shull, S.; Heintz, N.H.; Periasamy, M.; Manohar, M.; Janssen, Y.M.; Marsh, J.P.; Mossman, B.T. Differential regulation of antioxidant enzymes in response to oxidants. *J. Biol. Chem.* **1991**, *266*, 24398–24403.
55. Szymonik-Lesiuk, S.; Czechowska, G.; Stryjecka-Zimmer, M.; Słomka, M.; MĄldro, A.; Celiński, K.; Wielosz, M. superoxide dismutase, and glutathione peroxidase activities in various rat tissues after carbon tetrachloride intoxication. *J. Hepatobiliary Pancreat Surg.* **2003**, 309–315. [CrossRef]
56. Catherine, T.; Piquet-pellorce, L.M.G.C.; Samson, M. Chlordecone potentiates hepatic fibrosis in chronic liver injury induced by carbon tetrachloride in mice. *Toxicol. Lett.* **2016**. [CrossRef]
57. Li, D.; Friedman, S.L. Liver fibrogenesis and the role of hepatic stellate cells: New insights and prospects for therapy. *J. Gastroenterol. Hepatol.* **1999**, *14*, 618–633. [CrossRef]

58. Mejri, H.; Tir, M.; Feriani, A.; Ghazouani, L.; Allagui, M.S.; Saidani-Tounsi, M. Does Eryngium maritimum seeds extract protect against CCl 4 and cisplatin induced toxicity in rats: Preliminary phytochemical screening and assessment of its in vitro and in vivo antioxidant activity and antifibrotic effect. *J. Funct. Foods* **2017**, *37*, 363–372. [CrossRef]
59. Ogaly, H.A.; Eltablawy, N.A.; Abd-elsalam, R.M. Antifibrogenic influence of *Mentha piperita* L. essential Oil against CCl 4 -induced liver fibrosis in rats. *Oxid. Med. Cell. Longev.* **2018**, *2018*, 1–15. [CrossRef] [PubMed]

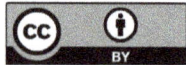

© 2020 by the authors. Licensee MDPI, Basel, Switzerland. This article is an open access article distributed under the terms and conditions of the Creative Commons Attribution (CC BY) license (http://creativecommons.org/licenses/by/4.0/).

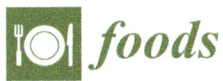 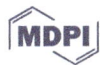

Article

Isolation, Gastroprotective Effects and Untargeted Metabolomics Analysis of *Lycium Minutifolium* J. Remy (Solanaceae)

Stephanie Rodriguez [1], Mariano Walter Pertino [2], Chantal Arcos [3], Luana Reichert [3], Javier Echeverria [4], Mario Simirgiotis [5], Jorge Borquez [6], Alberto Cornejo [7], Carlos Areche [1] and Beatriz Sepulveda [3,*]

1. Departamento de Química, Facultad de Ciencias, Universidad de Chile, 8320000 Santiago, Chile; funny.ddrpump@gmail.com (S.R.); areche@uchile.cl (C.A.)
2. Laboratorio de Química de Productos Naturales, Instituto de Química de Recursos Naturales, Universidad de Talca, 3460000 Talca, Chile; mwalter@utalca.cl
3. Departamento de Ciencias Químicas, Universidad Andres Bello, Campus Viña del Mar, Quillota 980, Viña del Mar, 2531098 Valparaiso, Chile; c.arcoscortez@gmail.com (C.A.); lureichert91@gmail.com (L.R.)
4. Departamento de Ciencias del Ambiente, Facultad de Química y Biología, Universidad de Santiago de Chile, 9170022 Santiago, Chile; javier.echeverriam@usach.cl
5. Instituto de Farmacia, Facultad de Ciencias, Universidad Austral de Chile, 5090000 Valdivia, Chile; mario.simirgiotis@gmail.com
6. Departamento de Química, Facultad de Ciencias Básicas, Universidad de Antofagasta, Av Coloso S-N, 1240000 Antofagasta, Chile; jorge.borquez@uantof.cl
7. Escuela de Tecnología Médica, Facultad de Medicina, Universidad Andres Bello, Sazié 2315, 8370092 Santiago, Chile; alberto.cornejo@unab.cl
* Correspondence: bsepulveda@uc.cl; Tel.: +56-063-2244369

Received: 4 April 2020; Accepted: 15 April 2020; Published: 3 May 2020

Abstract: *Lycium minutifolium* J. Remy (Solanaceae) is commonly used as an infusion in traditional medicine to treat stomach pain, meteorism, intestinal disorders, stomach ailments, and other severe problems including prostate cancer and stomach cancer. From the EtOAc extract of *L. minutifolium* bark five known metabolites were isolated using chromatographic techniques. The gastroprotective effects of the EtOAc fraction and edible infusion extract of the bark were assayed on the hydrochloric acid (HCl)/EtOH induced gastric ulcer model in mice to support the traditional use of the plant. The EtOAc extract and the edible infusion showed gastroprotective effect at dose of 100 mg/kg reducing lesions by 31% and 64%, respectively. The gastroprotective action mechanisms of the edible infusion at a single oral dose of 100 mg/kg were evaluated suggesting that prostaglandins, sulfhydryl groups, and nitric oxide are involved in the mode of gastroprotective action. The UHPLC analysis coupled to high-resolution mass spectrometry of the edible infusion showed the presence of twenty-three compounds. Our results can support the gastroprotective properties of the edible infusion extract, and at least can validate in part, the ethnopharmacological uses of the plant.

Keywords: coumarins; *Lycium*; metabolomic; HPLC-MS; orbitrap; secondary metabolites; endemic plants

1. Introduction

Peptic ulcer disease refers to a group of ulcerative disorders that occur only in those parts of the digestive tract exposed to acid and pepsin produced by gastric mucosa. Peptic ulcers are associated with fatal complications such as stomach perforation or stomach bleeding that may cause death [1]. So far, the complete pathogenesis of peptic ulceration is incompletely understood. Peptic ulcer disease is generally thought to be a breakdown in the balance between two opposing forces: the aggressive luminal factors and the gastric mucosal barrier. Hydrochloric acid (HCl) secreted by oxyntic cells and pepsin produced by chief cells in the gastric mucosa are well-known aggressive factors [1]. Among exogenous factors implicated in the pathogenesis of peptic ulcers, ethanol, steroid drugs, smoking, stress, non-steroidal anti-inflammatory drugs, genetic influences, viruses and bacteria such as *Helicobacter pylori* can be mentioned [1]. *H. pylori* has been implicated as the main agent of gastric cancer since it is related to chronic gastritis. In Chile, gastric cancer is a serious public health problem where the highest mortality index is in the regions of Maule, Bio-Bio and La Araucania [2]. An alternative for prevention of this condition is the use of combined strategies for the prevention of peptic ulcers with the use of natural gastroprotective agents.

The plant genus *Lycium* belongs to the Solanaceae family and is distributed in North and South America, Africa and Eurasia. According to Yao et al., 2018 [3], ninety-seven species and six varieties have been recognized: 32 are native to South America, 24 to North America, 24 to Africa and 12 to Eurasia. Among the mentioned species, *Lycium barbarum* L. and *L. chinensis* Mill. produce a famous edible fruit (goji), which is considered as a superfruit with well demonstrated bioactivity properties [3–5]. The chemistry of *Lycium* genus cover 355 components from different parts including fruits, root bark, leaves, seeds, and flowers according to Yao et al., 2018 [3]. Among the reported metabolites, coumarins, lignans, phenylpropanoids, flavonoids, amides, alkaloids, anthraquinones, organic acids, terpenoids, sterols, steroids, glycerolipids and peptides can be cited. Pharmacological reports have showed that the edible fruits and rootbarks display antioxidant, antimicrobial, antiaging, antiglaucoma, immunoregulatory, antitumor, hepatoprotective, hypotensive, neuroprotective, spermatogenesis, and blood sugar level-reducing activities, as well in some chronic diseases such as hemoptysis, cough, diabetes, hectic fever and night sweats [3–5]. From the point of view of traditional uses, fruits and root bark have been used in traditional Chinese medicine for the treatment of blurry vision, night sweat, fever, kidney deficiency, cough, asthma, diabetes, heart diseases, gynecopathy and neurasthenia [3–5]. In relation to *L. minutifolium* J. Remy, studies noticed that this species is endemically distributed in Chile [6], Argentina and Mauritius [3] without no reported use as food or medicine. In Chile, *L. minutifolium* (Figure 1), popularly known as "Caspiche" is endemic and distributed between the Atacama Desert (III Region) and Coquimbo (IV Region). It is commonly used as an infusion in traditional medicine to treat stomach pain, meteorism, intestinal disorders, stomach ailments, heal external wounds and ulcers, and proliferative problems including prostate and stomach cancer [7]. Surprisingly, no chemical or pharmacological studies on secondary metabolites have been performed for *L. minutifolium* so far.

Historically, secondary metabolite studies have been performed through the isolation of components of plants and structural elucidation using spectroscopic and spectrometric data. However, the scenario has changed with the arrival of hyphenated techniques. Liquid chromatography coupled to mass spectrometry (LC-MS) has become a dominant technique for targeted and untargeted metabolomics. Today, it is considered a powerful tool of analysis in food, hospitals, forensic laboratories as well as in basic research. Among LC-MS, high-resolution mass spectrometry has gained much popularity since it is able to discriminate ions based on their small mass difference, helping in detection of isobaric compounds [8].

As part of our studies on Atacama Desert plants, we inform in this work the isolation and structural elucidation of five known compounds plus UHPLC/ESI/MS/MS fingerprints of *L. minutifolium* for the first time. Furthermore, we discuss here the possible mode of gastroprotective action of the edible extract of this plant.

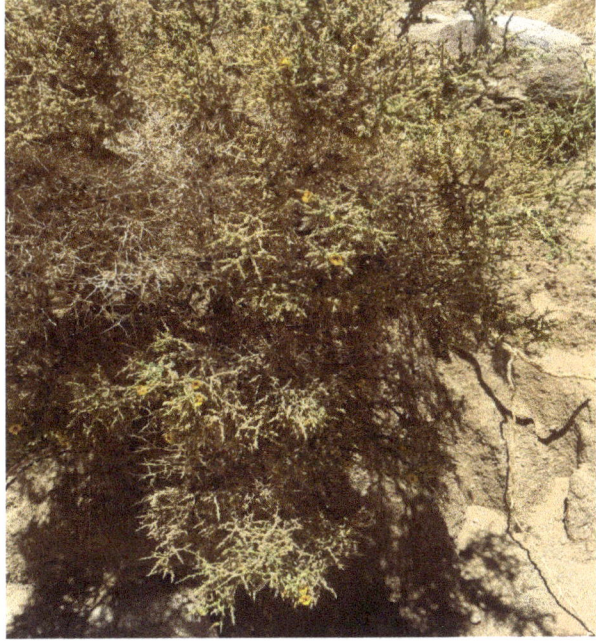

Figure 1. *L. minutifolium* plant.

2. Materials and Methods

2.1. Chemicals

TLC (Kieselgel 60 GF254, Merck) was conducted in *n*-hexane/EtOAc or DCM/MeOH mixtures and spots were sprayed with H_2SO_4-MeOH (1:9, *v/v*) and heated at 120 °C. Silica gel (Kieselgel 60, Merck 0.063–0.200 mm) and Sephadex (LH-20, Sigma) were used in column chromatography (CC). Technical solvents used in chromatography processes were previously distilled and dried according to standard procedures.

2.2. Plant Material

Lycium minutifolium J. Remy were collected in 2017 at "Cuesta el gato" (Copiapo, III Región, Chile) and identified by Prof. Dra Gloria Rojas from the Museo de Historia Natural, Santiago-Chile. A voucher specimen (N° LM120217) is kept at the Natural Product Lab. of the Universidad de Chile.

2.3. Extraction and Isolation

Dried and pulverized bark parts of *L. minutifolium* (1.2 kg) were macerated with ethyl acetate (3 times, 3.0 L, 3 day/extraction). Then, the organic solvent was concentrated under reduced pressure yielding 7.5 g of extract (EA-EXT). This organic extract (7.0 g) was submitted to flash chromatography on silica gel (63–200 μm, 150 g, column length 25 cm, i.d. 10 cm) and eluted with *n*-hexane/EtOAc mixtures (3.0 L each) of increasing polarity (9:1, 7:3, 1:1, 0:1; *v/v*) to give four fractions.

Fraction 1 (2.5 g, *n*-hexane/EtOAc 9:1) was chromatographed on a SiO_2 column (50 g) and eluted with *n*-hexane/EtOAc (1:0, 9:1, 8:2, 7:3, 6:4, 1:1 *v/v*) afforded 210 subfractions (25 mL each). These subfractions were combined based upon TLC monitoring obtaining three main fractions (1A–1C). Repeated CC (silica gel 63–200 μm, 30 g) on fraction 1A (1.0 g) eluted with *n*-hexane/EtOAc mixtures (0–10% EtOAc) led to the isolation of compound **1** (methyleugenol, 25 mg) [9,10] and compound **2** (sarisan, 40 mg) [11] (Figure 2). CC on fraction 1B (0.9 g) eluted with *n*-hexane/EtOAc mixtures (0–25% EtOAc) obtained compound **2** (sarisan, 15 mg) and compound **3** (eugenol, 5 mg) [9,10]. Fraction 1C (0.6 g) was submitted to Sephadex LH-20 (column length 40 cm, i.d. 6.5 cm, MeOH) and then to SiO_2 CC to afford eugenol **3** (13 mg), and lipids according to ^{1}H-NMR.

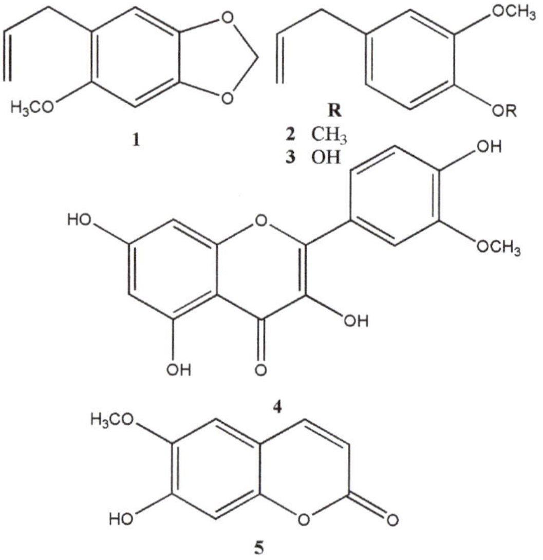

Figure 2. Secondary metabolites isolated from *L. minutifolium*.

Fraction 2 (1.5 g, *n*-hexane/EtOAc 7:3) was permeated on Sephadex LH-20 using MeOH as mobile phase allowing the separation of fatty acids and chlorophylls affording two fractions (2A–2B). Fraction 2A (0.4 g), after repeated CC on silica gel using *n*-hexane/EtOAc mixtures (9:1, 8:2, 7:3, 6:4 and 1:1 *v/v*), produced compound **4** (quercetin-3'-methylether, 2 mg) [5]. Further CC on Fraction 2B (1.1 g) using silica gel afforded compound **5** (scopoletin, 35 mg) [5].

Fraction 3 (2.0 g, *n*-hexane/EtOAc 1:1) was passed on Sephadex LH-20 using MeOH as mobile phase and then was chromatographed on 30 g silica gel with *n*-hexane/EtOAc mixtures (0% to 100%) affording scopoletin **5** and quercetin-3-methylether **4**.

Finally, Fraction 4 (1.0 g, *n*-hexane/EtOAc 0:1) was submitted to CC using Sephadex LH-20 (MeOH) allowing the separation of fats (discarded) and one coumarin according to TLC patron. Repeated CC on silica gel of this fraction afforded scopoletin **5** (20 mg) again (Figure 2).

2.4. UHPLC-ESI-MS/MS Studies

For this study, an infusion was prepared using 3 g of dried chopped bark parts adding deionized water (200 mL) at 100 °C. Then, the solution was lyophilised (Labconco) to obtain 98 mg of edible aqueous extract (EI-EXT).

A Thermo Scientific Dionex Ultimate 3000 UHPLC system, hyphenated with a Thermo high resolution Q-Exactive focus mass spectrometer (Thermo, Bremen, Germany) was used for the analysis. The chromatographic system was coupled to the MS with a Heated Electrospray Ionization Source II (HESI II). XCalibur 3.0 software (Thermo Fisher Scientific, Bremen, Germany) and Trace Finder 3.2 (Thermo Fisher Scientific, San José, CA, USA) were used for UHPLC control and data processing, respectively. Solvent delivery was performed at 1 mL/min using ultra-pure water supplemented with 1% formic acid (A) and acetonitrile with 1% formic acid (B). A program started with 5% B at zero time, then maintained 5% B for 5 min, then changed to 30% B within 10 min, then maintained 30% B for

15 min, then increased to 70% B for 5 min, then maintained 70% B for 10 min, and finally returned to 5% B in 10 min.

2.5. Animals

Mice weighing 30 ± 3 g were acquired from the Public Health Institute, Santiago, Chile. Standard conditions of Swiss albino mice were reported previously [12].

2.6. HCl/EtOH-Induced Lesions in Mice

The gastroprotective activity of the *Lycium minutifolium* extracts was tested at 100 mg/kg on the HCl/EtOH-induced lesion model as described previously [12].

2.7. HCl/Ethanol-Induced Gastric Lesions in Indomethacin-, NEM- and L-NAME-Pretreated Mice

To study the involvement of prostaglandins, sulfhydryl compounds, endogenous nitric oxide and vanilloid receptor in the gastroprotective activity of EI-EXT, Indomethacin s.c. (30 mg/kg), NEM s.c. (10 mg/kg), L-NAME i.p. (70 mg/kg) and RR s.c. (3.5 mg/kg) were injected 30 min before the administration of EI-EXT or vehicle as published previously [12,13].

2.8. Statistical Analysis

Our results were expressed as the mean ± S.D. Statistical differences between treatments and control were performed by one-way analysis of variance (ANOVA) followed by Dunnett's test. All statistical analyses were performed using the software GraphPad Prism 6 for Windows.

3. Results

3.1. Isolation of Secondary Metabolites

The bark of *L. minutifolium* was macerated with EtOAc for nine days at room temperature. The crude organic extract obtained after evaporation of the organic solvent was fractionated by flash column chromatography (SiO_2) yielding four fractions. Each fraction was subjected to repeated permeation with Sephadex LH-20 and chromatography over silica gel to yield five compounds (**1-5**). All compounds were isolated and identified using ^{1}H-NMR spectroscopic and HR-MS spectrometric techniques and belong to three different classes of compounds: phenylpropanes, flavonoids and coumarins. Among them sarisan **1**, methyleugenol **2**, eugenol **3**, quercetin-3'-methyl ether (isorhamnetin, **4**), and scopoletin **5** are reported for the first time in this species (Figure 2).

3.2. Metabolomic Profiling of the Infusion by Using UHPLC-ESI-MS/MS

Ten milligrams of the edible *L. minutifolium* aqueous extract (EI-EXT) was dissolved in fresh water, filtered and injected in the UHPLC-MS/MS machine (Figure 3 and Table 1). This infusion was chosen for metabolomic profiling due to the higher biological activity previously shown in comparison to that of ethyl acetate extract (EA-EXT) on the HCl/EtOH-induced gastric lesions model in mice.

Organic acids: Peak **1** with a molecular anion at m/z 191.0557 was identified as quinic acid ($C_7H_{11}O_6{}^-$) [14,15], while peak **2** was identified as citric acid (m/z 191.0199; $C_6H_7O_7{}^-$) [16]. Quinic acid is a cyclic polyol common in plants such as coffee, Tara, Eucalyptus, Urtica, and cinchona. Citric acid is common in citrus fruits and is used as flavoring and chelating agent.

Spermine alkaloids: Peak **3** presented a molecular anion at m/z 472.2447 and was identified as N^1, N^3-bis-dihydrocaffeoylspermidine ($C_{25}H_{34}N_3O_6{}^-$) and UV absorbance at dihydro caffeoyl structure (287 nm) (Figure 4). This structure was supported by the presence of two diagnostic fragments at m/z 308.1976 and 163.0393 [17]. Peak **3** was reported as constituent of *Scopolia tangutica* and *Iochroma cyaneum*, both belonging to Solanaceae family [18,19]. Peak **6** with a molecular ion at m/z 472.2453 was considered as a potential unknown with MS/MS fragmentation data closely related to a spermidine derivative such as the peak **3** and peak **7** (see Figure S1 in Supplementary Material). This peak showed two daughter fragments at *m/z* 308.1975 and 163.0392 considered typical daughter fragments for spermine alkaloids like the peak **3**. Peak **6** could be considered a new compound awaiting to be isolated. Peak **7** is a dehydrogenated derivative of peak **3** whose fragments were at *m/z* 334.1769; 308.1977; 306.1820 and 135.0443. Based on these data peak **7** was identified as N^1-caffeoyl-N^3-dihydrocaffeoylspermidine ($C_{25}H_{33}N_3O_6^-$). Peak **7** has been reported as metabolite in *Lycium barbarum* [3–5,19].

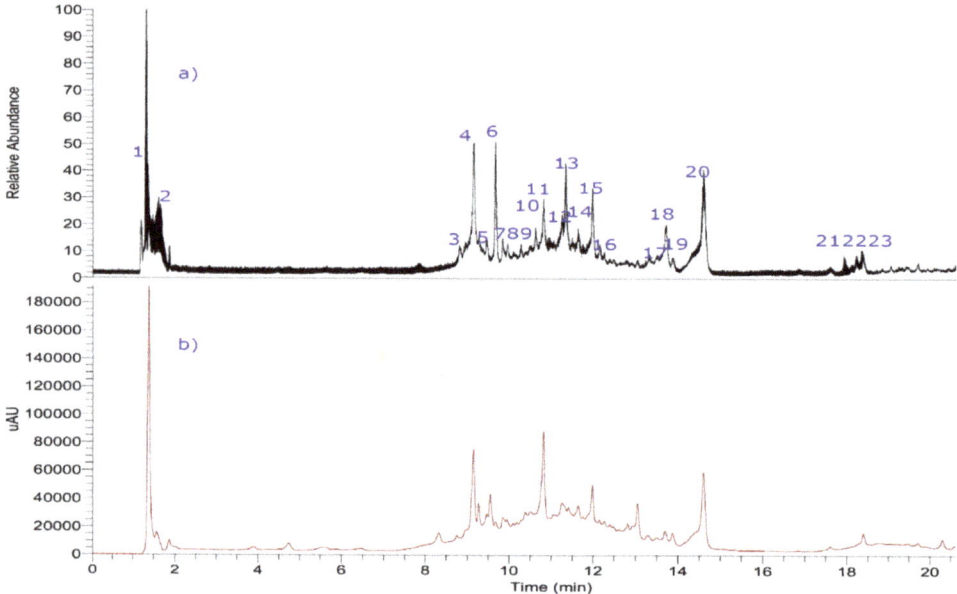

Figure 3. UHPLC-MS chromatograms of *Lycium minutifolium*. (**a**) TIC (total ion current) (**b**) UV at 280 nm.

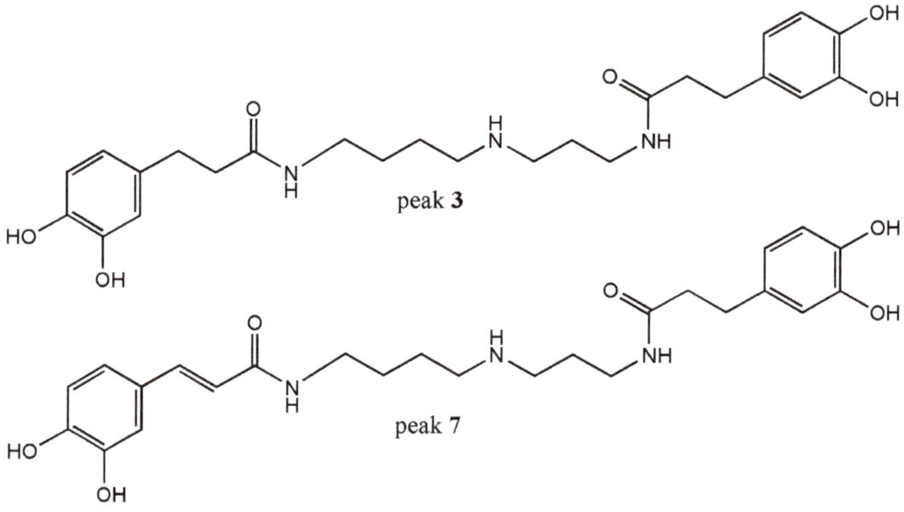

Figure 4. Spermine-type alkaloids detected by UHPLC/ESI/MS/MS from *L. minutifolium*.

Table 1. UHPLC-PDA-MS orbitrap mass spectral data of lyophilized infusion of *Lycium minutifolium*.

Peak	T_R (min.)	Tentative Identification	[M-H]$^-$	Theoretical Mass (m/z)	Measured Mass (m/z)	Accuracy (ppm)	MS^n Ions (ppm)
1	1.35	Quinic acid	$C_7H_{11}O_6^-$	191.0561	191.0557	−1.93	109.0286
2	1.87	Citric acid	$C_6H_7O_7^-$	191.0192	191.0199	3.36	111.0080
3	8.79	N1,N3-bis dihydrocaffeoyl spermidine	$C_{25}H_{34}N_3O_6^-$	472.2455	472.2447	−0.47	308.1976; 163.0393
4	9.13	Chlorogenic acid (5-Caffeoylquinic acid)	$C_{16}H_{17}O_9^-$	353.0876	353.0879	3.52	191.0557; 707.1813 (2M-H adduct)
5	9.24	Chlorogenic acid (4-Caffeoylquinic acid)	$C_{16}H_{17}O_9^-$	353.0876	353.0879	3.52	191.0557; 707.1813 (2M-H adduct)
6	9.65	N1,caffeoyl-N3-dihydrocaffeoyl spermidine bis dihydrocaffeoyl spermidine derivative	$C_{25}H_{34}N_3O_6^-$	472.2455	472.2453	−0.47	308.1975; 163.0392
7	9.82	N1,caffeoyl-N3-dihydrocaffeoyl spermidine	$C_{25}H_{33}N_3O_6^-$	470.2299	470.2293	1.11	334.1769; 308.1977; 306.1820; 135.0443
8	9.94	Chlorogenic acid (3-Caffeoylquinic acid)	$C_{16}H_{17}O_9^-$	353.0878	353.0881	0.90	191.0555
9	10.09	Atropine derivative	$C_{17}H_{18}NO_5^-$	316.1188	316.1192	−1.4	149.0601
10	10.25	Quercetin-3-O-hexoside-7-O-hexoside-hexoside	$C_{33}H_{39}O_{22}^-$	787.1938	787.1928	2.03	609.1457; 301.0341
11	10.78	Rutin	$C_{27}H_{29}O_{16}^-$	609.1455	609.1440	−2.8	301.0342; 300.0269; 179.0432
12	11.23	Kaempferol-3-O-hexoside-pentoside	$C_{27}H_{29}O_{15}^-$	593.1511	593.1501	1.62	285.0405; 255.0279
13	11.49	Isorhamnetin-hexoside-rhamnoside	$C_{28}H_{31}O_{16}^-$	623.1616	623.1611	1.28	477.1014; 315.0499; 300.0264
14	11.32	Kaempferol-3-O-hexoside	$C_{21}H_{19}O_{11}^-$	447.0933	447.0919	1.28	285.0401
15	11.63	esculin	$C_{15}H_{15}O_9^-$	339.0722	339.0714	0.46	177.0190
16	13.50	Eriodictyol	$C_{15}H_{11}O_6^-$	287.0556	287.0550	2.15	135.0442
17	13.67	Kaempferol or luteolin	$C_{15}H_9O_6^-$	285.0401	285.0393	2.90	179.0432; 151.0029
18	13.84	Quercetin	$C_{18}H_{15}O_7^-$	301.0342	301.0351	3.01	151.0034
19	14.57	Isorhamnetin	$C_{16}H_{11}O_7^-$	315.0510	315.0506	2.41	300.0273
20	17.92	Trihydroxyoleic acid	$C_{18}H_{33}O_5^-$	329.2333	329.2322	2.41	-
21	17.92	Trihydroxyoleic acid	$C_{18}H_{33}O_5^-$	329.2333	329.2321	2.23	-
22	18.19	Trihydroxyoleic acid	$C_{18}H_{33}O_5^-$	329.2333	329.2322	2.46	-
23	18.33	Methyl isorhamnetin	$C_{17}H_{13}O_7^-$	329.0665	329.0655	2.97	271.0243

Phenolic acids: Peak **4** was identified as chlorogenic acid (5-caffeoylquinic acid) [14,15]. Peak **5** as the isomer 4-caffeoylquinic acid, and peak **8** as the isomer 3-caffeoylquinic acid. Chlorogenic acid is the main phenolic compound in coffee, artichoke, carrot, kiwi fruit, pears, eggplant, peaches showing anti-inflammatory, antidiabetic, antioxidant, antibacterial, anti-obesity, cardioprotective, hepatoprotective, antipyretic, neuroprotective, antiviral, anti-hypertension and anti-microbial activities [20].

Flavonoids: Peak **10** was assigned as quercetin-3-O-hexoside-7-O-dihexoside based on its molecular ion (*m/z*: 787.1928) and their diagnostic fragments. Peak **11** with a molecular ion at *m/z*: 609.1440 was identified as rutin. Peaks **12–14**, **16–19** and **23** were assigned to kaempferol-3-O-hexoside-pentoside, isorhamnetin-hexoside-rhamnoside, kaempferol-3-O-hexoside, eriodictyol, kaempferol or luteolin, quercetin, isorhamnetin and methylisorhamnetin based on HR-MS and their respective diagnostic daughter fragments. All these flavonoids have been reported in *Lycium barbarum* and *L. chinensis* [3–5].

Coumarins: Only esculin was detected in *Lycium minutifolium* bark based on molecular ion at *m/z*: 339.0714 and their MS^2 fragment at *m/z*: 177.0190 (sculetin). This peak **15** has been reported as a constituent of *Lycium barbarum* [5].

Tropane alkaloids: Peak **9** was tentatively identified as an atropine derivative based on a diagnostic fragment at 149.0601 with a loss of atropine moiety. From *Lycium europaeum* L. fruits atropine, hyoscyamine and scopolamine have been identified. The presence of these alkaloids could question the safety of *Lycium* fruit for human consumption [5].

Fatty acids: Peaks **20–22** were tentatively identified as trihydroxyoleic acid and their isomers ($C_{18}H_{33}O_5$). Remarkably, the presence of oleic acid derivatives was found in *Lycium barbarum* fruits [5].

3.3. Gastroprotective Activity

The effects of the EtOAc extract (EA-EXT) and edible infusion (EI-EXT) in HCl/EtOH induced gastric lesion model in mice are shown in Table 2. The EA-EXT inhibited the gastric lesions by 31% while the EI-EXT by 64% at the dose of 100 mg/kg compared with control group. This dose is valid to show the ethnopharmacological properties of these extracts. In addition, we evaluated the possible mode of gastroprotective action of EI-EXT at a single oral dose of 100 mg/kg. The results of EI-EXT on the gastric lesions induced by HCl/EtOH in mice pretreated with Indometacin (IND, 10 mg/kg, s.c.), N-ethylmaleimide (NEM, 10 mg/kg, s.c.), NG-nitro-L-arginine methyl ester (L-NAME, 70 mg/kg, i.p.), or ruthenium red (RR, 3.5 mg/kg, s.c.) are shown in Table 3.

Table 2. Gastroprotective activity of the EA-EXT (organic extract) and EI-EXT (edible extract) on hydrochloric acid (HCl)/EtOH-induced gastric lesions in mice.

Treatment	n	Lesion Index (mm)	% Lesion Reduction	Dose (mg/Kg)
EA-EXT	7	31.3 ± 3.2 **	31 *	100
EI-EXT	7	16.2 ± 3.7	64 *	100
Lansoprazole	7	14.7 ± 4.8	69 *	30
Control	7	45.4 ± 4.5	-	-

The results were expressed as mean ± SD * $p < 0.01$; significantly different compared with the control and ** $p < 0.01$ significantly different compared with lansoprazole (analysis of variance (ANOVA) followed by Dunnett's test). n = number of mice.

Prostaglandins (PGs) are believed, through PGs production, to be involved in the protection of the stomach mucosa against chemical agents such as ethanol, HCl, and NaOH [21,22]. In our study, pre-treatment with indomethacin (an PGs inhibitor) reduced the gastric protection of EI-EXT (Table 3). This result indicates that PGs are involved in the gastroprotective effect of EI-EXT.

Table 3. Protective effect of edible infusion (EI-EXT) on the HCl/EtOH model in indomethacin-, NEM-, L-NAME, and RR-pretreated mice.

Treatment	Dose (mg/kg)	Lesion Index (mm)
Control	-	45.4 ± 4.5
EI-EXT	100	16.2 ± 3.7 *
IND + **EI-EXT**	10 + 100	39.8 ± 5.2
NEM + **EI-EXT**	10 + 100	36.1 ± 5.5
L-NAME + **EI-EXT**	70 + 100	40.0 ± 5.8 *
RR + **EI-EXT**	3.5 + 100	18.1 ± 3.5
Carbenoxolone	100	14.6 ± 4.2 *

Results were expressed as mean ± SD, $n = 7$. Analysis of variance followed by Dunnett's test. * $p < 0.01$ compared with the respective control.

The decrease of sulfhydryl (SH) groups have a relationship with gastric lesions induced by ethanol. Glutathione, a known endogenous sulfhydryl, preserves the integrity of the cell and acts as a scavenger of free radicals, an antioxidant, and maintains the immune system as well as protein synthesis and their surface [23]. In our study, pre-treatment with N-ethylmaleimide (NEM, SH-blocker) reduced the protection showed by EI-EXT. This evidence implies that endogenous SHs participate in the gastroprotective activity of this edible extract.

Nitric oxide (NO) is implied in gastric mucosa defense through the regulation of the gastric blood flow, angiogenesis and mucus secretion [24]. In our study, pre-treatment with N^G-nitro-L-arginine methyl ester (L-NAME, an inhibitor of NO synthase) reduced the gastroprotective activity of EI-EXT, suggesting that the protective effect of this edible extract is through the participation of endogenous NO (Table 3).

Capsaicin-sensitive sensory neurons through vanilloid receptors on the gastric mucosa protect via the regulation of acid secretion, gastric motility, gastric blood flow and mucus production [1]. In this study, pre-treatment with RR did not produce significant changes in the protection of EI-EXT suggesting that this extract did not imply VR.

Nature has provided many gastroprotective drugs during the last decades including carbenoxolone from *Glycyrrhiza glabra*, solon from sophoradin and gefarnate from cabbage (*Brassica oleracea* L.) as the most important gastroprotective agents [23]. So many crude drugs have been reported as gastroprotective agents and this information is summarized in some excellent reviews by Tundis et al., 2008 [25], Mota et al., 2009 [26], Sumbul et al., 2011 [27] and Khan et al., 2018 [28]. Regarding bioactive compounds, a polyssacharide fraction from traditional plant *Handroanthus heptaphyllus* constituted by arabinogalactans II has showed gastroprotective activity at 10 mg/kg on gastric lesions induced by ethanol. Moreover, this fraction at the same doses presented gastric ulcer healing in rats through the inhibition of mucus and GSH depletion. In another study, a polysaccharide fraction at 100 mg/kg from the medicinal plant *Bletilla striata* displayed a reduction in the formation of gastric lesions by the increase in PGE2 content, mitigating of oxidative stress, suppression of MAPK/NF-kB signaling pathway in gastric tissue and a reduction in the levels of pro-inflammatory agents as TNF-α, IL-1β, IL-6 and IL-18 [29]. Arunachalam et al., 2019 [30] reported that a hydroethanolic extract of *Cochlospermum regium* at 100 mg/kg showed preventive and curative activity in different gastric ulcer models supporting the traditional use of this plant. In the same study, it was demonstrated that the mechanism of gastroprotective action and antiulcer activity implied an increase in mucus production, gastric secretion inhibition, activation of K^+_{ATP} channels and α-2-adrenergic receptor, augmentation of antioxidant activity and stimulation of PGs and NO synthesis. In the case of *Lycium* species referred to gastroprotective and ulcerogenic activities, only *Lycium chinense* has been reported to have these properties [31,32]. An ethyl acetate extract of the aerial part of *L. chinense* showed gastroprotective activity based on its antioxidant, anti-inflammatory, anti-secretory and anti-apoptotic effects [32]. Pretreatment with ethyl acetate extract at 50–400 mg/kg attenuated the ethanol-induced gastric lesions either increasing oxidative stress markers (GSH and SOD), pH of gastric juice, and mucin soluble content, or decreasing MOP activity, MDA elevation, caspase-3-expresion and inflammatory markers (such as TNF-α, IL-1β, iNOS and COX-2). In a similar way, Cheng et al. 2016 [31] reported gastroprotective properties at doses of 50, 100, 200 and 400 mg/kg of the root bark of *L. chinense* suggesting that the mechanisms involved could be related to the scavenging of free radicals, antioxidant, anti-inflammatory and pro-inflammatory marker regulations. *Lycium barbarum*, a closely related plant to *Lycium chinense*, displayed anti-ulcer activity against water-immersion restraint stress, acetic acid and pylorus-ligation models in rats and this activity was related to the presence of polysaccharides isolated from water extract [33]. In our study, we have demonstrated that edible infusion (100 mg/kg) of *L. minutifolium* possesses gastroprotective properties against HCl/EtOH induced gastric lesion model in mice suggesting that this protective effect is through the participation of endogenous NO, endogenous SHs, and prostaglandins.

On the other hand, the mortality after peptic ulcer disease decreased significantly in the last few decades, due to treatment of *H. pylori* infections [34]. Several bioactive compounds were key defensive factors against this bacteria such as: arabinogalactanes (jambo, mangoes, and goji Lycium fruits), other polysaccharides obtained from fruits (*Maytenus ilicifolia* Mart. ex Reissek) and acidic heteroxylans, (for instance from Olea fruits), rhamnogalacturonanes (ubiquitous in several grapes and ginseng roots) and terpenoids, (such as pinene, lupeol, limonene, citral, nomiline and ursolic acid), and flavonoids such as flavonol derivatives have been showed to display this activity [28,35]. These compounds can prevent the invasion, colonization, and adherence of *H. pylori* into the cells of the stomach and prevent gastric cancer, suppressing cancer growth, which is very common in *H. pylori*-infected patients.

The potential bioactivity of this plant could be attributable to the chemical diversity found in the edible infusion such as phenolic acids, alkaloids and flavonoids detected by UHPLC/ESI/MS/MS. These compounds are believed to play an essential role in these bioassays as indicated in our study and others [26,27,36,37]. Further studies are required to isolate and evaluate the gastroprotection of all pure compounds.

4. Conclusions

In the present study, we isolated five known compounds named as methyl eugenol, sarisan, eugenol, quercetin-3′-methylether (isorhamnetin), and scopoletin for the first time from the ethyl acetate extract of *Lycium minutifolium*. Then, an edible infusion extract was prepared, and both extracts at 100 mg/kg displayed gastroprotective activity (31% and 64%) on the HCl/EtOH-induced gastric lesion model in mice. Our findings suggest that prostaglandins, sulfhydryl groups, and nitric oxide are involved in the mode of gastroprotective action of this edible extract. Finally, in the edible extract twenty-three compounds were tentatively detected by UHPLC/ESI/MS/MS including diverse compounds such as organic acids, spermine and tropane alkaloids, phenolic acids, flavonoids and fatty acids. Furthermore, peak **6** is considered an unknown spermine-type alkaloid. These results based on ethnomedicinal properties provide the basis for the utilization of *L. minutifolium* as a source of potential compounds or mixtures for the prevention of gastric ulcers.

Supplementary Materials: The following are available online at http://www.mdpi.com/2304-8158/9/5/565/s1, Figure S1: Full HR-orbitrap MS spectra and structures of some representative compounds, peaks 3, 4, 6, 7, 11 and 19.

Author Contributions: C.A. (Carlos Areche), M.S., J.E., and B.S. conceived and designed the experiments; A.C., S.R., and B.S., performed the gastroprotective experiments; C.A. (Chantal Arcos), L.R. and S.R., isolated the compounds; M.S., M.W.P., and J.B. analyzed the data of NMR and UHPLC/MS. All authors wrote the paper, read, and approved the final manuscript. All authors have read and agreed to the published version of the manuscript.

Funding: This research was funded by Fondecyt grant 1170871 and PAI/ACADEMIA No. 79160109. M.S. and J.B received financial support from Fondecyt, (Grant 1180059).

Conflicts of Interest: The authors do not have any conflict of interest.

References

1. Mozsik, G.Y.; Abdel-Salam, O.M.E.; Szolcsanyi, J. *Capsaicin-Sensitive Afferent Nerves in Gastric Mucosal Damage and Protection*; Budapest Akadémiai Kiadó: Budapest, Hungary, 1997.
2. Bellolio, E.; Riquelme, I.; Riffo-Campos, A.; Rueda, C.; Ferreccio, C.; Villaseca, M.; Brebi, P.; Muñoz, S.; Araya, J.C. Assessment of gastritis and gastric cancer risk in the Chilean population using the OLGA system. *Pathol. Oncol. Res.* **2019**, *25*, 1135–1142. [CrossRef] [PubMed]
3. Yao, R.; Heinrich, M.; Weckerle, C.S. The genus *Lycium* as food and medicine: A botanical, ethnobotanical and historical review. *J. Ethnopharm.* **2018**, *212*, 50–66. [CrossRef] [PubMed]
4. Potterat, O. Goji (*Lycium barbarum* and *L. chinense*): Phytochemistry, pharmacology and safety in the perspective of traditional uses and recent popularity. *Planta Med.* **2010**, *76*, 7–19. [CrossRef] [PubMed]
5. Qian, D.; Zhao, Y.; Yang, G.; Huang, L. Systematic review of chemical constituents in the genus *Lycium* (Solanaceae). *Molecules* **2017**, *22*, 911. [CrossRef]
6. Rodríguez, R.; Marticorena, C.; Alarcón, D.; Baeza, C.; Cavieres, L.; Finot, V.L.; Ruiz, E. Catálogo de las plantas vasculares de Chile. *Gayana Bot.* **2018**, *75*, 1–430. [CrossRef]
7. Moraga-Reyes, J. *Yerbas y Curanderos. Testimonios de Valle del Huasco*; La Calabaza del Diablo: Santiago, Chile, 2007.
8. Martins, C.P.B.; Bromirski, M.; Conaway, M.C.P.; Makarov, A.A. Orbitrap mass spectrometry: Evolution and Applicability. In *Comprensive Analitycal Chemistry*; Perez, S., Eichhorn, P., Barcelo, D., Eds.; Elsevier: Amsterdam, The Netherlands, 2016; Volume 71.
9. Alimuddin, A.H.; Mardjan, M.I.D.; Matsjeh, S.; Anwar, C.; Sholikhah, E.N. Synthesis 7-hydroxy-3′,4′-dimethoxyisoflavon from eugenol. *Indones. J. Chem.* **2011**, *11*, 163–168. [CrossRef]
10. Kaufman, T.S. The multiple faces of eugenol. A versatile starting material and building block for organic and bio-organic synthesis and a convenient precursor toward bio-based fine chemicals. *J. Braz. Chem. Soc.* **2015**, *26*, 1055–1085. [CrossRef]
11. Villegas, M.; Vargas, D.; Msonthii, J.D.; Marston, A.; Hostettmann, K. Isolation of the antifungal compounds falcarindiol and sarisan from *Heteromorpha trifoliate*. *Planta Med.* **1988**, *54*, 36–37. [CrossRef]
12. Areche, C.; Sepulveda, B.; Martin, A.S.; Garcia-Beltran, O.; Simirgiotis, M.; Cañete, A. An unusual mulinane diterpenoid from the Chilean plant *Azorella trifurcata* (Gaertn) Pers. *Org. Biomol. Chem.* **2014**, *12*, 6406–6413. [CrossRef]
13. Matsuda, H.; Pongpiriyadacha, Y.; Morikawa, T.; Kashima, Y.; Nakano, K.; Yoshikawa, M. Protective effects of polygodial and related compounds on ethanol-induced gastric mucosal lesions in rats: Structural requirements and mode of action. *Bioorg. Med. Chem. Lett.* **2002**, *12*, 477–482. [CrossRef]
14. Simirgiotis, M.J.; Benites, J.; Areche, C.; Sepúlveda, B. Antioxidant capacities and analysis of phenolic compounds in three endemic *Nolana* species by HPLC-PDA-ESI-MS. *Molecules* **2015**, *20*, 11490–11507. [CrossRef]
15. Simirgiotis, M.J.; Quispe, C.; Bórquez, J.; Areche, C.; Sepúlveda, B. Fast detection of phenolic compounds in extracts of easter pears (*Pyrus communis*) from the Atacama desert by ultrahigh-performance liquid chromatography and mass spectrometry (UHPLC-Q/Orbitrap/MS/MS). *Molecules* **2016**, *21*, 92. [CrossRef] [PubMed]
16. Brito, A.; Ramirez, J.E.; Areche, C.; Sepúlveda, B.; Simirgiotis, M.J. HPLC-UV-MS profiles of phenolic compounds and antioxidant activity of fruits from three citrus species consumed in Northern Chile. *Molecules* **2014**, *19*, 17400–17421. [CrossRef] [PubMed]
17. Parr, A.J.; Mellon, F.A.; Colquhoun, I.J.; Davies, H.V. Dihydrocaffeoyl polyamines (kukoamines and allies) in Potato (*Solanum tuberosum*) tubers detected during metabolite profiling. *J. Agric. Food Chem.* **2005**, *53*, 5461–5466. [CrossRef] [PubMed]
18. Sattar, E.A.; Glasl, H.; Nahrstedt, A.; Hilal, S.H.; Zaki, A.Y.; El-Zalabani, S.M.H. Hydroxycinnamic acid amides from *Iochroma cyaneum*. *Phytochemistry* **1990**, *29*, 3931–3933. [CrossRef]
19. Long, Z.; Zhang, Y.; Guo, Z.; Wang, L.; Xue, X.; Zhang, X.; Wang, S.; Wang, Z.; Civelli, O.; Liang, X. Amide alkaloids from *Scopolia tangutica*. *Planta Med.* **2014**, *80*, 1124–1130. [CrossRef]
20. Santana-Gálvez, J.; Cisneros-Zevallos, L.; Jacobo-Velázquez, D.A. Chlorogenic Acid: Recent Advances on Its Dual Role as a Food Additive and a Nutraceutical against Metabolic Syndrome. *Molecules* **2017**, *22*, 358. [CrossRef]

21. Borrelli, F.; Izzo, A.A. The plant kingdom as a source of anti-ulcer remedies. *Phytother. Res.* **2000**, *14*, 581–591. [CrossRef]
22. Wallace, J.L. Eicosanoids in the gastrointestinal tract. *Br. J. Pharmacol.* **2019**, *176*, 1000–1008. [CrossRef]
23. Lewis, D.A.; Hanson, P.J. Anti-Ulcer Drugs of Plant Origin. In *Progress in Medicinal Chemistry*; Elsevier: Amsterdam, The Netherlands, 1991; Volume 28, pp. 201–231.
24. Wallace, J.L. Nitric oxide in the gastrointestinal tract: Opportunities for drug development. *Br. J. Pharmacol.* **2019**, *176*, 147–154. [CrossRef]
25. Tundis, R.; Loizzo, M.R.; Bonesi, M.; Menichini, F.; Conforti, F.; Statti, G.; Menichini, F. Natural products as gastroprotective and antiulcer agents: Recent development. *Nat. Prod. Commun.* **2008**, *3*, 2129. [CrossRef]
26. Mota, K.S.; Dias, G.E.; Pinto, M.E.; Luis-Ferreira, A.; Souza-Brito, A.R.; Hiruma-Lima, C.A.; Barbosa-Filho, J.M.; Batista, L.M. Flavonoids with gastroprotective activity. *Molecules* **2009**, *14*, 979–1012. [CrossRef] [PubMed]
27. Sumbul, S.; Ahmad, M.A.; Asif, M.; Akhtar, M. Role of phenolic compounds in peptic ulcer: An overview. *J. Pharm. Bioallied Sci.* **2011**, *3*, 361–367. [PubMed]
28. Khan, M.S.A.; Khundmiri, S.U.K.; Khundmiri, S.R.; Al-Sanea, M.M.; Mok, P.L. Fruit-derived polysaccharides and terpenoids: Recent update on the gastroprotective effects and mechanisms. *Front. Pharmacol.* **2018**, *9*, 569. [CrossRef] [PubMed]
29. Zhang, C.; Gao, F.; Gan, S.; He, Y.; Chen, Z.; Liu, X.; Fu, C.; Qu, Y.; Zhang, J. Chemical characterization and gastroprotective effect of an isolated polysaccharide fraction from *Bletilla striata* against ethanol-induced acute gastric ulcer. *Food Chem. Toxicol.* **2019**, *131*, 110539. [CrossRef]
30. Arunachalam, K.; Damazo, A.S.; Pavan, E.; Oliveira, D.M.; Figueiredo, F.D.F.; Machado, M.T.M.; Balogun, S.O.; Soares, I.M.; Barbosa, R.D.S. *Cochlospermum regium* (Mart. Ex Schrank) Pilg: Evaluation of chemical profile, gastroprotective activity and mechanism of action of hydroethanolic extract of its xylopodium in acute and chronic experimental models. *J. Ethnopharmacol.* **2019**, *233*, 101–114. [CrossRef]
31. Chen, H.; Olatunji, O.J.; Zhou, Y. Anti-oxidative, anti-secretory and anti-inflammatory activities of the extract from the root bark of *Lycium chinense* (Cortex Lycii) against gastric ulcer in mice. *J. Nat. Med.* **2016**, *70*, 610–619. [CrossRef]
32. Olatunji, O.J.; Chen, H.; Zhou, Y. Antiulcerogenic properties of *Lycium chinense* Mill extracts against ethanol-induced acute gastric lesion in animal models and its active constituents. *Molecules* **2015**, *20*, 22553–22564. [CrossRef]
33. Li, P.; Xiao, B.; Chen, H.; Guo, J. Lycium Barbarum and Tumors in the Gastrointestinal Tract. In *Lycium Barbarum and Human Health*; Chang, R.C., So, K.F., Eds.; Springer: Dordrecht, The Netherlands, 2015.
34. Lau, J.Y.; Sung, J.; Hill, C.; Henderson, C.; Howden, C.W.; Metz, D.C. Systematic Review of the Epidemiology of Complicated Peptic Ulcer Disease: Incidence, Recurrence, Risk Factors and Mortality. *Digestion* **2011**, *84*, 102–113. [CrossRef]
35. Bonifácio, V.V.; dos Santos Ramos, A.A.; da Silva, B.B.; Bauab, M.M. Antimicrobial activity of natural products against *Helicobacter pylori*: A review. *Ann. Clin. Microbiol. Antimicrob.* **2014**, *13*, 54.
36. Alarcon de la Lastra, C.; Lopez, A.; Motilva, V. Gastroprotective and prostaglandin E2 generation in rats by flavonoids of *Dittrichia viscosa*. *Planta Med.* **1993**, *59*, 497–501. [CrossRef] [PubMed]
37. Alanko, J.; Riutta, A.; Holm, P.; Mucha, I.; Vapata, H.; Metsa-Ketela, T. Modulation of arachidonic acid metabolism by phenols: Relation to their structure and antioxidant/pro-oxidant properties. *Free Radic. Biol. Med.* **1999**, *26*, 193–201. [CrossRef]

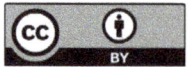

© 2020 by the authors. Licensee MDPI, Basel, Switzerland. This article is an open access article distributed under the terms and conditions of the Creative Commons Attribution (CC BY) license (http://creativecommons.org/licenses/by/4.0/).

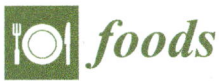

Article

Allelopathic Potential and Active Substances from *Wedelia Chinensis* (Osbeck)

Kawsar Hossen [1,2], Krishna Rany Das [1,2,3], Shun Okada [1,2], Arihiro Iwasaki [4], Kiyotake Suenaga [4] and Hisashi Kato-Noguchi [1,2,*]

1. Department of Applied Biological Science, Faculty of Agriculture, Kagawa University, Miki, Kagawa 761-0795, Japan; kwsarbau@gmail.com (K.H.); k_das007@yahoo.com (K.R.D.); oskhaudna.30@gmail.com (S.O.)
2. The United Graduate School of Agricultural Sciences, Ehime University, 3-5-7 Tarumi, Matsuyama 790-8566, Japan
3. Department of Entomology, Faculty of Agriculture, Bangladesh Agricultural University, Mymensingh 2202, Bangladesh
4. Department of Chemistry, Faculty of Science and Technology, Keio University, 3-14-1 Hiyoshi, Kohoku, Yokohama 223-8522, Japan; a.iwasaki@chem.keio.ac.jp (A.I.); suenaga@chem.keio.ac.jp (K.S.)
* Correspondence: kato.hisashi@kagawa-u.ac.jp

Received: 25 September 2020; Accepted: 30 October 2020; Published: 2 November 2020

Abstract: *Wedelia chinensis* (Asteraceae) is a wetland herb native to India, China, and Japan. It is a valuable medicinal plant recorded to have pharmaceutical properties. However, the phytotoxic potential of *Wedelia chinensis* has not yet been examined. Thus, we carried out this study to establish the allelopathic effects of *Wedelia chinensis* and to identify its phytotoxic substances. Extracts of *Wedelia chinensis* exhibited high inhibitory activity against the root and shoot growth of cress, alfalfa, rapeseed, lettuce, foxtail fescue, Italian ryegrass, timothy, and barnyard grass. The inhibition was varied with species and was dependent on concentrations. The extracts were separated through several purification steps, and the two effective substances were isolated and characterized as vanillic acid and gallic acid using spectral analysis. Vanillic acid and gallic acid significantly arrested the growth of cress and Italian ryegrass seedlings. The concentrations of vanillic acid and gallic acid needed for 50% inhibition (I_{50} values) of the seedling growth of the cress and Italian ryegrass were 0.04–15.4 and 0.45–6.6 mM, respectively. The findings suggest that vanillic acid and gallic acid may be required for the growth inhibitory activities of *Wedelia chinensis*.

Keywords: *Wedelia chinensis*; organic farming; phytotoxic substances; vanillic acid; gallic acid

1. Introduction

Organic farming emerged at the beginning of the 20th century as an alternative agricultural method to demote the hazardous effect of nonnatural herbicides on the environment and people [1,2]. Natural substances are used in organic farming, and at the same time, the use of synthetic substances is banned or severely restricted [3]. Organic farming needs various types of agricultural crop that help to sustain beneficial microorganisms in the soil and to enhance soil conservation to increase farm production. Accordingly, weeds should be controlled without applying chemical herbicides that cause enormous problems [4]. Thus, searching for nature-based product alternatives to synthetic herbicides is now a pressing issue to control weeds, which is a major impediment to crop production [5,6]. In light of these concerns, allelopathy can be explored and used as alternative weed management over synthetic herbicides [7]. Many studies have reported on the use of phytotoxic substances as a nature-friendly approach to weed management [7–9].

The perennial herb *Wedelia chinensis* from the Asteraceae family is usually named Wedelia in Chinese, bhringraj in Hindi, and manjal karisalanganni in Tamil [10]. *Wedelia chinensis* is a climbing herb that is introduced in submerged areas in Assam, Uttar, and Andhra Pradesh and in offshore areas of India. It is also grown in the Madras Presidency of India, Japan, and China [11,12]. The herb is a fragile, expanding, and hairy-type plant, with branches usually up to 50 cm long.

The leaf architecture is simple, arranged oppositely with subsessile leaflets and short, white hairs. Its flower is an axillary head and yellow. The fruits are nearly oval with hairs on the surface [13–15]. The literature reports that different parts (leaves, stems, and roots) of *Wedelia chinensis* are applied as hepatoprotection and a cholagogue and as folk medicine to treat various diseases such as diarrhea, jaundice, cough, diphtheria, headache, and pertussis; to help relieve mental stress; and to promote sleep [16,17]. Conventionally, the leaves, stems, and fruits are used in childbirth and to treat bites and stings, kidney dysfunction, fever, amenorrhea, infection, and wounds [18]. Leave extracts are a natural way to generally apply anti-inflammatory medicines such as Dolonex (Piroxicam) Brufen, and Voveran [13].

Pharmacological investigations have revealed that *Wedelia chinensis* had effects on diterpenoids, sesquiterpenes, triterpenoids, flavonoids, organic acids, and steroids [19,20] and has antioxidant [21,22], anti-inflammatory and antimicrobial [23], and anticancer effects [24]. Moreover, *Wedelia chinensis* is a common garden herb that tends to form a community, and field investigations have shown that there are few weeds in its community [25]. Although *Wedelia chinensis* is known to contain many pharmaceutical features, the allelopathic effects of this plant have not yet been recorded in the literature. Therefore, the study was conducted to explore the allelopathy and to identify the allelochemicals from *Wedelia chinensis*.

2. Materials and Methods

2.1. Plant Material Collection

The *Wedelia chinensis* is a perennial climbing-type herb that is grown in the submerged and seashore areas of subtropical regions. The whole plants (except roots) of *Wedelia chinensis* were collected from the Botanical Garden of Bangladesh Agricultural University (BAU), Mymensingh, Bangladesh in August and September 2016. The species was identified by Sarwar Abul Khayer Mohammad Golam (Department of Crop Botany, BAU) at voucher number BGBAU 16MP-0003 deposited in the Medicinal Plant Herbarium, Botanical Garden, BAU. All of the plant parts were cleaned under running water, dried in the shade to prevent scorching from sunshine, and then ground into powder with a grinder. The plant powder was put into a polybag and kept at 2 °C before extraction.

2.2. Test Plant Species

Eight test plants (including both crop and weed species) were used in this experiment for biological assay: lettuce (*Lactuca sativa* L.), alfalfa (*Medicago sativa* L.), cress (*Lepidium sativum* L.), rapeseed (*Brassica napus* L.), Italian ryegrass (*Lolium multiflorum* Lam.), barnyard grass (*Echinochloa crus-galli* (L.) P. Beauv.), foxtail fescue (*Vulpia myuros* (L.) C.C. Gmel.), and timothy (*Phleum pratense* L.). These species were selected based on their noted growth pattern (alfalfa, lettuce, cress, and rapeseed), susceptibility to allelopathic substances, and abundance (Italian ryegrass, foxtail fescue, timothy, and barnyard grass) in crop fields as weeds.

2.3. Extraction

The *Wedelia chinensis* powder (1.60 kg) was extracted utilizing 8 L of 70% (*v/v*) aqueous methanol. The plant extracts were filtered onto a single layer of filter paper (No. 2; Toyo Roshi Ltd., Tokyo, Japan). Plant residues were extracted again for one day with the equivalent amount of methanol (100%) and filtered. Both filtrates were mixed and evaporated until dry using a rotary evaporator at 40 °C.

2.4. Growth Bioassay

The extracts of *Wedelia chinensis* were diluted into 300 mL of methanol to make six test concentrations as 1, 3, 10, 30, 100, and 300 mg DW (dry weight) equivalent extract/mL. Aliquots of the extract were applied to the single sheet of filter paper (No. 02) into Petri dishes (28 mm) at assay concentrations and kept in a draft chamber to desiccate the methanol. The filter paper was then soaked with 0.6 mL (*v/v*) aqueous solution of Tween 20 (polyoxyethylene sorbitan monolaurate; Nacalai, Kyoto, Japan) in each Petri dish to serve as a surfactant. Ten seeds of lettuce, alfalfa, cress, and, rapeseed, and 10 pre-emergence seeds of timothy, Italian ryegrass, barnyard grass, and foxtail fescue (incubated in dark condition for 68 h, 48 h, 46 h, and 72 h, respectively, at the temperature of 25 °C) were placed onto the filter paper in the Petri dishes. The control treatments were prepared for the seeds and pre-emergence seeds with an aqueous mixture of polyoxyethylene sorbitan monolaurate without the extracts. After two days of incubation in dark condition at 25 °C, the growth of the all tested plants were estimated. The seedling percentage length of seedlings was determined based on the length of the control seedlings. The concentration needed for 50% growth inhibition (I_{50} values) was determined for each species using a logistic regression equation of the concentration–response curves. Throughout this experiment, the assay was performed with three replications for each model plant and replicated twice (10 seeds or pre-germinated seeds/replication).

2.5. Extract Partitions

The *Wedelia chinensis* extracts were evaporated at 40 °C with a rotary evaporator to make an aqueous residue, and pH of the residues was modified to 7.0 by using 1 Molar (M) phosphate buffer. The plant extracts were then partitioned eight times with an equivalent amount of EtOAc (ethyl acetate) and divided into H_2O (aqueous) and EtOAc fractions. A bioassay was set with cress seeds to measure the phytotoxic effects of H_2O and EtOAc fractions.

2.6. Isolation and Purification of the Active Substances

After saturating overnight with sodium sulphate, the EtOAc (ethyl acetate) fraction was evaporated to dryness. The extract residues were loaded into a silica gel column (60 g of silica gel 60, 70–230 mesh; Nacalai Tesque, Kyoto, Japan) and eluted with *n*-hexane with increasing quantities of EtOAc (increased 10%/step (*v/v*), in 150 mL/step) and 300 mL methanol. The repressing effects of all fractions were calculated through the cress assay, as previously stated. In the column of silica gel, the most active fractions were obtained from 60, 70, and 80% EtOAc in *n*-hexane and EtOAc, which were mixed together and then evaporated until complete dryness; purified through a column of Sephadex LH-20 (GE Healthcare Bio-Science AB, SE-75184, Uppsala, Sweden); and rinsed with 20, 30, 40, 50, 60, and 80% (*v/v*) aqueous methanol (150 mL/step) and 300 mL methanol. The highest active fraction was eluted with 40% aqueous methanol (Figure 1), then evaporated until dry, diluted in 20% (*v/v*) aqueous methanol, and burdened into a reverse-phase C_{18} cartridge (YMC Co. Ltd., Kyoto, Japan). The C_{18} cartridge was rinsed with 20, 30, 40, 50, 60, and 80% (*v/v*) aqueous methanol and cold methanol. The highest active fraction was rinsed with 50% aqueous methanol, which was then refined with reverse phase high-performance liquid chromatography (HPLC) (5 µm, 4.6 × 250 mm I.D., Inertsil® ODS-3; GL Science Inc., Tokyo, Japan). The HPLC column was rinsed with 20% (*v/v*) aqueous methanol at a flow rate of 0.8 mL/min. The active substances were determined at the wavelength of 220 nm and at the oven temperature of 40 °C from 62 to 100 min retention time as a colorless substance (substance 1) and from 65 to 70 min retention time as a whitish substance (substance 2). Both substances were characterized using high resolution electrospray ionisation mass spectrometry (HRESIMS), proton nuclear magnetic resonance (^{1}H-NMR), and specific rotation.

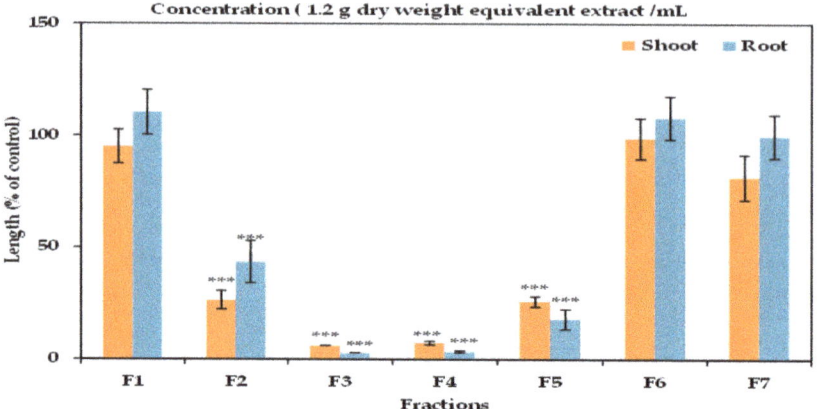

Figure 1. Effect on the seedling growth of cress of all fractions of the extracts of *Wedelia chinensis* that has been obtained from the column of Sephadex LH-20: cress seeds were exposed to the concentration equivalent of the extracts gained from 1.2 g DW (dry weight) of *Wedelia chinensis*/mL for F1 (20% aqueous methanol), F2 (30% aqueous methanol), F3 (40% aqueous methanol), F4 (50% aqueous methanol), F5 (60% aqueous methanol), F6 (80% aqueous methanol), and F7 (methanol). The values are mean ± SE for each treatment from the two independent experiments with 10 seedlings. Asterisks show major variations between treatments and control: *** $p < 0.001$ (ANOVA one way and least significant difference (LSD) test post hoc).

2.7. Bioassay of the Isolated Substances

The extracted compounds were diluted in methanol to make final bioassay concentrations: 0.003, 0.01, 0.03, 0.1, 0.3, and 1 mM of substance 1 and 0.03, 0.1, 0.3, 1, 3, 10, and 30 mM of substance 2 were applied to filter paper (No. 2, 28 mm; Toyo Roshi Ltd., Tokyo, Japan) in Petri dishes (28 mm) and kept in a draft chamber to desiccate the solvent. The growth inhibitory activity of the isolated compounds, as previously described, were calculated using cress and Italian ryegrass. The I_{50} values for these compounds against the tested plant species were determined as mentioned above.

2.8. Statistics

Each assay experiment was conducted with three replications and replicated twice in a completely randomized block design. The resulting data were analyzed using SPSS software version 16.0 (SPSS Inc., Chicago, IL, USA). The data that were obtained from each experiment were then subjected to analysis of variance (ANOVA), and the significant differences between the mean of treatments and control were calculated using a post hoc Tukey's test with least significant difference (LSD) test at 5% level of probability.

3. Results

3.1. Allelopathic Effects of Wedelia chinensis on the Seedling Growth of the Tested Plant Species

The aqueous methanol extracts of *Wedelia chinensis* suppressed the seedling growth of the tested plants (lettuce, cress, rapeseed, alfalfa, barnyard grass, Italian ryegrass, timothy, and foxtail fescue) at various concentrations (Figure 2). The growth seedlings of all the tested plants (other than barnyard grass) were completely arrested (100%) in the concentration of 300 mg DW equivalent extract of *Wedelia chinensis*/mL. When the tested plants were exposed to the concentration of 100 mg DW equivalent extract of *W. chinensis*/mL, the lettuce seedlings were completely inhibited and the shoot and root growth of alfalfa, rapeseed, cress, barnyard grass, Italian ryegrass, timothy, and foxtail fescue were restricted to 9, 2.9, 6, 10.6, 12.1, 14.3, 7.4, and 0.2% growth compared with the control shoots and 8.7, 1.3,

4.1, 4.4, 0.1, 5.7, and 5.6% growth compared with the control roots, respectively. The growth inhibition of the tested plants was different at other concentrations (Figure 2). These findings indicated that the *Wedelia chinensis* extracts suppressed the seedling growth of both the dicots and monocots species, and the inhibition of growth increased when the concentration of the extracts increased. The I_{50} values varied at 3.3–42.2 (for shoots) and 8.7–48 mg (for roots) DW equivalent extract/mL for tested species (Table 1). The lettuce seedling was the most susceptible to the extracts based on I_{50} values, and the least sensitive was the barnyard grass shoots and alfalfa roots. These findings suggest that the growth inhibition by the *Wedelia chinensis* extract varied among the tested plants. The concentration-dependent and species-specific inhibitory effects of *Wedelia chinensis* extracts indicate that this plant might contain an allelopathic potential and might therefore possess allelochemicals.

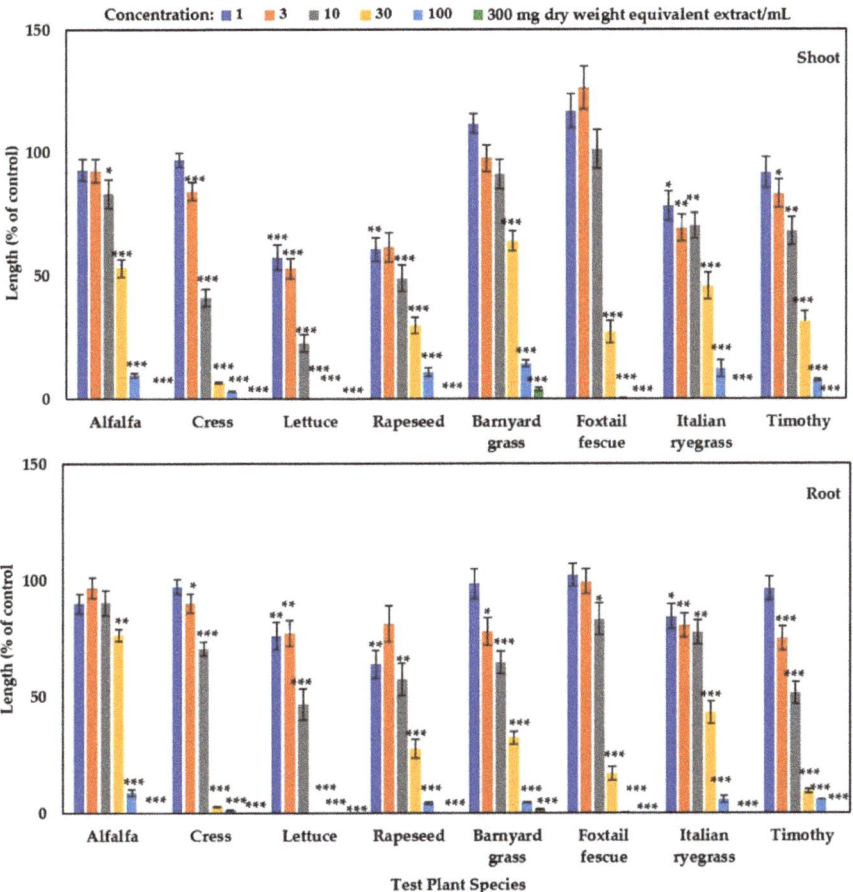

Figure 2. Growth inhibitory effects of *Wedelia chinensis* plant extracts on the shoot and root growth of lettuce, alfalfa, cress, rapeseed, barnyard grass, timothy, Italian ryegrass, and foxtail fescue: the tested species were exposed to the concentrations of 1, 3, 10, 30, 100, and 300 mg DW equivalent extracts of *Wedelia chinensis*/mL. The values are mean ± SE for each treatment from the two independent experiments with 3 replications (10 seedlings for each replication) for every experiment ($n = 60$) that is displayed. Asterisks signify important variations between treatments and control: * $p < 0.05$, ** $p < 0.01$, and *** $p < 0.001$ (ANOVA one-way and LSD test by post hoc).

Table 1. The I_{50} values of the aqueous methanol extracts of *Wedelia chinensis* against shoot and root growth of the tested species.

Tested Species		I_{50} Values (mg DW Equivalent Extract/mL)	
		Shoot	Root
Dicot	Alfalfa	32.6	48.0
	Cress	7.8	13.9
	Lettuce	3.3	8.7
	Rapeseed	8.9	13.1
Monocot	Barnyard grass	42.2	16.4
	Foxtail fescue	21.3	17.3
	Italian ryegrass	24.7	23.9
	Timothy	17.1	10.4

3.2. Identification of the Phytotoxic Substances

In the partitioning purification step, the H_2O and EtOAc fraction of the *Wedelia chinensis* extracts displayed concentration-dependent growth inhibitory effects against the growth of cress seedlings, but a higher inhibitory effect was found in the EtOAc fraction (Figure 3). Thus, the EtOAc fraction was again purified using various chromatographic proceedings (column of silica gel, Sephadex LH-20 column, and reverse-phase C_{18} cartridges), and for each purification proceeding, the inhibitory activity was measured using a cress bioassay. Using the reverse-phase of HPLC in the bottommost purification step, two phytotoxic compounds were isolated. The phytotoxic substances were identified based on NMR and spectral analysis of the data and by comparison with the previously recorded data.

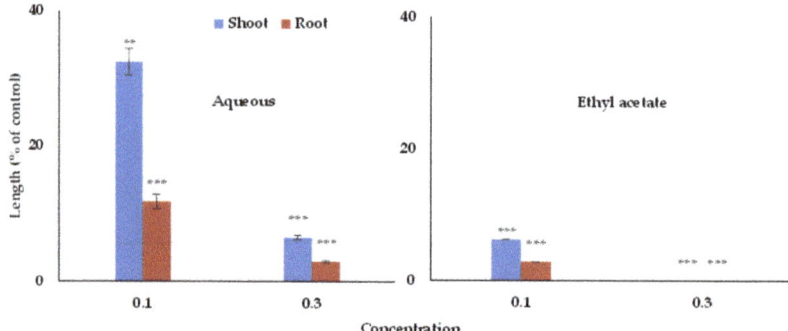

Figure 3. Effect on the seedling growth of cress of the aqueous and ethyl acetate fractions that has been obtained by partitioning of *Wedelia chinensis* extracts: cress was subjected to concentrations equal to 0.1 and 0.3 g DW extracts of *Wedelia chinensis*/mL. The values are mean ± SE for each treatment from the two independent experiments with 10 seedlings. Asterisks show major variations between treatments and control: ** $p < 0.01$ and *** $p < 0.001$ (ANOVA one way and LSD test post hoc).

The molecular formula of substance 1 was determined as $C_8H_7O_4$ using HRESIMS *m/z* 167.0348 [M-H]⁻ (calcd for $C_8H_7O_4$, 167.0348, Δ = +0.4 mmu); ^{1}H NMR (400 MHz, CD_3OD) δ_H 7.56 (d, *J* = 1.6 Hz, 1 H, H3), 7.55 (dd, *J* = 9.4, 1.6 Hz, 1 H, H7), 6.83 (d, *J* = 9.4 Hz, 1 H, H6), 3.89 (s, 3 H, H8). Substance 1 was identified as vanillic acid (Figure 4) by comparing the data with those of the previously reported in the literature [26].

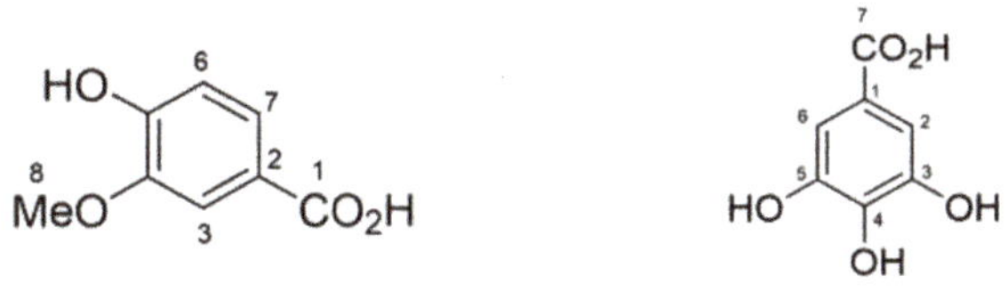

Vanillic Acid   **Gallic Acid**

Figure 4. The chemical structures of vanillic acid and gallic acid obtained from the extracts of *Wedelia chinensis*.

The molecular formula of substance 2 was determined as $C_7H_5O_5$ using HRESIMS *m/z* 169.0749 [M-H]$^-$ (calcd for $C_7H_5O_5$, 169.0749); ^{1}H NMR (400 MHz, CD$_3$OD) δ_H 7.05 (s, 2 H, H2, 6); ^{13}C NMR (100 MHz, CD$_3$OD) δ_C 170.4 (C–7), 146.4 (C–3, 5), 139.6 (C–4), 122.0 (C–1), 110.3 (C–2, 6). Substance 2 was identified as gallic acid (Figure 4) by comparing the data with those of the previously reported in the literature [27].

3.3. Biological Activity of the Isolated Substances

The biological activity of vanillic acid and gallic acid were tested against cress and Italian ryegrass. The obtained results of the assay exhibited that the growth of the cress and Italian ryegrass seedlings was significantly impaired by both compounds (Figures 5 and 6). The level of inhibition by the isolated compounds increased with increasing concentration, suggesting that the inhibition was dose dependent. Vanillic acid and gallic acid significantly restricted the growth of the cress seedlings at concentrations of 0.03 and 3 mM, respectively (Figures 5 and 6). Vanillic acid had the highest inhibition (12% of control) against the growth of the cress shoots and roots at a concentration of 1 mM, whereas gallic acid exhibited maximum suppression of the growth of the cress shoots and roots at 12.8 and 7.8% of control growth, respectively, at a concentration of 30 mM (Figures 5 and 6). In contrast, vanillic acid and gallic acid significantly arrested the seedling growth of Italian ryegrass at concentrations of 0.1 and 3 mM, respectively (Figures 5 and 6). At 1 mM, vanillic acid showed maximum inhibition against the growth of the Italian ryegrass shoots and roots at 39.4 and 38.9% of control, respectively, while gallic acid displayed maximum suppression against the growth of the shoots and roots at 16.9 and 2.8%, respectively, compared with control growth at a concentration of 30 mM.

The I_{50} values of vanillic acid against cress shoot and root were 0.04 and 0.05 mM, respectively, (Table 2) which are about 12- and 9-times higher, respectively than that for the Italian ryegrass shoots (0.47 mM) and roots (0.45 mM). In contrast, the I_{50} values of gallic acid against Italian ryegrass shoot and root were 6.6 and 2.3 mM, respectively, (Table 2) which are roughly 2.3- and 6-times lower, respectively, than that for the cress shoot (15.4 mM), and root (13.8 mM). The I_{50} values show that vanillic acid had greater growth inhibitory effects against both tested species compared with gallic acid. In addition, the cress shoot and root displayed greater susceptibility to vanillic acid than that of Italian ryegrass, and the Italian ryegrass showed higher sensitivity to gallic acid than cress.

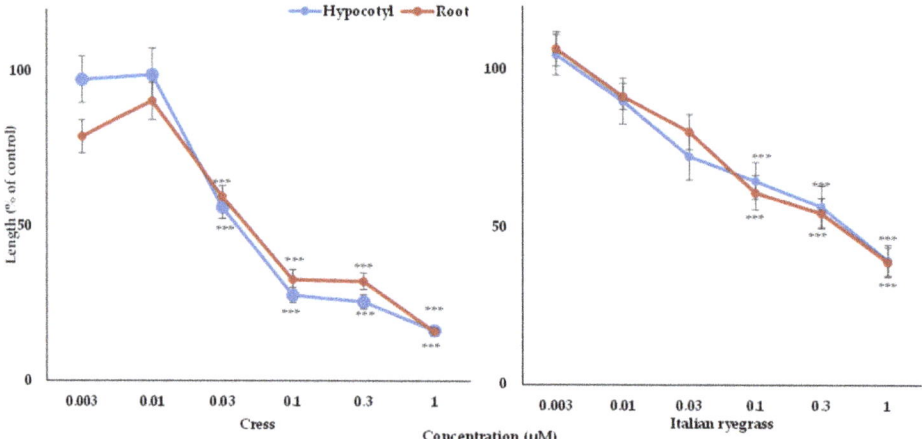

Figure 5. Effect of vanillic acid on the seedling's growth of cress and Italian ryegrass: mean ± SE from the two separate experiments with three replications (10 seedlings for each replication) for every experiment that is displayed. Asterisks signify important variations between treatments and control: *** $p < 0.001$ (ANOVA one-way and LSD test by post hoc).

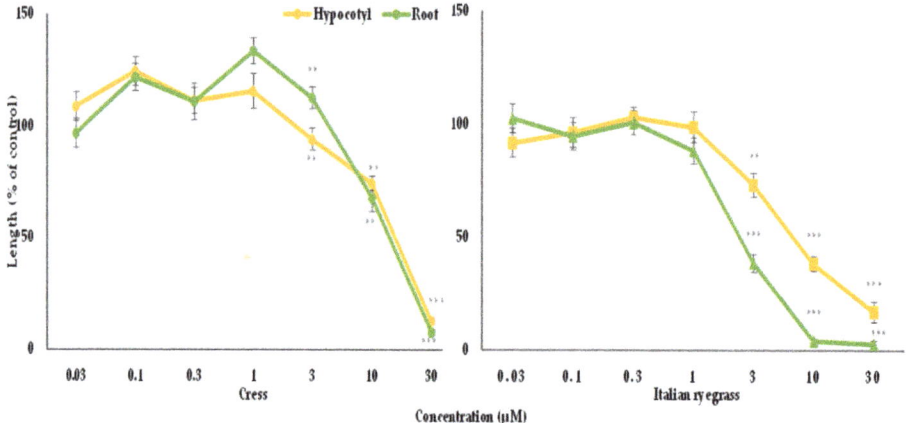

Figure 6. Effect of gallic acid on the seedling's growth of cress and Italian ryegrass: mean ± SE from the two separate experiments with three replications (10 seedlings for each replication) for every experiment that is displayed. Asterisks signify important variations between treatments and control: ** $p < 0.01$, and *** $p < 0.001$ (ANOVA one-way and LSD test by post hoc).

Table 2. The I_{50} values of vanillic acid and gallic acid from *Wedelia chinensis* against the shoot and root growth of cress and Italian ryegrass.

Tested Species		Vanillic Acid	Gallic Acid
		(mM)	
Cress	Shoot	0.04	15.4
	Root	0.05	13.8
Italian ryegrass	Shoot	0.47	6.6
	Root	0.45	2.3

3.4. Discussion

The present study showed the phytotoxic activities of aqueous methanol extracts of *Wedelia chinensis*, which significantly restricted the seedlings growth of eight tested species: lettuce, alfalfa, cress, rapeseed, barnyard grass, Italian ryegrass, timothy, and foxtail fescue (Figure 2). Phytotoxic effects increased with increasing extract concentration. Our results corroborate other research studies [28–33], which reported the concentration-dependent and species-specific growth inhibitory activities of various plant extracts. These findings suggested that the growth inhibitory effects of the plant extracts indicate the presence of phytotoxic substances. The extracts in this study were subjected to chromatographic fractionations, and two substances were isolated and characterized using spectral analysis as vanillic acid and gallic acid. These two substances are phenolic compounds. Phenolic substances are the most common classes of phytochemicals that have important morphophysiological significance in various plants and exhibit various biological activities like anti-inflammatory, antimicrobial, and antioxidant effects [34]. Phenolic substances are the most significant phytochemicals that are involved in allelopathy [35,36]. The development of secondary metabolites, particularly phenolic substances, is important for the survival of plants and help to improve their self-defense and plant protection [37].

Vanillic acid is present in various fruits, cereal grains, olives, and different plants, along with beer, cider, wine [38,39], *Gardeniae fructus* [40], potato [41], red propolis [42], palm plant [43], *Juglans regia* [44], *Angelica sinensis* [45,46], *Chenopodium murale* [47], pumpkin seeds [48], *Melilotus messanensis* [49], orchard grass [50], and *Poliomintha longiflora* [51]. Vanillic acid is commonly used in different food preservatives, additives and flavoring agents and in the perfume industry [52]. It also plays an important role in protein and fatty acid biosynthesis [53]. Vanillic acid is applied as an antibacterial agent [54,55]; is a natural antioxidant in vegetables, fruits, and other plants [44,56]; is also used in antiapoptotic, hypotensive, hepatoprotective, cardioprotective roles and in the regulation of genes [57–59]. It is also commonly used in prescriptive Chinese drug [60]. Although vanillic acid has been identified in different plants and its allelopathic activity is well documented [61–65], this is the first report on vanillic acid from *Wedelia chinensis*.

Gallic acid is present in fruits and vegetables [66]; gallnuts, grapes, and blackberries [67]; eucalyptus species and *Picea schrenkiana* [68]; tea [69]; chestnuts and several berries [51]; *Myriophyllum spicatum*, *Cynomorium coccineum*, and *Microcystis aeruginosa* [70,71]; and black tea [72]. It has many medicinal uses such as antimicrobial [73], neuroprotection [74], antioxidant [75,76], anticancer [77,78], and antiulcer [79] uses and for cardiovascular diseases (CVDs) [80]. Furthermore, gallic acid has lipid homeostasis [81] and antihyperglycemic effects [82] and acts as a cardioprotective agent [83,84]. Gallic acid is also used in the food industry; in manufacturing inks, paints, and dyes; and in cinematography [85]. Gallic acid has been identified in various plants, and its allelopathic potential has also been shown in many studies [86–89], but this is the first report on gallic acid in *Wedelia chinensis* so far.

The I_{50} values show that the inhibitory activity of vanillic acid against the growth of cress and Italian ryegrass was stronger than that of gallic acid. The disparity in phytotoxic activity might be due to the difference between their chemical structures as the phytotoxic activity of allelopathic compounds is determined based on their structural variations [90,91]. Vanillic acid and gallic acid (a derivative of benzoic acid) contain a benzene ring. In vanillic acid, an OH group, an OCH_3 group, and a COOH group are found on the benzene ring, and gallic acid has three OH groups and one COOH group but no OCH_3 group. Research on the relationships between structure and activity showed that the number and location of OH and OCH_3 groups determine the phytotoxic effects of benzoic acid [92]. In addition, hydroxy and methoxy substituents in the benzene ring have been reported to either decrease or increase the phytotoxic effects of benzoic acid [93]. However, a compound to drug should have amphipathic characteristics, including aqueous solubility and sufficient lipid solubility. Vanillic acid and gallic acid both have excellent aqueous solubility due to their COOH group. However, the methoxy group in vanillic acid increases more lipid solubility than that of the hydroxyl group present in gallic acid, which may be the reason that vanillic acid shows stronger inhibitory effects compared to the gallic acid.

Therefore, the growth inhibitory potential of vanillic acid and gallic acid lead to the phytotoxicity of *Wedelia chinensis*. Hence, the phytotoxic effects of *Wedelia chinensis* allow this plant to develop vigorously with minimal weed infestation because it inhibits nearby plants by releasing allelopathic substances.

4. Conclusions

The obtained results from the study suggested that *Wedelia chinensis* possesses potent phytotoxic effects, repressing the growth of lettuce, alfalfa, cress, rapeseed, barnyard grass, Italian ryegrass, timothy, and foxtail fescue. Two phytotoxic compounds, vanillic acid and gallic acid, were isolated from the aqueous methanol extracts of *Wedelia chinensis*. Vanillic acid and gallic acid significantly impeded the growth of cress and Italian ryegrass seedlings. This is the first report on the phytotoxic activity of *Wedelia chinensis*. Our research indicated that *Wedelia chinensis* can be used for the biological control of weeds, which may help to develop organic farming.

Author Contributions: Conceptualization, K.H. and H.K.-N.; methodology, K.H., A.I., K.S., K.R.D., S.O., and H.K.-N.; software, K.H. and K.R.D.; validation, A.I., K.S., K.R.D., S.O., and H.K.-N.; formal analysis, K.H. and K.R.D.; investigation, K.H.; Resources, H.K.-N.; data curation, H.K.-N.; writing—original draft preparation, K.H.; writing—review and editing, H.K.-N.; visualization, K.H.; supervision, H.K.-N. All authors have read and agreed to the published version of the manuscript.

Funding: This study was funded by a MEXT scholarship, grant number MEXT-193490, from the government of Japan to carry out the research in Japan.

Acknowledgments: The authors are thankful to Dennis Murphy, The United Graduate School of Agricultural Sciences, Ehime University, Japan, for editing the English of the manuscript.

Conflicts of Interest: The authors declare no conflict of interest.

References

1. Jabran, K.; Mahajan, G.; Sardana, V.; Chauhan, B.S. Allelopathy for weed control in agricultural systems. *Crop. Prot.* **2015**, *72*, 57–65. [CrossRef]
2. Santos, P.C.; Santos, V.H.M.; Mecina, G.F.; Andrade, A.R.; Fegueiredo, P.A.; Moraes, V.M.O.; Silva, L.P.; Silva, R.M.G. Phytotoxicity of *Tegetes erecta L.* and *Tegetes patula L.* on plant germination and growth. *S. Afr. J. Bot.* **2015**, *100*, 114–121.
3. Crowder, D.W.; Reganold, J.P. Financial competitiveness of organic agriculture on a global scale. *Proc. Natl. Acad. Sci. USA* **2015**, *112*, 7611–7616. [CrossRef] [PubMed]
4. Mahmood, I.; Imadi, S.R.; Shazadi, K.; Gul, A.; Hakeem, K.R. Effects of Pesticides on Environment. In *Plant, Soil and Microbes*; Springer Science and Business Media LLC: Berlin/Heidelberg, Germany, 2016; pp. 253–269.
5. Chai, M.; Zhu, X.; Cui, H.; Jiang, C.; Zhang, J.; Shi, L. Lily Cultivars Have Allelopathic Potential in Controlling *Orobanche aegyptiaca Persoon*. *PLoS ONE* **2015**, *10*, e0142811. [CrossRef]
6. Das, K.R.; Iwasaki, A.; Suenaga, K.; Kato-Noguchi, H. Evaluation of phytotoxic potential and identification of phytotoxic substances in *Cassia alata Linn*. leaves. *Acta Agric. Scand. Sect. B Plant Soil Sci.* **2019**, *69*, 1–10. [CrossRef]
7. Suwitchayanon, P.; Suenaga, K.; Iwasaki, A.; Kato-Noguchi, H. Myrislignan, a Growth Inhibitor from the Roots of Citronella grass. *Nat. Prod. Commun.* **2017**, *12*, 1077–1078. [CrossRef]
8. Gomaa, N.H.; AbdElgawad, H.R. Phytotoxic effects of *Echinochloa colona* (L.) Link. (*Poaceae*) extracts on the germination and seedling growth of weeds. *Span. J. Agric. Res.* **2012**, *10*, 492. [CrossRef]
9. Asaduzzaman, M.; An, M.; Pratley, J.E.; Luckett, D.J.; Lemerle, D. Canola (*Brassica napus*) germplasm shows variable allelopathic effects against annual ryegrass (*Lolium rigidum*). *Plant Soil* **2014**, *380*, 47–56. [CrossRef]
10. Chopra, R.N.; Nayar, S.L.; Chopra, I.C.; Asolkar, L.V.; Kakkar, K.K.; Chakre, O.J.; Varma, B.S. *Glossary of Indian Medicinal Plants*; Council of Scientific & Industrial Research: New Delhi, India, 1956; p. 258.
11. Kirtikar, K.R.; Basu, B.D. *Indian Medicinal Plants*; Bishen Singh Mahendra Pal Singh: Dehradun, India, 2006; pp. 1364–1365.
12. Sharma, A.; Anand, K.; Pushpangadan, P.; Chandan, B.; Chopra, C.; Prabhakar, Y.S.; Damodaran, N. Hepatoprotective effects of *Wedelia calendulacea*. *J. Ethnopharmacol.* **1989**, *25*, 93–102. [CrossRef] [PubMed]

13. Agarwala, B.; Azam, F.M.S.; Khatun, M.A.; Rahman, F.; Rahmatullah, M. Simultaneous shoot regeneration and rhizogenesis of *Wedelia chinensis* for In Vitro clonal propagation. *Am. Eurasian J. Sustain. Agric.* **2010**, *4*, 65–69.
14. Kumar, R.M.; Suresh, V.; Rajesh, S.V.; Kumar, N.S.; Arunachalam, G. Pharmacognostical studies of the plant *Wedelia chinensis* (Osbeck) MERR. *Int. J. Pharm. Res. Dev.* **2011**, *2*, 53–57.
15. Meena, A.K.; Rao, M.M.; Meena, R.P.; Panda, P. Pharmacological and phytochemical evidences for the plants of Wedelia Genus–A review. *Asian J. Pharm. Res.* **2011**, *1*, 7–12.
16. Umasankar, K.; Kumar, R.M.; Suresh, A.; Kumar, N.S.; Arunachalam, G.; Suresh, V. CNS activity of ethanol extract of *Wedelia chinensis* in experimental animals. *Int. J. Pharm. Sci. Nanotechnol.* **2010**, *3*, 881–886.
17. Nomani, I.; Mazumder, A.; Chakrabarthy, G.S. *Wedelia chinensis* (*Asteraceae*)—An overview of a potent medicinal herb. *Int. J. Pharm. Tech. Res.* **2013**, *5*, 957–964.
18. Mathew, K.M. *Flora of Tamilnadu-Carnatic*; The Rapinat Herbarium—St. Joseph's College: Trichirapalli, India, 1983; Volume 2, p. 392.
19. Li, X.; Wang, Y.-F.; Shi, Q.; Sauriol, F. A New 30-Noroleanane Saponin from *Wedelia chinensis*. *Helvetica Chim. Acta* **2012**, *95*, 1395–1400. [CrossRef]
20. Qiu, Q.; Wu, X.; Li, G.Q.; Li, Y.L.; Wang, G.C. Chemical constituents from *Wedelia chinensis*. *Chin. Tradit. Pat. Med.* **2014**, *36*, 1000–1004.
21. Manjamalai, A.; Grace, V.B. Antioxidant Activity of Essential Oils from *Wedelia chinensis* (Osbeck) In Vitro and In Vivo Lung Cancer Bearing C57BL/6 Mice. *Asian Pac. J. Cancer Prev.* **2012**, *13*, 3065–3071. [CrossRef]
22. Talukdar, T.; Talukdar, D. Response of antioxidative enzymes to arsenic-induced phytotoxicity in leaves of a medicinal daisy, *Wedelia chinensis* Merrill. *J. Nat. Sci. Biol. Med.* **2013**, *4*, 383–388. [CrossRef]
23. Manjamalai, A.; Jiflin, G.J.; Grace, V.M.B. Study on the effect of essential oil of *Wedelia chinensis* (Osbeck) against microbes and inflammation. *Asian J. Pharm. Clin. Res.* **2012**, *5*, 155–163.
24. Tsai, C.-H.; Tzeng, S.-F.; Hsieh, S.C.; Lin, C.-Y.; Tsai, C.-J.; Chen, Y.-R.; Yang, Y.-C.; Chou, Y.-W.; Lee, M.-T.; Hsiao, P.-W. Development of a standardized and effect-optimized herbal extract of *Wedelia chinensis* for prostate cancer. *Phytomedicine* **2015**, *22*, 406–414. [CrossRef]
25. Rensen, Z.; Xianglian, L.; Shiming, L.; Qiang, Z.; Huifen, T. Allelopathic potential of *Wedelia chinensis* and its allelochemicals. *Acta Ecol. Sinica* **1996**, *16*, 20–27.
26. Chang, S.W.; Kim, K.H.; Lee, I.K.; Choi, S.U.; Ryu, S.Y.; Lee, K.R. Phytochemical Constituents of *Bistorta manshuriensis*. *Nat. Prod. Sci.* **2009**, *15*, 234–240.
27. Al-Majmaie, S.; Nahar, L.; Sharples, G.P.; Wadi, K.; Sarker, S.D. Isolation and Antimicrobial Activity of Rutin and Its Derivatives from *Ruta chalepensis* (*Rutaceae*) Growing in Iraq. *Rec. Nat. Prod.* **2018**, *13*, 64–70. [CrossRef]
28. Kato-Noguchi, H.; Suzuki, M.; Noguchi, K.; Ohno, O.; Suenaga, K.; Laosinwattana, C. A Potent Phytotoxic Substance in *Aglaia odorata* Lour. *Chem. Biodivers.* **2016**, *13*, 549–554. [CrossRef]
29. Islam, S.; Iwasaki, A.; Suenaga, K.; Kato-Noguchi, H. Isolation and identification of two potential phytotoxic substances from the aquatic fern *Marsilea crenata*. *J. Plant Biol.* **2017**, *60*, 75–81. [CrossRef]
30. Appiah, K.S.; Mardani, H.K.; Omari, R.A.; Eziah, V.Y.; Ofosu-Anim, J.; Onwona-Agyeman, S.; Amoatey, C.A.; Kawada, K.; Katsura, K.; Oikawa, Y.; et al. Involvement of Carnosic Acid in the Phytotoxicity of *Rosmarinus officinalis* Leaves. *Toxins* **2018**, *10*, 498. [CrossRef]
31. Boonmee, S.; Iwasaki, A.; Suenaga, K.; Kato-Noguchi, H. Evaluation of phytotoxic activity of leaf and stem extracts and identification of a phytotoxic substance from *Caesalpinia mimosoides* Lamk. *Theor. Exp. Plant Physiol.* **2018**, *30*, 129–139. [CrossRef]
32. Islam, M.S.; Zaman, F.; Iwasaki, A.; Suenaga, K.; Kato-Noguchi, H. Phytotoxic potential of *Chrysopogon aciculatus* (Retz.) Trin. (*Poaceae*). *Weed Biol. Manag.* **2019**, *19*, 51–58. [CrossRef]
33. Rob, M.; Hossen, K.; Iwasaki, A.; Suenaga, K.; Kato-Noguchi, H. Phytotoxic Activity and Identification of Phytotoxic Substances from *Schumannianthus dichotomus*. *Plants* **2020**, *9*, 102. [CrossRef]
34. Đorđević, T.; Sarić-Krsmanović, M.; Umiljendić, J.G. Phenolic Compounds and Allelopathic Potential of Fermented and Unfermented Wheat and Corn Straw Extracts. *Chem. Biodivers.* **2019**, *16*, e1800420. [CrossRef]
35. Chon, S.-U.; Jang, H.-G.; Kim, D.-K.; Kim, Y.-M.; Boo, H.-O. Allelopathic potential in lettuce (*Lactuca sativa* L.) plants. *Sci. Hortic.* **2005**, *106*, 309–317. [CrossRef]

36. Benković, V.; Orsolić, N.; Knezević, A.H.; Ramić, S.; Dikić, D.; Basić, I.; Kopjar, N. Evaluation of the radioprotective effects of propolis and flavonoids in gamma-irradiated mice: The alkaline comet assay study. *Biol. Pharm. Bull.* **2008**, *31*, 167–172. [CrossRef]
37. ArrayExpress—A Database of Functional Genomics Experiments. Available online: http://www.ebi.ac.uk/arrayexpress/ (accessed on 12 November 2012).
38. European Medicinal Agency. *Assessment Report on Angelica sinensis (Oliv.) Diels, Radix*; EMA/HMPC/614586/2012; European Medicinal Agency: Amsterdam, The Netherlands, 2013.
39. Siriamornpun, S.; Kaewseejan, N. Quality, bioactive compounds and antioxidant capacity of selected climacteric fruits with relation to their maturity. *Sci. Hortic.* **2017**, *221*, 33–42. [CrossRef]
40. Bevilacqua, A.; D'Amato, D.; Sinigaglia, M.; Corbo, M.R. Combination of Homogenization, Citrus Extract and Vanillic Acid for the Inhibition of Some Spoiling and Pathogenic Bacteria Representative of Dairy Microflora. *Food Bioprocess Technol.* **2012**, *6*, 2048–2058. [CrossRef]
41. Kim, J.; Soh, S.Y.; Bae, H.; Nam, S. Antioxidant and phenolic contents in potatoes (*Solanum tuberosum* L.) and micropropagated potatoes. *Appl. Biol. Chem.* **2019**, *62*, 17. [CrossRef]
42. Espinosa, R.R.; Inchingolo, R.; Alencar, S.M.; Rodriguez-Estrada, M.T.; Castro, I.A. Antioxidant activity of phenolic compounds added to a functional emulsion containing omega-3 fatty acids and plant sterol esters. *Food Chem.* **2015**, *182*, 95–104. [CrossRef] [PubMed]
43. Pacheco-Palencia, L.A.; Mertens-Talcott, S.; Talcott, S.T. Chemical Composition, Antioxidant Properties, and Thermal Stability of a Phytochemical Enriched Oil from Açai (*Euterpe oleracea* Mart.). *J. Agric. Food Chem.* **2008**, *56*, 4631–4636. [CrossRef]
44. Zhang, Z.; Liao, L.; Moore, J.; Wu, T.; Wang, Z. Antioxidant phenolic compounds from walnut kernels (*Juglans regia* L.). *Food Chem.* **2009**, *113*, 160–165. [CrossRef]
45. Kim, M.-C.; Kim, S.-J.; Kim, D.-S.; Jeon, Y.-D.; Park, S.J.; Lee, H.S.; Um, J.-Y.; Hong, S.-H. Vanillic acid inhibits inflammatory mediators by suppressing NF-κB in lipopolysaccharide-stimulated mouse peritoneal macrophages. *Immunopharmacol. Immunotoxicol.* **2011**, *33*, 525–532. [CrossRef]
46. Zhao, C.; Jia, Y.; Lu, F. Angelica Stem: A Potential Low-Cost Source of Bioactive Phthalides and Phytosterols. *Molecules* **2018**, *23*, 3065. [CrossRef]
47. Batish, D.R.; Lavanya, K.; Singh, H.P.; Kohli, R.K. Root-mediated Allelopathic Interference of Nettle-leaved Goosefoot (*Chenopodium murale*) on Wheat (*Triticum aestivum*). *J. Agron. Crop. Sci.* **2007**, *193*, 37–44. [CrossRef]
48. Mitić, M.; Janković, S.; Mašković, P.; Arsić, B.; Mitić, J.; Ickovski, J. Kinetic models of the extraction of vanillic acid from pumpkin seeds. *Open Chem.* **2020**, *18*, 22–30. [CrossRef]
49. Macías, F.A.; Simonet, A.M.; Galindo, J.C.G.; Castellano, D. Bioactive phenolics and polar compounds from *Melilotus messanensis*. *Phytochemistry* **1999**, *50*, 35–46. [CrossRef]
50. Parveen, I.; Winters, A.; Threadgill, M.D.; Hauck, B.; Morris, P.; Shah, I.P. Extraction, structural characterisation and evaluation of hydroxycinnamate esters of orchard grass (*Dactylis glomerata*) as substrates for polyphenol oxidase. *Phytochemistry* **2008**, *69*, 2799–2806. [CrossRef]
51. Zheng, W.; Wang, S.Y. Antioxidant Activity and Phenolic Compounds in Selected Herbs. *J. Agric. Food Chem.* **2001**, *49*, 5165–5170. [CrossRef] [PubMed]
52. Almeida, I.V.; Cavalcante, F.; Vicentini, V. Different responses of vanillic acid, a phenolic compound, in HTC cells: Cytotoxicity, antiproliferative activity, and protection from DNA-induced damage. *Genet. Mol. Res.* **2016**, *15*, 1–12. [CrossRef]
53. Sethupathy, S.; Ananthi, S.; Selvaraj, A.; Shanmuganathan, B.; Vigneshwari, L.; Balamurugan, K.; Mahalingam, S.; Pandian, S.K. Vanillic acid from *Actinidia deliciosa* impedes virulence in *Serratia marcescens* by affecting S-layer, flagellin and fatty acid biosynthesis proteins. *Sci. Rep.* **2017**, *7*, 1–17. [CrossRef] [PubMed]
54. Yemiş, G.P.; Pagotto, F.; Bach, S.; Delaquis, P. Effect of Vanillin, Ethyl Vanillin, and Vanillic Acid on the Growth and Heat Resistance of Cronobacter Species. *J. Food Prot.* **2011**, *74*, 2062–2069. [CrossRef]
55. Yemiş, G.P.; Pagotto, F.; Bach, S.; Delaquis, P. Thermal Tolerance and Survival of Cronobacter sakazakii in Powdered Infant Formula Supplemented with Vanillin, Ethyl Vanillin, and Vanillic Acid. *J. Food Sci.* **2012**, *77*, M523–M527. [CrossRef] [PubMed]
56. Robards, K.; Prenzler, P.D.; Tucker, G.; Swatsitang, P.; Glover, W. Phenolic compounds and their role in oxidative processes in fruits. *Food Chem.* **1999**, *66*, 401–436. [CrossRef]

57. Huang, S.-M.; Hsu, C.-L.; Chuang, H.-C.; Shih, P.-H.; Wu, C.-H.; Yen, G.-C. Inhibitory effect of vanillic acid on methylglyoxal-mediated glycation in apoptotic Neuro-2A cells. *NeuroToxicology* **2008**, *29*, 1016–1022. [CrossRef]
58. Itoh, A.; Isoda, K.; Kondoh, M.; Kawase, M.; Kobayashi, M.; Tamesada, M.; Yagi, K. Hepatoprotective Effect of Syringic Acid and Vanillic Acid on Concanavalin A-Induced Liver Injury. *Biol. Pharm. Bull.* **2009**, *32*, 1215–1219. [CrossRef] [PubMed]
59. Kim, S.-J.; Kim, M.-C.; Um, J.-Y.; Hong, S.-H. The Beneficial Effect of Vanillic Acid on Ulcerative Colitis. *Molecules* **2010**, *15*, 7208–7217. [CrossRef]
60. Duke, J.A. *Handbook of Phytochemical Constituents of Gras Herbs and Other Economic Plants*; CRC Press: Boca Raton, FL, USA, 1992; pp. 254–255.
61. Kalinova, J.; Vrchotová, N.; Tříska, J. Exudation of Allelopathic Substances in Buckwheat (*Fagopyrum esculentum* Moench). *J. Agric. Food Chem.* **2007**, *55*, 6453–6459. [CrossRef]
62. Shankar, S.R.M.; Girish, R.; Karthik, N.; Rajendran, R.; Mahendran, V.S. Allelopathic effects of phenolics and terpenoids extracted from *Gmelina arborea* on germination of black gram (*Vigna mungo*) and green gram (*Vigna radiata*). *Allelopath. J.* **2009**, *23*, 323–331.
63. Zhang, T.-T.; Zheng, C.-Y.; Hu, W.; Xu, W.-W.; Wang, H.-F. The allelopathy and allelopathic mechanism of phenolic acids on toxic *Microcystis aeruginosa*. *Environ. Boil. Fishes* **2009**, *22*, 71–77. [CrossRef]
64. Ghareib, H.R.A.; Abdelhamed, M.S.; Ibrahim, O.H. Antioxidative effects of the acetone fraction and vanillic acid from *Chenopodium muraleon* tomato plants. *Weed Biol. Manag.* **2010**, *10*, 64–72. [CrossRef]
65. Khang, D.T.; Anh, L.H.; Ha, P.T.T.; Tuyen, P.T.; Van Quan, N.; Minh, L.T.; Quan, N.T.; Minh, T.N.; Xuan, T.D.; Khanh, T.D.; et al. Allelopathic Activity of Dehulled Rice and its Allelochemicals on Weed Germination. *Int. Lett. Nat. Sci.* **2016**, *58*, 1–10. [CrossRef]
66. Kawada, M.; Ohno, Y.; Ri, Y.; Ikoma, T.; Yuugetu, H.; Asai, T.; Watanabe, M.; Yasuda, N.; Akao, S.; Takemura, G.; et al. Anti-tumor effect of gallic acid on LL-2 lung cancer cells transplanted in mice. *Anti Cancer Drugs* **2001**, *12*, 847–852. [CrossRef]
67. Choubey, S.; Varughese, L.R.; Kumar, V.; Beniwal, V. Medicinal importance of gallic acid and its ester derivatives: A patent review. *Pharm. Pat. Anal.* **2015**, *4*, 305–315. [CrossRef]
68. Li, Z.-H.; Wang, Q.; Ruan, X.; Pan, C.-D.; Jiang, D.-A. Phenolics and Plant Allelopathy. *Molecules* **2010**, *15*, 8933–8952. [CrossRef] [PubMed]
69. Pandurangan, A.K.; Mohebali, N.; Norhaizan, M.E.; Looi, C.Y. Gallic acid attenuates dextran sulfate sodium-induced experimental colitis in BALB/c mice. *Drug Des. Dev. Ther.* **2015**, *9*, 3923–3934. [CrossRef]
70. Zucca, P.; Rosa, A.; Tuberoso, C.I.G.; Piras, A.; Rinaldi, A.; Sanjust, E.; Dessì, M.A.; Rescigno, A.; Sanjust, E. Evaluation of Antioxidant Potential of "Maltese Mushroom" (*Cynomorium coccineum*) by Means of Multiple Chemical and Biological Assays. *Nutrients* **2013**, *5*, 149–161. [CrossRef]
71. Liu, Y.; Carver, J.A.; Calabrese, A.N.; Pukala, T.L. Gallic acid interacts with α-synuclein to prevent the structural collapse necessary for its aggregation. *Biochim. Biophys. Acta Proteins Proteom.* **2014**, *1844*, 1481–1485. [CrossRef]
72. Souza, M.C.; Santos, M.P.; Sumere, B.R.; Silva, L.C.; Cunha, D.T.; Martínez, J.; Barbero, G.F.; Rostagno, M.A. Isolation of gallic acid, caffeine and flavonols from black tea by on-line coupling of pressurized liquid extraction with an adsorbent for the production of functional bakery products. *LWT* **2020**, *117*, 108661. [CrossRef]
73. Chanwitheesuk, A.; Teerawutgulrag, A.; Kilburn, J.D.; Rakariyatham, N. Antimicrobial gallic acid from *Caesalpinia mimosoides* Lamk. *Food Chem.* **2007**, *100*, 1044–1048. [CrossRef]
74. Mansouri, S.M.T.; Farbood, Y.; Sameri, M.J.; Sarkaki, A.; NaghiZadeh, B.; Rafeirad, M. Neuroprotective effects of oral gallic acid against oxidative stress induced by 6-hydroxydopamine in rats. *Food Chem.* **2013**, *138*, 1028–1033. [CrossRef]
75. Rafiee, S.A.; Farhoosh, R.; Sharif, A. Antioxidant Activity of Gallic Acid as Affected by an Extra Carboxyl Group than Pyrogallol in Various Oxidative Environments. *Eur. J. Lipid Sci. Technol.* **2018**, *120*. [CrossRef]
76. Wang, Y.; Wu, C.; Zhou, X.; Zhang, M.; Chen, Y.; Nie, S.; Xie, M. Combined application of gallate ester and α-tocopherol in oil-in-water emulsion: Their distribution and antioxidant efficiency. *J. Dispers. Sci. Technol.* **2019**, *41*, 909–917. [CrossRef]
77. Wang, K.; Zhu, X.; Zhang, K.; Zhu, L.; Zhou, F. Investigation of Gallic Acid Induced Anticancer Effect in Human Breast Carcinoma MCF-7 Cells. *J. Biochem. Mol. Toxicol.* **2014**, *28*, 387–393. [CrossRef]

78. Kim, S.-H.; Jun, C.-D.; Suk, K.; Choi, B.-J.; Lim, H.; Park, S.; Lee, S.H.; Shin, H.-Y.; Kim, D.-K.; Shin, T.-Y. Gallic Acid Inhibits Histamine Release and Pro-inflammatory Cytokine Production in Mast Cells. *Toxicol. Sci.* **2005**, *91*, 123–131. [CrossRef]
79. Sen, S.; Asokkumar, K.; Umamaheswari, M.; Sivashanmugam, A.T.; SubhadraDevi, V. Antiulcerogenic Effect of Gallic Acid in Rats and its Effect on Oxidant and Antioxidant Parameters in Stomach Tissue. *Indian J. Pharm. Sci.* **2013**, *75*, 149–155. [PubMed]
80. Akbari, G. Molecular mechanisms underlying gallic acid effects against cardiovascular diseases: An update review. *Avicenna J. Phytomed.* **2020**, *10*, 11–23.
81. Chao, J.; Huo, T.-I.; Cheng, H.-Y.; Tsai, J.-C.; Liao, J.-W.; Lee, M.-S.; Qin, X.-M.; Hsieh, M.-T.; Pao, L.-H.; Peng, W.-H. Gallic Acid Ameliorated Impaired Glucose and Lipid Homeostasis in High Fat Diet-Induced NAFLD Mice. *PLoS ONE* **2014**, *9*, e96969. [CrossRef]
82. Huang, D.-W.; Chang, W.-C.; Wu, J.S.-B.; Shih, R.-W.; Shen, S.-C. Gallic acid ameliorates hyperglycemia and improves hepatic carbohydrate metabolism in rats fed a high-fructose diet. *Nutr. Res.* **2016**, *36*, 150–160. [CrossRef]
83. Kee, H.J.; Cho, S.-N.; Kim, G.R.; Choi, S.Y.; Ryu, Y.; Kim, I.K.; Hong, Y.J.; Park, H.W.; Ahn, Y.; Cho, J.G.; et al. Gallic acid inhibits vascular calcification through the blockade of BMP2–Smad1/5/8 signaling pathway. *Vasc. Pharmacol.* **2014**, *63*, 71–78. [CrossRef]
84. Jin, L.; Lin, M.Q.; Piao, Z.H.; Cho, J.Y.; Kim, G.R.; Choi, S.Y.; Ryu, Y.; Sun, S.; Kee, H.J.; Jeong, M.H. Gallic acid attenuates hypertension, cardiac remodeling, and fibrosis in mice with NG-nitro-L-arginine methyl ester-induced hypertension via regulation of histone deacetylase 1 or histone deacetylase 2. *J. Hypertens.* **2017**, *35*, 1502–1512. [CrossRef] [PubMed]
85. Saeed, S.; Aslam, S.; Mehmood, T.; Naseer, R.; Nawaz, S.; Mujahid, H.; Firyal, S.; Anjum, A.A.; Sultan, A. Production of Gallic Acid Under Solid-State Fermentation by Utilizing Waste from Food Processing Industries. *Waste Biomass Valoris.* **2020**, 1–9. [CrossRef]
86. Dziga, D.; Suda, M.; Bialczyk, J.; Lechowski, Z.; Czaja-Prokop, U. The alteration of *Microcystis aeruginosa* biomass and dissolved microcystin-LR concentration following exposure to plant-producing phenols. *Environ. Toxicol.* **2007**, *22*, 341–346. [CrossRef]
87. Techer, D.; Fontaine, P.; Personne, A.; Viot, S.; Thomas, M. Allelopathic potential and ecotoxicity evaluation of gallic and nonanoic acids to prevent cyanobacterial growth in lentic systems: A preliminary mesocosm study. *Sci. Total Environ.* **2016**, *547*, 157–165. [CrossRef]
88. Liu, Y.; Li, F.; Huang, Q. Allelopathic effects of gallic acid from *Aegiceras corniculatum* on *Cyclotella caspia*. *J. Environ. Sci.* **2013**, *25*, 776–784. [CrossRef]
89. Vitalini, S.; Orlando, F.; Palmioli, A.; Alali, S.; Airoldi, C.; De Noni, I.; Vaglia, V.; Bocchi, S.; Iriti, M. Different phytotoxic effect of *Lolium multiflorum* Lam. leaves against *Echinochloa oryzoides* (Ard.) Fritsch and *Oriza sativa* L. *Environ. Sci. Pollut. Res.* **2020**, *27*, 33204–33214. [CrossRef]
90. DellaGreca, M.; Fiorentino, A.; Monaco, P.; Previtera, L.; Temussi, F.; Zarrelli, A. New dimeric phenanthrenoids from the rhizomes of *Juncus acutus*. Structure determination and antialgal activity. *Tetrahedron* **2003**, *59*, 2317–2324. [CrossRef]
91. Macías, F.A.; Marín, D.; Oliveros-Bastidas, A.; Molinillo, J.M.G. Optimization of Benzoxazinones as Natural Herbicide Models by Lipophilicity Enhancement. *J. Agric. Food Chem.* **2006**, *54*, 9357–9365. [CrossRef] [PubMed]
92. DellaGreca, M.; Fiorentino, A.; Monaco, P.; Previtera, L.; Zarrelli, A. A new dimeric 9,10-dihydrophenanthrenoid from the rhizome of *Juncus acutus*. *Tetrahedron Lett.* **2002**, *43*, 2573–2575. [CrossRef]
93. Michalowicz, J.; Duda, W. Phenols sources and toxicity. *Pol. J. Environ. Stud.* **2007**, *16*, 347–362.

Publisher's Note: MDPI stays neutral with regard to jurisdictional claims in published maps and institutional affiliations.

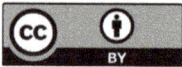

© 2020 by the authors. Licensee MDPI, Basel, Switzerland. This article is an open access article distributed under the terms and conditions of the Creative Commons Attribution (CC BY) license (http://creativecommons.org/licenses/by/4.0/).

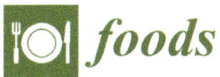

Article

Phenolic and Carotenoid Profile of Lamb's Lettuce and Improvement of the Bioactive Content by Preharvest Conditions

Virginia Hernández [1], M. Ángeles Botella [2], Pilar Hellín [1], Juana Cava [1], Jose Fenoll [1], Teresa Mestre [3], Vicente Martínez [3] and Pilar Flores [1,*]

1 Instituto Murciano de Investigación y Desarrollo Agrario (IMIDA), c/Mayor s/n, La Alberca, 30150 Murcia, Spain; virginia.hernandez5@carm.es (V.H.); mariap.hellin@carm.es (P.H.); juana.cava@carm.es (J.C.); jose.fenoll@carm.es (J.F.)
2 Departamento de Biología Aplicada, Escuela Politécnica Superior de Orihuela (EPSO), Universidad Miguel Hernández, Ctra de Beniel km 3.2, 03312 Orihuela, Spain; mangeles.botella@umh.es
3 Centro de Edafología y Biología Aplicada del Segura (CEBAS), CSIC, Campus Universitario de Espinardo, 30100 Murcia, Spain; tmestre@cebas.csic.es (T.M.); vicente@cebas.csic.es (V.M.)
* Correspondence: mpilar.flores@carm.es

Citation: Hernández, V.; Botella, M.Á.; Hellín, P.; Cava, J.; Fenoll, J.; Mestre, T.; Martínez, V.; Flores, P. Phenolic and Carotenoid Profile of Lamb's Lettuce and Improvement of the Bioactive Content by Preharvest Conditions. *Foods* **2021**, *10*, 188. https://doi.org/10.3390/foods10010188

Received: 14 December 2020
Accepted: 14 January 2021
Published: 18 January 2021

Publisher's Note: MDPI stays neutral with regard to jurisdictional claims in published maps and institutional affiliations.

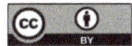

Copyright: © 2021 by the authors. Licensee MDPI, Basel, Switzerland. This article is an open access article distributed under the terms and conditions of the Creative Commons Attribution (CC BY) license (https://creativecommons.org/licenses/by/4.0/).

Abstract: This study characterizes the phenolic, carotenoid and chlorophyll profile of lamb's lettuce, a vegetable whose consumption in salads and ready-to-eat products is constantly growing. The MS/MS analysis allowed the identification of thirty-five phenolic compounds including hydroxybenzoic and hydroxycinnamic acids, flavanones, flavanols and flavanones, many of which are reported here in lamb's lettuce for the first time. Chlorogenic acid was the principal phenolic compound found (57.1% of the total phenolic concentration) followed by its isomer *cis*-5-caffeoylquinic. Other major phenolic compounds were also hydroxycinnamic acids (coumaroylquinic, dicaffeoylquinic and feruloylquinic acids) as well as the flavones luteolin-7-rutinoside, diosmetin-apiosylglucoside and diosmin. Regarding carotenoids, seven xanthophyll and four carotenes, among which β-carotene and lutein were the major compounds, were detected from their UV-Vis absorption spectrum. In addition, chlorophylls a and b, their isomers and derivatives (pheophytin) were identified. Preharvest factors such as reduced fertilization levels or salinity increased some secondary metabolites, highlighting the importance of these factors on the final nutritional value of plant foods. Lamb's lettuce was seen to be a good potential source of bioactive compounds, and fertilization management might be considered a useful tool for increasing its nutritional interest.

Keywords: corn salad; leafy vegetables; phytochemicals; liquid chromatography; mass spectrometry

1. Introduction

The regular consumption of fruit and vegetables has many benefits for human health in terms of reducing the possibility of developing chronic diseases [1]. It has been estimated that a high intake of fruit and vegetables can reduce the risk of developing cardiovascular diseases [2] and several types of cancer [3]. Most of these health-promoting effects are related to the vegetable bioactive content. Phenolics are the most abundant antioxidants in the human diet [4], of which approximately a third correspond to phenolic acids and two thirds to flavonoids [1]. Several reports indicate that polyphenolic compounds are effective in the prevention of diseases caused by long-term diabetes such as cardiovascular disease, neuropathy, nephropathy and retinopathy [5]. Moreover, phenolic compounds seem to inhibit cell proliferation and tumor metastasis and induce apoptosis in various types of cancer cells, including colon, lung, prostate, hepatocellular, breast cancer or multiple myeloma [6,7]. While many plants contain phenolic compounds, their concentration and chemical forms depend on individual plant species. Vegetables and fruits are also rich in carotenoids, molecules with a high antioxidant capacity, and the consumption of a diet rich in carotenoids is thought to reduce the risk of cancer, cardiovascular diseases, age-related maculopathy and cataracts [8]. The influence of chlorophylls on human health has not been as widely studied as that of phenolic compounds and carotenoids, although evidence of their benefits has been reported [9].

Due to their importance in human health, the characterization of bioactive compounds contained in fruits and vegetables and their related beneficial effects need to be studied in greater depth. Specifically, green leafy vegetables can be a source of ascorbic acid, flavonoids, phenolic acids and carotenoids, besides minerals, fiber and many trace elements. Lettuce and escarole have long been the most common vegetables used in salads, partly due to their healthy attributes, and several studies about characterization of polyphenols in lettuce can be found in the literature [10,11]. However, new leafy vegetables are increasingly consumed in salads, especially as ready to eat products. Among them lamb's lettuce (*Valerianella locusta* L. Laterr.) has special relevance due to its pleasant taste and texture and nutritional value. However, information on *V. locusta* in the literature is scarce and mostly focuses on the shelf-life and quality changes that may take place during postharvest storage [12] or by some preharvest conditions [13–16]. Plant development and yield are strongly affected by mineral nutrition and environmental stresses that reallocate resources from primary to secondary metabolism with a direct effect on product quality [15]. In some species it has been shown that salt stress induced the synthesis of substances in proportion to the increase in NaCl concentrations, confirming the important role of these molecules for the tolerance to stress conditions in plants and salinity as an efficient technique for increasing the secondary metabolite content in plants [17]. However, little information on the phytochemical profile of *V. locusta* can be found, with the exception of some recent works [18]. Moreover, despite the well-documented impact that mineral nutrition and irrigation water quality have on the biochemical composition of plants, and hence on the nutritional value of vegetables, there is hardly any information about how these preharvest aspects can affect lamb's lettuce quality.

The main objective of the present study was the characterization of the phenolic, carotenoid and chlorophyll profile of lamb's lettuce. Taking into consideration mineral nutrition and salinity as two of the preharvest factors that most affect the quality of plant foods, the impact of fertilization and salinity (NaCl content) on the bioactive compound content of lamb's lettuce was also evaluated.

2. Materials and Methods

2.1. Plant Material

Lamb's lettuce (*Valerianella locusta* L. Laterr. cv. Favor) plants were grown in a greenhouse equipped with a dynamic root floating system that pumped the nutrient solution from a tank into different containers (trays). Plants were supported through a floating board made of high-density polyethylene. The roots were fully submerged in the nutrient solution that circulated back to the tank through a drain for reuse. The pH of each nutrient solution was adjusted to between 5.5 and 6.0 every day. Water lost by transpiration was replaced every two days and nutrients were added every week to restore their initial concentrations. In order to study the impact of fertilization and salinity on the bioactive compound content, the control nutrient solution [½ Hoagland solution, electrical conductivity (EC)1 dS cm^{-1}, 7 mM N, 2 mM Ca and 3.5 mM K] was modified to obtain different treatments in four consecutive experiments with different levels of nitrogen (0.1, 1 and 7 mM N), calcium (0.5, 2, and 5 mM Ca), potassium (0.1, 0.5 and 3.5 mM K), and salinity (0, 15, 30 and 60 mM NaCl), respectively. In every experiment, the plants were distributed in two blocks with three replicates per treatment and block. Each replicate consisted of a tray (3.6 m^{-2}) containing 100 plants m^{-2}. Salinity treatments consisted of applying 15 mM NaCl on one, two or four days (for the 15, 30 and 60 mM NaCl treatments, respectively) in order to avoid an osmotic shock. Final ECs of the different saline treatments were 1 (control), 2.7, 4.0 and 6.5 dS cm^{-1}. Thirty days after transplanting (DAT), when the plant had five fully expanded leaves, fifty plants per replicate were harvested and weighed after being washed and gently dried. They were then powdered with liquid N_2 and kept at $-80\ °C$ until subsequent analysis. Each sample was analyzed in triplicate.

2.2. Metabolite Analyses

2.2.1. Phenolic Compounds

Phenolic compounds were extracted with methanol:formic acid (97:3) according to Cantos et al. [19] and analyzed using an Agilent 1200 liquid chromatograph (Santa Clara, CA, USA) equipped with a G6410A triple quadrupole mass spectrometer detector (MS/MS) equipped with an electrospray ionization (ESI) interface, operating in negative ion mode. A Lichrosphere C_{18} analytical column of 250 mm × 4 mm and 5 μm particle size was used (Agilent Technologies, Waldbronn, Germany). The mobile phase was 0.1% formic acid in water (solvent A) and 0.1% formic acid in acetonitrile (solvent B) at a flow rate of 1 mL·min^{-1}. The gradient began with 5% B, raised to 10% B in 9 min, 30% in 50 min, and 100% in 2 min and held at 100% B for an additional 3 min before returning to initial conditions in 1 min and remaining isocratic for 6 min. The following operation parameters were used: 2000 V capillary voltage, 60 psi nebulizer pressure, 13 L/min drying gas flow and 350 °C drying gas temperature. Fragmentor voltages (F) from 20 to 200 V and collision energies (CE) from 2 to 50 V were used for optimizing selective reaction monitoring (SRM) transitions. Myricetin (Sigma-Aldrich, St. Louis, MO, USA) was used as internal standard. The phenolic compounds were identified by MS/MS experiments: full scan and neutral loss (NL), precursor ion (PreI) and product ion (ProdI) scan modes. Protocatechuic, luteolin−7-O-glucoside, diosmetin, diosmin, apigenin−7-O-glucoside, hesperidin (hesperetin−7-O-rutinoside) (Extrasynthese, Genay, France) and chlorogenic acid (5-O-caffeoylquinic acid), caffeic acid, p-coumaric acid, luteolin, and quercetin were quantified with respect to their standards (Sigma-Aldrich, Steinheim, Germany). Chlorogenic isomers were quantified with respect to chlorogenic acid; caffeic acid-O-hexosides, dicaffeoylquinic and caffeoylferuloylquinic acid with respect to caffeic acid; sinapic-hexose with respect to sinapic acid (Sigma-Aldrich, Steinheim, Germany); coumaroylquinic isomers with respect to p-coumaric acid; feruloylquinic isomers with respect to ferulic acid (Sigma-Aldrich, Steinheim, Germany); isorhamnetin-rutinoside with respect to isorhamnetin (Sigma-Aldrich, Steinheim, Germany); luteolin-apiosylglucoside and luteolin−7–rutinoside with respect to lutein-7-O-glucoside; quercetin-glucuronide, quercetin-glucoside with respect to quercetin; apigenin-rutinoside and acacetin-rutinoside with respect to apigenin−7-O-glucoside; diosmetin-apiosylglucoside with respect to diosmin.

2.2.2. Carotenoids

Carotenoids and chlorophylls were extracted with methanol/tetrahydrofuran (1:1, v/v) containing MgO (Merck, Darmstadt, Germany) and 0.1% (w/v) butylated hydroxytoluene (BHT) (Sigma-Aldrich, St. Louis, MO, USA) following the methodology validated by Motilva et al. [20]. For that, an Agilent Series 1100 liquid chromatograph (Santa Clara, CA, USA) equipped with a photodiode array detector (DAD) and a 250 mm × 4.6 mm i.d., 3 μm two serially coupled Prontosil C_{30} columns Bischoff (Leonberg, Germany) were used. The mobile phase was methanol (solvent A) and methyl tert-butyl ether (solvent B) eluted at a flow rate of 1.0 mL/min, as follows: (1) initial conditions 15% solvent B and 85% solvent A, maintained for 20 min (2) a 20-min linear gradient to 30% solvent B, then maintained for 10 min (3) a 80-min linear gradient to 90% solvent B. Compounds were eluted and recorded for 70 min and the subsequent gradient allowed the column to be cleaned. All-*trans*-violaxanthin, 9 *cis*-neoxanthin, antheraxanthin, all-*trans*-lutein, zeaxanthin, β-cryptoxanthin, all-*trans*-β-carotene and all-*trans*-α-carotene were quantified using commercially available external standards (DHI LAB, Hoersholm, Denmark). Luteoxanthin was quantified with respect to antheraxanthin. The *cis* isomers of β-carotene were quantified with respect to all-*trans*-β-carotene. β-apo-8′-carotenal (Sigma-Aldrich, St. Louis, MO, USA) was added as internal standard.

2.2.3. Vitamin C

For the study of the impact of fertilization and salinity on the bioactive composition, the vitamin C concentration was determined according to Fenoll et al. [21], using HPLC with an MS/MS detector.

2.2.4. Statistical Analysis

The results were statistically analyzed using IBM SPSS Statistic 21 by analysis of variance (ANOVA) and Tukey's test for differences between means.

3. Results and Discussion

3.1. Phenolic Compounds

3.1.1. Hydroxybenzoic Acid

Protocatechuic acid (compound 1) was directly identified by comparing its retention time and mass spectrum with those of the corresponding standard, with $[M - H]^-$ at m/z 153 and a main fragment at m/z 109 due to the loss of CO_2 from the carboxylic acid [22] (Table 1). It is a widely distributed, naturally occurring phenolic acid, which is frequently found in commonly consumed products of plant origin such as onion, plum, grapes, nuts and spices [23]. In lamb's lettuce protocatechuic acid was detected in very low concentrations compared with other phenolic compounds.

Table 1. Phenolic compounds identified in lamb's lettuce by MS/MS approaches. Retention time (RT, min), precursor ion ($[M - H]^-$), base peak (100% relative abundance) (bp) and other fragments (and their relative abundances) detected in the product ion mode and concentration (C) of each compound ($\mu g\ g^{-1}$ fresh weight).

	Compound	RT	$[M - H]^-$	bp	Product Ions	C [a]
1	Protocatechuic	11.65	153	109		0.015
2	3-Caffeoylquinic acid	12.31	353	191	179(55), 135(6)	0.15
3	Caffeic acid-O-hexoside 1	14.28	341	179	135(10)	0.093
4	Caffeic acid-O-hexoside 2	16.71	341	179	135(4)	0.036
5	Caffeic acid-O-hexoside 3	17.33	341	179	135(14)	0.011
6	5-Caffeoylquinic acid	18.06	353	191	179(2), 173(1)	367.6
7	4-Caffeoylquinic acid	18.46	353	173	191(55), 179(85), 135(40)	3.2
8	Sinapic acid-hexoside 1	19.18	385	223	208(3), 179(5), 164(5)	7.4
9	Caffeic acid	20.47	179	135		2.3
10	cis-5-Caffeoylquinic acid	20.96	353	191	179(7), 173(1)	55.5
11	Sinapic acid-hexoside 2	21.89	385	223	208(5), 179(3), 164(2)	5.2
12	cis 5-O-p-Coumaroylquinic	23.48	337	191	173(6), 163(4)	35.1
13	trans 5-O-p-Feruloylquinic acid	25.73	367	191	173(8)	20.1
14	trans 5-O-p-Coumaroylquinic acid	25.93	337	191	173(1), 163(1)	27.1
15	p-Coumaric acid	27.53	163	119		0.056
16	cis 5-O-p-Feruloylquinic acid	28.01	367	191	173(3)	10.0
17	Luteolin-7-O-apiosylglucoside	32.80	579	285		1.2
18	Luteolin-7-rutinoside	33.72	593	285		27.9
19	Isorhamnetin-rutinoside	34.18	623	315		1.5
20	Quercetin-glucuronide	34.51	477	301		0.01
21	Luteolin-7-O-glucoside	34.99	447	285		0.20
22	Quercetin-3-O-glucoside	35.09	463	300	301(35)	0.031
23	3,4-Dicaffeoylquinic acid	35.98	515	353	191(6), 179(5), 173(2)	3.1
24	3,5-Dicaffeoylquinic acid	37.61	515	353	191(5), 179(4)	26.1
25	Apigenin-rutinoside	38.12	577	269		0.25
26	Hesperidin	38.48	609	301		1.1
27	Diosmetin-apiosylglucoside	39.75	593	299	284(1)	23.9
28	4,5-Dicaffeoylquinic acid	40.50	515		191(15), 179(50), 173(65)	1.5
29	Apigenin-7-O-glucoside	40.69	431	269		0.012
30	Diosmin	40.80	607	299	284(1)	21.6
31	Feruloyl-caffeoylquinic acid	43.91	529	353	367(55), 191(10), 179(17)	0.043
32	Acacetin-rutinoside	50.00	591	283		1.1
33	Quercetin	50.99	301	151	179(24), 121(42), 107(33)	0.15
34	Luteolin	51.14	285	133	175(10), 151(10)	0.051
35	Diosmetin	54.78	299	284	256(11)	0.16

[a] Mean values of plants (edible part) grown in standard conditions (½ Hoagland).

3.1.2. Hydroxycinnamic Acids and Derivatives

Chlorogenic (5-O-caffeoylquinic acid) (compound **6**), caffeic (compound **9**) and *p*-coumaric (compound **15**) acids were directly identified by comparing their retention times with those of their corresponding standards and confirmed by MS/MS experiments. In the mass spectrum of compounds **9** and **15**, characteristic m/z values of 135 and 119, respectively, were observed, indicating the loss of CO_2. In addition to 5-O-caffeoylquinic acid, the presence of another three caffeoylquinic acid isomers (compounds **2**, **7** and **10**) was confirmed by the loss of 162 Da (caffeic acid units) and their characteristic product ion patterns. Compound **2** was identified as neochlorogenic (3-O-caffeoylquinic acid) due to its relative retention time, its base peak at m/z 191 (quinic) and the intensity of fragment ions at m/z 179 and 135 [24]. Compound **7** was identified as cryptochlorogenic (4-O-caffeoylquinic acid) according to its base peak m/z 173 [quinic–H–H_2O]$^-$ and the typical less abundant fragment ions m/z 179, 191 and 135. Compound **10** was tentatively identified as cis-5-caffeoylquinic acid according to its retention time and fragmentation pattern, which was identical to 5-caffeoylquinic acid [25]. In agreement with previous studies in the study by V. locusta [18], chlorogenic acid was the principal phenolic compound found, to account, in our case, for 57.1% of the total phenolic concentration. Similarly to lamb's lettuce, both lettuce and escarole have a high chlorogenic acid content, but in both the main hidroxycinnamic acid derivatives are O-caffeoylmalic acid and dicaffeoyltartaric acid [11]. Chlorogenic acid is a major phenolic compound in the leaves of other plant species, such as some Ericacea species [26] and many herbs [27]. Chlorogenic acid is one of the main polyphenols in the human diet, and it has been reported to have a variety of beneficial effects: for example, antioxidant [28], antidiabetic [29], antihypertensive [30] and anticancer [31] activities. It has been proposed as a nutraceutical for the prevention and treatment of the metabolic syndrome and associated disorders and as a food additive due to its potential to prevent the degradation of other bioactive compounds, and its prebiotic activity in humans [27].

Three compounds with fragment ions at m/z 341 (compounds **3**, **4** and **5**) were identified as caffeic acid O-hexoside derivatives and their identities were confirmed by a neutral loss scan of 162 Da and precursor scan experiments of 179 (caffeic). In addition, a product ion experiment revealed the characteristic loss of CO_2 (m/z 135). As previously described, the glycosides eluted before their aglycone (caffeic acid) [32]. Although these and other caffeic derivatives are the main polyphenols in green leafy vegetables [11], they were found at relatively low concentrations in lamb's lettuce.

The presence of three dicaffeoylquinic acids (compounds **23**, **24** and **28**) was confirmed by a parent ion at m/z 515 and a main product ion at m/z 353 (−162 Da, loss of caffeoyl moiety). The elution order of these compounds and the relative abundance of fragments at m/z 191, 179 173 and 135 led us to tentatively identify the compounds as 3,4-dicaffeoylquinic, 3,5-dicaffeoylquinic and 4,5-dicaffeoylquinic acids [25]. After chlorogenic acid, dicaffeoylquinic was the most abundant caffeoyl derivative in lamb's lettuce. It is also present in lettuce [33] and in wild rosemary (*Eriocephalus africanus* L.), in which mono- and dicaffeolquinic acids were seen to represent 90% and 74%, respectively, of the total phenolics [34].

The product scan MS mode was used to monitor the fragmentation patterns of the ions with m/z 337 for coumaroylquinic (compounds **12** and **14**) and m/z 367 for feruloylquinic (compounds **13** and **16**) acids. All these hydroxycinnamoylquinic acids produce an intense ion at m/z 191 [quinic acid−H]$^-$. Coumaroyl quinic acids also showed fragment ions at m/z 173 (loss of H_2O) and 163 (loss of coumaroyl moiety). As both isomers (compounds **12** and **14**) showed identical fragmentation patterns, they were identified as cis 5-O-p-coumaroylquinic and trans 5-O-p-coumaroylquinic acids, according to the mass spectral characteristics reported by Baeza et al. [25]. Similarly, feruloylquinic acids (compounds **13** and **16**) presented mass spectral characteristic compatible with the isomer 5-O-p-feruoylquinic acid [25]. Once again, both compounds showed identical fragmentation so that they were tentatively identified as trans and cis 5-O-p-feruloylquinic acids.

Coumaroylquinic acid was the second most common phenolic compound in lamb's lettuce (9.7% of the total). It has also been found in lettuce [33], broccoli [35] and in several aromatic herbs [36]. Feruloylquinic acid was the fifth-ranked major compound in lamb's lettuce. It can be found in a number of fruits such as blackcurrant, apricot, peach and plum [37], but few references have been found for leafy vegetables. In particular, feruloylquinic acid has been found Cichorium endivia [38] and recently it has been reported in *Artemisia annua* L. leaves [39].

Compound **31** was identified as feruloyl-caffeoylquinic acid based on its precursor ion at m/z 529, the base compound at m/z 353, produced by the loss of the feruloyl unit, and another intense ion at m/z 367 resulting from the loss of a caffeoyl unit [40]. This compound was found in lamb's lettuce at low concentration.

Two compounds (compounds **8** and **11**) with an ion mass signal at m/z 385 were detected and identified as sinapic acid-hexoside according to their MS spectrum and previous data described by other authors in tronchuda cabbage [41]. In both compounds, the main fragment was found at m/z 223 (sinapic acid). In addition, minor product ions were observed at m/z 265 (loss of a part of hexose ring), 208 (methyl radical loss), 179 (decarboxylation), and 164 (combined methyl radical loss and decarboxylation). Sinapic acid and its derivatives have not received so much attention as other hydroxycinnamic acids, but their antioxidant and antibacterial effects are interesting for their application as natural food preservatives and for developing functional foods [42].

3.1.3. Flavones

The aglycone luteolin (compound **34**) was identified by comparing its mass spectrum with that of the standard, which presented the expected fragmentation patterns with a precursor ion at m/z 285 and a characteristic fragment ion at m/z 133 and other fragment ions at m/z 175 and 151. Luteolin−7-O-glucoside (compound **21**) was identified by comparison of its retention time and mass spectrum with those of the corresponding standard. In addition, two more luteolin derivatives (compounds **17** and **18**) were detected and tentatively identified as luteolin−7-O-apiosylglucoside ([M − H]$^-$ at m/z 579) and luteolin-7-rutinoside ([M − H]$^-$ at m/z 593), both presenting the main fragment ion at m/z 285 (luteolin). Their identities were confirmed by their precursor ion spectra and neutral losses of 294 Da (162 + 132 Da) (apiosylglucoside moiety), 308 Da (146 + 162 Da) (rhamnosylglucoside moiety) and 162 Da (hexoside moiety) for compounds **17**, **18** and **21**, respectively. Luteolin is a flavone that usually occurs in its glycosylated forms in camomile and other species belonging to the Asteraceae family among others [43]. In lamb's lettuce (thepresent study), luteolin-7-rutinoside was the main flavonoid found (4.3% of total phenolics). Several epidemiological studies have shown that luteolin possesses antioxidant, anti-inflammatory, antimicrobial and anticancer activities [43]. Luteolin-7-rutinoside has been previously identified in lettuce [11] and Mentha piperita [44] and luteolin-7-O-apiosylglucoside in celery [45].

The identification of compound **35** (diosmetin) and compound **30** (diosmin) was confirmed by comparing their retention times and mass spectra with their standards. Diosmetin presented the base compound ion at m/z 284 as a result of the loss of a methyl unit and further fragment ion at m/z 256 [M − H − CH$_3$−CO]$^-$. Diosmin showed the base peak ion at m/z 299 as a result of the loss of 308 Da (162 + 146). Compound **27** exhibited the [M − H]$^-$ ion at m/z 593, and a neutral loss of 294 Da (apiosylglucoside moiety), yielding fragment ions at m/z 299 (diosmetin), so that it was identified as diosmetin-apiosylglucoside. Diosmetin and its derivatives are mainly found in citrus fruits [46] but they have also been identified in parsley [47]. In lamb's lettuce, the major forms were diosmin and diosmetin-apiosylglucoside. Diosmetin and its derivatives have been seen to possess potential biological activity with anticancer anti-inflammatory, antioxidant, antimicrobial and oestrogenic activities [48].

Other flavones found in lamb's lettuce were two apigenin derivatives: by comparison with its standard, compound **29** with [M − H]$^-$ ion at m/z 431 and a fragment at m/z

269 (resulting from the loss of a glucoside moiety) identified as apigenin−7-O-glucoside, while compound **25** with [M − H]⁻ ion at m/z 577 was identified as apigenin-rutinoside, since it exhibited the fragment at m/z 269, which is related to the loss of 308 Da (162 + 146). Apigenin−7-O-glucoside has been found as major polyphenol in chamomile flowers [49], while apigenin-rutinoside has been isolated from *Mentha longifolia* L. for use as condiment and a herbal tea [50]. In lamb's lettuce, apigenin derivatives were found as minor polyphenolic compounds.

The precursor ion of compound **32** was detected at m/z 591 and a characteristic MS/MS fragment ion at m/z 283 (−308 Da), so it was tentatively identified as acacetin-rutinoside. This flavone has been identified in Compositae species [51].

3.1.4. Flavonols

Quercetin (compound **33**) was directly identified by comparison of its retention time with the corresponding standard and confirmed by MS/MS experiments. It showed a precursor ion at m/z 301, a characteristic fragment ion at m/z 151 and other fragment ions at m/z 179, 121 and 107. As regards quercetin derivatives, compound **20** was identified as quercetin-glucuronide with an [M − H]⁻ ion at m/z 477 and the main fragment ions at m/z 301 due to the loss of a glucuronyl (176 Da) unit. Compound **22** with an [M − H]⁻ ion at m/z 463, presented two high intensity fragments at m/z 301 [M − H − 162]⁻ and 300 [M − H − 162]⁻•. The radical aglycone was the most abundant fragment for collision energies from 5 to 30 eV and presented similar abundance to that of the aglycone at higher collision energies. The higher intensity of the radical aglycone compared with the aglycone suggested 3-OH was the glycosylation site [52], so this compound was attributed to quercetin−3-O-glucoside. The concentrations of both quercetin and its derivatives were low in lamb's lettuce compared to other polyphenols.

Compound **19** was identified as isorhamnetin-rutinoside with an [M − H]⁻ ion at m/z 623 and a characteristic product ion at m/z 315 corresponding to isorhamnetin aglycone and a loss of 308 Da (rutinose). This compound is commonly extracted from marigold for medicinal purposes (*Calendula officinalis* L.) [53] but is also found in other vegetables such as *Asparagus acutifolius* [54].

3.1.5. Flavanones

The mass spectral characteristics of compound **26**, with [M − H]⁻ at m/z 609 and the main fragment at m/z 301 as a result of the loss of a rutinoside moiety (−308 Da), corresponded to hesperetin−7-O-rutinoside (hesperidin), which is a common flavanone in citrus fruits [55] but the only one we detected in lamb's lettuce.

3.2. Carotenoid and Chlorophyll Profiling
3.2.1. Carotenoids

The chromatographic behavior and UV-Vis absorption spectrum allowed identification of seven xanthophyll and four carotene pigments in lamb's lettuce leaves (Table 2). All-trans-violaxanthin (compound **1**), 9 cis-neoxanthin (compound **2**), antheraxanthin (compound **4**), all-trans-lutein (compound **7**), zeaxanthin (compound **8**) and β-cryptoxanthin (compound **12**) were identified based on a comparison of their retention times and spectra with those of the corresponding standard. Taking into consideration its chromatographic and spectroscopic properties, compound **3** was identified as luteoxanthin [56]. In agreement with the results reported for other leafy vegetables, lutein was the major xanthophyll found in lamb's lettuce (28% of total carotenoid content), with values in the range of those described for different types of lettuce [57]. As expected for a green leafy vegetable, neoxanthin was found in the 9 or 9′ cis isomer form [58] since this isomer is present in the chloroplasts, while the all-trans-neoxanthin is found only in non-photosynthetic organs [59]. However, contrarily to the results reported for other species [57], the neoxanthin concentration was higher than that of violaxanthin. Minor xanthophylls such as zeaxanthin and β-cryptoxanthin were present in concentrations well over the values reported for other leafy vegetables [60]. Antheraxanthin has previously been found in commonly consumed leafy vegetables such as spinach [61], chicory, dandelion, garden rocket wild rocket [62]. The presence of luteoxanthin has been reported in spinach [63] and medical herbs [1], but our study identified it, for the first time, in lamb's lettuce. The role of xanthophylls in vision health has been extensively studied. Zeaxanthin and lutein, particularly, play an important role in photoprotection against macular degeneration and there is also evidence that zeaxanthin and lutein play a role in visual and auditory processing, general mental acuity, and protection against various chronic diseases [64].

Table 2. Tentative identification, retention time (RT, min) spectral characteristic (absorbance maxima and Q-ratios found in the present study and those reported in the literature) and concentration (C, µg g^{-1} fresh weight) of carotenoids and chlorophylls in lamb's lettuce. Wavelengths given in parenthesis denote shoulders.

	Compound	RT		λ (nm)			Q_{ratio} Found	Q_{ratio} Reported	C [a]
1	all-*trans*-violaxanthin	10.68		416	440	468			5.5
2	9 or 9'-*cis*-neoxanthin	11.58	328	412	436	464	0.11	0.13 [56]	8.1
3	luteoxanthin	12.44		398	422	448			3.3
4	antheraxanthin	14.72		422	444	472			3.8
5	chlorophyll b	15.42		468	602	652			
6	chlorophyll b'	17.26		468	602	652			
7	all-*trans*-lutein	17.96		(422)	444	472			27.2
8	zeaxanthin	22.24		(428)	450	478			0.62
9	chlorophyll a	23.45		432	618	666			
10	chlorophyll a'	27.09		432	618	666			
11	β-apo-8'-carotenal [b]	28.38			466				
12	β-cryptoxanthin	38.52		(426)	452	478			0.41
13	13-*cis*-β-carotene	44.59	338	(424)	446	470	0.39	0.35 [62]	1.9
14	all-*trans*-α-carotene	47.55		(426)	446	474			1.2
15	pheophytin a	53.22	408	506	538	610	666		
16	all-*trans*-β-carotene	54.93		(428)	452	478			57.4
17	pheophytin a'	56.85	408	506	538	610	666		
18	9-*cis*-β-carotene	59.81	342	(426)	446	474	0.08	0.10 [63]	3.2

[a] Mean values of plants (edible part) grown in standard conditions (½ Hoagland). [b] Internal standard.

The identification of both all-trans-β-carotene and all-trans-α-carotene was based on the use of their standards. In the case of cis-isomers, their spectral fine structure and peak cis intensity were considered (Table 2). Compounds **13** and **18** were identified as 13-cis- and 9-cis-β-carotene, respectively, according to their order of elution, the hypsochromic shift of 9 and 5 nm, and the Q-ratios similar to those previously reported [65,66]. Carotenes represented 66% of the total carotenoid content, all-trans-β-carotene being the major carotene (accounting for 58% of total carotenoids), as previously has been previously reported for lamb's lettuce and other leafy vegetables [67]. Among carotenes, β-carotene exhibits the highest pro-vitamin A potential, although α-carotene and β-cryptoxanthin play a similar role. In addition to many other fundamental functions in human health, β-carotene helps prevent the progression of eye diseases by quenching free radicals and thus attenuating oxidative stress [68].

3.2.2. Chlorophylls

Chromatographic analysis with two serially coupled C_{30} columns allowed the simultaneous separation of chlorophylls and carotenoids (Table 2). According to their characteristic UV-Vis spectra, compounds **5** and **9** corresponded to chlorophylls a and b, respectively [69]. In additions, compounds **6** and **10** were identified as chlorophylls a' and b'. These two chlorophyll epimeric isomers have identical absorption spectra to those of chlorophylls a and b, which eluted before their corresponding epimers due to their higher polarity [70]. Finally, the absorbance spectra and the chromatographic behavior of compounds **15** and **17** were in agreement with those reported for pheophytin a and pheophytin a' [70].

As the role of carotenoids as bioactive compounds has been widely investigated, studies on chlorophylls are relatively scarce. There have been some reports on the antioxidant capacity of chlorophylls [71,72]. Ferruzzi et al. [8] have suggested that chlorophylls may play a role in human health and disease prevention. Indeed, the potential bioactivity of dietary chlorophyll derivatives with antioxidant and antimutagenic activities has been suggested. The antioxidant action of chlorophyll has been observed in vivo, providing protection to the liver and kidneys from the oxidative stress caused by sodium nitrate [73]. However, compared with carotenoids, little is known about chlorophyll metabolites, their absorption, transport, metabolic pathways and their oxidation mechanisms [72], and more studies are needed.

3.3. Effect of Mineral Nutrition and Salinity on Lamb's Lettuce Composition

In order to know the effect of mineral nutrition on the different phenolic compounds, they were grouped into phenolic families. The calcium (Ca) concentration and salinity of the nutrient solution had no effect on the main phenolic families (Table 3), while potassium (K) and nitrogen (N) levels had a significant effect on most of the families. The lowest K concentration (0.1 mM) significantly increased flavone (37%), and flavanone (46%) concentrations compared to treatment with 3.5 mM K. The flavanone content was also significantly higher (45%) in the 0.5 mM K treatment than in the presence of the highest K concentration. Reducing the concentration of N from 7 mM to 1 or 0.1 mM had a similar effect, leading to significantly higher hydroxycinnamic acid (40–48%), flavonol (40–44%) and flavanone (2.6–3.6-fold) concentrations. In addition, treatment with 0.1 mM N increased the flavone content to a greater extent (3.5-fold) than 1 mM N (2.3-fold). In agreement with the results for lamb's lettuce, a K deficiency in spinach increased total phenolic and flavonoid contents in non-saline conditions [74]. Similarly, in lettuce and other leafy vegetables, previous studies have also shown that a reduction in the N supply enhances the phenolic content and antioxidant capacity [75,76]. Moreover, the extracts from lettuce plants grown under low nitrogen conditions had a more pronounced anti-proliferative effect on colorectal cancer than those from lettuce grown with an adequate nitrogen supply, which was attributed to enhanced phenolic concentrations [77]. For this reason, the authors suggested that vegetables with improved health-related properties could be developed by increasing the phenolic content through a reduction in nitrogen nutrition.

Table 3. Concentration of main phenolic families ($\mu g\ g^{-1}$ fresh weight) in lamb's lettuce under different nutritional conditions. Values are means $\pm$ SE (n = 4).

	mM	Hydroxicinamic	Flavones	Flavonols	Flavanones
Ca	0.5	838 ± 90	113 ± 9	3.54 ± 0.54	4.27 ± 0.67
	2	771 ± 12	119 ± 7	3.96 ± 0.21	3.70 ± 0.12
	5	779 ± 20	130 ± 9	4.50 ± 0.48	4.90 ± 0.31
		n.s.	n.s.	n.s.	n.s.
K	0.1	302 ± 49	44 ± 1 [b]	0.46 ± 0.15	1.66 ± 0.13 [b]
	0.5	259 ± 17	37 ± 2 [a]	0.21 ± 0.10	1.64 ± 0.20 [b]
	3.5	235 ± 29	32 ± 1 [a]	0.30 ± 0.24	1.13 ± 0.12 [a]
		n.s.	**	n.s.	*
N	0.1	840 ± 18 [b]	263 ± 4 [c]	2.32 ± 0.16 [b]	3.09 ± 0.26 [b]
	1	791 ± 85 [b]	173 ± 29 [b]	2.38 ± 0.24 [b]	3.73 ± 0.67 [b]
	7	565 ± 12 [a]	76 ± 4 [a]	1.65 ± 0.14 [a]	1.05 ± 0.06 [a]
		**	***	*	**
NaCl	C	479 ± 16	63 ± 2	2.10 ± 0.18	0.92 ± 0.12
	15	471 ± 25	60 ± 2	1.99 ± 0.32	0.87 ± 0.07
	30	480 ± 56	52 ± 2	1.87 ± 0.34	0.74 ± 0.05
	60	397 ± 116	46 ± 13	2.19 ± 0.41	0.75 ± 0.19
		n.s.	n.s.	n.s.	n.s.

*, **, *** Significant differences between means at 5, 1 or 0.1% level of probability, respectively; n.s., non-significant at p = 5%. For each stage, different letters in the same column indicate significant differences between means according to Duncan's test at the 5% level.

The carotenoid content of lamb's lettuce was significantly affected by K and N levels and salinity, but not by Ca (Table 4). The lowest level of K (0.1 mM) significantly increased total carotenoids (82%), mainly as a result of the increase in β-carotene and lutein, the major carotenoids identified in the present work (data not shown). Similar results in relation to K have been found in spinach, a deficiency increasing the carotenoid and flavonoid contents, as mentioned [74]. By contrast, low N (0.1 and 1 mM) concentrations led to a lower total carotenoids content. In spinach, N deficiency enhanced the phenolic and anthocyanin contents but drastically reduced the carotenoid content [74]. As regards the effect of salinity, only the highest concentration of NaCl (60 mM) led to a significant increase of 58% in total carotenoids. A similar increase in carotenoids under salinity has been found in spinach [74].

Table 4. Concentration of vitamin C, β-carotene and lutein (µg g^{-1} fresh weight) in lamb's lettuce grown under different nutritional conditions. Values are means ± SE (n = 4).

Treatments	mM	Total Carotenoids	Total Chlorophyll	Vitamin C
Ca	0.5	130 ± 10	125 ± 8 [b]	376 ± 4
	2	150 ± 7	86 ± 5 [a]	364 ± 6
	5	154 ± 18	89 ± 9 [a]	356 ± 10
		n.s.	**	n.s.
K	0.1	148 ± 16 [b]	205 ± 22 [b]	454 ± 8
	0.5	100 ± 8 [a]	140 ± 13 [a]	397 ± 21
	3.5	82 ± 4 [a]	114 ± 7 [a]	425 ± 26
		**	**	n.s.
N	0.1	91 ± 4 [a]	94 ± 3 [a]	661 ± 20
	1	86 ± 9 [a]	87 ± 8 [a]	682 ± 55
	7	109 ± 3 [b]	116 ± 3 [b]	624 ± 3
		*	**	n.s
NaCl	0	83 ± 3 [a]	100 ± 4 [b]	515 ± 10 [a]
	15	113 ± 7 [ab]	101 ± 6 [b]	541 ± 17 [ab]
	30	121 ± 8 [ab]	88 ± 4 [ab]	540 ± 20 [ab]
	60	132 ± 16 [b]	80 ± 1 [a]	597 ± 20 [b]
		*		*

*, ** Significant differences between means at 5, 1% level of probability, respectively; n.s., non-significant at p = 5%. For each stage, different letters in the same column indicate significant differences between means according to Duncan's test at the 5% level.

The total chlorophyll content increased as the concentration of Ca and K in the nutrient solution decreased (Table 4). Contrarily to Ca and K, low levels of N and the highest level of salinity (60 mM NaCl) lowered the chlorophyll content. A decrease in N levels also decreased the total chlorophyll content of lamb's lettuce cv. Princess [78] and similarly, in spinach [79]

Lamb's lettuce was seen to be a good source of vitamin C with similar or even higher values than those reported for other commonly consumed leafy vegetables such as lettuce or spinach [54]. Its content in lamb's lettuce was not affected by the reduction in any of the studied plant mineral nutrients. However, in other salad species, including lettuce, changes in ascorbic acid have been related with mineral nutrition [80]. Regarding salinity, the highest concentration of NaCl (60 mM) significantly increased the vitamin C content, as has been found in *Amaranthus* leafy vegetables [81] and tomato fruits [82]. Our results agree with those of El-Nakel et al. [80], who indicated that nutritional chemical stress (e.g., mild to moderate salinity and nutrient stress) can improve the nutritional value of vegetables through the accumulation of certain metabolites as a response in their adaptation to suboptimal conditions.

4. Conclusions

Chromatographic analysis of the phenolic profile revealed the presence of 35 phenolic compounds in lamb's lettuce. The main compounds were chlorogenic, coumaroylquinic, dicaffeoylquinic and feruloylquinic acids, and luteolin-7-rutinoside, disometin-apiosylglucoside, diosmin and sinapic acid-hexoside. The major carotenoids identified were β-carotene and lutein. According to our results, lamb's lettuce can be considered a good option as a salad ingredient due to its phenolic, carotenoid, chlorophyll and vitamin C content. Many of the identified secondary metabolites are reported here in lamb's lettuce for the first time. Variations in the concentrations of some of these compounds were observed as a result of different fertilization doses and salinity levels. Low levels of K increased flavones, flavanones, carotenoids and chlorophylls, while a reduction in the N concentration led to an even greater increase in all the phenolic families but reduced the carotenoid and chlorophyll content. Finally, salinity increased the carotenoid and vitamin C contents, but decreased that of chlorophylls. These results highlight the impact of plant mineral nutrition on the accumulation of bioactive compounds and point to the management of fertilization or saline conditions as a useful tool for increasing the phytochemical content and functional quality of lamb's lettuce. More studies are needed to explore the impact of other genetic (cultivar) and preharvest factors on secondary metabolite content as future strategies to improve the functional value of lamb's lettuce.

Author Contributions: Conceptualization, P.F., V.M. and P.H.; methodology, V.H., T.M., P.H. and P.F.; software V.H. and T.M.; validation V.M., P.H., M.Á.B. and P.F.; formal analysis, V.H. and J.C.; investigation, V.H., J.C., M.Á.B., V.M., P.H. and P.F.; resources, V.M., P.H., P.F.; data curation, V.H., M.Á.B.; writing—original draft preparation, M.A.B. and P.F.; writing—review and editing, M.Á.B., P.F. and V.H.; visualization, M.Á.B., P.H. and J.F.; project administration, V.M. and P.F.; funding acquisition, P.F., P.H., J.F. and V.M. All authors have read and agreed to the published version of the manuscript.

Funding: This research was funded by Fundación Séneca—Agencia de Ciencia y Tecnología de la Región de Murcia.

Data Availability Statement: The data presented in this study are available on request from the corresponding author.

Acknowledgments: The authors are grateful to Inmaculada Garrido González, María V. Molina Menor and Elia Molina Menor for technical assistance.

Conflicts of Interest: The authors declare no conflict of interest. The funders had no role in the design of the study; in the collection, analyses, or interpretation of data; in the writing of the manuscript, or in the decision to publish the results.

References

1. Liu, H.L.; Kao, T.H.; Chen, B.H. Determination of carotenoids in the chinese medical herb jiao-gu-lan (*Gynostemma pentaphyllum* MAKINO) by liquid chromatography. *Chromatographia* **2004**, *60*, 411–417. [CrossRef]
2. Bazzano, L.A.; He, J.; Ogden, L.G.; Loria, C.M.; Vupputuri, S.; Myers, L.; Whelton, P.K. Fruit and vegetable intake and risk of cardiovascular disease in US adults: The first National Health and Nutrition Examination Survey Epidemiologic Follow-up Study. *Am. J. Clin.* **2002**, *76*, 93–99. [CrossRef] [PubMed]
3. Benetou, V.; Orfanos, P.; Lagiou, P.; Trichopoulos, D.; Boffetta, P.; Trichopoulou, A. Vegetables and fruits in relation to cancer risk: Evidence from the Greek EPIC cohort study. *Cancer Epidemiol. Biomark. Prev.* **2008**, *17*, 387–392. [CrossRef] [PubMed]
4. Villatoro-Pulido, M.; Priego-Capote, F.; Alvarez-Sanchez, B.; Saha, S.; Philo, M.; Obregon-Cano, S.; De Haro-Bailon, A.; Font, R.; Del Rio-Celestino, M. An approach to the phytochemical profiling of rocket *Eruca sativa* (Mill.) Thell. *J. Sci. Food Agr.* **2013**, *93*, 3809–3819. [CrossRef]
5. Lin, D.; Xiao, M.; Zhao, J.; Li, Z.; Xing, B.; Li, X.; Kong, M.; Li, L.; Zhang, Q.; Liu, Y.; et al. An overview of plant phenolic compounds and their importance in human nutrition and management of type 2 diabetes. *Molecules* **2016**, *21*, 1374. [CrossRef] [PubMed]
6. Baena, R.; Salinas, P. Diet and cancer: Risk factors and epidemiological evidence. *Maturitas* **2014**, *77*, 202–208. [CrossRef]
7. Pellegrina, C.D.; Padovani, G.; Mainente, F.; Zoccatelli, G.; Bissoli, G.; Mosconi, S.; Veneri, G.; Peruffo, A.; Andrighetto, G.; Rizzi, C.; et al. Anti-tumour potential of a gallic acid-containing phenolic fraction from *Oenothera biennis*. *Cancer Lett.* **2005**, *226*, 17–25. [CrossRef]
8. Mayne, S.T. β-carotene, carotenoids, and disease prevention in humans. *FASEB J.* **1996**, *10*, 690–701. [CrossRef]
9. Ferruzzi, M.G.; Bohm, V.; Courtney, P.D.; Schwartz, S.J. Antioxidant and antimutagenic activity of dietary chlorophyll derivatives determined by radical scavenging and bacterial reverse mutagenesis assays. *J. Food Sci.* **2002**, *67*, 2589–2595. [CrossRef]

10. Ferreres, F.; Gil, M.I.; Castaner, M.; TomasBarberan, F.A. Phenolic metabolites in red pigmented lettuce (*Lactuca sativa*). Changes with minimal processing and cold storage. *J. Agr. Food Chem.* **1997**, *45*, 4249–4254. [CrossRef]
11. Llorach, R.; Martinez-Sanchez, A.; Tomas-Barberan, F.A.; Gil, M.I.; Ferreres, F. Characterisation of polyphenols and antioxidant properties of five lettuce varieties and escarole. *Food Chem.* **2008**, *108*, 1028–1038. [CrossRef] [PubMed]
12. Ferrante, A.; Martinetti, L.; Maggiore, T. Biochemical changes in cut vs. intact lamb's lettuce (*Valerianella olitoria*) leaves during storage. *Int. J. Food Sci. Technol.* **2009**, *44*, 1050–1056.
13. Dalla Costa, L.; Tomasi, N.; Gottardi, S.; Iacuzzo, F.; Cortella, G.; Manzocco, L.; Pinton, R.; Mimmo, T.; Cesco, S. The effect of growth medium temperature on corn salad *Valerianella locusta* (L.) Laterr baby leaf yield and quality. *Hortscience* **2011**, *46*, 1619–1625. [CrossRef]
14. Manzocco, L.; Foschia, M.; Tomasi, N.; Maifreni, M.; Costa, L.D.; Marino, M.; Cortella, G.; Cesco, S. Influence of hydroponic and soil cultivation on quality and shelf life of ready-to-eat lamb's lettuce (*Valerianella locusta* L. Laterr). *J. Sci. Food Agr.* **2011**, *91*, 1373–1380. [CrossRef]
15. Ceglie, F.G.; Amodio, M.L.; de Chiara, M.L.V.; Madzaric, S.; Mimiola, G.; Testani, E.; Tittarelli, F.; Colelli, G. Effect of organic agronomic techniques and packaging on the quality of lamb's lettuce. *J. Sci. Food Agr.* **2018**, *98*, 4606–4615. [CrossRef]
16. Dlugosz-Grochowska, O.; Wojciechowska, R.; Kruczek, M.; Habela, A. Supplemental lighting with leds improves the biochemical composition of two *Valerianella locusta* (L.) cultivars. *Hortic. Environ. Biotechnol.* **2017**, *58*, 441–449. [CrossRef]
17. Pappalardo, H.D.; Toscano, V.; Puglia, G.D.; Genovese, C.; Raccuia, S.A. *Cynara cardunculus* L. as a multipurpose crop for plant secondary metabolites production in marginal stressed lands. *Front. Plant Sci.* **2020**, *11*, 240. [CrossRef]
18. Ramos-Bueno, R.P.; Rincon-Cervera, M.A.; Gonzalez-Fernandez, M.J.; Guil-Guerrero, J.L. Phytochemical composition and antitumor activities of new salad greens: Rucola (*Diplotaxis tenuifolia*) and corn salad (*Valerianella locusta*). *Plant Foods Hum. Nutr.* **2016**, *71*, 197–203. [CrossRef]
19. Cantos, E.; Espin, J.C.; Tomas-Barberan, F.A. Varietal differences among the polyphenol profiles of seven table grape cultivars studied by LC-DAD-MS-MS. *J. Agr. Food Chem.* **2002**, *50*, 5691–5696. [CrossRef]
20. Motilva, M.J.; Macia, A.; Romero, M.P.; Labrador, A.; Dominguez, A.; Peiro, L. Optimisation and validation of analytical methods for the simultaneous extraction of antioxidants: Application to the analysis of tomato sauces. *Food Chem.* **2014**, *163*, 234–243. [CrossRef]
21. Fenoll, J.; Martinez, A.; Hellin, P.; Flores, P. Simultaneous determination of ascorbic and dehydroascorbic acids in vegetables and fruits by liquid chromatography with tandem-mass spectrometry. *Food Chem.* **2011**, *127*, 340–344. [CrossRef]
22. Navarro, M.; Moreira, I.; Arnaez, E.; Quesada, S.; Azofeifa, G.; Vargas, F.; Alvarado, D.; Chen, P. Polyphenolic characterization and antioxidant activity of *Malus domestica* and *Prunus domestica* cultivars from Costa Rica. *Foods* **2018**, *7*, 15. [CrossRef] [PubMed]
23. Kakkar, S.; Bais, S. A review on protocatechuic acid and its pharmacological potential. *ISRN Pharmacol.* **2014**, *23*, 952943. [CrossRef] [PubMed]
24. Clifford, M.N.; Knight, S.; Kuhnert, N. Discriminating between the six isomers of dicaffeoylquinic acid by LC-MSn. *J. Agr. Food Chem.* **2005**, *53*, 3821–3832. [CrossRef]
25. Baeza, G.; Sarria, B.; Bravo, L.; Mateos, R. Exhaustive qualitative LC-DAD-MSn analysis of arabica green coffee beans: Cinnamoyl-glycosides and cinnamoylshikimic acids as new polyphenols in green coffee. *J. Agr. Food Chem.* **2016**, *64*, 9663–9674. [CrossRef] [PubMed]
26. Stefanescu, B.E.; Szabo, K.; Mocan, A.; Crisan, G. Phenolic compounds from five ericaceae species leaves and their related bioavailability and health benefits. *Molecules* **2019**, *24*, 2046. [CrossRef]
27. Santana-Gálvez, J.; Cisneros-Zevallos, L.; Jacobo-Velázquez, D.A. Chlorogenic acid: Recent advances on its dual role as a food additive and a nutraceutical against metabolic syndrome. *Molecules* **2017**, *22*, 358. [CrossRef]
28. Liang, N.; Kitts, D.D. Role of chlorogenic acids in controlling oxidative and inflammatory stress conditions. *Nutrients* **2016**, *8*, 16. [CrossRef]
29. Meng, S.; Cao, J.; Feng, Q.; Peng, J.; Hu, Y. Roles of chlorogenic acid on regulating glucose and lipids metabolism: A review. *Evid. Based Complement. Alternat. Med.* **2013**, *6778*, 801457. [CrossRef]
30. Zhao, Y.; Wang, J.; Ballevre, O.; Luo, H.; Zhang, W. Antihypertensive effects and mechanisms of chlorogenic acids. *Hypertens. Res.* **2012**, *35*, 370–374. [CrossRef]
31. Belkaid, A.; Currie, J.-C.; Desgagnes, J.; Annabi, B. The chemopreventive properties of chlorogenic acid reveal a potential new role for the microsomal glucose-6-phosphate translocase in brain tumor progression. *Cancer Cell Int.* **2006**, *6*, 7. [CrossRef] [PubMed]
32. Kramberger, K.; Barlic-Maganja, D.; Bandelj, D.; Arbeiter, A.B.; Peeters, K.; Visnjevec, A.M.; Praznikar, Z.J. HPLC-DAD-ESI-QTOF-MS Determination of bioactive compounds and antioxidant activity comparison of the hydroalcoholic and water extracts from two *Helichrysum Ital.* species. *Metabolites* **2020**, *10*, 403. [CrossRef] [PubMed]
33. Lee, J.H.; Felipe, P.; Yang, Y.H.; Kim, M.Y.; Kwon, O.Y.; Sok, D.E.; Kim, H.C.; Kim, M.R. Effects of dietary supplementation with red-pigmented leafy lettuce (*Lactuca sativa*) on lipid profiles and antioxidant status in C57BL/6J mice fed a high-fat high-cholesterol diet. *Br. J. Nutr.* **2009**, *101*, 1246–1254. [CrossRef] [PubMed]
34. Catarino, M.D.; Silva, A.M.S.; Saraiva, S.C.; Sobral, A.J.F.N.; Cardoso, S.M. Characterization of phenolic constituents and evaluation of antioxidant properties of leaves and stems of Eriocephalus africanus. *Arab. J. Chem.* **2018**, *11*, 62–69. [CrossRef]
35. Flores, P.; Hernández, V.; Fenoll, J.; Hellín, P. Pre-harvest application of ozonated water on broccoli crops: Effect on head quality. *J. Food Compos. Anal.* **2019**, *83*, 103260. [CrossRef]

36. Csernatoni, F.; Socaciu, C.; Pop, R.M.; Ranga, F.; Bunghez, F.; Romanciuc, F. Comparative fingerprint of aromatic herbs and yeast alcoholic extracts used as ingredients for promen, a prostate preventive nutraceutical. *Food Sci. Technol.* **2013**, *70*, 45–52. [CrossRef]
37. Schuster, B.; Herrmann, K. Hydroxybenzoic and hydroxycinnamic acid-derivatives in soft fruits. *Phytochemistry* **1985**, *24*, 2761–2764. [CrossRef]
38. Papetti, A.; Daglia, M.; Aceti, C.; Sordelli, B.; Spini, V.; Carazzone, C.; Gazzani, G. Hydroxycinnamic acid derivatives occurring in *Cichorium endivia* vegetables. *J. Pharm. Biomed. Anal.* **2008**, *48*, 472–476. [CrossRef]
39. El-Askary, H.I.; Mohamed, S.S.; El-Gohari, H.M.A.; Ezzat, S.M.; Meselhy, M.R. Quinic acid derivatives from *Artemisia annua* L. leaves; biological activities and seasonal variation. *S. Afr. J. Bot.* **2020**, *128*, 200–208. [CrossRef]
40. Poleti Martucci, M.E.; De Vos, R.C.H.; Carollo, C.A.; Gobbo-Neto, L. Metabolomics as a potential chemotaxonomical tool: Application in the genus vernonia schreb. *PLoS ONE* **2014**, *9*, e93149. [CrossRef]
41. Ferreres, F.; Sousa, C.; Vrchovska, V.; Valentao, P.; Pereira, J.A.; Seabra, R.M.; Andrade, P.B. Chemical composition and antioxidant activity of tronchuda cabbage internal leaves. *Eur. Food Res. Technol.* **2006**, *222*, 88–98. [CrossRef]
42. Niciforovic, N.; Abramovic, H. Sinapic acid and its derivatives: Natural sources and bioactivity. *Compr. Rev. Food Sci. Saf.* **2014**, *13*, 34–51. [CrossRef] [PubMed]
43. López-Lázaro, M. Distribution and biological activities of the flavonoid luteolin. *Mini-Rev. Med. Chem.* **2009**, *9*, 31–59. [CrossRef] [PubMed]
44. Inoue, T.; Sugimoto, Y.; Masuda, H.; Kamei, C. Antiallergic effect of flavonoid glycosides obtained from *Mentha piperita* L. *Biol. Pharm. Bull.* **2002**, *25*, 256–259. [CrossRef]
45. Lin, L.Z.; Lu, S.; Harnly, J.M. Detection and quantification of glycosylated flavonoid malonates in celery, Chinese celery, and celery seed by LC-DAD-ESI/MS. *J. Agr. Food Chem.* **2007**, *55*, 1321–1326. [CrossRef]
46. Brito, A.; Ramirez, J.E.; Areche, C.; Sepulveda, B.; Simirgiotis, M.J. HPLC-UV-MS profiles of phenolic compounds and antioxidant activity of fruits from three citrus species consumed in northern chile. *Molecules* **2014**, *19*, 17400–17421. [CrossRef]
47. Justesen, U. Negative atmospheric pressure chemical ionisation low-energy collision activation mass spectrometry for the characterisation of flavonoids in extracts of fresh herbs. *J. Chromatogr. A* **2000**, *902*, 369–379. [CrossRef]
48. Patel, K.; Gadewar, M.; Tahilyani, V.; Patel, D.K. A review on pharmacological and analytical aspects of diosmetin: A concise report. *Chin. J. Integr. Med.* **2013**, *19*, 792–800. [CrossRef]
49. Guzelmeric, E.; Vovk, I.; Yesilada, E. Development and validation of an HPTLC method for apigenin 7-O-glucoside in chamomile flowers and its application for fingerprint discrimination of chamomile-like materials. *J. Pharm. Biomed.* **2015**, *107*, 108–118. [CrossRef]
50. Gulluce, M.; Orhan, F.; Adiguzel, A.; Bal, T.; Guvenalp, Z.; Dermirezer, L.O. Determination of antimutagenic properties of apigenin-7-O-rutinoside, a flavonoid isolated from *Mentha longifolia* (L.) Huds. ssp longifolia with yeast DEL assay. *Toxicol. Ind. Health* **2013**, *29*, 534–540. [CrossRef]
51. Hwang, S.H.; Paek, J.H.; Lim, S.S. Simultaneous ultra performance liquid chromatography determination and antioxidant activity of linarin, luteolin, chlorogenic acid and apigenin in different parts of compositae species. *Molecules* **2016**, *21*, 1609. [CrossRef] [PubMed]
52. Hvattum, E.; Ekeberg, D. Study of the collision-induced radical cleavage of flavonoid glycosides using negative electrospray ionization tandem quadrupole mass spectrometry. *J. Mass Spectrom.* **2003**, *38*, 43–49. [CrossRef] [PubMed]
53. Olennikov, D.N.; Kashchenko, N.I.; Chirikova, N.K.; Akobirshoeva, A.; Zilfikarov, I.N.; Vennos, C. Isorhamnetin and quercetin derivatives as anti-acetylcholinesterase principles of marigold (*Calendula officinalis*) flowers and preparations. *Int. J. Mol. Sci.* **2017**, *18*, 1685. [CrossRef]
54. Sergio, L.; Boari, F.; Pieralice, M.; Linsalata, V.; Cantore, V.; Di Venere, D. Bioactive phenolics and antioxidant capacity of some wild edible greens as affected by different cooking treatments. *Foods* **2020**, *18*, 1320. [CrossRef] [PubMed]
55. Cebadera, L.; Dias, M.I.; Barros, L.; Fernández-Ruiz, V.; Cámara, R.M.; Del Pino, A.; Santos-Buelga, C.; Ferreira, I.C.F.R.; Morales, P.; Camara, M. Characterization of extra early spanish clementine varieties (*Citrus clementina* Hort ex Tan) as a relevant source of bioactive compounds with antioxidant activity. *Foods* **2020**, *9*, 642. [CrossRef] [PubMed]
56. Petry, F.C.; Mercadante, A.Z. Composition by LC-MS/MS of new carotenoid esters in mango and citrus. *J. Agr. Food Chem.* **2016**, *64*, 8207–8224. [CrossRef] [PubMed]
57. López, A.; Javier, G.A.; Fenoll, J.; Hellín, P.; Flores, P. Chemical composition and antioxidant capacity of lettuce: Comparative study of regular-sized (Romaine) and baby-sized (Little Gem and Mini Romaine) types. *J. Food Compos. Anal.* **2014**, *33*, 39–48. [CrossRef]
58. Gupta, P.; Sreelakshmi, Y.; Sharma, R. A rapid and sensitive method for determination of carotenoids in plant tissues by high performance liquid chromatography. *Plant Methods* **2015**, *11*, 5. [CrossRef]
59. Takaichi, S.; Mimuro, M. Distribution and geometric isomerism of neoxanthin in oxygenic phototrophs: 9′-cis, a sole molecular form. *Plant Cell Physiol.* **1998**, *39*, 968–977. [CrossRef]
60. Moloto, M.R.; Phan, A.D.T.; Shai, J.L.; Sultanbawa, Y.; Sivakumar, D. Comparison of phenolic compounds, carotenoids, amino acid composition, in vitro antioxidant and anti-diabetic activities in the leaves of seven cowpea (*Vigna unguiculata*) cultivars. *Foods* **2020**, *9*, 1285. [CrossRef]

61. Pandey, D.M.; Kang, K.H.; Yeo, U.D. Effects of excessive photon on the photosynthetic pigments and violaxanthin de-epoxidase activity in the xanthophyll cycle of spinach leaf. *Plant Sci.* **2005**, *168*, 161–166. [CrossRef]
62. Znidarcic, D.; Ban, D.; Sircelj, H. Carotenoid and chlorophyll composition of commonly consumed leafy vegetables in Mediterranean countries. *Food Chem.* **2011**, *129*, 1164–1168. [CrossRef] [PubMed]
63. Zeb, A.; Nisar, P. Effects of high temperature frying of spinach leaves in sunflower oil on carotenoids, chlorophylls, and tocopherol composition. *Front. Chem.* **2017**, *5*, 19. [CrossRef] [PubMed]
64. Demmig-Adams, B.; Lopez-Pozo, M.; Stewart, J.J.; Adams, W.W., III. Zeaxanthin and lutein: Photoprotectors, anti-inflammatories, and brain food. *Molecules* **2020**, *25*, 3607. [CrossRef]
65. Chen, J.P.; Tai, C.Y.; Chen, B.H. Improved liquid chromatographic method for determination of carotenoids in Taiwanese mango (*Mangifera indica* L.). *J. Chromatogr. A* **2004**, *1054*, 261–268. [CrossRef]
66. Lin, C.H.; Chen, B.H. Determination of carotenoids in tomato juice by liquid chromatography. *J. Chromatogr. A* **2003**, *1012*, 103–109. [CrossRef]
67. Müller, H. Determination of the carotenoid content in selected vegetables and fruit by HPLC and photodiode array detection. *J. Food Sci. Technol.* **1997**, *204*, 88–94. [CrossRef]
68. Johra, F.T.; Bepari, A.K.; Bristy, A.T.; Reza, H.M. A mechanistic review of β-carotene, lutein, and zeaxanthin in eye health and disease. *Antioxidants* **2020**, *9*, 1046. [CrossRef]
69. Lichtenthaler, H.K.; Buschmann, C. *Chlorophylls and Carotenoids: Measurement and Characterization by UV-VIS Spectroscopy*; Wrolstad, R.E., Acree, T.E., An, H., Decker, E.A., Penner, M.H., Reid, D.S., Schwartz, S.J., Shoemaker, C.F., Sporns, P., Eds.; Current Protocols in Food Analytical Chemistry (CPFA), John Wiley and Sons: New York, NY, USA, 2001; pp. F4.3.1–F4.3.8.
70. Milenković, S.M.; Zvezdanović, J.; Anđelković, T.; Dejan, Z. The identification of chlorophyll and its derivatives in the pigment mixtures: HPLC-chromatography, visible and mass spectroscopy studies. *Adv. Technol.* **2012**, *1*, 16–24.
71. Lanfer-Marquez, U.M.; Barros, R.M.C.; Sinnecker, P. Antioxidant activity of chlorophylls and their derivatives. *Food Res. Int.* **2005**, *38*, 885–891. [CrossRef]
72. Pérez-Gálvez, A.; Viera, I.; Roca, M. Carotenoids and chlorophylls as antioxidants. *Antioxidants* **2020**, *9*, 505. [CrossRef] [PubMed]
73. Suparmi, S.; Fasitasari, M.; Martosupono, M.; Mangimbulude, J.C. Comparisons of curative effects of chlorophyll from *Sauropus androgynus* (L) merr leaf extract and cu-chlorophyllin on sodium nitrate-induced oxidative stress in rats. *J. Toxicol.* **2016**, *5*, 1–7. [CrossRef] [PubMed]
74. Xu, C.; Mou, B. Responses of spinach to salinity and nutrient deficiency in growth, physiology, and nutritional value. *J. Am. Soc. Hortic. Sci.* **2016**, *141*, 12–21. [CrossRef]
75. Tsouvaltzis, P.; Kasampalis, D.S.; Aktsoglou, D.C.; Barbayiannis, N.; Siomos, A.S. Effect of reduced nitrogen and supplemented amino acids nutrient solution on the nutritional quality of baby green and red lettuce grown in a floating system. *Agronomy* **2020**, *10*, 922. [CrossRef]
76. El-Nakhel, C.; Petropoulos, S.A.; Pannico, A.; Kyriacou, M.C.; Giordano, M.; Colla, G.; Troise, A.D.; Vitaglione, P.; De Pascale, S.; Rouphael, Y. The bioactive profile of lettuce produced in a closed soilless system as configured by combinatorial effects of genotype and macrocation supply composition. *Food. Chem.* **2020**, *309*, 125713. [CrossRef]
77. Zhou, W.; Liang, X.; Dai, P.; Chen, Y.; Zhang, Y.; Zhang, M.; Lu, L.; Jin, C.; Lin, X. Alteration of phenolic composition in lettuce (*Lactuca sativa* L.) by reducing nitrogen supply enhances its anti-proliferative effects on colorectal cancer cells. *Int. J. Mol. Sci.* **2019**, *20*, 4205. [CrossRef]
78. Di Mola, I.; Cozzolino, E.; Ottaiano, L.; Nocerino, S.; Rouphael, Y.; Colla, G.; El-Nakhel, C.; Mori, M. Nitrogen use and uptake efficiency and crop performance of baby spinach (*Spinacia oleracea* L.) and lamb's lettuce (*Valerianella locusta* L.) grown under variable sub-optimal n regimes combined with plant-based biostimulant application. *Agronomy* **2020**, *10*, 278. [CrossRef]
79. Nemadodzi, L.E.; Araya, H.; Nkomo, M.; Ngezimana, W.; Mudau, N.F. Nitrogen, phosphorus, and potassium effects on the physiology and biomass yield of baby spinach (*Spinacia oleracea* L.). *J. Plant Nutr.* **2017**, *40*, 2033–2044. [CrossRef]
80. El-Nakhel, C.; Pannico, A.; Kyriacou, M.C.; Giordano, M.; De Pascale, S.; Rouphael, Y. Macronutrient deprivation eustress elicits differential secondary metabolites in red and green-pigmented butterhead lettuce grown in a closed soilless system. *J. Sci. Food Agr.* **2019**, *99*, 6962–6972. [CrossRef]
81. Sarker, U.; Oba, S. Salinity stress enhances color parameters, bioactive leaf pigments, vitamins, polyphenols, flavonoids and antioxidant activity in selected *Amaranthus* leafy vegetables. *J. Sci. Food Agr.* **2019**, *99*, 2275–2284. [CrossRef]
82. Flores, P.; Hernández, V.; Hellín, P.; Fenoll, J.; Cava, J.; Mestre, T.; Martínez, V. Metabolite profile of the tomato dwarf cultivar Micro-Tom and comparative response to saline and nutritional stresses with regard to a commercial cultivar. *J. Sci. Food Agr.* **2016**, *96*, 1562–1570. [CrossRef] [PubMed]

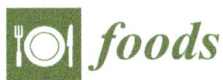 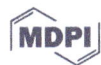

Article

The Quality of Greek Oregano (*O. vulgare* L. subsp. *hirtum* (Link) Ietswaart) and Common Oregano (*O. vulgare* L. subsp. *vulgare*) Cultivated in the Temperate Climate of Central Europe

Zenon Węglarz, Olga Kosakowska *, Jarosław. L. Przybył, Ewelina Pióro-Jabrucka and Katarzyna Bączek

Department of Vegetable and Medicinal Plants, Institute of Horticultural Sciences, Warsaw University of Life Sciences–SGGW, 02-787 Warsaw, Poland; zenon_weglarz@sggw.edu.pl (Z.W.); jaroslaw_przybyl@sggw.edu.pl (J.L.P.); ewelina_pioro_jabrucka@sggw.edu.pl (E.P.-J.); katarzyna_baczek@sggw.edu.pl (K.B.)
* Correspondence: olga_kosakowska@sggw.edu.pl; Tel.: +48-22-593-2247

Received: 23 October 2020; Accepted: 13 November 2020; Published: 15 November 2020

Abstract: The purpose of the study was to determine the differences between two subspecies: *O. vulgare* L. subsp. *hirtum* (Link) Ietswaart (Greek oregano) and *O. vulgare* L. subsp. *vulgare* (common oregano) growing in cultivation conditions within temperate climate of Central Europe. The characteristic of the subspecies was undertaken in terms of selected morphological parameters and the quality of the raw material. The herb of both subspecies was evaluated on the content and composition of essential oil by hydrodistillation followed by GC-MS and GC-FID (gas chromatography coupled with mass spectrometry and flame ionization detector), the total content of phenolic acids (according to PP 6th ed.) and the content of rosmarinic acid (by HPLC). The sensory evaluation (QDA) was performed, as well. Greek oregano was distinguished by visibly higher number of glandular trichomes on the leaves (up to 4.85 per 1 mm^2) followed by higher content of essential oil in the herb (up to 3.36 g × 100 g^{-1} DW) in comparison to common oregano. Based on the essential oil composition, Greek oregano was classified as mixed carvacrol/γ-terpinene chemotype, while common oregano as mixed sabinyl/cymyl type rich in sesquiterpenes. Greek oregano was also characterized by higher total content of phenolic acids (up to 6.16 g × 100 g^{-1} DW) and rosmarinic acid (up to 6787.2 mg × 100 g^{-1} DW) than common oregano. Essential oil content reached the maximum at the beginning of blooming (common oregano) and at the full blooming stage (Greek oregano). In turn, the amount of phenolic acids followed by rosmarinic acid was the highest at the beginning of seed-setting stage, in the case of both subspecies. The differences between subspecies concerning chemical composition (especially essential oil) were reflected in the sensory attributes, where both odor and taste notes were found at higher level for Greek oregano. Results of our work indicate that Greek oregano is well adapted to grow in the temperate zone conditions. Such adaptation was reflected mainly in the satisfied yield and maintaining characters typical for the Mediterranean plant, e.g., a high essential oil content followed by high carvacrol share, traits the most important from practice viewpoint.

Keywords: *Origanum* subspecies; morphological traits; glandular trichomes; essential oil composition; rosmarinic acid; sensory evaluation

---

1. Introduction

Plants belonging to *Origanum* genus (*Lamiaceae* family) have been known as culinary and medicinal plants since ancient times. This genus contains 49 taxa belonging to 10 sections. Some species, including *Origanum vulgare* L., are rich in essential oil and commonly known as "oregano" [1]. *Origanum vulgare* L., an aromatic, perennial sub-shrub, is widely distributed all over Eurasia and North Africa [2]. The species is regarded to be extremely variable, both in its morphological features and chemical composition. Given its specific biological character and significant economic importance, *O. vulgare* has been placed in the List of Priority Species in Europe [3]. According to the widely accepted taxonomy, six subspecies of *O. vulgare* have been recognized [2,4]. Among them, *O. vulgare* L. subsp. *hirtum* (Link) Ietswaart so-called Greek oregano, endemic to the Mediterranean area, is cultivated almost all over the world and regarded as the most valuable one [5]. Another subspecies important from economic point of view, is *Origanum vulgare* L. subsp. *vulgare* (common oregano). It frequently occurs on the region of Northern and Central Europe and is the only representative of *O. vulgare* in Poland [6,7]. The upper, not woody parts of flowering shoots (herb) of both subspecies is commonly used and traded raw material. Besides the range of occurrence, these two subspecies differ in terms of many features, whereas the content and composition of essential oil seems to be the most important, because it determines medicinal properties of the herb and its sensory value [2]. Greek oregano is rich in essential oil (about 5%), while common oregano contains less amount (up to 2%) of this substance. Subspecies create few various chemotypes defined on the basis of the dominant compound in essential oil. Greek oregano accumulates mainly phenolic monoterpenes (thymol and carvacrol) followed by its precursors (*p*-cymene and γ-terpinene). In turn, common oregano is distinguished by less active biosynthesis of "cymyl" compounds in favor of the bicyclic "sabinyl" (i.e. sabinene, *cis/trans* sabinene hydrate and its acetates) or acyclic once (i.a., β-ocimene, β-myrcen, linalyl acetate, linalool). This kind of chemotype is often accompanied by high content of sesquiterpenes (i.a. germacrene D, β-caryophyllene and caryophyllene oxide) [1,7–18]. Both *Origanum* subspecies contain also considerable amounts of non-volatile phenolic compounds such as flavonoids and phenolic acids. Rosmarinic acid followed by caffeic, vanillic, *o*-coumaric and protocatechuic acids dominate in common oregano herb [7,19,20]. When given Greek oregano, rosmarinic and lithospermic acids are the present in the highest amounts [13,21,22]. In both subspecies, flavonoids are represented mainly by derivatives of luteoline and apigenine [7,13,20–24]. In relation with such a wide range of biologically active compounds, both *Origanum* subspecies indicate various pharmacological activities, especially antimicrobial, choleretic and antioxidant. Common oregano herb reveals also diuretic and expectorant properties, while Greek oregano—stimulative, carminative, antispasmodic, and anticancer [25,26]. It is worth noting that Greek oregano is listed in the European Pharmacopeia and is recommended as a remedy for gastrointestinal disorders treatment, temporary loss of appetite and to stimulate bile secretion [25–27]. Common oregano, even though not mentioned in European Pharmacopeia, used to be applied in the same way in both modern and folk medicine [28]. Both *Origanum* subspecies are widely used not only in pharmaceutical industry but also as a food preservative and flavoring, cosmetic ingredient, and, most importantly—as a culinary herb [29,30].

Despite abovementioned intraspecific diversity, *O. vulgare* is still treated as a collective taxon [31–34]. Moreover, many varieties, landraces, forms, ecotypes, and cultivars are nowadays available for stakeholders, creating possibility of subspecies misleading [35]. This altogether may lead to decrease homogeneity and the quality of raw material. It is especially important, since herbal products standardization requirements are taken into consideration [36].

Up to now, Greek oregano cultivation areas have been located mainly within a warmer climate. Recent studies have showed that this subspecies may be cultivated in temperate zone of Central Europe, as well [13,37,38]. However, in Poland, the cultivation of this subspecies is at its infancy [18]. In turn, common oregano used to be collected in Poland both from natural sites and cultivation [28]. However, the harvest from the wild may result in heterogeneous raw material. Moreover, the number of wild growing common oregano populations has recently significantly decreased what can lead to genetic erosion. Thus, the collection of common oregano herb exclusively from cultivation would provide natural resources protection as well as ensure high quality of raw material [39].

The aim of the study was to determine the differences between Greek oregano and common oregano in cultivation conditions within temperate climate of Central Europe. The characteristic of the subspecies was undertaken in terms of selected morphological parameters and the quality of raw material, reflected in the content of biologically active compounds (the total content and composition of essential oil and phenolic acids) and sensory evaluation.

2. Materials and Methods

2.1. Plant Material

The experiment was carried out at the experimental field of the Department of Vegetable and Medicinal Plants, Warsaw University of Life Sciences (WULS-SGGW) (5210180 N; 2105234 E), on heavy alluvial soil. Seeds of Greek oregano and common oregano originated from Polish Gene Bank collection (accession numbers: 406735 and 401291, respectively). Seeds were sown in the first week of February (2020) into multi-pots filled with a peat substrate, in a greenhouse. A total of 180 seedlings of each subspecies were randomly selected and planted out into the field in the last week of April. The randomized block design (60 seedlings per plot; in 3 replications) was applied, with a spacing of 40 × 60 cm. The harvest of the herb (upper, not woody parts of shoots) was performed on 1-year old plants, at three stages of plant's development: at the beginning of blooming (fourth week of June), at the full blooming (third week of July) and at the beginning of seed-setting (second week of August). The herb was cut at a height of about 15 cm above ground. The fresh and dry weight of the herb was determined (g per plant). After drying at 35 °C, the herb was ground and prepared for chemical analysis. Climatic parameters were recorded (Table 1).

Table 1. Climatic parameters in the vegetation season of 2020.

Months	Temperature (°C)	Rainfall (mm)	Air Humidity (%)	Sun Hours	Sun Days
April	12	13.1	53	210	17
May	15	127.1	64	157.5	4
June	22	108.2	68	179	3
July	22	43.2	61	225	6
August	24	70.1	62	295	12

2.2. Morphological Observations

Morphological characters were evaluated according to the List of Descriptors for *Origanum vulgare* L. elaborated by the Medicinal and Aromatic Plants Working Group of European Cooperative Programme for Plant Genetic Resources (MAPs WG ECP/GR) [40]. Observations were carried out directly before the first harvest of raw material, on 10 plants per subspecies. Following traits were determined: plant growth habit, plant height (cm), number of shoots per plant, number of internodes per shoots, color of petals, branching density, stem pubescence, color of stem, degree of lignification, foliage density, shape of leaf blade, leaf area, leaf margin and shape of leaf apex. Moreover, microscopic observations concerning density of glandular trichomes on abaxial and adaxial surface of the leaves were evaluated, according to the method described by Kosakowska et al. [41]. Photographic documentation was performed (Figures 1 and 2).

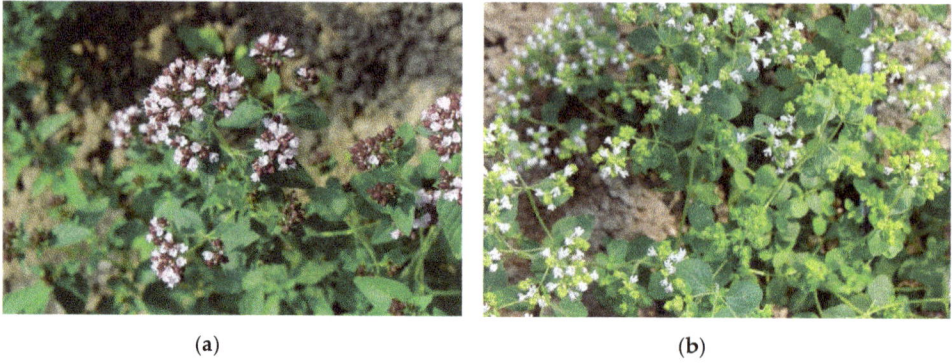

Figure 1. Common oregano (**a**) and Greek oregano (**b**).

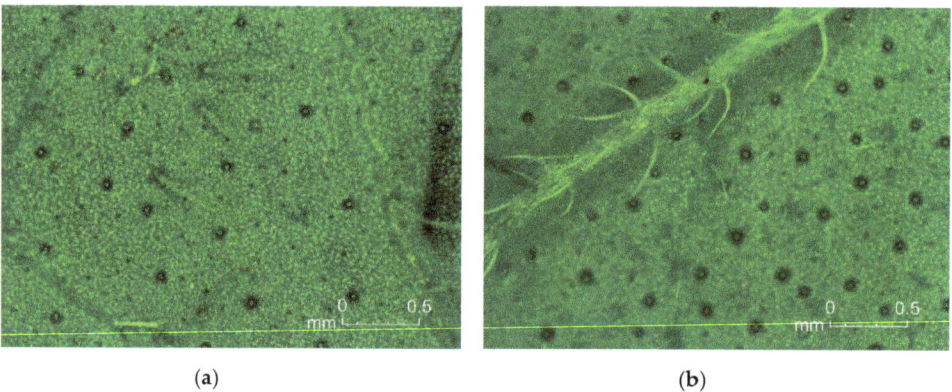

Figure 2. Glandular trichomes on abaxial leaf surface of common oregano (**a**) and Greek oregano (**b**).

2.3. Chemical Analysis

2.3.1. Content of Essential Oil

A total of 50 g of air-dried herb was subjected for hydrodistillation for 3 h using a Clevenger-type apparatus. The content of essential oil was expressed as g × 100 g^{-1} of dry weight (DW). Essential oils were collected and stored in amber vials, at 4 °C.

2.3.2. Analysis of Essential Oils by GC-MS and GC-FID (Gas Chromatography Coupled with Mass Spectrometry and Flame Ionization Detector)

The analysis was carried out by usage of an Agilent Technologies 7890A gas chromatograph coupled with a flame ionization detector (FID) and MS Agilent Technologies 5975C Inert XL_MSD with Triple Axis Detector (Agilent Technologies, Wilmington, DE, USA). Polar, capillary, HP 20M column (25 m × 0.32 mm × 0.3 μm film thickness) (Agilent Technologies, Wilmington, DE, USA) was used. Separation conditions were given previously by Bączek et al. [42].

2.3.3. Total Content of Phenolic Acids

The analyses (Arnov's method) was performed in accordance with Polish Pharmacopeia 6th ed. [43]. A total of 1 g of air-dry, grounded herb was extracted twice with portions of 25 mL of distilled water (a total of 50 mL), with shaking for 30 min each time at room temperature (a total of 1 h). Collected extract was filled to 50 mL with distilled water. A total of 1 mL of extract was mixed with 5 mL of distilled water, 1 mL 0.5 M HCl, 1 mL of Arnov reagent (10 g of sodium molybdate and 10 g of sodium nitrite dissolved in 100 mL of distilled water) and 1 mL 1 M NaOH and subsequently completed to 10 mL with distilled water. The absorbance of both basic (with extract) and comparison (without extract) solutions were measured at 490 nm. The total phenolic acid content was recalculated and given as caffeic acid equivalent (g $\times$ 100 g^{-1} DW).

2.3.4. Analysis of Phenolic Acids by HPLC-DAD (High Pressure Liquid Chromatography Coupled with Diode Array Detector)

The sample preparation, parameters of chromatographic separation and integration as well as validation procedure was given earlier by Kosakowska et al. [41]. The content of rosmarinic acid was calculated in mg $\times$ 100 g^{-1} DW.

2.4. Sensory Analysis

Sensory evaluation was carried out in the sensory laboratory of the Department of Vegetables and Medicinal Plants, WULS-SGGW. Quantitative descriptive analysis (QDA) was used. The evaluation was determined on the fresh herb of both subspecies, collected in the first cut (at the beginning of blooming). Attributes of its taste and odor were selected and estimated. In order to select attributes, 'brainstorming' sessions were done by an expert panel consisting of a minimum of 10 assessors. Evaluation was performed in two independent sessions. The description of method has already been given by Kosakowska et al. [18].

2.5. Statistical Analysis

Data were subjected to statistical analysis using Statistica 12 software (Cracov, Poland). The mean values were compared by using the one way analysis of variance (ANOVA) followed by Tukey's multiple range test. The differences between individual means were deemed to be significant at $p < 0.05$. Standard deviation ($\pm$SD) was estimated.

3. Results and Discussion

Investigated subspecies differed in both morphological and chemical traits (Tables 2–6). Common oregano was characterized by erect type of growth and ligneous, slightly hairy stems. The color of stems was dark green and red, while petals were pink. The plant height was at a level of 36.11 cm. In turn, Greek oregano was distinguished by semi-erect type of growth, and green, slightly ligneous but hairy stems. This subspecies was characterized by white color of petals. Greek oregano plants grown in Poland were about 10 cm lower than common oregano plants. The foliage density was described as medium (in common oregano) and dense (in Greek oregano). The branching density was sparse in both subspecies. Number of shoots per plant achieved values 27.59 in the case of common oregano, and 22.77 in Greek oregano. The number of internodes per shoot was similar in both subspecies (8.44; 7.60, respectively) (Tables 2 and 3). Obtained results indicate on significant differences between examined *Origanum* subspecies and correspond well with the literature data [14,17,19,44–49]. However, it should be underlined that each subspecies is very variable itself and its morphological features strongly depend on the population/accession origin. For instance, common oregano plant's height ranged from 18 to 59 cm [46], while Greek oregano—from 67.8 to 79.9 cm [49]. Observed phenotypical plasticity may be related to allogamous way of this plant's reproduction as well as its heterozygous character. Traits such as type of growth habit, lignification degree as well as branching and foliar density can be important from the practical viewpoint, since they affect the yield of herb and enable its mechanical harvest [17]. In the present study, the fresh and dry weight of common oregano herb was slightly higher (63.81; 16.71 g $\times$ plant^{-1}) in comparison to Greek oregano (49.17; 13.28 g $\times$ plant^{-1}) (Table 3). Such results may be related to high temperature requirements of Greek oregano resulting from its Mediterranean origin. Taking into consideration the possible response of this subspecies to climatic parameters, its cultivation under covers may be effective. Results obtained by Kosakowska et al. [18] showed that Greek oregano plants cultivated under foil were distinguished by almost twice the mass of the herb when compared to those grown without covers. In general, Greek oregano cultivation is widely presented in literature, however the majority of these data concerns warm climate zones [50–53].

Table 2. Morphological traits of investigated plants.

	Common Oregano *O. vulgare* ssp. *vulgare*	Greek Oregano *O. vulgare* ssp. *hirtum*
Plant habit	erect	semi-erect
Color of petals	pink	white
Branching density	sparse	sparse
Stem pubescence	slightly hairy	hairy
Color of stem	dark green and red	green
Degree of lignification	ligneous	slightly ligneous
Foliage density	medium	dense
Shape of leaf blade	ovate	rhomboid
Leaf margin	denticulate	denticulate
Shape of leaf apex	acute	rounded

Table 3. Morphological traits of investigated plants cd.

	Common Oregano *O. vulgare* ssp. *vulgare*	Greek Oregano *O. vulgare* ssp. *hirtum*
Plant height (cm)	36.11 ± 1.93 *	26.15 ± 1.86
Number of shoots per plant	27.59 ± 2.32 *	22.77 ± 1.53
Number of internodes per shoot	8.44 ± 1.56	7.60 ± 0.95
Fresh weight of herb (g × plant^{-1})	63.81 ± 13.0	49.17 ± 13.55
Dry weight of herb (g × plant^{-1})	16.71 ± 2.73	13.28 ± 3.22

Values marked in rows with '*' differ at $p < 0.05$.

Examined *Origanum* subspecies cultivated in Poland varied also in terms of leaves parameters. Leaves of common oregano were characterized by higher area of blade than Greek oregano (78.27 and 61.76 mm^2, respectively) (Table 4). Moreover, they were distinguished by ovate shape and acute apex, while in the case of Greek oregano, the shape of leaf blade was rhomboid with rounded apex. Leaves of both subspecies had denticulate leaf margin (Table 2). Another feature that strongly differentiated common oregano and Greek oregano leaves was the density of glandular trichomes situated on the upper and down leaf surface (Table 4). In *Origanum* subspecies (as well as in other Lamiaceae), glandular trichomes are multicellular epidermal glands responsible for storage of essential oil. Two different types of these glands were recognized on the epidermis of *Origanum* species: peltate and capitate glands. The glandular trichomes are built of one basal cell, one stalk cell and a multi-cellular head, where essential oil is synthesized before being transferred to subcuticular area [54–56]. Svidenko et al. [56] claim that the location of glandular trichomes have valuable taxonomic significance at the species level. In the present work, the number of glandular trichomes per 1 mm^2 was significantly higher when given Greek oregano leaves (4.78 on adaxial and 4.85 on abaxial surface) in comparison to common oregano (0.78 and 1.17, respectively) (Table 4). This pattern corresponds with studies undertaken earlier by Shafiee-Hajiabad et al. [57]. However, the author showed higher number of glands in both subspecies: up to 17 per 1 mm^2 in Greek oregano and up to 9.67 per 1 mm^2 in common oregano. This inaccuracy may be related to the phenomenon that the formation of glandular trichomes is variable and can be controlled by both genetic and environmental factors [54,58].

Table 4. Leaves area and density of glandular trichomes (GT) on the leaves.

	Common Oregano *O. vulgare* ssp. *vulgare*	**Greek Oregano** *O. vulgare* ssp. *hirtum*
Leaf area (mm^2)	78.27 ± 5.50 *	61.76 ± 5.84
Density of GT on adaxial surface of leaf (number per 1 mm^2)	0.78 ± 0.05	4.78 ± 0.65 *
Density of GT on abaxial surface of leaf (number per 1 mm^2)	1.17 ± 0.19	4.85 ± 0.59 *

Values marked in rows with '*' differ at $p < 0.05$.

When given aromatic plants, including oregano, the problem concerning the content and composition of essential oil seems to be one of the most important, because this substance is responsible for both sensory value and pharmacological activity of the raw material. In the present work, in the case of common oregano, the essential oil content ranged from 0.27 to 0.49 g × 100 g^{-1} DW, with the maximum noticed at the beginning of plant's blooming. In turn, in Greek oregano the amount of this substance varied from 2.75 g × 100 g^{-1} DW (beginning of blooming) to 3.36 (full blooming stage) (Table 5). These results support the thesis that common oregano belongs to essential oil-poor group of *Origanum* subspecies, while Greek oregano represents the essential oil-rich group [2]. It is worth noting that the relationship between the number of glandular trichomes and essential oil content has been found (Tables 4 and 5), what refers to results shown by Shafiee-Hajiabad et al. [57]. Moreover, obtained results correspond with the phenomenon that the oregano essential oil fluctuates during vegetation season and usually reaches the maximum level at the full blooming stage of plant's development, therefore this time used to be regarded as the best for harvest [13,38]. It is known that many various factors can affect the content and composition of essential oils in aromatic plants, where the most seem to be: genetic, physiological and environmental including temperature, intensity of solar and radiation humidity [59–61].

In the present study, 25 compounds were identified in the common oregano essential oil, forming up to 98.11% of total identified fraction. In the case of Greek oregano, 24 constituents were detected, accounting up to 98.89%. The monoterpenes created the fundamental part in both essential oils, with a domination of monoterpene hydrocarbons comprising up to 53.43% and 53.27%, respectively. In Greek oregano, phenolic monoterpenes were also present in the considerable amounts (up to 32.75%). Carvacrol took the majority of this fraction (up to 32.02%), while monoterpene hydrocarbons part was formed mainly by γ-terpinene (up to 28.00%). The domination of above listed compounds let to qualify investigated Greek oregano essential oil as mixed carvacrol/γ-terpinene chemotype. According to literature data, this subspecies is able to create various chemotypes (pure or mixed), based on the dominant compound, such as: carvacrol, tymol, *p*-cymene and γ-terpinene [8,18,38,57]. In present work it was observed that the percentage share of carvarol in Greek oregano essential oil increased from the beginning of blooming to the beginning of the seed-setting stage of plant's development (28.35, 32.02% respectively), in parallel with γ-terpinene decrease (from 28.00 to 19.62%) (Table 5). These results agree with those shown by Grevsen et al. [13] and correspond to Hudaib et al. [62] studies, indicating that phenolic monoterpenes (thymol and carvacrol) and their precursors (γ-terpinene and *p*-cymene) show synchronized patterns of variations during vegetation season. Taking into consideration that the synthesis of monoterpenes can be affected by temperature, obtained results may be related to the plant's physiological response for this climatic parameter [61].

The results of our work indicate on the domination of sabinene in common oregano essential oil. This compound represents monoterpene hydrocarbons fraction. Its content was at the similar level during plant's vegetation: 27.16% at the beginning of blooming, 27.60% at the full blooming and 26.42%—at the beginning of seed-setting. Sabinene was accompanied by other monoterpenes present in amounts not exceeding 10%, i.a.: *p*-cymene, 1.8 cyneol, linalool, terpinolene, etc. Interestingly, there was also a high content of phenolic monoterpenes (carvacrol and thymol) in analyzed common oregano samples (up to 15.89 and 3.57%, respectively). Besides monoterpens, the sesquiterpenes fraction was found in considerable amounts, with β-caryophyllene and its oxide as dominants (Table 5). Thus, such a chemical composition allows to classify this essential oil as mixed sabinyl/cymyl type rich in sesquiterpenes. Sabinyl chemotypes are regarded to be the most frequent within common oregano subspecies, while the occurrence of phenolic monoterpenes is rather rare [7,16]. Based on the literature data, it seems that common oregano is more polymorphic than Greek oregano, since a lot of different chemotypes have been distinguished, as following: *p*-cymene + β-caryophyllene, germacrene D + β-caryophyllene, sabinene, cis-sabinene hydrate, terpinen 4-ol, etc. [9–11,17,44]. Irrespectively of the subspecies, carvacrol or/and thymol chemotypes are considered to be the most valuable in the view of medicinal activities (especially antimicrobial) of these phenolic monoterpenes [25]. Moreover, these substances are responsible for sensory properties of the raw material, in particular: its herbal and spicy aroma [63,64]. According to European Pharmacopeia 9th, the sum of thymol and carvacrol in Greek oregano should not be lower than 60% [27]. Thus, phenolic chemotypes seem to be interesting for industrial purposes, especially pharmaceutical and food. Obtained results indicate that investigated Greek oregano accession doesn't meet EP requirements. However, acyclic (e.g., rich in linalool) or sesquiterpenes (e.g., rich in β-caryophyllene) as well as sabinyl chemotypes can be valuable from practical point of view, as well. For instance, due to pleasant floral aroma of linalool, chemotypes rich in this constituent (occurring in common oregano) may be used in cosmetic and perfumery industry [65].

Table 5. The total content (g × 100 g^{-1} DW) and gas chromatographic composition (% peak area) of essential oil samples.

No	Compound	RI^a	RI^b	Common Oregano *O. vulgare* ssp. *vulgare*			Greek Oregano *O. vulgare* ssp. *hirtum*		
				Beginning of Blooming	Full Blooming	Beginning of Seed-Setting	Beginning of Blooming	Full Blooming	Beginning of Seed-Setting
1	α-thujene	1023	1012–1039	1.30	1.85	1.46	4.11	4.39	1.73
2	α-pinene	1028	1008–1039	0.44	0.57	0.42	0.29	0.28	2.45
3	camphene	1076	1043–1086	0.03	0.04	0.05	0.78	0.80	2.04
4	β-pinene	1113	1085–1130	2.58	2.57	1.73	4.01	3.23	3.20
5	sabinene	1125	1098–1140	27.16	27.60	26.42	0.12	0.51	2.61
6	3-carene	1145	1122–1169	0.00	0.00	0.00	0.17	0.16	0.06
7	α-terpinene	1183	1154–1195	1.01	1.53	1.29	5.30	4.28	3.43
8	D-limonene	1206	1178–1219	0.87	1.10	0.75	0.33	0.32	3.72
9	α-phellandrene	1210	1148–1186	0.00	0.00	0.00	0.43	0.41	0.88
10	1.8 cyneol	1213	1186–1231	3.62	3.34	2.66	0.00	0.00	0.00
11	trans β-ocimene	1235	1211–1251	0.77	1.48	1.44	0.09	0.13	0.10
12	γ-terpinene	1248	1222–1266	2.46	4.20	3.51	28.00	22.99	19.62
13	*p*-cymene	1273	1246–1291	6.85	8.53	6.29	8.88	14.53	9.13
14	*m*-cymene	1277	1244–1279	0.41	0.62	0.43	0.00	0.00	0.00
15	terpinolene	1284	1261–1300	3.62	3.34	2.66	0.34	1.24	0.00
16	1-octen-3-ol	1445	1411–1465	1.98	2.62	2.33	1.01	0.43	1.73
17	linalool	1542	1507–1564	4.06	4.78	3.84	0.75	3.45	0.86
18	β-caryophyllene	1596	1570–1685	7.84	8.19	8.49	2.80	1.18	2.70
19	terpinen-4-ol	1597	1564–1630	4.04	5.09	3.22	3.68	2.42	3.13
20	cis-terpineol	1620	1616–1644	0.20	0.39	0.69	0.80	0.22	0.75
21	trans-terpineol	1670	-	0.21	0.15	0.36	0.30	0.85	0.30
22	borneol	1684	1653–1728	0.00	0.05	0.00	2.86	2.74	3.02
23	β-bisabolene	1741	1698–1748	0.00	0.00	0.00	1.90	2.54	2.19
24	β-ionone	1845	1892–1958	0.21	0.15	0.07	0.00	0.00	0.00
25	caryophyllene oxide	1976	1936–2023	9.95	9.04	10.19	0.20	0.09	0.44
26	humulene oxide II	2017	1992–2083	1.19	0.67	0.71	0.00	0.00	0.00
27	thymol	2165	2100–2205	3.57	2.47	2.40	0.79	0.83	0.73
28	carvacrol	2214	2140–2246	10.63	5.68	15.89	28.35	30.87	32.02
29	α-cadinol	2228	2180–2255	1.14	1.06	0.81	0.00	0.00	0.00
	Total identified			94.84	97.11	98.11	96.29	98.89	96.84
	Monoterpene hydrocarbons			47.5	53.43	46.45	52.85	53.27	48.97
	Oxygenated monoterpenes			12.34	13.95	10.84	8.39	9.68	8.06
	Phenolic monoterpenes			14.2	8.15	18.29	29.14	31.7	32.75
	Sesquiterpene hydrocarbons			7.84	8.19	8.49	4.7	3.72	4.89
	Oxygenated sesquiterpenes			12.28	10.77	11.71	0.2	0.09	0.44
	Other compounds			1.98	2.62	2.33	1.01	0.43	1.73
	Essential oil content			0.49	0.27	0.40	2.75	3.36	3.10

RI^a—experimental retention index on polar HP 20M column, RI^b—range of retention indexes on polar column reported by Babushok et al. [66].

Another group of metabolites conditioning medicinal and sensory value of oregano herb are phenolics. Phenolic acids and flavonoids reveal various pharmacological activities as well as contribute to the color and flavor profile of plants [67,68]. Within phenolic acids, rosmarinic acid is a dominant compound in the Lamiaceae species, including *O. vulgare* [7,20,22,23,69]. This acid belongs to cinnamic acids derivatives. It is a depside, built on the basis of caffeic and 3, 4-dihydroxyphenyl lactic acids. Taking into consideration its extremely high antioxidant and antimicrobial activity, it may be used as a raw material quality marker [70,71]. In the present work, the content of rosmarinic acid in common oregano herb ranged from 2370.0 to 4998.9 mg $\times$ 100 g^{-1} DW, while in Greek oregano from 4569.0 to 6787.2 mg $\times$ 100 g^{-1} DW (Table 6). In both subspecies, the consequent increase of this compound (from the beginning of blooming until the beginning of the seed-setting phase) was noticed. Interestingly, a similar pattern was observed in the case of phenolic acids total content (2.65–4.89 and 4.63–6.16 g $\times$ 100 g^{-1} DW, respectively) (Table 6). Such phenomenon can be associated with the physiological function of these metabolites, which as natural antioxidants, are generally involved in mechanisms of plant protection and defense [72]. Moreover, as lignin's components, phenolic acids make cell walls stronger [73]. Thus, plants being at the beginning of the seed-setting period may be more resistant to various stresses, than the younger ones, what is reflected in higher phenolic acids content.

Table 6. The total content of phenolic acids (g $\times$ 100 g^{-1} DW) and rosmarinic acid content (mg $\times$ 100 g^{-1} DW).

Compound	Common Oregano *O. vulgare* ssp. *vulgare*			Greek Oregano *O. vulgare* ssp. *hirtum*		
	Beginning of Blooming	Full Blooming	Beginning of Seed-Setting	Beginning of Blooming	Full Blooming	Beginning of Seed-Setting
Total content	2.65 ± 0.28 a	2.52 ± 0.26 a	4.89 ± 0.83 b	4.63 ± 0.52 A	4.97 ± 0.42 A	6.16 ± 0.30 B
Rosmarinic acid	2370.0 ± 258.6 a	4762.3 ± 415.0 b	4998.9 ± 263.0 b	4569.0 ± 249.5 A	4992.5 ± 301.5 A	6787.2 ± 608.4 B

Values marked in rows with different letters differ at $p < 0.05$.

In the case of culinary herbs, the organoleptic characteristic and their acceptance by consumers are important issues. Unpleasant flavor may be a reason of the rejection of the product, even though its quality meets Pharmacopeia or ISO (International Organization for Standardization) specifications [74]. Therefore, the sensory evaluation seems to be a crucial factor affecting the overall quality of spices. Results of sensory analysis, carried out in the present work, indicate on visible differences between odor and taste attributes of common oregano and Greek oregano (Figures 3 and 4). Following notes were selected for odor: minty, coniferous, turpenic, herbaceous (bitter), oregano-like, majoram-like, sweet, spicy, floral, oil-like and medicinal. General intensity of odor was estimated, as well. When given taste: bitter, pungent, coniferous, astringent, minty, herbaceous, spicy, acidic, sweet and salty attributes were chosen. With regards to odor, it was observed that notes of Greek oregano herb were higher in comparison to common oregano, expect from sweet and floral ones (Figure 3). Similarly, when taste attributes were concerned: they were noticed at higher level for Greek oregano herb, apart from the sweet note. However, acidic and salty taste was described at the similar level for herb of both examined subspecies (Figure 4). In the case of *Origanum* plants, the sensory profile is conditioned mainly by its essential oil content and composition. As it was mentioned before, in our work, common oregano was qualified as mixed sabinyl/cymyl type rich in sesquiterpenes, while Greek oregano as mixed carvacrol/γ-terpinene chemotype (Table 5). Here, the more intense odor and taste of Greek oregano was probably related to carvacrol domination in its essential oil. Sensory attributes of carvacrol are defined as spicy, herbal, medicinal, phenolic, woody, cedar and pungent [64]. Other volatiles present in Greek oregano essential oil in the considerable amounts, such as γ-terpinene and *p*-cymene, also may affect its sensory profile. Odor of both substances is regarded as gasoline and citrus, while γ-terpinene is additionally described as herbaceous and turpentine [75]. The results obtained in our previous work showed that sensory profile of Greek oregano may be affected by the cultivation method [18].

According to Bonfanti et al. [29] and Asensio et al. [76], it may be related with methods of raw material conservation, as well.

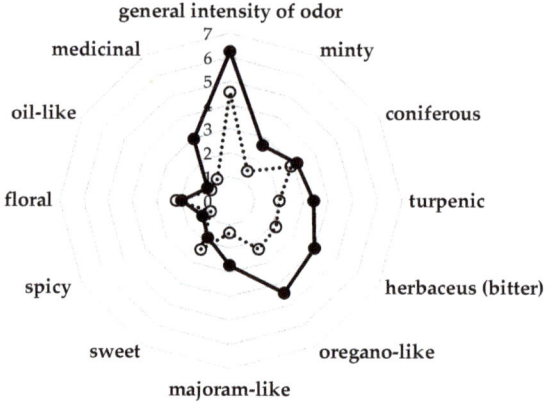
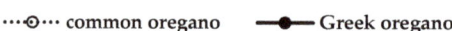

Figure 3. Sensory profile of herb odor of common oregano and Greek oregano.

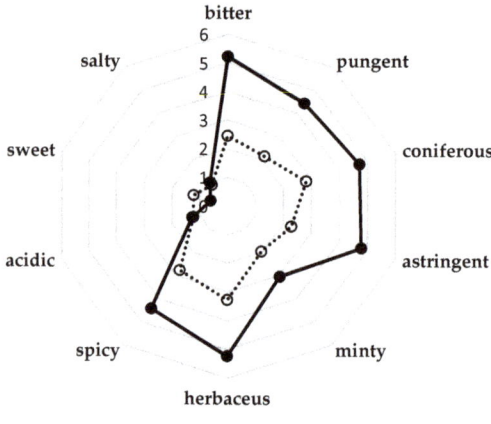
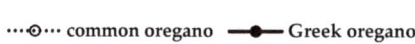

Figure 4. Sensory profile of herb taste of common oregano and Greek oregano.

4. Conclusions

Results obtained in the present work indicate on quite good adaptation of Greek oregano to climatic conditions of Central Europe. This subspecies, grown in the temperate zone, is able to create satisfied yield and still keeps its typical characters of the Mediterranean plant. Among them, a high amount of essential oil followed by a high percentage share of carvacrol seem to be the most important from the practice point of view. Common oregano also presented interesting features, especially when its chemotype (sabinyl/cymyl type rich in sesquiterpenes) and sensory value (floral, sweet) are concerned. Herb of both subspecies appeared to be a rich source of rosmarinic acid, a compound known for its extremely high antioxidant properties. It was shown that the content of this substance fluctuated during plant's development: increased from the beginning of blooming to the beginning of seed-setting, both in Greek oregano and common oregano. With regards to the obtained results, it seems that Greek oregano can be successfully cultivated in the temperate climate of Central Europe. The production of this herb on site, which usually results in its lower price, may increase its availability and utilization, not only as a spice but also as natural medicine.

Author Contributions: Conceptualization, Z.W, K.B. and O.K.; methodology of chemical analysis, O.K., J.L.P.; validation, J.L.P.; investigation, O.K., K.B., J.L.P., Z.W.; writing—original draft preparation, O.K.; references, and statistics—E.P.-J., writing—review and editing, Z.W. and O.K.; supervision, Z.W. and K.B.; project administration, K.B.; funding acquisition, K.B. All authors have read and agreed to the published version of the manuscript.

Funding: The studies were supported by the Polish Ministry of Agriculture and Rural Development, within the Multiannual Programme "Creating the Scientific Basis of the Biological Progress and Conservation of Plant Genetic Resources as a Source of Innovation to Support Sustainable Agriculture and Food Security of the Country"—Task 1.6.

Acknowledgments: The technical help of Analytical Centre (WULS-SGGW) is gratefully acknowledged.

Conflicts of Interest: The authors declare no conflict of interest.

References

1. Skoula, M.; Harborne, J.B. The taxonomy and chemistry of *Origanum*. In *Oregano: The Genera Origanum and Lippia*; Kintzios, S., Ed.; Taylor and Francis: London, UK; New York, NY, USA, 2002; pp. 67–108.
2. Kokkini, S. Taxonomy, diversity and distribution of *Origanum* species. In *Proceedings of the IPGRI International Workshop on Oregano*; Padulosi, S., Ed.; CIHEAM Valenzano: Bari, Italy, 1997; pp. 122–132.
3. Asdal, A.; Galambosi, B.; Bjorn, G.; Olsson, K.; Pihlik, U.; Radušiene, J. Spice—And medicinal plants in the Nordic and Baltic countries. In *Report from a Project Group at the Nordic Gene Bank*; Conservation of Genetic Resources; NGB: Alnarp, Norway, 2006; p. 157.
4. Ietswaart, J.H. *A Taxonomic Revision of the Genus Origanum*; Leiden University Press: The Hague, The Netherlands; Boston, MA, USA; London, UK, 1980.
5. Oliwier, G.W. The world market of oregano. In *Proceedings of the IPGRI International Workshop on Oregano*; Padulosi, S., Ed.; CIHEAM Valenzano: Bari, Italy, 1996; pp. 141–146.
6. Matuszkiewicz, W. *Przewodnik do Oznaczania Zbiorowisk Roślinnych Polski*; Państwowe Wydawnictwo Naukowe: Warsaw, Poland, 2011.
7. Lukas, B.; Schmiderer, C.; Novak, J. Phytochemical diversity of *Origanum vulgare* L. subsp. vulgare (Laminaceae) from Austria. *Bioch. Syst. Ecol.* **2013**, *50*, 106–113. [CrossRef]
8. D'antuono, L.; Galletti, G.; Bocchini, P. Variability of essential oil content and composition of *Origanum vulgare* L. populations from a north Mediterranean area (Liguria region, Northern Italy). *Ann. Bot.* **2000**, *86*, 471–478. [CrossRef]
9. Mockute, D.; Bernotiene, G.; Judzentiene, A. The essential oil of *Origanum vulgare* L. ssp. *vulgare* growing wild in Vilnius district (Lithuania). *Phytochemistry* **2001**, *57*, 65–69. [CrossRef]
10. Mockute, D.; Bernotiene, G.; Judzentiene, A. The β-ocimene chemotype of essential oils of the inflorescences and the leaves with stems from *Origanum vulgare* ssp. *vulgare* growing wild in Lithuania. *Bioch. Syst. Ecol.* **2003**, *31*, 269–278. [CrossRef]
11. Mockute, D.; Bernotiene, G.; Judzentiene, A. Chemical composition of essential oils of *Origanum vulgare* L. growing in Lithuania. *Biologija* **2004**, *4*, 44–49.
12. De Martino, L.; De Feo, V.; Formisano, C.; Mignola, E.; Senatore, F. Chemical composition and antimicrobial activity of the essential oils from three chemotypes of *Origanum vulgare* L. ssp. *hirtum* (Link) Ietswaart growing wild in Campania (Southern Italy). *Molecules* **2009**, *14*, 2735–2746. [CrossRef] [PubMed]
13. Grevsen, K.; Fretté, X.C.; Christensen, L.P. Content and composition of volatile terpenes, flavonoids and phenolic acids in Greek oregano (*Origanum vulgare* L. ssp. *hirtum*) at different development stages during cultivation in cool temperate climate. *Eur. J. Hortic. Sci.* **2009**, *74*, 193–203.
14. Azizi, A.; Hadian, J.; Gholami, M.; Friedt, W.; Honermeier, B. Correlations between genetic, morphological and chemical diversities in a germplasm collection of the medicinal plant *Origanum vulgare* L. *Chem. Biodivers.* **2012**, *9*, 2784–2801. [CrossRef]

15. Kosakowska, O.; Bączek, K.; Geszprych, A.; Węglarz, Z. Ocena składu chemicznego olejku eterycznego dziko rosnących populacji lebiodki pospolitej (*Origanum vulgare* L.). *Pol. J. Agron.* **2013**, *15*, 67–71.
16. Lukas, B.; Schmiderer, C.; Novak, J. Essential oil diversity of European *Origanum vulgare* L. (*Lamiaceae*). *Phytochemistry* **2015**, *119*, 32–40. [CrossRef]
17. Kosakowska, O.; Czupa, W. Morphological and chemical variability of common oregano (*Origanum vulgare* L. subsp. *vulgare*) occurring in eastern Poland. *Herba Pol.* **2018**, *64*, 11–21. [CrossRef]
18. Kosakowska, O.; Węglarz, Z.; Bączek, K. Yield and quality of 'Greek oregano' (*Origanum vulgare* L. subsp. hirtum) herb from organic production system in temperate climate. *Ind. Crop Prod.* **2019**, *141*, 111782. [CrossRef]
19. Węglarz, Z.; Osińska, E.; Geszprych, A.; Przybył, J. Intraspecific variability of wild marjoram (*Origanum vulgare* L.) naturally occurring in Poland. *Braz. J. Med. Plants* **2006**, *8*, 23–26.
20. Radusiene, J.; Ivanauskas, L.; Janulis, V.; Jakstas, V. Composition and variability of phenolic compounds in *Origanum vulgare* from Lithuania. *Biologija* **2008**, *54*, 45–49. [CrossRef]
21. Skoula, M.; Grayer, J.; Kite, G.C.; Veitch, N.C. Exudate flavones and flavanones in *Origanum* species and their interspecific variation. *Biochem. Syst. Ecol.* **2008**, *36*, 646–654. [CrossRef]
22. González, M.D.; Lanzelotti, P.L.; Luis, C.M. Chemical fingerprinting by HPLC-DAD to differentiate certain subspecies of *Origanum vulgare* L. *Food Anal. Methods* **2017**, *10*, 1460–1468. [CrossRef]
23. Gulluce, M.; Karadayi, M.; Guvenalp, Z.; Ozbek, H.; Arasoglu, T.; Baris, O. Isolation of some active compounds from *Origanum vulgare* L. ssp. *vulgare* and determination of their genotoxic potentials. *Food Chem.* **2012**, *130*, 248–253.
24. Gutierrez-Grijalva, E.; Picos-Salas, M.A.; Leyva-Lopez, N.; Criollo-Mendoza, M.S.; Vazquez-Olivo, G.; Heredia, J.B. Flavonoids and phenolic acids from oregano: Occurrence, biological activity and health benefits. *Plants* **2017**, *7*, 2. [CrossRef]
25. Baricevic, D.; Bartol, T. The biological/pharmacological activity of the *Origanum* genus. In *Medicinal and Aromatic Plants—Industrial Profiles*; Kintzios, S., Ed.; Taylor and Francis: London, UK; New York, NY, USA, 2002; pp. 176–213.
26. Chishti, S.; Kaloo, Z.A.; Sultan, P. Medicinal importance of genus *Origanum*: A review. *J. Pharmacogn. Phytother.* **2013**, *5*, 170–177.
27. Senderski, M.E. *Praktyczny Poradnik o Ziołach i Ziołolecznictwie*; Liber: Warsaw, Poland, 2009.
28. Uerpmann-Wittzack, R. European Pharmacopoeia. In *European Directorate for the Quality of Medicines and Health Care (EDQM)*, 9th ed.; Council of Europe: Strasbourg, France, 2017.
29. Bonfanti, C.; Iannì, R.; Mazzaglia, A.; Lanza, C.M.; Napoli, E.M.; Ruberto, G. Emerging cultivation of oregano in Sicily: Sensory evaluation of plants and chemical composition of essential oils. *Ind. Crop Prod.* **2012**, *35*, 160–165. [CrossRef]
30. Cattelan, M.G.; de Castilhos, M.B.M.; da Silva, D.C.; Conti-Silva, C.; Hoffmann, F. Oregano essential oil: Effect on sensory acceptability. *Nutr. Food Sci.* **2015**, *45*, 574–582. [CrossRef]
31. Bisht, D.; Chanotiya, C.; Rana, M.; Semwa, M. Variability in essential oil and bioactive chiral monoterpenoid compositions of Indian oregano (*Origanum vulgare* L.) populations from northwestern Himalaya and their chemotaxonomy. *Ind. Crop Prod.* **2009**, *30*, 422–426. [CrossRef]
32. Elezi, F.; Plaku, F.; Ibraliu, A.; Stefkov, G.; Karapandzova, M.; Kulevanova, S.; Aliu, S. Genetic variation of oregano (*Origanum vulgare* L.) for etheric oil in Albania. *Agric. Sci.* **2013**, *4*, 449–453.
33. Gong, H.Y.; Liu, W.H.; Lv, G.Y.; Zhou, X. Analysis of essential oils of *Origanum vulgare* from six production areas of China and Pakistan. *Bras. J. Pharm.* **2014**, *24*, 25–32. [CrossRef]
34. Zhang, X.L.; Guo, Y.S.; Wang, C.H.; Li, G.Q.; Xu, J.J.; Chung, H.Y.; Ye, W.C.; Li, Y.L.; Wang, G.C. Phenolic compounds from *Origanum vulgare* and their antioxidant and antiviral activities. *Food Chem.* **2014**, *152*, 300–306. [CrossRef] [PubMed]
35. Pasquier, B. Selection work on *Origanum vulgare* in France. In *Proceedings of the IPGRI International Workshop on Oregano*; Padulosi, S., Ed.; CIHEAM: Valenzano (Bari), Italy, 1997; pp. 93–99.
36. Soares, L.A.L.S.; Ferreira, M.R.A. Standardization and quality control of herbal medicines. In *Recent Developments in Phytomedicine Technology*; New Developments in Medical Research; de Freitas, L.A.P., Teixeira, C.C.C., Zamarioli, C.M., Eds.; Nova Science Publisher: Hauppauge, NY, USA, 2017.

37. Berghold, H.S.; Wagner, M.M.; Thaller, A.; Müller, M.; Rakowitz, M.; Pasteiner, S.; Boechzelt, H. Ertrag, gehalt und zusammensetzung des ätherischen öls von fünf oregano-zuchtstämmen (*Origanum vulgare* L.) in abhängigkeitvom entwicklungsstadium. *Z. Arzn. Gew. Pfl.* **2008**, *13*, 36–43.
38. Baranauskiene, R.; Venskutonis, P.; Dambrauskiene, E.; Viškelis, P. Harvesting time influences the yield and oil composition of *Origanum vulgare* L. ssp. *vulgare* and ssp. *hirtum*. *Ind. Crop Prod.* **2013**, *49*, 43–51. [CrossRef]
39. Angielczyk, M.; Bączek, K.; Geszprych, A.; Kosakowska, O.; Mirgos, M.; Pióro-Jabrucka, E.; Węglarz, Z. *Ekologiczna Uprawa Ziół—Rośliny Lecznicze i Aromatyczne ze Stanowisk Naturalnych i z Uprawy w Ekologicznym Systemie Produkcji*; Węglarz, Z., Bączek, K., Eds.; Ministry of Agriculture and Rural Development: Warsaw, Poland, 2013.
40. Žukauska, I.; Sivicka, I. *Draft Descriptor List Origanum Vulgare L.*; European Cooperative Programme for Plant Genetic Resources: Rome, Italy, 2011.
41. Kosakowska, O.; Bączek, K.; Przybył, J.; Pawełczak, A.; Rolewska, K.; Węglarz, Z. Morphological and chemical traits as quality determinants of common thyme (*Thymus vulgaris* L.) on the example of Standard Winter cultivar. *Agronomy* **2020**, *10*, 909. [CrossRef]
42. Bączek, K.; Kosakowska, O.; Przybył, J.L.; Kuźma, P.; Ejdys, M.; Obiedziński, M.; Węglarz, Z. Intraspecific variability of yarrow (*Achillea millefolium* L. s.l.) in respect of developmental and chemical traits. *Herba Pol.* **2015**, *61*, 37–52. [CrossRef]
43. Polish Pharmacopoeia. *Office of Registration of Medicinal Products, Medical Devices and Biocidal Products*, 6th ed.; Polish Pharmaceutical Society: Warsaw, Poland, 2002.
44. Chalchat, J.C.; Pasquier, B. Morphological and chemical studies of *Origanum* clones: *Origanum vulgare* L. ssp. *vulgare*. *J. Essent. Oil Res.* **1998**, *11*, 143–144. [CrossRef]
45. Franz, C.; Novak, J. Breeding of oregano. In *Oregano: The Genera Origanum and Lippia; Medicinal and Aromatic Plants—Industrial Profiles Series*; Kintzios, S.E., Ed.; Taylor and Francis: London, UK; New York, NY, USA, 2004; Volume 25, pp. 163–175.
46. Radusiene, J.; Stakeviciene, D.; Venskutonis, R. Morphological and chemical variation of *Origanum vulgare* L. from Lithuania. *Acta Hort.* **2005**, *675*, 197–203.
47. Azizi, A.; Wagner, C.; Honermeier, B.; Friedt, W. Intraspecific diversity and relationships among subspecies of *Origanum vulgare* revealed by comparative AFLP and SAMPL marker analysis. *Plant Syst. Evol.* **2009**, *281*, 151–160. [CrossRef]
48. Sivicka, I.; Žukauska, I.; Adamovičs, A. Aspects of morphological diversity of oregano in Latvia. *Mod. Phytomor.* **2013**, *4*, 61–64.
49. Sarrou, E.; Tsivelika, N.; Chatzopoulou, P.; Tsakalidis, G.; Menexes, G.; Mavromatis, A. Conventional breeding of Greek oregano (*Origanum vulgare* ssp. *hirtum*) and development of improved cultivars for yield potential and essential oil quality. *Euphytica* **2017**, *213*, 104. [CrossRef]
50. Azizi, A.; Yan, F.; Honermeier, B. Herbage yield, essential oil content and composition of three oregano (*Origanum vulgare* L.) populations as affected by soil moisture regimes and nitrogen supply. *Ind. Crop Prod.* **2009**, *29*, 554–561. [CrossRef]
51. Dordas, C. 2009. Application of calcium and magnesium improves growth yield and essential oil yield of oregano (*Origanum vulgare* ssp. *hirtum*). *Ind. Crop Prod.* **2009**, *29*, 599–608. [CrossRef]
52. Tibaldi, G.; Fontana, E.; Nicola, S. Growing conditions and postharvest management can affect the essential oil of *Origanum vulgare* L. ssp. *hirtum* (Link) Ietswaart. *Ind. Crop Prod.* **2011**, *34*, 1516–1522. [CrossRef]
53. Karamanos, A.J.; Sotiropoulou, D. Field studies of nitrogen application on Greek oregano (*Origanum vulgare* ssp. *hirtum* (Link) Ietswaart) essential oil during two cultivation seasons. *Ind. Crop Prod.* **2013**, *46*, 246–252. [CrossRef]
54. Bosabalidis, A.; Garieli, C.; Niopas, I. Flavone aglycones in glandular hairs of *Origanum x intercedens*. *Phytochemistry* **1998**, *49*, 1549–1553. [CrossRef]
55. Hazzoumi, Z.; Moustakime, Y.; Joutei, K.A. Essential oil and glandular hairs: Diversity and roles. In *Essential Oils—Oils of Nature*; InTech Open: London, UK, 2019. [CrossRef]
56. Svidenko, L.; Grygorieva, O.; Vergun, O.; Hudz, N.; Horčinová, E.; Sedláčková, V.; Šimková, J.; Brindza, J. Characteristic of leaf peltate glandular trichomes and their variability of some *Lamiaceae* family species. *Agrobiodiversity* **2018**, 124–131. [CrossRef]

57. Shafiee-Hajiabad, M.; Hardt, M.; Honermeier, B. Comparative investigation about the trichome morphology of Common oregano (*Origanum vulgare* L. subsp. *vulgare*) and Greek oregano (*Origanum vulgare* L. subsp. *hirtum*). *J. Appl. Res. Med. Aromat. Plants* **2014**, *1*, 50–58. [CrossRef]
58. Roy, B.; Stanton, M.; Eppley, S. Effect of environmental stress on leaf hair density and consequences for selection. *J. Evol. Biol.* **1999**, *12*, 1089–1103. [CrossRef]
59. Rohloff, J. Essential oil drugs—Terpene composition of aromatic herbs. In *Production Practices and Quality Assessment of Food Crops*; Dris, R., Jain, S.M., Eds.; Quality Handling and Evaluation, Kluwer Academic Publishers: Dordrecht, The Netherlands, 2004; Volume 3, pp. 73–128.
60. Figueiredo, A.C.; Barroso, J.G.; José, G.; Pedro, L.G.; Scheffer, J.J.C. Factors affecting secondary metabolite production in plants: Volatile components and essential oils. *Flavour Frag. J.* **2008**, *23*, 213–226. [CrossRef]
61. Başer, K.H.C.; Bouchbauer, G. *Handbook of Essential Oils: Science, Technology and Applications*; Chemical Rubber Company Press: London, UK, 2009.
62. Hudaib, M.; Speroni, E.; Maria, A.; Pietra, D.; Cavrini, V. GC/MS evaluation of thyme (*Thymus vulgaris* L.) oil composition and variations during the vegetative cycle. *J. Pharm. Biomed. Anal.* **2002**, *29*, 691–700. [CrossRef]
63. Clark, G.S. An aroma chemical profile. *Perfum. Flavorist* **1995**, *20*, 41–44.
64. Wang, H.; Chambers, E.; Kan, J. Sensory characteristics of combinations of phenolic compounds potentially associated with smoked aroma in foods. *Molecules* **2018**, *23*, 1867. [CrossRef]
65. Aprotosoaie, A.C.; Hancianu, M.; Costache, I.I.; Miron, A. Linalool: A review on a key odorant molecule with valuable biological properties. *Flavour Fragr. J.* **2014**, *29*, 193–219. [CrossRef]
66. Babushok, V.I.; Linstrom, P.J.; Zenkevich, I.G. Retention Indices for Frequently Reported Compounds of Plant Essential Oils. *J. Phys. Chem. Ref. Data* **2011**, *40*. [CrossRef]
67. Andersen, R.M.; Markham, K.R. *Flavonoids: Chemistry, Biochemistry, and Applications*; Taylor and Francis: Boca Raton, FL, USA; London, UK; New York, NY, USA, 2006.
68. He, J.; Carvalho, A.R.; Mateus, N.; De Freitas, V. Spectral features and stability of oligomeric pyranoanthocyanin-flavanol pigments isolated from red wines. *J. Agric. Food Chem.* **2010**, *58*, 9249–9258. [CrossRef]
69. Janicsák, G.; Máthé, I.; Miklóssy-Vári, V.; Blunden, G. Comparative studies of the rosmarinic and caffeic acid contents of *Lamiaceae* species. *Biochem. Syst. Ecol.* **1999**, *27*, 733–738. [CrossRef]
70. Petersen, M.; Simmons, M.J. Rosmarinic acid. *Mol. Interest* **2003**, *62*, 121–125. [CrossRef]
71. Adomako-Bonsu, A.G.; Chan, S.L.F.; Pratten, M.; Fry, J.R. Antioxidant activity of rosmarinic acid and its principal metabolites in chemical and cellular systems: Importance of physico-chemical characteristics. *Toxicol. In Vitro* **2017**, *40*, 248–255. [CrossRef] [PubMed]
72. Goleniowski, M.; Bonfill, M.; Cusido, R.; Palazon, J. Phenolic Acids. In *Natural Products*; Ramawat, K.G., Merillon, J.M., Eds.; Springer: Berlin/Heidelberg, Germany, 2013.
73. Weng, J.K.; Chapple, C. The origin and evolution of lignin biosynthesis. *New Phytol.* **2010**, *187*, 273–285. [CrossRef] [PubMed]
74. Sárosi, S.; Sipos, L.; Kókai, Z.; Pluhár, Z.; Szilvássy, B.; Novák, I. Effect of different drying techniques on the aroma profile of *Thymus vulgaris* analyzed by GC–MS and sensory profile methods. *Ind. Crop Prod.* **2013**, *46*, 210–216. [CrossRef]
75. Baranauskiene, R.; Kazernavičiute, R.; Pukalskiene, M.; Maždžieriene, R.; Venskutonis, P.R. Agrorefinery of *Tanacetum vulgare* L. into valuable products and evaluation of their antioxidant properties and phytochemical composition. *Ind. Crop Prod.* **2014**, *60*, 113–122. [CrossRef]
76. Asensio, C.M.; Grosso, N.R.; Juliani, H.R. Quality characters, chemical composition and biological activities of oregano (*Origanum* spp.) essential oils from Central and Southern Argentina. *Ind. Crop Prod.* **2015**, *63*, 203–213. [CrossRef]

Publisher's Note: MDPI stays neutral with regard to jurisdictional claims in published maps and institutional affiliations.

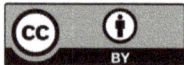

© 2020 by the authors. Licensee MDPI, Basel, Switzerland. This article is an open access article distributed under the terms and conditions of the Creative Commons Attribution (CC BY) license (http://creativecommons.org/licenses/by/4.0/).

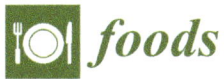

Article

Stem Lettuce and Its Metabolites: Does the Variety Make Any Difference?

Janusz Malarz, Klaudia Michalska and Anna Stojakowska *

Maj Institute of Pharmacology, Polish Academy of Sciences, Department of Phytochemistry, Smętna Street 12, 31-343 Kraków, Poland; malarzj@if-pan.krakow.pl (J.M.); klaudiaz@if-pan.krakow.pl (K.M.)
* Correspondence: stoja@if-pan.krakow.pl; Tel.: +48-1-26-623-254

Abstract: The objective of the present study was to characterize chemical composition of hitherto unexamined aerial parts of *Lactuca sativa* var. *angustana* cv. Grüner Stern. In contrast to leafy and head varieties of the lettuces, asparagus lettuce grown in Europe is much less studied. Fractionation of a methanolic extract from leaves of *L. sativa* cv. Grüner Stern, supported with HPLC/DAD and ^{1}H NMR analysis, led to the isolation and/or identification of numerous terpenoid and phenolic compounds, including five apocarotenoids—(-)-loliolide, (+)-dehydrovomifoliol, blumenol A, (6S,9S)-vomifoliol, and corchoionoside C; three sesquiterpene lactones; two lignans—((+)-syringaresinol and its 4-O-β-glucoside); five caffeic acid derivatives; and three flavonoids. Some of the compounds, to the best of our knowledge, have never been isolated from *L. sativa* before. Moreover, monolignols, phenolic acids and a tryptophan-derived alkaloid were found in the analyzed plant material. Stems, leaves and shoot tips of the asparagus lettuce were examined to assess their phenolics and sesquiterpene lactone content as well as DPPH scavenging activity. Another stem lettuce—*L. sativa* var. *angustana* cv. Karola, two cultivars of leafy lettuces and one species of wild lettuce—*L. serriola*, were also examined as a reference material using HPLC/DAD. The results have been discussed regarding our previous studies and the literature data available.

Keywords: apocarotenoid; caffeic acid derivative; flavonoid; *Lactuca sativa*; lignan; megastigmane; sesquiterpene lactone; 1,2,3,4-tetrahydro-β-carboline-3-carboxylic acid

Citation: Malarz, J.; Michalska, K.; Stojakowska, A. Stem Lettuce and Its Metabolites: Does the Variety Make Any Difference?. *Foods* 2021, *10*, 59. https://doi.org/10.3390/foods10010059

Received: 26 November 2020
Accepted: 24 December 2020
Published: 29 December 2020

Publisher's Note: MDPI stays neutral with regard to jurisdictional claims in published maps and institutional affiliations.

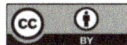

Copyright: © 2020 by the authors. Licensee MDPI, Basel, Switzerland. This article is an open access article distributed under the terms and conditions of the Creative Commons Attribution (CC BY) license (https://creativecommons.org/licenses/by/4.0/).

1. Introduction

Lettuce (*Lactuca sativa* L.), one of the most popular leafy vegetables, is present in the market in a wide variety of cultivars, which differ from one another in their taste, color, texture, pathogen resistance, and value as a functional food. This diversity is connected with an array of specialized metabolites produced by the plants. Rapid development of hyphenated analytical techniques brought about an increase in number of metabolomic studies devoted to crop plants, including popular vegetables like lettuce [1–8]. The studies have been chiefly focused on polyphenols, especially flavonoids and hydroxycinnamates, which are believed to carry some health benefits [9]. Another group of widely investigated specialized metabolites produced by the plant are terpenoids, including carotenoids, pentacyclic triterpenes, and sesquiterpene lactones. The last ones are responsible for the bitter taste of lettuce as well as, to some extent, for inhibition of insect feeding [10–13]. Pharmacological studies proved that lactucin-type guaianolides isolated from lettuce demonstrated anti-inflammatory and antinociceptive activity [14,15]. Metabolomic studies on the cultivated lettuce plants revealed also the occurrence of lignans [2–4,6]. The group of specialized plant metabolites seems to be of importance as an estrogenic component of human diet. However, their content in some lettuce cultivars is probably too low to exert any significant effect on the consumer's health [16].

Stem lettuce, also called asparagus lettuce (*Lactuca sativa* L. var. *angustana* Irish, synonym—var. *asparagina* Bailey) is popular in China as both vegetable and medicinal plant (Chinese lettuce, celtuce or "wosun") [17]. The vegetable is currently much less known in European countries, although it has a history of cultivation in our region [18,19]. Until the middle of the 20th century, a local cultivar of the plant (*L. sativa* L. var. *angustana* cv. Cracoviensis; "głąbiki krakowskie") was popular in Kraków and the surrounding area.

Specialized metabolites accumulated by aerial parts of the asparagus lettuce have not been examined in detail. To the best of our knowledge, only two studies concerning secondary metabolites from edible parts of celtuce have been published so far [17,20]. The paper by Han et al. [17] dealt with sesquiterpenoids from stalks of a Chinese cultivar of the vegetable (purchased on local market). Starkenmann et al. [20] investigated the compounds responsible for the specific smell of the cooked stalks of celtuce. The only paper on constituents of *L. sativa* var. *angustana* cv. Grüner Stern [21] revealed a great structural diversity of sesquiterpene lactones accumulated in roots of the plant. Some of the isolated lactones were new for the cultivated lettuces.

Not only the stalks but also the fresh leaves, which could be used as a component of salads, are the edible parts of the asparagus lettuce [19]. Thus, we decided to study chemical constituents of the leaves from *L. sativa* var. *angustana* cv. Grüner Stern and compare their phytochemical profile to those of the two contemporary cultivars of *L. sativa* and to that of its wild predecessor—*L. serriola* [22]. Moreover, we were interested in chemical differences in composition of extracts from different organs of the celtuce plant.

The present study was aimed at identification of hitherto not described specialized metabolites in the leaves of asparagus lettuce (cv. Grüner Stern) that are of putative value for both consumers and breeders. An attempt was also made to find chemical traits specific for this old cultivar.

2. Materials and Methods

2.1. Chemicals and Solvents

Chlorogenic acid (5-CQA, purity > 97% by HPLC), cichoric acid (DCTA, purity > 98%), luteolin-7-O-β-D-glucoside (purity ≥ 98%), and a standard sample of cynarin (1,3-DCQA, purity > 99% by HPLC) were purchased from Roth (Karlsruhe, Germany). Caftaric acid (CTA, purity > 97%), quercetin-3-O-glucuronide (miquelianin, purity ≥ 95%), Folin–Ciocalteu reagent, gallic acid (GA), 2.2-diphenyl-1-picrylhydrazyl (DPPH), and 6-hydroxy-2,5,7,8-tetramethylchroman-2-carboxylic acid (Trolox) were obtained from Sigma-Aldrich Co. (St. Louis, MO, USA). Luteolin-7-O-glucuronide (purity > 95%) was supplied by HWI pharma services GmbH (Ruelzheim, Germany). Samples of luteolin, quercetin-3-O-β-glucoside (isoquercitrin), quercetin-3-O-β-galactoside (hyperoside), 3,5-dicaffeoylquinic acid (3,5-DCQA), lactucin-type and zaluzanin C-type sesquiterpene lactones, (-)-loliolide, protocatechuic, and caffeic acids as well as monolignols were isolated in our laboratory from different plants of the Asteraceae family and identified by comparison of their spectral data with those found in the literature. CHCl$_3$, EtOAc BuOH, and MeOH of analytical grade were purchased from Avantor Performance Materials S.A. (Gliwice, Poland). Water was purified by a Milli-Q system (Millipore Corp., Bedford, MA, USA). MeOH and MeCN of HPLC grade as well as formic acid and glacial acetic acid of analytical grade were purchased from Merck (Darmstadt, Germany).

2.2. General Experimental Procedures

Optical rotation was determined on a PolAAr31 polarimeter (Optical Activity Ltd., Ramsey, UK). NMR spectra were recorded either in CDCl$_3$ or in CD$_3$OD on a Bruker AVANCE III HD 400 (resonance frequency—400.17 MHz for ^{1}H) (Bruker Corp., Billerica, MA, USA). Analytical RP-HPLC separations were performed either at 25 °C, on a Zorbax Eclipse XDB-C18 column 4.6 × 150 mm (Agilent Technologies, Santa Clara, CA, USA) or at 40 °C on a on a Kinetex XB-C18 column (4.6 × 250 mm, 5 µm; Phenomenex, CA, USA) using an Agilent 1200 Series HPLC system (Agilent Technologies) equipped with a Rheodyne manual sample injector, quaternary pump, degasser, column oven, and a diode array detector. Semipreparative RP-HPLC was performed on a Vertex Plus column (Eurospher II 100-5 C18, 8 × 250 mm) (Knauer GmbH, Berlin, Germany) eluted with H$_2$O-

MeOH mixtures at a flow rate of 1.0–2.0 mL min^{-1}, using Knauer P4.1S pump coupled to a dual wavelength UV/VIS detector operating at 210 and 260 nm. Conventional column chromatography (CC) was carried out using Merck silica gel 60 (0.063–0.2 mm), Polyamide 6 (Sigma-Aldrich Co.), and Sephadex LH-20 (GE Healthcare, Uppsala, Sweden). Thin layer chromatography (TLC) was performed on Merck silica gel 60 (0.25 mm) precoated plates.

2.3. Plant Material

Aerial parts of *L. sativa* L. var. *angustana* cv. Grüner Stern were collected three times. First, in July 2014, the raw material for isolation work was harvested (leaves, stalks, and shoot tops from the flowering plants; voucher No 03/2014). Next, in June and July 2020, the plant material for HPLC/DAD analyses (leaves from 8 and 15 weeks old plants; voucher No 02/2020) was collected concomitantly with the leaves of three other *L. sativa* cultivars and the leaves of *L. serriola*. Seeds of *L. sativa* L. var. *angustana* cv. Grüner Stern were obtained from the Botanical Garden of the Bonn University (Germany). Seeds of *L. sativa* var. *angustana* cv. Karola, *L. sativa* cv. Great Lakes, and *L. sativa* var. *crispa* cv. Amerikanischer Brauner were purchased from the commercial growers. Seeds of *L. serriola* L., collected from the wild, were delivered by the Botanical Gardens in Münster (Westfälische Wilhelms-Universität, Münster, Germany; voucher No 05/2020) and Nantes (Ville de Nantes, France; voucher No 04/2020). All plants were grown in the Garden of Medicinal Plants, Maj Institute of Pharmacology, Polish Academy of Sciences, Kraków, Poland, where the voucher specimens were deposited. Data on cultivation conditions (type of soil, average annual temperature, annual rainfall, and agrotechnical procedures applied) are described elsewhere [23]. The collected plant material was dried at room temperature under shade.

2.4. Isolation of Chemical Constituents from Leaves of L. sativa L. var. angustana cv. Grüner Stern

The dried plant material (378 g) was powdered and exhaustively extracted with 70% MeOH (4 × 1.5 L) at room temperature with shaking. The combined extracts were concentrated in vacuo providing c. 500 mL of an aqueous suspension. The suspension was successively extracted with *n*-hexane, CHCl$_3$, EtOAc, and *n*-BuOH. The obtained organic extracts were evaporated under the reduced pressure to yield 3.62, 1.60, 1.76, and 8.56 g of the dry residue, respectively.

The CHCl$_3$ extract (1.60 g) was subjected to CC on silica (28.0 g) using gradients of EtOAc in hexane (up to 100% EtOAc) and subsequently, MeOH in EtOAc (up to 50% MeOH) as elution systems. The separated fractions (50 mL each) were monitored by TLC and the relevant ones were combined. Elution with hexane-EtOAc (4:1, *v/v*) gave fractions 52–59 that were further separated by the preparative TLC on silica using hexane-EtOAc (3:2, *v/v*) as a mobile phase (two developments) to yield **1** (2.7 mg). Fractions 60–65, after preparative TLC (hexane-EtOAc, 3:2 *v/v*, two developments) were subjected to semipreparative RP-HPLC (H$_2$O-MeOH, 2:3, *v/v*, 2 mL min^{-1}) to give **2** (2.0 mg). From the fractions 93–97, eluted with hexane-EtOAc 7:3 (*v/v*) and initially purified by TLC (hexane:EtOAc, 1:1, *v/v*), after semipreparative RP-HPLC (H$_2$O-MeOH, 2:3, *v/v*, 2 mL min^{-1}), **3** (1.3 mg) and **4** (0.9 mg) were obtained. Fractions 103–111 (eluted with hexane-EtOAc 1:1 (*v/v*)) were further separated by preparative TLC (CHCl$_3$-MeOH, 19:1, *v/v*) to furnish **5** (3.9 mg), and a mixture that was subjected to semipreparative RP-HPLC (H$_2$O-MeOH, 3:7, *v/v*, 2 mL min^{-1}) to yield **6** and **7** in a mixture (2:1, 1.3 mg). Elution with EtOAc-MeOH (9:1, *v/v*) gave fractions 175–184 that after preparative TLC (CHCl$_3$-MeOH, 9:1, *v/v*) and subsequent semipreparative RP-HPLC (H$_2$O-MeOH, 3:2, *v/v*, 2 mL min^{-1}) yielded **8** (1.7 mg).

The EtOAc soluble part of the methanolic extract was partitioned by the conventional CC on silica gel. As an eluent, a gradient solvent system composed of MeOH in CHCl$_3$ (up to 100% MeOH) was used. Fractions 12–29 (eluted with CHCl$_3$-MeOH, 19:1, *v/v*) were subjected to preparative TLC to give subfractions A and B. The subfraction A was further separated by semipreparative RP-HPLC (H$_2$O-MeOH-HCOOH-CH$_3$COOH, 69:30:0.9:0.1,

$v/v/v/v$, 2 mL min^{-1}) to yield **9** (2.4 mg) and **10** (13.8 mg). The subfraction B after purification by semipreparative RP-HPLC (H$_2$O-MeOH-HCOOH-CH$_3$COOH, 49:50:0.9:0.1, $v/v/v/v$, 2 mL min^{-1}) furnished **11** (2.6 mg). Fractions eluted with CHCl$_3$-MeOH 9:1 (v/v) were submitted to preparative TLC (CHCl$_3$-MeOH, 17:3, v/v) to give **12** (13.7 mg).

The n-BuOH part of the methanolic extract was initially separated by CC on polyamide to give fractions P1-P65 (100 mL each). The separated fractions were monitored by analytical RP-HPLC/DAD, and the relevant ones were combined. The fractions that contained commonly known *L. sativa* metabolites, easily detectable by HPLC/DAD (protocatechuic acid, caffeic acid, 5-CQA, luteolin-7-*O*-β-glucopyranoside, and isoquercitrin), as major constituents, were not further separated.

Fraction P1 (2.46 g), eluted with H$_2$O, was subjected to CC on Sephadex LH-20 using H$_2$O as an eluent. The obtained subfractions, P1S1–P1S2 (50 mL each) and P1S3-P1S12 (25 mL each), were monitored by RP-HPLC/DAD. The subfraction P1S4 was subjected to semipreparative RP-HPLC (H$_2$O-MeOH-HCOOH-CH$_3$COOH, 74:25:0.9:0.1, $v/v/v/v$, 1 mL min^{-1}) to give a complex mixture of compounds containing (based on ^{1}H NMR) benzyl glucoside, syringin, dihydrosyringin, roseoside, and cichorioside B (14.4 mg, t_R = 12.0 min) and a mixture of **13** and **14** (1:4, 8.8 mg, t_R = 24.2 min).

Fraction P2 (1.27 g), eluted with H$_2$O, was separated on Sephadex LH-20, with H$_2$O, to give subfractions P2S1–P2S12 (25 mL each). The subfraction P2S5 (23.4 mg), based on ^{1}H NMR, contained esculetin glucoside (**15**) and syringaresinol glucoside as major constituents. The subfractions P2S7–P2S11 (13.8 mg) contained a tryptophan derivative (**16**).

Fractions P52–P55 (0.08 g), after semipreparative RP-HPLC (H$_2$O-MeOH-HCOOH-CH$_3$COOH, 59:40:0.9:0.1, $v/v/v/v$, 1 mL min^{-1}), yielded luteolin-7-*O*-glucuronide butyl ester (4.5 mg). The compound, most likely, was an artifact formed during the separation process, as the corresponding peak was absent from the hydroalcoholic extract from leaves.

Fractions P57–P65 (0.16 g) were further purified by semipreparative RP-HPLC (H$_2$O-MeOH-HCOOH-CH$_3$COOH, 59:40:0.9:0.1, $v/v/v/v$, 2 mL min^{-1}) to furnish a mixture of caffeoylquinic derivatives (**17** and **18**, 7.0 mg, 4:1, t_R = 15.2 min) and pure **18** (18.8 mg, t_R = 25.0 min).

2.5. Assessment of the Reducing Capacity of the Plant Material

The reducing capacity of the plant material, referred to as "total phenolic content" (TPC), was estimated using Folin–Ciocalteu colorimetric method, as described earlier [24]. Measurements were done using 20 mg of the dry plant material per sample. Leaves of 8- and 15-week-old plants of asparagus lettuce (cv. Karola and cv. Grüner Stern) and *L. serriola* (two accessions) were collected and dried separately for each individual plant. Results (means of three samples, each prepared from one plant) were expressed as gallic acid equivalents (mg GA g^{-1} DW).

2.6. DPPH Radical Scavenging Assay

Portions of dried and pulverized leaves, stalks, and shoot tops of *L. sativa* var. angustana cv. Grüner Stern (100 mg each) were extracted twice with 12.5 mL of 50% MeOH at room temperature. The solutions from two subsequent extractions were pooled together and evaporated in vacuo. The obtained residues were dissolved in 1 mL of 70% MeOH each, left to stand overnight, at 4 °C, centrifuged (11,340× g, 5 min), and the supernatant was diluted 10 times to obtain concentration corresponding to 10 mg of the dry plant material per 1 mL of the sample. DPPH was dissolved in methanol to obtain the stable free radical solution (100 μM). Solution (4 mM) of Trolox (reference compound) was prepared by dissolving of 100 mg of the compound in 100 mL of methanol. To a spectrophotometric cuvette (1 cm pathlength) containing 480 μL of the methanolic DPPH solution, 20 μL of the diluted plant extract (final concentration 10 mg DW mL^{-1}) was added. A decrease in absorbance at λ = 517 nm was measured by UV/VIS CE 2021 spectrophotometer (Cecil, UK) after 0.5, 1, 2, 3, 4, 5, 10, 15, 20, and 30 min.

2.7. Sesquiterpene Lactone Analysis

Methanol extracts from the dry and pulverized plant tissues (200 mg) were subjected to RP-HPLC/DAD analysis, as it was described before [25]. Lactucin-like guaianolides could be easily detected in the extracts due to their distinctive chromophore (λ_{max}—258 nm).

2.8. Quantification of Major Caffeic Acid Derivatives

The dry and pulverized plant tissue (50 mg) was extracted twice with 10 mL of 70% MeOH at room temperature for 3 h on a rotary shaker (100 r.p.m.). The extracts were combined and evaporated to dryness under reduced pressure to give a residue that was redissolved in 1 mL of 70% MeOH and centrifuged ($11,340 \times g$, 5 min) prior to HPLC analysis. Analytical RP-HPLC separations of the samples were performed as it was described earlier [26]. Quantification was carried out using an external standard method. The calibration curves were constructed using four concentration levels (0.001, 0.01, 0.1, and 1.0 mg mL^{-1}) of 5-CQA, caffeic acid, CTA, and DCTA. Peak areas, measured at 325 nm, were referred to the corresponding calibration curve.

3. Results

Eighteen known natural compounds (**1–18**) were isolated from the leaves of *L. sativa* var. *angustana* cv. Grüner Stern, collected at the beginning of flowering. Structures of the compounds (some shown in Figure 1) were confirmed by direct comparison of their spectral data (UV, ^{1}H NMR) and optical activity with either that of the standard samples or that found in the literature (^{1}H NMR spectra of the newly isolated compounds are available as the Supplementary Material attached to this paper). (+)-Dehydrovomifoliol (=(6*S*,7*E*)-6-hydroxy-4,7-megastigmadien-3,9-dione, **1**) [27], (-)-loliolide (**2**) [28], (6*S*,9*R*) vomifoliol (=blumenol A, **3**), (6*S*,9*S*)-vomifoliol (**4**) [29], and (6*S*,9*S*)-roseoside (=corchoionoside C, **14**) [30,31] (see Figure 1), as far as we are aware, have not been found in cultivated lettuce plants until now. Lignans: (+)-syringaresinol (**5**) and (±)-syringaresinol-4-*O*-β-glucopyranoside (**8**) [32,33] as well as a tryptophan-derived alkaloid—1,2,3,4-tetrahydro-β-carboline-3-carboxylic acid (=lycoperodine-1, **16**) [34–36] were tentatively identified in some cultivars of *L. sativa* using advanced analytical techniques [2–6]. A sesquiterpene lactone-9α-hydroxy-11β,13-dihydrozaluzanin C (**6**) [37] has been previously isolated from roots of *L. laciniata* Makino (synonym of *L. sativa* L.) [38] and roots of *Lactuca altaica* Fisch. & C.A. Mey (currently regarded as a synonym of *L. serriola* L.) [39], but has not been found neither in stalks of Chinese celtuce [17] nor in roots of *L. sativa* cv. Grüner Stern [21]. Thus, the compound **6** has been isolated from the commercial cultivar of lettuce for the first time. A dihydroderivative of **6**—9α-hydroxy-4β,11β,13,15-tetrahydrozaluzanin C (**7**) [40] has been described as a constituent of celtuce stalks [17], and it has been the only report on its occurrence in cultivated lettuce plants.

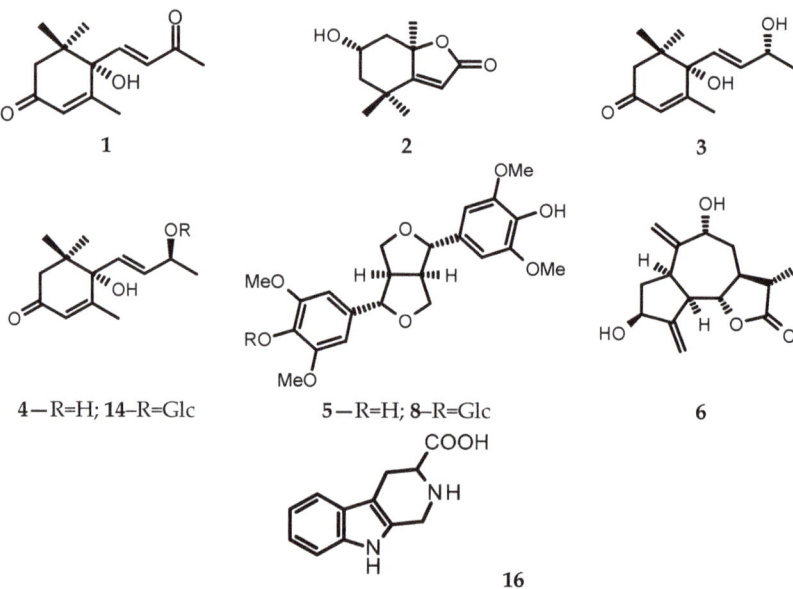

Figure 1. Chemical structures of some compounds isolated from leaves of the asparagus lettuce cv. Grüner Stern. Compounds **1–4** ((+)-Dehydrovomifoliol, (-)-loliolide, blumenol A, (6S,9S)-vomifoliol), **6** (9α-hydroxy-11β,13-dihydrozaluzanin C), and **14** (corchoionoside C) were known natural products newly found in the cultivated lettuce, whereas compounds **5** ((+)-syringaresinol), **8** ((±)-syringaresinol-4-O-β-glucopyranoside), and **16** (1,2,3,4-tetrahydro-β-carboline-3-carboxylic acid) were previously tentatively identified in various commercial cultivars of lettuce by means of ultra-high-performance liquid chromatography (UHPLC) with photodiode array (DAD) and mass detection (ESI/QTOF/MS – electrospray ionization/quadrupole time-of-flight mass spectrometry).

The remaining compounds: protocatechuic acid (=3,4-dihydroxybenzoic acid, **9**), caffeic acid (**10**), luteolin (**11**), isoquercitrin (=quercetin-3-O-β-glucopyranoside, **12**), benzyl-O-β-glucopyranoside (**13**), cichoriin (**15**), 3,5-DCQA (**17**), and 4,5-DCQA (**18**) [2,41–43] are commonly known metabolites of wild and cultivated lettuces. Moreover, the presence of syringin, dihydrosyringin, and cichorioside B, in the analyzed plant material, was confirmed based on the ^{1}H NMR spectra of some partially purified fractions.

The reducing capacities of extracts from leaves of *L. sativa* var. asparagina cv. Grüner Stern, cv. Karola, and *L. serriola* plants of different provenience (all 8 weeks old) ranged from 36.363 ± 2.78 to 43.27 ± 1.79 mg g^{-1} GA eq for cv. Grüner Stern and *L. serriola* from France, respectively (Table 1). Statistically significant differences in TPC (one-way ANOVA, $p < 0.05$) between *L. serriola* and the two examined cultivars of stem lettuce were not found neither in 8 weeks old nor in 15 weeks old plants.

In order to roughly assess radical-quenching activities of extracts from different parts of the asparagus lettuce, DPPH radical scavenging measurements were done. The experiments revealed substantial differences in activity of the examined extracts. The extract from leaves (10 mg DW mL^{-1}) scavenged 72.7% ± 5.8% of the DPPH radical, whereas the extracts from stalks caused quenching of only 7.4% of the available free radical, after 30 min reaction (Figure 2).

Table 1. Reducing capacities (total phenolic contents) of extracts from leaves of *Lactuca sativa* var. *asparagina* and *Lactuca serriola* plants harvested after 8 and 15 weeks of growth in the open field. Results, expressed as gallic acid equivalents (GA eq), are means of three measurements (±SD).

Plant Material	Total Phenolic Content (mg g^{-1} Dry Weight) GA eq
L. sativa cv. Grüner Stern, 8 weeks	36.36 ± 2.78
15 weeks	44.09 ± 3.83
L. sativa cv. Karola, 8 weeks	41.55 ± 1.55
15 weeks	44.46 ± 3.82
L. serriola Münster, 8 weeks	36.38 ± 5.58
15 weeks	46.03 ± 4.47
L. serriola Nantes, 8 weeks	43.27 ± 1.79
15 weeks	46.81 ± 4.21

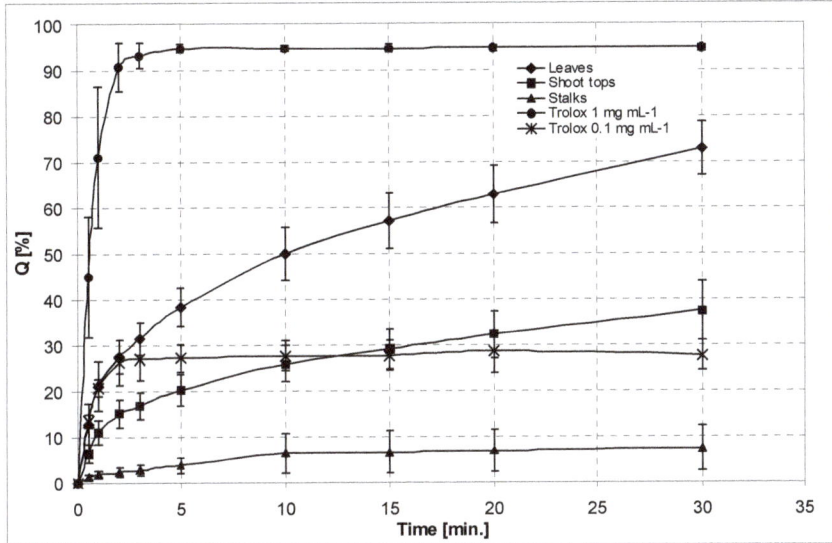

Figure 2. DPPH radical scavenging activity of 0.1 and 1 mg mL^{-1} solutions of Trolox (reference compound) and hydroalcoholic extracts from stalks, shoot tops, and leaves of *L. sativa* var. *asparagina* cv. Grüner Stern (10 mg of the dried plant material per 1 mL of extract).

Except for cichorioside B, identified as one of the components of the complex mixture of compounds from the butanolic fraction, we did not find any lactucin-like guaianolide during the fractionation of the extract from leaves of asparagus lettuce. Roots of the plant, investigated earlier [20], yielded mainly glucosides of **6** and 9α-hydroxyzaluzanin C accompanied by minor amounts of lactucin-like guaianolides, of which cichorioside B was the most abundant one. As 11β,13-dihydrolactucopicrin, another lactucin-like sesquiterpene lactone, was isolated from the celtuce stalks [17], its presence in the material under study was checked by HPLC/DAD method.

To assess the content of 11β,13-dihydrolactucopicrin/lactucopicrin (one of the most characteristic and easily detectable pairs of sesquiterpene lactones from *L. sativa*) in the analyzed plant material, a series of extracts was prepared from different organs of the asparagus lettuce (Figure 3a), leaves of *L. serriola*, and leaves of various cultivars of *L. sativa* (Figure 3b). The aerial parts of *L. sativa* cv. Grüner Stern, collected in July, contained c. 0.003% DW of 11β,13-dihydrolactucopicrin/lactucopicrin. The content was two times smaller than that found in roots of the plant. In general, *L. serriola* leaves, and leaves of the analyzed *L. sativa* cultivars, did not accumulate detectable amounts of the compounds until the eighth week of growth. The exceptions were two individual plants of *L. serriola* (Nantes) and one plant of the Amerikanischer Brauner cultivar (c. 0.005–0.009% DW). After 15 weeks of growth, 11β,13-dihydrolactucopicrin/lactucopicrin was not detected in leaves of asparagus lettuce (cv. Grüner Stern and cv. Karola), but was present in leaves of both *L. serriola* accessions (0.087–0.123% DW) and leafy cultivars of *L. sativa* (0.008–0.014% DW).

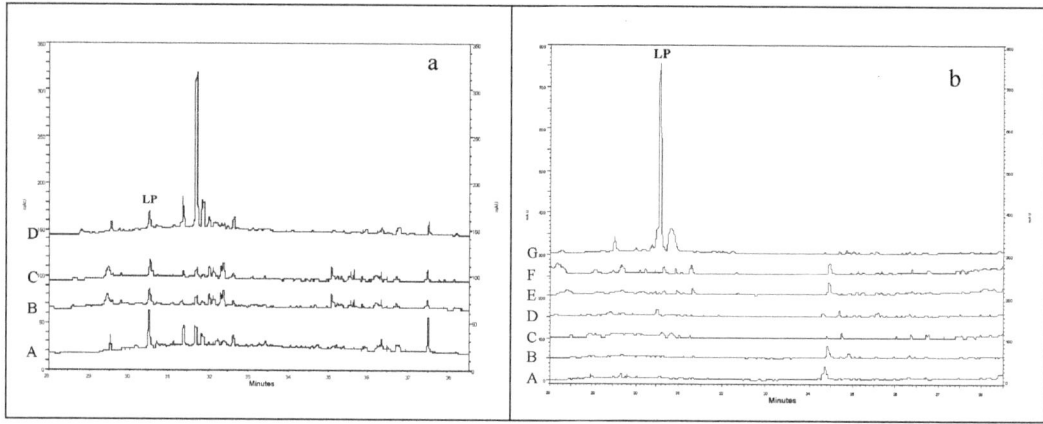

Figure 3. Chromatographic separations (HPLC/DAD, λ = 260 nm) of extracts from: (**a**) different parts/organs of *L. sativa* var. *angustana* cv. Grüner Stern, harvested in the beginning of flowering (A—roots, B—shoot tops, C—leaves, and D—stalks); (**b**) leaves of 8-week-old *L. sativa* and *L. serriola* plants (A—*L. sativa* cv. Grüner Stern, B—*L. sativa* cv. Karola, C—*L. sativa* cv. Great Lakes, D—*L. sativa* cv. Amerikanischer Brauner, E—*L. serriola* (Münster), F—*L. serriola* (Nantes), and G—leaves of *L. serriola* in flowering). Signals corresponding to 11β,13-dihydrolactucopicrin/lactucopicrin were marked as LP.

To investigate the diversity in polyphenolic profile among the analyzed plant species and cultivars, a series of hydroalcoholic extracts from leaf samples was prepared and chromatographically analyzed. Six major hydroxycinnamate signals (Figure 4) could be observed in the analyzed samples, i.e., CTA (t_R = 5.5 min), 5-CQA (t_R = 6.7 min), caffeic acid (t_R = 7.4 min), DCTA (t_R = 13.0 min), and two unidentified caffeates (t_R = 8.9 min and t_R = 15.1 min). The compounds were quantified according to the previously described procedure. The results are summarized in Table 2.

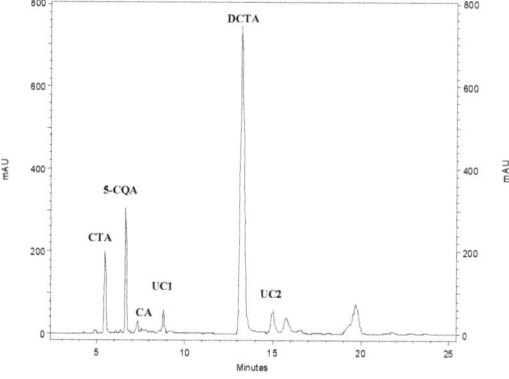

Figure 4. HPLC/DAD chromatogram of hydroalcoholic extract from leaves of 8-week-old *L. sativa* var. *asparagina* cv. Grüner Stern plant (50 mg of the dried plant material per 1 mL of extract, detection wavelength—325 nm). CTA—caftaric acid, 5-CQA—chlorogenic acid, CA—caffeic acid, UC1 and UC2—unidentified caffeic acid derivatives, DCTA—cichoric acid.

Table 2. Results of the assessment of major hydroxycinnamate constituents in the leaves of 8-week-old *Lactuca sativa* and *Lactuca serriola* plants. CTA—caftaric acid, 5-CQA—chlorogenic acid, DCTA—cichoric acid. Results are means of three independent measurements ± SD (results denoted with the same letter were not statistically different, $p < 0.05$).

Plant Material	CTA	5-CQA	Caffeic Acid	DCTA
L. sativa cv. Grüner Stern	0.121 ± 0.087 [a]	0.108 ± 0.023 [a]	0.018 ± 0.03 [a]	1.023 ± 0.124 [a]
L. sativa cv. Karola	0.185 ± 0.037 [a]	0.246 ± 0.036 [b]	0.021 ± 0.007 [a]	1.733 ± 0.101 [a]
L. sativa cv. Great Lakes	0.142 ± 0.01 [a]	0.176 ± 0.047 [a]	0.038 ± 0.001 [a]	1.234 ± 0.026 [a]
L. sativa cv. Amerikanischer Brauner	0.161 ± 0.02 [a]	0.622 ± 0.035 [c]	0.047 ± 0.01 [a]	2.069 ± 0.075 [a]
L. serriola Münster	0.560 ± 0.027 [b]	0.062 ± 0.004 [a]	0.029 ± 0.007 [a]	1.888 ± 0.483 [a]
L. serriola Nantes	0.363 ± 0.055 [b]	0.243 ± 0.007 [a]	0.027 ± 0.002 [a]	2.267 ± 0.537 [a]

Looking at the obtained chromatograms, distinctly higher content of CTA in leaves of *L. serriola* in comparison with that in *L. sativa* cultivars could be noticed in the 8 weeks old plants. Statistical analysis (one-way ANOVA, $p < 0.05$ followed by Tukey's HSD test) of the quantitative results obtained for caffeic acid derivatives (CTA, 5-CQA, caffeic acid, DCTA) confirmed significant differences in CTA content between *L. serriola* and cultivated lettuces (irrespectively of the cultivar). Seven weeks later, however, no differences in the major caffeate contents could be found (data not shown).

Major flavonoid signals were localized at t_R = 15.9 min (quercetin-3-O-β-glucoside, λ_{max}—351 and luteolin-7-O-β-glucoside, λ_{max}—345 nm, a pair of poorly separated compounds), t_R = 16.7 min (luteolin-7-O-glucuronide, λ_{max}—345), and at t_R = 19.9 min (unidentified compound, λ_{max}—351 nm). Virtually the same set of polyphenolics could be observed in every sample.

4. Discussion

Numerous factors regulate production and accumulation of secondary metabolites in lettuce including light, temperature, availability of nutrients, and presence of pathogens and pests. Accumulation of particular compounds in the plant organs could be also affected by the stage of a plant life cycle [20–24]. Moreover, colonizing microorganisms, e.g., mycorrhizal fungi, can affect secondary metabolism of the host plant [25]. The multiplicity of factors that affect the plant metabolome makes direct comparison of results obtained in different experiments difficult, though some general conclusions can be drawn on the basis of the available data.

The apocarotenoids 1–4 and 14 have not been found previously in cultivated lettuces. Comprehensive metabolomic fingerprints obtained by different HPLC/DAD/MS methods [2,5–8] did not reveal the presence of these compounds. Their absence from the investigated plant material, however, is very unlikely. The compounds originated from degradation of carotenoids and are widely distributed within the plant kingdom. Loliolide and β-damascenone are known metabolites of *L. serriola*, a wild predecessor of the cultivated lettuces [44,45]. Its plausible that the minute amounts of apocarotenoids were difficult to detect in a very complex matrix submitted to metabolomic analysis. Their isolation from the asparagus lettuce may suggest higher contents of the metabolites in the plant material under study in comparison with other lettuce cultivars. It is worth to note that lettuce is frequently used as a model plant to investigate allelopathic activity of apocarotenoids [46–48]. The compounds demonstrate diverse biological effects of ecological and pharmacological significance. (+)-Dehydrovomifoliol (**1**) inhibited germination of *L. sativa* cv. Roman and *Allium cepa* L. seeds and inhibited development of *L. sativa* cv. Napoli V.F. plants, but stimulated shoot and root elongation in *Hordeum vulgare* L. [46,47]. It moderately inhibited LPS-induced NO production in mouse RAW264.7 cells, after 24 h, by Griess reagent-based assay [49] and expressed cytotoxic effect against some cancer cell lines in vitro [50]. (-)-Loliolide (**2**), formerly identified as a potent ant repellent [51], recently has been postulated to be an endogenous inducer of herbivore resistance in plants [52]. The compound inhibited cellular senescence in human dermal fibroblasts [53], exerted antimelanogenic and oxidative stress-protective effects in mouse melanoma and human keratinocyte cells [54], inhibited HCV virus entry in vitro [55], and, similarly to **1**, LPS-induced NO generation in RAW264.7 cells [56]. Blumenol A (**3**) and its isomer (6*S*,9*S*)-vomifoliol (**4**) demonstrated anti-inflammatory activity in different types of in vitro assays [57–59]. Recently, neuroprotective function of vomifoliol in amyloid-*beta*$_{1-42}$-treated neuroblastoma cells has been also studied [60]. Blumenol A moderately inhibited elongation of shoots and roots of *L. sativa* cv. Napoli V.F. and growth of some monocots [47,48]. Compound **5** (corchoionoside C, a glucoside of **4**) is one of the four stereoisomers of roseoside. Corchoionoside C inhibited histamine release, induced by antigen–antibody reaction, from rat peritoneal exudate cells [61]. Roseoside of unspecified stereostructure inhibited production of hypertension-related molecules by the rat myocardial cells stimulated with angiotensin II [62] and delayed carcinogenesis induced by peroxynitrite and TPA treatment in mice [63]. (+)-Roseoside caused vasorelaxation of the precontracted aortic rings from Sprague–Dawley rats (in endothelium-dependent manner) [64] and demonstrated insulinotropic activity [65].

Phenolic compounds are the most extensively studied lettuce metabolites. Their dietary intake is promoted as they are generally considered beneficial to human health [9]. According to van Treuren et al. [7], wild relatives of *L. sativa*, as well as primitive forms of domesticated lettuce, contain more polyphenols than modern cultivars. The main groups of the lettuce polyphenols are flavonoids (including anthocyanins from red varieties) and hydroxycinnamic acids derivatives and lignans. Although flavonoids and hydroxycinnamates are major constituents of lettuce plants (see DCTA content in leaves, Table 2), lignans are usually present in minute amounts. Up to 16 μg of lignans in 100 g of fresh lettuce leaves was reported by Milder et al. [16]. Isolation yield of lignans from the leaves of asparagus lettuce (c. 1.4 mg per 100 g dry weight) suggested relatively high content of the compounds in the investigated plant material. Metabolomic studies disclosed lignan accumulation patterns in some cultivated lettuces with syringaresinol and its glycosides as major representatives of this subclass of plant phenolics [2–4]. The asparagus lettuce investigated in the present study seems to follow the same scheme. In addition, major flavonoids detected in leaves of *L. sativa* cv. Grüner Stern corresponded to those found in leafy cultivars of the species. Significant qualitative and quantitative differences in the contents of the major hydroxycinnamates were not observed as well. The reducing capacity (TPC) of extracts from *L. serriola* and the two examined cultivars of the asparagus lettuce, Karola and Grüner Stern (Table 1), was comparable and falls within the range of TPC values estimated for different leaf cultivars of *L. sativa* [66]. The DPPH scavenging activity of extracts from different parts of *L. sativa* cv. Grüner Stern (Figure 2) suggests that the leaves of the plant are the richest in antioxidant compounds.

Sesquiterpene lactones are the most distinctive terpenoid constituents of lettuces. They are responsible for the bitter taste and, to some extent, for the insect resistance of the plants [10–13]. The compounds are usually present in very small amounts in the plant material intended for consumption (due to their bitterness) and their contents markedly increase at the bolting stage [67]. In the extract from leaves of the asparagus lettuce only 9α-hydroxy-11β,13-dihydrozaluzanin C (**6**) and 9α-hydroxy-4β,11β,13,15-tetrahydrozaluzanin C (**7**) were present in quantities that allow successful isolation of the lactones. The former compound was a novel constituent of the cultivated lettuce. Cichorioside B (dihydrolactucin glucoside) was identified as a component of a complex fraction from the butanolic part of the extract. Lactucopicrin and/or its dihydroderivative could not be detected in leaves of the asparagus lettuce collected in the initial phase of cultivation (until the 15th week). The compound was accumulated by the plants that enter the flowering stage albeit in small quantities.

Though metabolomic analyses of selected *L. sativa* cultivars [2,5,6] revealed the presence of tryptophan-derived alkaloids (including **16**), this is the first report on isolation of 1,2,3,4-tetrahydro-β-carboline-3-carboxylic acid (**16**) from the commercial cultivar of lettuce. The compound was first isolated from the leaves of *Allium tuberosum* [34]. Later on, it was purified from aged garlic, tomato, and some Asteraceae plants including *Cichorium endivia*

L. [36]. 1,2,3,4-Tetrahydro-β-carboline-3-carboxylic acid induced apoptosis in colorectal cancer cell line HCT-8, in a dose-dependent manner [36], and was identified as one of the main antioxidants in aged garlic extracts [68].

5. Conclusions

Our findings concerning secondary metabolites from leaves of the old cultivar of stem lettuce (cv. Grüner Stern) broaden the knowledge on the chemistry of the garden lettuce—one of the most popular leafy vegetables. Among the newly identified constituents of the plant, apocarotenoids may have been of importance, taking into consideration both their ecological role and their pharmacological activity. It is worth to note that the apocarotenoids (compounds **1–4** and **14**) and 9α-hydroxyzaluzanin C derivatives (9α-hydroxy-11β,13-dihydrozaluzanin C and 9α-hydroxy-4β,11β,13,15-tetrahydrozaluzanin C) have not been found before in any of the commercial cultivars of the lettuce. The investigated plant material, in terms of polyphenolic content and antioxidative activity, was similar to modern leafy cultivars of *L. sativa*.

Supplementary Materials: The following are available online at https://www.mdpi.com/2304-8158/10/1/59/s1, Supplementary material (Figures S1–S8, ^{1}H NMR spectra of compounds **1–3**, **5–8**, **14**, and **16**).

Author Contributions: Conceptualization, A.S.; methodology, J.M., K.M., and A.S.; investigation, J.M., K.M., and A.S.; resources, J.M., K.M., and A.S.; data curation, J.M. and A.S.; writing—original draft preparation, J.M. and A.S.; writing—review and editing, A.S; project administration, A.S. All authors have read and agreed to the published version of the manuscript.

Funding: This research received no external funding.

Institutional Review Board Statement: Not applicable.

Informed Consent Statement: Not applicable.

Data Availability Statement: Data is contained within the article or supplementary material.

Conflicts of Interest: The authors declare no conflict of interest.

References

1. Sobolev, A.P.; Brosio, E.; Gianferri, R.; Segre, A.L. Metabolite profile of lettuce leaves by high-field NMR spectra. *Magn. Reson. Chem.* **2005**, *43*, 625–638. [CrossRef] [PubMed]
2. Abu-Reidah, L.M.; Contreras, M.M.; Arráez-Román, D.; Segura-Carretero, A.; Fernández-Gutiérrez, A. Reversed-phase ultra-high-performance liquid chromatography coupled to electrospray ionization-quadrupole-time-of-flight mass spectrometry as a powerful tool for metabolomic profiling of vegetables: *Lactuca sativa* as an example of its application. *J. Chromatogr. A* **2013**, *1313*, 212–227. [CrossRef] [PubMed]
3. Viacava, G.E.; Roura, S.I.; Berrueta, L.A.; Iriondo, C.; Gallo, B.; Alonso-Salces, R.M. Characterization of phenolic compounds in green and red oak-leaf lettuce cultivars by UHPLC-DAD-ESI-QtoF/MS using MS^E scan mode. *J. Mass. Spectrom.* **2017**, *52*, 873–902. [CrossRef]
4. Viacava, G.E.; Roura, S.I.; López-Márquez, D.M.; Berrueta, L.A.; Gallo, B.; Alonso-Salces, R.M. Polyphenolic profile of butterhead lettuce cultivar by ultrahigh performance liquid chromatography coupled online to UV-visible spectrophotometry and quadrupole time-of-flight mass spectrometry. *Food Chem.* **2018**, *260*, 239–273. [CrossRef] [PubMed]
5. Yang, X.; Wei, S.; Liu, B.; Guo, D.; Zheng, B.; Feng, L.; Liu, Y.; Thomás-Barberán, F.A.; Luo, L.; Huang, D. A novel integrated non-targeted metabolomic analysis reveals significant metabolite variations between different lettuce (*Lactuca sativa* L.) varieties. *Hortic. Res.* **2018**, *5*, 33. [CrossRef] [PubMed]
6. Ismail, H.; Gillespie, A.L.; Calderwood, D.; Iqbal, H.; Gallagher, C.; Chevallier, O.P.; Elliott, C.T.; Pan, X.; Mirza, B.; Green, B.D. The health promoting bioactivities of *Lactuca sativa* can be enhanced by genetic modulation of plant secondary metabolites. *Metabolites* **2019**, *9*, 97. [CrossRef]
7. Van Treuren, R.; Van Eekelen, H.D.L.M.; Wehrens, R.; De Vos, R.C.H. Metabolite variation in the lettuce gene pool: Towards healthier crop varieties and food. *Metabolomics* **2018**, *14*, 146. [CrossRef]
8. Qin, X.-X.; Zhang, M.-Y.; Han, Y.-Y.; Hao, J.-H.; Liu, C.-J.; Fan, S.-X. Beneficial phytochemicals with anti-tumor potential revealed through metabolic profiling of new red pigmented lettuces (*Lactuca sativa* L.). *Int. J. Mol. Sci.* **2018**, *19*, 1165. [CrossRef]
9. Crozier, A.; Jaganath, I.B.; Clifford, M.N. Dietary phenolics: Chemistry, bioavailability and effects on health. *Nat. Prod. Rep.* **2009**, *26*, 1001–1043. [CrossRef]

10. Van Beek, T.A.; Maas, P.; King, B.M.; Leclercq, E.; Voragen, A.G.J.; De Groot, A. Bitter sesquiterpene lactones from chicory roots. *J. Agric. Food Chem.* **1990**, *38*, 1035–1038. [CrossRef]
11. Mai, F.; Glomb, M.A. Structural and sensory characterization of novel sesquiterpene lactones from iceberg lettuce. *J. Agric. Food Chem.* **2016**, *64*, 295–301. [CrossRef] [PubMed]
12. Rees, S.B.; Harborne, J.B. The role of sesquiterpene lactones and phenolics in the chemical defence of the chicory plant. *Phytochemistry* **1985**, *24*, 2225–2231. [CrossRef]
13. Daniewski, W.M.; Gumułka, M.; Drożdż, B.; Grabarczyk, H.; Błoszyk, E. Sesquiterpene lactones. XXXVIII. Constituents of *Picris echioides* L. and their antifeedant activity. *Acta Soc. Bot. Pol.* **1989**, *58*, 351–354.
14. Cavin, C.; Delannoy, M.; Malnoe, A.; Debefve, E.; Touche, A.; Courtois, D.; Schilter, B. Inhibition of the expression and activity of cyclooxygenase-2 by chicory extract. *Biochem. Biophys. Res. Commun.* **2005**, *327*, 742–749. [CrossRef]
15. Wesołowska, A.; Nikiforuk, A.; Michalska, K.; Kisiel, W.; Chojnacka-Wójcik, E. Analgesic and sedative activities of lactucin and some lactucin-like guaianolides in mice. *J. Ethnopharm.* **2006**, *107*, 254–258. [CrossRef]
16. Milder, I.E.J.; Arts, I.C.W.; van de Putte, B.; Venema, D.P.; Hollman, P.C.H. Lignan contents of Dutch plant foods: A database including lariciresinol, pinoresinol, secoisolariciresinol and matairesinol. *Br. J. Nutr.* **2005**, *93*, 393–402. [CrossRef]
17. Han, Y.F.; Cao, G.X.; Gao, X.J.; Xia, M. Isolation and characterization of the sesquiterpene lactones from *Lactuca sativa* L. var. anagustata. *Food Chem.* **2010**, *120*, 1083–1088. [CrossRef]
18. Lissek-Wolf, G.; Lehmann, C.; Huyskens-Keil, S. *Die Vielfalt alter Salatsorten—Eine Dokumentation*; Bundesministerium für Ernährung, Landwirtschaft und Verbraucherschutz: Bonn, Germany, 2009; pp. 122–141. (In German)
19. Kotlińska, T.; Rutkowska-Łoś, A.; Pająkowski, J.; Podyma, W. *Informator nt. Starych Odmian Roślin Rolniczych i Ogrodniczych Występujących na Terenie Rzeczpospolitej Polskiej i Możliwościach ich Introdukcji Do Uprawy Jako Odmiany Regionalne i Amatorskie. Ministerstwo Rolnictwa i Rozwoju Wsi*; Ministry of Agriculture and Rural Development: Warsaw, Poland, 2015; pp. 27–29. (In Polish)
20. Starkenmann, C.; Niclass, I.; Vuichoud, B.; Schweizer, S.; He, X.-F. Occurrence of 2-acetyl-1-pyrroline and its nonvolatile precursors in celtuce (*Lactuca sativa* L. var. augustana). *J. Agric. Food Chem.* **2019**, *67*, 1710–11717. [CrossRef]
21. Michalska, K.; Michalski, O.; Stojakowska, A. Sesquiterpenoids from roots of *Lactuca sativa* var. angustana cv. Grüner Stern. *Phytochem. Lett.* **2017**, *20*, 425–428. [CrossRef]
22. De Vries, J.M. Origin and domestication of *Lactuca sativa* L. *Gen. Resour. Crop. Evol.* **1997**, *44*, 165–174. [CrossRef]
23. Piszczek, P.; Kuszewska, K.; Błaszkowski, J.; Sochacka-Obruśnik, A.; Stojakowska, A.; Zubek, S. Associations between root-inhabiting fungi and 40 species of medicinal plants with potential applications in the pharmaceutical and biotechnological industries. *Appl. Soil Ecol.* **2019**, *137*, 69–77. [CrossRef]
24. Velioglu, Y.S.; Mazza, G.; Gao, L.; Oomah, B.D. Antioxidant activity and total phenolics in selected fruits, vegetables, and grain products. *J. Agric. Food Chem.* **1998**, *46*, 4113–4117. [CrossRef]
25. Beharav, A.; Stojakowska, A.; Ben-David, R.; Malarz, J.; Michalska, K.; Kisiel, W. Variation of sesquiterpene lactone contents in *Lactuca georgica* natural populations from Armenia. *Gen. Resour. Crop. Evol.* **2015**, *62*, 431–441. [CrossRef]
26. Malarz, J.; Stojakowska, A.; Kisiel, W. Long-Term Cultured Hairy Roots of Chicory—A Rich Source of Hydroxycinnamates and 8-Deoxylactucin Glucoside. *Appl. Biochem. Biotechnol.* **2013**, *171*, 1589–1601. [CrossRef]
27. Kisiel, W.; Michalska, K.; Szneler, E. Norisoprenoids from aerial parts of *Cichorium pumilum*. *Biochem. Syst. Ecol.* **2004**, *32*, 343–346. [CrossRef]
28. Sung, P.J.; Chen, B.-Y.; Chen, Y.-H.; Chiang, M.Y.; Lin, M.-R. Loliolide: Occurrence of a carotenoid metabolite in the octocoral *Briareum excavatum* (Briareidae). *Biochem. Syst. Ecol.* **2010**, *38*, 116–118. [CrossRef]
29. Yamano, Y.; Ito, M. Synthesis of Optically Active Vomifoliol and Roseoside Stereoisomers. *Chem. Pharm. Bull.* **2005**, *53*, 541–546. [CrossRef]
30. Çalış, I.; Kuruüzüm-Uz, A.; Lorenzetto, P.A.; Rüedi, P. (6S)-Hydroxy-3-oxo-α-ionol glucosides from *Capparis spinosa* fruits. *Phytochemistry* **2002**, *59*, 451–457. [CrossRef]
31. Yajima, A.; Oono, Y.; Nakagawa, R.; Nukada, T.; Yabuta, G. A simple synthesis of four stereoisomers of roseoside and their inhibitory activity on leukotriene release from mice bone marrow-derived cultured mast cells. *Bioorg. Med. Chem.* **2009**, *17*, 189–194. [CrossRef]
32. Xiong, J.; Bui, V.-B.; Liu, X.-H.; Hong, Z.-L.; Yang, G.-X.; Hu, J.-F. Lignans from the stems of *Clematis armandii* ("Chuan-Mu-Tong") and their anti-neuroinflammatory activities. *J. Ethnopharmacol.* **2014**, *153*, 737–743. [CrossRef]
33. Shahat, A.A.; Abdel-Azim, N.S.; Pieters, L.; Vlietinck, A.J. Isolation and NMR spectra of syringaresinol-β-D-glucoside from *Cressa cretica*. *Fitoterapia* **2004**, *75*, 771–773. [CrossRef]
34. Choi, J.S.; Kim, J.Y.; Woo, W.S.; Young, H.S. Isolation of a β-carboline alkaloid from the leaves of *Allium tuberosum*. *Arch. Pharm. Res.* **1988**, *11*, 270–272. [CrossRef]
35. Ke, R.; Zhu, E.-Y.; Chou, G.-X. A new phenylpropanoid glycoside from *Cirsium setosum*. *Acta Pharm. Sin.* **2010**, *45*, 879–882.
36. Wang, F.-X.; Deng, A.-J.; Li, M.; Wei, J.-F.; Qin, H.-L.; Wang, A.-P. (3S)-1,2,3,4-Tetrahydro-β-carboline-3-carboxylic acid from *Cichorium endivia* L. induces apoptosis of human colorectal cancer HCT-8 cells. *Molecules* **2013**, *18*, 418–429. [CrossRef]
37. Kisiel, W.; Kohlmünzer, S. Ixerin F from *Crepis biennis*. *Planta Med.* **1987**, *53*, 390. [CrossRef] [PubMed]
38. Nishimura, K.; Miyase, T.; Ueno, A.; Noro, T.; Kuroyanagi, M.; Fukushima, S. Sesquiterpene lactones from *Lactuca laciniata*. *Phytochemistry* **1986**, *25*, 2375–2379. [CrossRef]

39. Michalska, K.; Szneler, E.; Kisiel, W. *Lactuca altaica* as a rich source of sesquiterpene lactones. *Biochem. Syst. Ecol.* **2010**, *38*, 1246–1249. [CrossRef]
40. Kisiel, W.; Barszcz, B. Sesquiterpene lactones from *Crepis rhoeadifolia*. *Phytochemistry* **1996**, *43*, 823–825. [CrossRef]
41. Kisiel, W.; Michalska, K. A new coumarin glucoside ester from *Cichorium intybus*. *Fitoterapia* **2002**, *73*, 544–546. [CrossRef]
42. Lee, E.J.; Kim, J.S.; Kim, H.P.; Lee, J.-H.; Kang, S.S. Phenolic constituents from the flower buds of *Lonicera japonica* and their 5-lipoxygenase inhibitory activities. *Food Chem.* **2010**, *120*, 134–139. [CrossRef]
43. Luyen, B.T.T.; Tai, B.H.; Thao, N.P.; Cha, J.Y.; Lee, H.Y.; Lee, Y.M.; Kim, Y.H. Anti-inflammatory components of *Chrysanthemum indicum* flowers. *Bioorg. Med. Chem. Lett.* **2015**, *25*, 266–269. [CrossRef] [PubMed]
44. Marco, J.A.; Sanz, J.F.; Albiach, R. A sesquiterpene ester from *Lactuca serriola*. *Phytochemistry* **1992**, *31*, 2539–2540. [CrossRef]
45. Abd-ElGawad, A.M.; Elshamy, A.I.; El Gendy, A.E.-N.; Al-Rowaily, S.L.; Assaeed, A.M. Preponderance of oxygenated sesquiterpenes and diterpenes in the volatile oil constituents of *Lactuca serriola* L. revealed antioxidant and allelopathic activity. *Chem. Biodiv.* **2019**, *16*, e1900278. [CrossRef] [PubMed]
46. Macias, F.A.; Oliva, R.M.; Varela, R.M.; Torres, A.; Molinillo, J.M.G. Allelochemicals from sunflower leaves cv. Peredovick. *Phytochemistry* **1999**, *52*, 613–621. [CrossRef]
47. DellaGreca, M.; Di Marino, C.; Zarrelli, A.; D'Abrosca, B. Isolation and phytotoxicity of apocarotenoids from *Chenopodium album*. *J. Nat. Prod.* **2004**, *67*, 1492–1495. [CrossRef]
48. Macias, F.A.; Lacret, R.; Varela, R.M.; Nogueiras, C.; Molinillo, J.M.G. Bioactive apocarotenoids from *Tectona grandis*. *Phytochemistry* **2008**, *69*, 2708–2715. [CrossRef] [PubMed]
49. Jin, Q.; Lee, C.; Lee, J.W.; Yeon, E.T.; Lee, D.; Han, S.B.; Hong, J.T.; Kim, Y.; Lee, M.K.; Hwang, B.Y. 2-Phenoxychromones and prenylflavonoids from *Epimedium koreanum* and their inhibitory effects on LPS-induced nitric oxide and interleukin-1β production. *J. Nat. Prod.* **2014**, *77*, 1724–1728. [CrossRef] [PubMed]
50. Ren, Y.; Shen, L.; Zhang, D.-W.; Dai, S.-J. Two new sesquiterpenoids from *Solanum lyratum* with cytotoxic activities. *Chem. Pharm. Bull.* **2009**, *57*, 408–410. [CrossRef]
51. Okunade, A.L.; Wiemer, D.F. (-)-Loliolide, an ant-repellent compound from *Xanthoxyllum setulosum*. *J. Nat. Prod.* **1985**, *48*, 472–473. [CrossRef]
52. Murata, M.; Nakai, Y.; Kawazu, K.; Ishizaka, M.; Kajiwara, H.; Abe, H.; Takeuchi, K.; Ichinose, Y.; Mitsuhara, I.; Mochizuki, A.; et al. Loliolide, a carotenoid metabolite, is a potential endogenous inducer of herbivore resistance. *Plant Physiol.* **2019**, *179*, 1822–1833. [CrossRef]
53. Yang, H.H.; Hwangbo, K.; Zheng, M.S.; Cho, J.H.; Son, J.-K.; Kim, H.Y.; Baek, S.H.; Choi, H.C.; Park, S.Y.; Kim, J.-R. Inhibitory effects of (-)-loliolide on cellular senescence in human dermal fibroblasts. *Arch. Pharm. Res.* **2015**, *38*, 876–884. [CrossRef] [PubMed]
54. Park, S.H.; Choi, E.; Kim, S.; Kim, D.S.; Kim, J.H.; Chang, S.G.; Choi, J.S.; Park, K.J.; Roh, K.-B.; Lee, J.; et al. Oxidative stress-protective and anti-melanogenic effects of loliolide and ethanol extract from fresh water green algae, *Prasiola japonica*. *Int. J. Mol. Sci.* **2018**, *19*, 2825. [CrossRef] [PubMed]
55. Chung, C.-Y.; Liu, C.-H.; Burnouf, T.; Wang, G.-H.; Chang, S.P.; Jassey, A.; Tai, C.-J.; Tai, C.-J.; Huang, C.-J.; Richardson, C.D.; et al. Activity based and fraction guided analysis of *Phyllanthus urinaria* identifies loliolide as a potent inhibitor of hepatitis C virus entry. *Anivir. Res.* **2016**, *130*, 58–68. [CrossRef]
56. Ren, J.; Qin, J.J.; Cheng, X.R.; Yan, S.K.; Jin, H.Z.; Zhang, W.D. Five new sesquiterpene lactones from *Inula hupehensis*. *Arch. Pharm. Res.* **2013**, *36*, 1319–1325. [CrossRef] [PubMed]
57. Qin, J.-J.; Jin, H.-Z.; Zhu, J.-X.; Fu, J.-J.; Zeng, Q.; Cheng, X.-R.; Zhu, Y.; Shan, L.; Zhang, S.-D.; Pan, Y.-X.; et al. New sesquiterpenes from *Inula japonica* Thunb. with their inhibitory activities against LPS-induced NO production in RAW264.7 macrophages. *Tetrahedron* **2010**, *66*, 9379–9388. [CrossRef]
58. Dat, N.T.; Jin, X.; Hong, Y.-S.; Lee, J.J. An isoaurone and other constituents from *Trichosanthes kirilowii* seeds inhibit hypoxia-inducible factor-1 and nuclear factor-κB. *J. Nat. Prod.* **2010**, *73*, 1167–1169. [CrossRef] [PubMed]
59. Zhou, D.; Wei, H.; Jiang, Z.; Li, X.; Jiao, K.; Jia, X.; Hou, Y.; Li, N. Natural potential neuroinflammatory inhibitors from *Alhagi sparsifolia* Shap. *Bioorg. Med. Chem. Lett.* **2017**, *27*, 973–978. [CrossRef] [PubMed]
60. Tan, M.A.; Gonzalez, S.J.B.; Alejandro, G.J.D.; An, S.S.A. Neuroprotective effect of vomifoliol, isolated from *Tarenna obtusifolia* Merr. (Rubiaceae), against amyloid-beta$_{1-42}$-treated neuroblastoma SH-SY5Y cells. *3 Biotech.* **2020**, *10*, 424. [CrossRef]
61. Yoshikawa, M.; Shimada, H.; Saka, M.; Yoshizumi, S.; Yamahara, J.; Matsuda, H. Medicinal foodstuffs. V. Moroheiya. (1): Absolute stereostuctures of corchoionosides A, B, and C, histamine release inhibitors from the leaves of Vietnamese *Corchorus olitorius* L. (Tiliaceae). *Chem. Pharm. Bull.* **1997**, *45*, 464–469. [CrossRef]
62. Hong, E.Y.; Kim, T.Y.; Hong, G.U.; Kang, H.; Lee, J.-Y.; Park, J.Y.; Kim, S.-C.; Kim, Y.H.; Chung, M.-H.; Kwon, Y.-I.; et al. Inhibitory effects of roseoside and icariside E4 isolated from a natural product mixture (No-ap) on the expression of angiotensin II receptor 1 and oxidative stress in angiotensin II-stimulated H9C2 cells. *Molecules* **2019**, *24*, 414. [CrossRef]
63. Ito, H.; Kobayashi, E.; Li, S.-H.; Hatano, T.; Sugita, D.; Kubo, N.; Shimura, S.; Itoh, Y.; Tokuda, H.; Nishino, H.; et al. Antitumor activity of compounds isolated from leaves of *Eriobotrya japonica*. *J. Agric. Food Chem.* **2002**, *50*, 2400–2403. [CrossRef] [PubMed]
64. Lee, T.-H.; Wang, G.-J.; Lee, C.-K.; Kuo, Y.-H.; Chou, C.-H. Inhibitory effects of glycosides from the leaves of *Melaleuca quinquenervia* on vascular contraction of rats. *Planta Med.* **2002**, *68*, 492–496. [CrossRef] [PubMed]

65. Frankish, N.; de Sousa Menezes, F.; Mills, C.; Sheridan, H. Enhancement of insulin release from the β-cell line INS-1 by an ethanolic extract of *Bauhinia variegata* and its major constituent roseoside. *Planta Med.* **2010**, *76*, 995–997. [CrossRef] [PubMed]
66. Liu, X.; Ardo, S.; Bunning, M.; Parry, J.; Zhou, K.; Stushnoff, C.; Stoniker, F.; Yu, L.; Kendall, P. Total phenolic content and DPPH radical scavenging activity of lettuce (*Lactuca sativa* L.) grown in Colorado. *LWT* **2007**, *40*, 552–557. [CrossRef]
67. Assefa, A.D.; Choi, S.; Lee, J.E.; Sung, J.-S.; Hur, O.-S.; Ro, N.-Y.; Lee, H.-S.; Jang, S.-W.; Rhee, J.-H. Identification and quantification of selected metabolites in differently pigmented leaves of lettuce (*Lactuca sativa* L.) cultivars harvested at mature and bolting stages. *BMC Chem.* **2019**, *13*, 56. [CrossRef]
68. Wang, X.; Liu, R.; Yang, Y.; Zhang, M. Isolation, purification and identification of antioxidants in an aqueous aged garlic extract. *Food Chem.* **2015**, *187*, 37–43. [CrossRef]

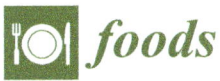 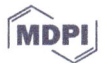

Article

Analysis of Total Phenols, Sugars, and Mineral Elements in Colored Tubers of *Solanum tuberosum* L.

Piret Saar-Reismaa [1], Katrin Kotkas [2], Viive Rosenberg [2], Maria Kulp [1], Maria Kuhtinskaja [1] and Merike Vaher [1,*]

[1] School of Science, Tallinn University of Technology, Akadeemia tee 15, 12618 Tallinn, Estonia; piret.saar1@taltech.ee (P.S.-R.); maria.kulp@taltech.ee (M.K.); maria.kuhtinskaja@taltech.ee (M.K.)
[2] Estonian Crop Research Institute, J. Aamissepa 1, 48309 Jõgeva, Estonia; katrin.kotkas@etki.ee (K.K.); viiverosenberg@gmail.com (V.R.)
* Correspondence: merike.vaher@taltech.ee; Tel.: +372-620-4359

Received: 25 November 2020; Accepted: 12 December 2020; Published: 14 December 2020

Abstract: The use of colored tubers of *Solanum tuberosum* L. is growing worldwide due to their health benefits and attractive color. The positive health effects of purple-fleshed tubers are a result of anthocyanins and various phenolic compounds. The aim of this study was to evaluate and compare variety Blue Congo and its cross-breeds of Desiree and Granola to yellow-fleshed tubers. The concentration of total phenols, anthocyanins, sugars, and mineral elements were evaluated in all tubers. The results showed differences between all tested materials, with largest differences in sugar content. Moreover, the results confirmed the preservation of health improving compounds of Blue Congo when cross-bred with yellow-fleshed tubers. The total phenolic content and anthocyanin concentrations of all analyzed tubers were above the comparison yellow ones.

Keywords: colored potato tubers; total phenols; anthocyanins; antioxidants; saccharides; nutrition; microelements

1. Introduction

Worldwide, potatoes (*Solanum tuberosum* L.) are the fourth important food crop after wheat, rice, and maize. Potatoes are grown in cool-temperature regions, in mountainous areas as well as at higher altitudes in the tropic. Potato tubers are a rich source of high-value protein, carbohydrates, essential vitamins, minerals, and trace elements. The average range of a potato tuber composition is as follows: starch (10–18%) having 22–30% amylose content, total sugars (1–7%), protein (1–2%), fiber (0.5%), lipids (0.1–0.5%), vitamin A (trace/100 g of fresh weight (FW)), vitamin C (30 mg/100 g of FW), various trace minerals, and glycoalkaloids (1–3 mg/100 g of FW) [1].

Potato tubers are known to be naturally high in potassium, up to 400 mg per 100 g fresh tubers [2], or 1.7% of dry matter [3]. The potassium from potatoes can help lower blood pressure due to its vasodilation effect [4]. The tubers also contain other essential microelements like iron and calcium, that are responsible for bone structure and strength, in addition, zinc, manganese, copper, and magnesium are represented, that regulate cell renewal, energy production, and are responsible for over-all immunity [5]. Consumption of potato tubers with high nutritional content contributes to fulfilling of the daily recommended intake of several essential elements.

Over the past decade or so, colored-flesh potatoes have become more widely available to home gardeners, including potato tubers of blue, red, yellow, and white flesh. Purple-fleshed potatoes give the possibility to add color to the menu and additional nutrients to human diet. The addition of colored tubers adds the benefits from healthy antioxidants. Colored-flesh potatoes get their color from various pigments, which are antioxidants. Purple and rose-flesh potatoes contain the anthocyanin pigments, while yellow-colored flesh varieties contain carotenoids [6]. Purple-fleshed potatoes like

Blue Congo get their color from common anthocyanins malvidin, peonidin, delphinidin, cyanidin, and petunidin [7]. Epidemiological evidence indicates health benefits from anthocyanins include improved eyesight and circulatory system function, benefits for diabetics, and anti-inflammatory, antiviral, and antimicrobial activity [8–10].

Potato tubers are also a great source of carbohydrates, which occur mainly in starch form [11] and are also used for industrial starch production. The starch content is directly related to the sugar content of tubers. As most potatoes are consumed after processing at high temperatures, the asparagine and glycose or fructose from the tubers can lead to acrylamide formation. This is due to Maillard reaction—a reaction between amino acid and sugar [12]. Moreover, higher levels of reducing sugars (glucose and fructose) as well as non-reducing sucrose in potato tubers may result in unfavorable browning or even a bitter taste [13]. Therefore, it is important to evaluate the sugar content in raw potato tubers, to determine if new varieties would produce high levels of acrylamide in processing. Moreover, potato tubers additionally contain myo-inositol, which is a sugar-like carbohydrate produced by most plants. Myo-inositol is important for phosphate storage and normal cell-to-cell communication and its metabolism is associated to diabetes [14].

The aim of the study was to evaluate the content of total phenols (TPs), anthocyanins, mineral elements, and sugars in tubers from variety Blue Congo, its seedlings, and cross-breeds with Granola and Desiree using various selective methods to create the plant material.

2. Materials and Methods

2.1. Studied Plant Material

The plant material, created by different methods in vitro was grown in a test-field in Saku, Estonia (local latitude 57°25′). The soil type of the experimental area was Calcaric cambisols according to the World Reference Base classification (EAO 2014) where the agrochemical indicators were as follows: pH 6.3 (ISO 10,390 [15]); soil carbon content Corg 3.3% (Tyurin method [16]) and concentration of soluble P and K being 114 and 161 mg/kg (Mehlich III method [17]). In spring time, before the cultivation, in the field the complex fertilizer Cropcare 8-11-23 500 kg/ha was used.

Detailed description of tubers is given in Table 1. Initial mini-tubers of the variety Blue Congo were received from Sweden by the potato grower in 1991. Mini-tubers grown in green-house were eradicated on virus infection by using thermotherapy and meristem-plants were created in vitro [18].

Table 1. Descriptors for tubers of the variety Blue Congo seedlings and cross-breeds between Blue Congo with Desiree and Blue Congo with Granola.

Sample No	Material Number	Descriptors of Tubers		
		Skin Color	Flesh Color	Tuber's Shape
Botanical Seeds				
1	25	Violet	Oak leaf form with white border around	Ovate
2	34	Violet	Violet with white border	Elongate, big
3	51	Dark violet	Dark violet marble	Ovate
4	53	Dark violet	Dark violet marble	Elongate
5	76	Pale violet	Pale reddish violet, white border	Ovate
6	89	Pale violet	White border, beautiful violet oak form	Round
7	116	Reddish violet	Pale reddish violet with white border	Ovate
Cross-Breeding Blue Congo and Desiree				
8	41	Dark violet	White border, violet vary-colored oak leaf form	Ovate
9	47	Dark pink	Pale pink border white in middle	Ovate

Table 1. Cont.

Sample No	Material Number	Descriptors of Tubers		
		Skin Color	Flesh Color	Tuber's Shape
Cross-Breeding Blue Congo and Granola				
10	9	Dark violet	Dark violet pale border	Elongate big
11	16	Dark violet	Strong white border violet vary-color	Elongate big
12	28	Dark violet	Vary-color violet narrow border	Elongate-ovate
13	30	Dark pink	Netting pink violet	Uniform ovate
14	36	Dark pink	Netting blanched yellow middle	Ovate
15	41	Dark violet	Violet netting	Uniform ovate
Meristem Clones of Blue Congo				
16	40	Dark violet netting	Pale violet middle with pale border	Round
17	195	Dark violet netting	Dark violet with white border	Ovate
18	197	Dark violet netting	Pale violet with wider white border	Round
Commercial Varieties				
19	Teele	Yellow netting	Yellow	Round-ovate
20	Laura	Smooth dark red	Dark yellow	Round-ovate
21	Sweet Potato	Purple	Purple	Elongate

Botanical seeds of the variety Blue Congo (1–7 in Table 1) were cultivated into the test-tubes in sterile condition, regenerated plants were multiplied in vitro and grown in the test-field. In 2013, the plants of the variety Blue Congo were pollinated in field conditions with the variety Desiree (8, 9) and with the variety Granola (10–15). The tubers of the variety Desiree are red skinned with yellow flesh, and the tubers of the variety Granola are yellow skinned with blanched yellow flesh.

New tissue cultures from the plants preserved in vitro were created on years 2004–2007. On the base of field results, three best meristem clones were selected (16–18).

As a comparing variety group, two commercial varieties were included. Variety Teele tubers are with bright yellow skin and yellow flesh and variety Laura tubers are with red skin with dark yellow flesh. Comparison with super-market purple-fleshed sweet potato tubers (*Ipomoea batatas* L.) were also included.

2.2. Extraction and Dry-Weight

From each genotype (plant material type) (Table 1) 5 tubers were selected. The tubers were washed with distilled water, dried at room temperature and homogenized (Nutribullet, Los Angeles, CA, USA). The homogenates were divided into aliquots and stored at 4 °C for further analysis. The aliquots were used for determination of dry weights (DW), microelements, and for making extracts for analysis of total phenols (TPs), anthocyanins, and naturally occurring sugars.

For evaluation of TPs and anthocyanins the following extraction procedure was conducted: 5 g of tuber homogenate was mixed with 25 mL 80% (v/v) methanol in a 50 mL graduated tube. The mixture was allowed to stand with intermittent shaking for 1 h at room temperature in the dark. After that the mixture was subjected to ultrasonication (Sonorex digital 10P, Bandelin, Berlin, Germany) for 30 min at 30 °C. After which it was centrifugated (EBA 200S, Hettich, Westphalia, Germany) at 8000 rpm/min for 15 min and the supernatant was filtered through 0.45 µm Minisart® Syringe Filter (Sartorius, Goettingen, Germany) and stored at 4 °C. The carbohydrate extraction was achieved in the ultrasonic bath with 50% (v/v) aqueous methanol from 5 g of homogenate using the same procedure as in case of extraction of polyphenols.

The dry weight of the tubers was measured by drying ~1 g of the homogenate at 105 °C until constant weight using an Ohaus Moisture Analyzer MB90 (Parsippany, NJ, USA) in triplicates. The content of dry matter ranged from 15.8 to 31.5% for examined potato tubers and was 34.9% for the purple sweet potato tuber.

2.3. Determination of Total Phenols and Anthocyanins

The concentration of the total phenolic compounds was determined for each extract by an adapted micro-scale protocol for the Folin–Ciocalteu colorimetric method [19,20]. In brief, phenolic groups are oxidized by phosphomolybdic and phosphotungstic acids in Folin–Ciocalteu reagent, forming a green–blue complex detectable at 765 nm. 50 µL of each tuber extract solution of an appropriate concentration was mixed with 1350 µL of water, 100 µL Folin–Ciocalteu reagent and 500 µL of Na_2CO_3 (20% w/w). The absorbance at 765 nm was measured after 2 h reaction at room temperature (in the dark) with a Cary 50 Bio UV–vis spectrophotometer (Palo Alto, Varian, CA, USA). The hydro-methanolic gallic acid solution was freshly prepared in a series of concentrations (0.3–3 mM) and tested in parallel to establish the calibration curve. The total phenolic content of each potato extract was calculated as milligrams of gallic acid equivalent per g dry sample (mg GAE/g of DW).

The total content of non-hydrolyzed anthocyanins was measured using the pH differential method described by Albishi et al. [21] with minor modification. Monomeric anthocyanin pigments reversibly change color with change in pH. The colored oxonium form exist at pH 1.0, and the colorless hemiketal form predominates at pH 4.5. The difference in the absorbance at 520 nm is proportional to the pigment concentration. 400 µL of potato tuber or 200 µL of sweet potato tuber extract and 600 or 800 µL of 25 mM potassium chloride buffer (pH 1.0) and 400 mM sodium acetate buffer (pH 4.5) respectively were mixed. The mixtures were left at room temperature for 1 h (in the dark). The absorbance was measured at 520 nm and 700 nm against a blank cell filled with 80% MeOH in buffer. The results were expressed as mg of cyanidin-3-glucoside equivalents per kg dry sample (mg CGE/kg of DW).

The experiments were carried out in triplicates, and the results are reported as the mean ± standard deviation.

2.4. Capillary Electrophoretic Analysis of Natural Sugars

Capillary electrophoresis (CE) was performed using an Agilent 3D CE instrument (Agilent Technologies, Santa Clara, CA, USA) equipped with a diode array UV/Vis detector. Uncoated fused silica capillary with effective length of 71.5 cm and i.d. of 50 µm was employed. The optimized conditions for the analysis: temperature of the capillary was 16 °C, applied voltage was +17 kV and samples were injected under 35 mbar pressure for 10 s. 130 mM NaOH containing 36 mM Na_2HPO_4 (pH 12.6) was used as a background electrolyte (BGE). The wavelength for detection was 270 nm [22]. Identification of the sugars was done by standard addition method, the standard solutions of sucrose, D-(+)-maltose, D-(+)-glucose, D-(−)-fructose, sugar alcohol myo-inositol, and sodium hydroxide were from Sigma (Darmstadt, Germany). Milli-Q water (Millipore S. A, Molsheim, France) was used for all solutions of standards, background electrolyte (BGE), and dilution of samples.

2.5. Atomic Absobrance Analysis of Microelements

The stock atomic spectroscopy standard solutions (1000 mg/L) Cu, Zn, Mn, Fe, Mg, Ca, Se, and K were purchased from Fluka, Buchs, Switzerland. Spectra AA 220F and 220Z atomic absorption spectrometers (Varian, Mulgrave, Australia) equipped with a side-heated GTA-110Z graphite atomizer, a Zeeman effect background correction, and an integrated autosampler were used. Graphite tubes with coating and platforms made of pyrolytic graphite were used throughout the work. Argon of 99.99% purity (AGA, Helsinki, Finland) was used as the purge gas. Acetylene of 99.99% purity (AGA, Helsinki, Finland) was used as the fuel gas in flame atomic absorption spectroscopy. For the determination of total mineral element constituents ~1 g of potato tubers homogenate was mineralized with 4 mL of concentrated nitric acid and 1 mL of concentrated hydrogen peroxide in 50 mL plastic tubes at temperature 80 °C for 5 h. After cooling down, the solution was transferred to volumetric flasks (15 mL) with ultrapure water. All the experiments were made in triplicates. The concentrated nitric acid and hydrogen peroxide were from Sigma (Darmstadt, Germany).

2.6. Statistical Analysis

The statistical analysis was conducted using Microsoft Excel and R version 4.0.2. The significant variations were evaluated using the Excel built-in data analysis package (t-test two samples, $p = 0.05$) and the principal component analysis (PCA) was carried out and visualized in R 4.0.2 x64.

3. Results and Discussion

3.1. Total Phenlos and Anthocyanins

To evaluate the possible positive health influences of colored tubers, the total phenols (TPs) and anthocyanin concentrations were evaluated compared to sweet potato and two yellow-fleshed tubers. The total phenols were evaluated in all tubers and compared as concentration of gallic acid equivalents mg/g of dry weight (mg GAE/g of DW). All sample tubers (Sample 1–20) as well as the sweet potato sample (Sample 21) showed TP concentrations between 0.8 and 3.1 mg GAE/g of DW as shown in Figure 1.

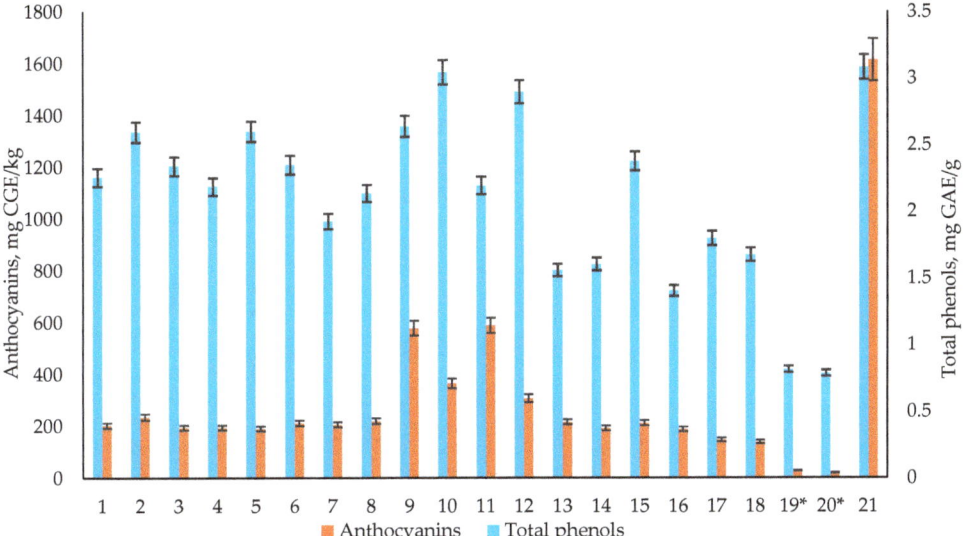

Figure 1. The concentrations of anthocyanins and total phenols in samples 1–21. All concentrations are given for dry weight. * $p < 0.05$ for total phenols and anthocyanin concentration between yellow-fleshed and colored potato tubers.

The biggest difference occurred between all colored tubers (Samples 1–18) and the yellow varieties (Samples 19–20), where the yellow-fleshed tubers had significantly ($p < 0.05$) lower TP concentrations. The values for all the colored potato tubers were from 1.4 to 3.1 mg GAE/g of DW, but for the yellow fleshed tubers only 0.8 mg GAE/g of DW, showing an increase of 75–175% of TPs for purple-fleshed varieties. These results are in accordance with previous studies of colored tubers, that show an increase of various phenolic acids, coumarins, and flavonoids in purple fleshed potatoes compared to yellow or white tubers [6,23]. The results also show that crossbreeding with potatoes with yellow flesh do not significantly decrease the variation of TPs in tubers, allowing for more versatile and specific breeding. The TP concentration in the purple sweet potato tuber did not have a remarkable difference compared to all other purple-fleshed tubers.

Another important evaluation criterion for the health-benefit of the purple-flesh potato is the content of anthocyanins. The same samples were analyzed for anthocyanins with results shown in

Figure 1. As anthocyanins are directly linked to the coloration of the flesh, the concentrations of anthocyanins in yellow-fleshed sample tubers, samples 19–20, were the smallest, showing a statistical difference to all other tubers ($p < 0.05$). All colored potato tubers had anthocyanin concentrations from 138.6 to 588.5 mg CGE/kg of DW, compared to yellow fleshed tubers concentrations around 20 mg CGE/kg of DW. Such results are to be expected as Jansen and Flamme [24] have previously shown, that whole violet and violet/white fleshed tubers had anthocyanin concentrations from 181 to 1570 mg/kg of FW, while white and yellow fleshed tubers only had 4–82 mg/kg of FW of anthocyanins. The purple sweet potato had over six times higher concentration of 1613.4 mg CGE/kg of DW compared the average of 254.9 mg CGE/kg of DW from Blue Congo and its examined accessions varieties. Unlike TPs, the anthocyanins had a small increase in the average concentration in Blue Congo cross-breeds with Granola, implying the positive effect from the breed Granola.

3.2. Analysis of Sugars

The sugar content of potatoes is an important quality indicator. It has been shown that the tuber sugar content can vary by genotype, but is largely influenced by the storage and treatment, even more so at temperatures below 10 °C [13]. All analyzed samples were therefor stored at similar temperature to avoid any environment factor as a variable.

The analysis was carried out using a CE with UV detection and lactose was used as an internal standard (IS). All samples were analyzed for myo-inositol, sucrose, maltose, glucose, and fructose. Examples of analyzed tuber electropherograms are shown in Figure 2.

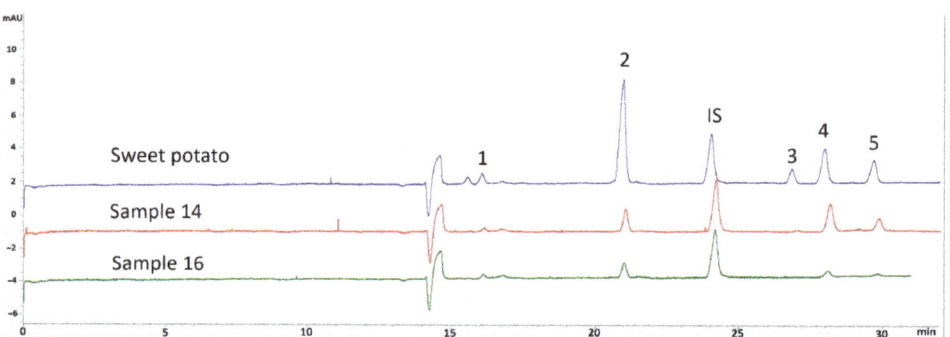

Figure 2. Electropherograms of sugar analysis from sweet potato tuber Sample 21 (blue), purple-fleshed cross-breed with Granola Sample 14 (red) and a meristem clone of Blue Congo sample 16 (green). Identification 1—myo-inositol, 2—sucrose, IS—internal standard, 3—maltose, 4—glucose, 5—fructose.

None of the potato tuber samples contained maltose above the detection limit. The only sample to contain maltose was the purple sweet potato tuber, which was to be expected as the sweet taste of the tuber is due to maltose concentration [25]. To better evaluate the overall sugar content of all analyzed tubers, the fructose, glucose, sucrose, and myo-inositol concentrations were summed in a bar chart shown in Figure 3.

The overall sugar content in all potato tubers ranged from 10.3 mg/g to 47.1 mg/g with an average of 21.6 mg/g. These results are in accordance with other published reports of total sugar concentrations in potato tubers that ranged from 7.5 to 74.1 mg/g of DW [26], and are also in accordance to climatically similarly grown potato tubers, where sucrose, glucose, and fructose ranged from 6.4 to 21.8, 2.3 to 29.7, and 1.2 to 25.4 mg/g of DW, respectively [27]. The sweet potato tuber total sugar concentration was 95.0 mg/g, which was mainly due to high concentration of sucrose. The lowest sugar concentrations were observed in the Blue Congo meristem clones, that averaged only 11.0 mg/g of total sugars.

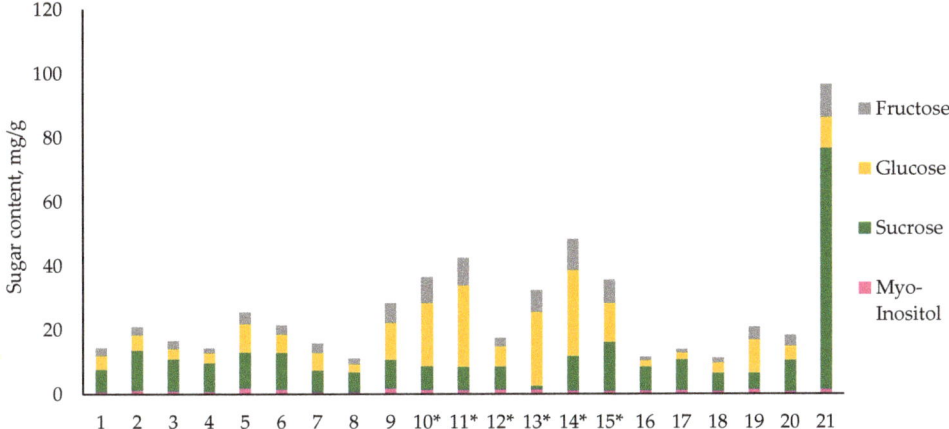

Figure 3. The total content of sugars from analyzed potato tubers Samples 1–18 correspond to purple-fleshed tubers, samples 19–20 to yellow-fleshed tubers and sample 21 to a purple sweet potato tuber. * $p < 0.05$ for total sugars between cross-breeds of Blue Congo with Granola compared to all other potato tubers.

Additionally, there was a significant difference ($p < 0.05$) in the samples 9–15 corresponding mainly to the cross-breeds of Blue Congo and Granola with an average sugar content of 34.1 mg/g, while all other potato tubers had an average of only 16.3 mg/g. As the sugar content is used as a quality factor, the higher sugar concentration may result in unacceptably brown and bitter food products. Thus, the higher amounts found in Granola cross-breeds make such cultures less-favorable compared to the original Blue Congo variety for fried products. The cross-breeds with Desiree did not show such tendencies.

3.3. Microelements in Tubers

The dispersion of various elements throughout the potato tubers is mixed, as some elements have higher concentration in the skins, while others in the flesh; moreover, there is some research that shows heterogeneous distribution between the stem and distal end of the tubers [28]. To better evaluate overall concentrations, whole tubers were washed and grounded for the analysis. Selected microelements essential for living organisms were evaluated using atomic absorbance spectroscopy (AAS). In total, eight elements were measured from all samples including copper, zinc, manganese, iron, magnesium, calcium, potassium, and selenium. All levels of Se were below the detection limit of the method (<20 mg/kg of DW). The results for all other elements are presented in Table 2 below.

Potato tubers are best-known for their high potassium content as it is an essential element for the acid–base regulation as well as heart, liver, nerve, and muscle functioning [29]. The potassium concentration was the highest, ranging from 10.35 to 22.83 g/kg of DW, with an average of 16.4 g/kg of DW. These results are comparable to non-organic K levels determined in potato tubers [30].

The zinc concentration varied from 9.8 to 26.0 mg/kg of DW, matching with previous results of fertilized and organic Zn concentrations [5,31,32]. The concentrations did not vary depending on the flesh coloration of the tuber, but the purple sweet potato tuber had a significantly lower Zn concentration of only 8.2 mg/kg of DW.

The Fe concentrations of analyzed tubers varied from 48.3 to 133 mg/g of DW, which is similar to works by Andre et al. [28]. The Fe levels in samples 19 and 20 as well as in the sweet potato were the lowest compared to colored-flesh tubers. The Fe found in potato tubers is considered to be non-heme iron and therefor considered a valuable source of iron for the human diet. The lack of iron can cause severe health problems, including impaired development in adolescence and reduced work capacity, making potatoes useful sources for such nutrients. Moreover, as potatoes also contain vitamin C, which increases the iron uptake from potatoes, the health benefits are significant against anemia.

Table 2. Mineral composition of the tubers as determined by atomic absorbance spectroscopy (AAS) per dry weight ($n = 3$).

Sample No	Cu, mg/kg	Zn, mg/kg	Mn, mg/kg	Fe, mg/kg	Mg, mg/kg	Ca, mg/kg	K, g/kg
1	2.477	11.02	8.68	77.2	973.6	349.2	19.49
2	3.212	17.02	7.21	80.3	880.8	437.5	17.05
3	4.000	14.11	8.02	57.0	1253.6	554.1	22.83
4	2.146	12.14	7.18	61.2	921.4	583.0	17.36
5	3.016	17.31	8.63	109.9	1264.3	508.8	21.54
6	2.793	13.51	7.16	74.3	926.6	466.7	17.19
7	4.244	12.64	8.73	70.6	976.1	375.6	14.27
8	2.952	10.91	8.56	85.6	1082.8	623.9	17.78
9	4.116	26.01	9.25	86.1	865.3	331.8	11.81
10	4.335	15.69	12.04	85.0	1004.8	668.9	16.53
11	5.390	14.53	7.30	115.1	1138.4	591.8	18.86
12	1.994	14.64	9.89	133.0	1240.2	316.8	18.84
13	3.708	14.74	9.82	82.5	1087.7	377.8	14.19
14	5.937	18.35	9.37	120.3	1225.3	729.1	18.67
15	4.689	14.95	6.75	54.4	1029.6	392.2	13.71
16	3.943	9.81	10.29	56.2	692.4	319.4	10.35
17	4.688	14.20	6.74	58.9	921.0	501.3	14.47
18	3.153	13.32	7.86	77.7	1045.0	517.5	15.11
19	3.353	12.41	5.26	48.3	867.7	489.2	13.06
20	4.385	14.62	10.60	53.4	922.2	270.5	15.81
21	9.630	8.17	6.79	45.8	988.8	679.1	8.37

Calcium is needed for skeletal and neural functioning, as well as metabolism. Although, the Ca content is insufficient for marginal dietary benefits, the tuber quality and storage capacity is evaluated on the basis of it [33]. The Ca levels averaged at 470 mg/kg of DW, being similar to previously reported values, with the highest concentration of 729 mg/kg of DW and lowest of 270 mg/kg of DW. There were no significant variances between different breeding varieties or colored and yellow-fleshed tubers, nor sweet potato tuber.

Mn concentrations were relatively low, similar to organic cultivars, with the levels being from 5.3 to 12.0 mg/kg of DW. In general, higher magnesium levels were detected in the tubers of cross-breeds of Blue Congo and Granola. The overall levels varied from 629 to 1264 mg/kg of DW with an average of 1015 mg/kg of DW, which is comparable to both conventional and organically cultivated potato tubers, that averaged from 1183 to 1646 mg/kg of DW [5,32].

No obvious differences were seen between breeding varieties and cross-breeds of Blue Congo tubers. The differences were observed with a purple sweet potato tuber as well as yellow-fleshed tubers compared to purple-fleshed tubers. Most of the results correlate to each other as the main source of mineral concentrations is due to the soil and fertilization processes used, which were similar for all the tubers analyzed, except for the purple sweet potato tuber and store-bought varieties.

3.4. Principal Component Analysis

A principal component analysis (PCA) was done to better evaluate the correlations between different breeding varieties and concentrations of mineral elements, natural sugars, and total phenols as well as anthocyanins. The sweet potato tuber results were excluded from the PCA analysis sweet potato is from another genus and it would be an outlier due to too different profile. The results of principal components 1 and 2 (PC1 and PC2) showed obvious groupings of all varieties as is seen in

Figure 4. As the PC1 and PC2 had a total explained variance of 65.5%, the PCA was determined to be successful.

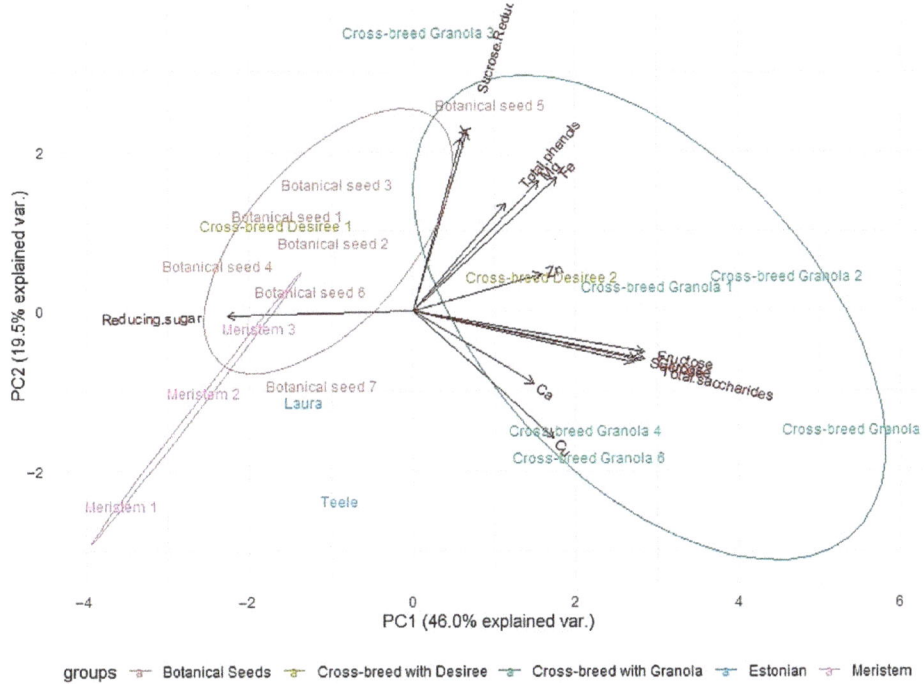

Figure 4. Principal component analysis (PCA) results of all analyzed 20 potato varieties and their mineral composition, natural sugars, total phenols, and anthocyanin content. Pink—meristem clones of Blue Congo, green—Blue Congo cross-breeds with Granola, blue—yellow-fleshed tubers, orange—Blue Congo botanical seeds, yellow—Blue Congo cross-breeds with Desiree.

There were five main groups of potato tubers: botanical seeds of Blue Congo, meristem clones of Blue Congo, Blue Congo cross-breeds with Granola, Blue Congo cross-breeds with Desiree, and commercial varieties (Laura, Teele). The main distinguishable groupings were of botanical seeds of Blue Congo, which showed similarities to the meristem clones, but had almost no overlapping with cross-breeds with Granola. The main differences in the meristem clones and cross-breeds can be attributed to the reducing sugars, which make the Granola cross-breeds sugar rich as previously determined. Unfortunately, the high sugar content has links with higher copper and calcium concentrations, meaning that the possible benefits of Ca and Cu will not be obtained if the variety is deemed unsuitable as the sugar content may lead to cancerogenic acrylamide. To overcome this, there are studies that demonstrate the possibility to reduce the concentration of acrylamide formation even up to 93% by pretreatment of tubers [34]. The multi-step pretreatment may unfortunately diminish other nutrients. Moreover, the anthocyanin concentration is also in correlation with total saccharides, proving the value of such variety.

Additionally, there was a correlation between higher concentration of Fe and total phenol concentration, which is in accordance with Brown's previous results [31] where colored-flesh tubers have higher concentrations of TPs and Fe. The correlation of Fe and TPs also includes the higher concentration of Mg. The concentration of potassium was slightly correlated, showing cross-breeds with Desiree and some botanical seeds presenting with both positive characteristics. Interestingly, the botanical seeds of Blue Congo showed differences to the meristem clones of Blue Congo, with the botanical seeds having higher levels of nutrients. The yellow-fleshed tubers of Teele and Laura separated from all other tested material and had the smallest levels of anthocyanins, total phenols and additionally microelements, proving further that the purple-fleshed tubers have higher potential for a healthier alternative in the human diet.

4. Conclusions

The results of this work demonstrate differences of various potato tubers depending on their genotypes and varieties. Mainly Blue Congo tubers and their purple-fleshed cross-breeds were compared to yellow-fleshed potato tubers and purple sweet potato tubers. The levels of total phenolic compounds and anthocyanins found in purple-fleshed tubers were significantly higher compared to yellow-fleshed ones. Although, the Blue Congo and Granola cross-breed showed highest levels of sugars, the PCA analysis showed that additional beneficial anthocyanin concentration was in correlation with higher sugar content. In addition, the results confirmed that cross-breeding Blue Congo with a yellow-fleshed tuber does not diminish the positive benefits of high levels of phenolic compounds and anthocyanins.

The results showed great potential to create versatile plant material with increased levels of specific TPs or anthocyanins, as well as adding to the knowledge of correlations of micronutrients to TPs, sugars, and anthocyanin concentrations. Thus, providing health benefits for various consumers to help with essential microelements as well as overall improvement of immune system and health.

Author Contributions: Conceptualization, M.V. and V.R.; field tests, K.K.; analysis, M.V., P.S.-R., M.K. (Maria Kulp) and M.K. (Maria Kuhtinskaja); writing—original draft preparation, P.S.-R.; writing—review and editing, M.V., K.K. and P.S.-R.; project administration, M.V.; funding acquisition, M.V. All authors have read and agreed to the published version of the manuscript.

Funding: This study was supported by the Estonian Ministry of Education and Research (Grant No. IUT 3320) and SA Archimedes (Development of additional analytical capabilities for Estonian Center of Analytical Chemistry, AKKI).

Conflicts of Interest: The authors declare no conflict of interest.

References

1. De Meulenaer, B.; Medeiros, R.; Mestdagh, F. *Chapter 18 Acrylamide in Potato Products*; Singh, J., Kaur, L.B.T., Second, E., Eds.; Academic Press: San Diego, CA, USA, 2016; pp. 527–562. ISBN 978-0-12-800002-1.
2. White, P.J.; Broadley, M.R. Biofortification of crops with seven mineral elements often lacking in human diets-Iron, zinc, copper, calcium, magnesium, selenium and iodine. *New Phytol.* **2009**, *182*, 49–84. [CrossRef] [PubMed]
3. Schilling, G.; Eißner, H.; Schmidt, L.; Peiter, E. Yield formation of five crop species under water shortage and differential potassium supply. *J. Plant Nutr. Soil Sci.* **2016**, *179*, 234–243. [CrossRef]
4. Usmani, A.; Mishra, A. The Globe's Healthiest Food with Numerous Medicinal Properties—Solanum tuberosum. *Res. Rev. A J. Pharmacol.* **2016**, *6*, 1–10.
5. Wierzbowska, J.; Rychcik, B.; Światły, A. The effect of different production systems on the content of micronutrients and trace elements in potato tubers. *Acta Agric. Scand. Sect. B Soil Plant Sci.* **2018**, *68*, 701–708. [CrossRef]
6. Murniece, I.; Kruma, Z.; Skrabule, I.; Vaivode, A. Carotenoids and Phenols of Organically and Conventionally Cultivated Potato Varieties. *Int. J. Chem. Eng. Appl.* **2013**, *4*, 342–348. [CrossRef]
7. Kita, A.; Bakowska-Barczak, A.; Hamouz, K.; Kułakowska, K.; Lisińska, G. The effect of frying on anthocyanin stability and antioxidant activity of crisps from red- and purple-fleshed potatoes (*Solanum tuberosum* L.). *J. Food Compos. Anal.* **2013**, *32*, 169–175. [CrossRef]
8. Choi, J.H.; Kim, S. Investigation of the anticoagulant and antithrombotic effects of chlorogenic acid. *J. Biochem. Mol. Toxicol.* **2017**, *31*, 1–6. [CrossRef]

9. Strugała, P.; Dzydzan, O.; Brodyak, I.; Kucharska, A.Z.; Kuropka, P.; Liuta, M.; Kaleta-Kuratewicz, K.; Przewodowska, A.; Michałowska, D.; Gabrielska, J.; et al. Antidiabetic and antioxidative potential of the blue Congo variety of purple potato extract in streptozotocin-induced diabetic rats. *Molecules* **2019**, *24*, 3126. [CrossRef]
10. Brown, C.R.; Wrolstad, R.; Durst, R.; Yang, C.P.; Clevidence, B. Breeding studies in potatoes containing high concentrations of anthocyanins. *Am. J. Potato Res.* **2003**, *80*, 241–249. [CrossRef]
11. Cummings, J.H.; Beatty, E.R.; Kingman, S.M.; Bingham, S.A.; Englyst, H.N. Digestion and physiological properties of resistant starch in the human large bowel. *Br. J. Nutr.* **1996**, *75*, 733–747. [CrossRef]
12. Zyzak, D.V.; Sanders, R.A.; Stojanovic, M.; Tallmadge, D.H.; Eberhart, B.L.; Ewald, D.K.; Gruber, D.C.; Morsch, T.R.; Strothers, M.A.; Rizzi, G.P.; et al. Acrylamide formation mechanism in heated foods. *J. Agric. Food Chem.* **2003**, *51*, 4782–4787. [CrossRef] [PubMed]
13. Kumar, D.; Singh, B.P.; Kumar, P. An overview of the factors affecting sugar content of potatoes. *Ann. Appl. Biol.* **2004**, *145*, 247–256. [CrossRef]
14. Clements, R.S.; Darnell, B. Myo-inositol content of common foods: Development of a high-myo-inositol diet. *Am. J. Clin. Nutr.* **1955**, *33*, 1954–1967. [CrossRef] [PubMed]
15. ISO Standard no. 10390:2005. *Soil Quality—Determination of pH*; International Organization for Standardization: Geneva, Switzerland, 2005.
16. Jankauskas, B.; Jankauskiene, G.; Slepetiene, A.; Fullen, M.A.; Booth, C.A. International comparison of analytical methods of determining the soil organic matter content of Lithuanian Eutric Albeluvisols. *Commun. Soil Sci. Plant Anal.* **2006**, *37*, 707–720. [CrossRef]
17. AgroEcoLab Mehlich 3 Extraction Protocol. Available online: http://www.agroecologylab.com/uploads/2/7/2/8/27281831/mehlich3_extraction.pdf (accessed on 9 September 2020).
18. Kotkas, K.; Rosenberg, V. The Methods for Potato Virus Eradication and Creation of Meristem Clones with Improved Traits, Virus-Free Potato Meristem Plants and Virus-Free Potato. International Patent WO 2009/143856 A1, 3 December 2009.
19. Waterhouse, A.L. Determination of Total Phenolics. *Curr. Protoc. Food Anal. Chem.* **2002**, *6*, I1.1.1–I1.1.8. [CrossRef]
20. Vaher, M.; Borissova, M.; Seiman, A.; Aid, T.; Kolde, H.; Kazarjan, J.; Kaljurand, M. Automatic spot preparation and image processing of paper microzone-based assays for analysis of bioactive compounds in plant extracts. *Food Chem.* **2014**, *143*, 465–471. [CrossRef]
21. Albishi, T.; John, J.A.; Al-Khalifa, A.S.; Shahidi, F. Phenolic content and antioxidant activities of selected potato varieties and their processing by-products. *J. Funct. Foods* **2013**, *5*, 590–600. [CrossRef]
22. Vaher, M.; Helmja, K.; Käsper, A.; Kurašin, M.; Väljamäe, P.; Kudrjašova, M.; Koel, M.; Kaljurand, M. Capillary electrophoretic monitoring of hydrothermal pre-treatment and enzymatic hydrolysis of willow: Comparison with HPLC and NMR. *Catal. Today* **2012**, *196*, 34–41. [CrossRef]
23. Ru, W.; Pang, Y.; Gan, Y.; Liu, Q.; Bao, J. Phenolic compounds and antioxidant activities of potato cultivars with white, yellow, red and purple flesh. *Antioxidants* **2019**, *8*, 419. [CrossRef]
24. Jansen, G.; Flamme, W. Coloured potatoes (*Solanum tuberosum* L.)-Anthocyanin content and tuber quality. *Genet. Resour. Crop Evol.* **2006**, *53*, 1321–1331. [CrossRef]
25. Wang, S.; Nie, S.; Zhu, F. Chemical constituents and health effects of sweet potato. *Food Res. Int.* **2016**, *89*, 90–116. [CrossRef] [PubMed]
26. Duarte-Delgado, D.; Ñústez-López, C.E.; Narváez-Cuenca, C.E.; Restrepo-Sánchez, L.P.; Melo, S.E.; Sarmiento, F.; Kushalappa, A.C.; Mosquera-Vásquez, T. Natural variation of sucrose, glucose and fructose contents in Colombian genotypes of Solanum tuberosum Group Phureja at harvest. *J. Sci. Food Agric.* **2016**, *96*, 4288–4294. [CrossRef] [PubMed]
27. Piikki, K.; Vorne, V.; Ojanperä, K.; Pleijel, H. Potato tuber sugars, starch and organic acids in relation to ozone exposure. *Potato Res.* **2003**, *46*, 67–79. [CrossRef]
28. Andre, C.M.; Ghislain, M.; Bertin, P.; Oufir, M.; Herrera, M.D.R.; Hoffmann, L.; Hausman, J.F.; Larondelle, Y.; Evers, D. Andean potato cultivars (Solarium tuberosum L.) as a source of antioxidant and mineral micronutrients. *J. Agric. Food Chem.* **2007**, *55*, 366–378. [CrossRef] [PubMed]
29. Navarre, D.A.; Goyer, A.; Shakya, R. Chapter 14-Nutritional Value of Potatoes: Vitamin, Phytonutrient, and Mineral Content. In *Advances in Potato Chemistry and Technology*; Singh, J., Kaur, L.B.T.-A., Eds.; Academic Press: San Diego, CA, USA, 2009; pp. 395–424. ISBN 978-0-12-374349-7.

30. Wszelaki, A.L.; Delwiche, J.F.; Walker, S.D.; Liggett, R.E.; Scheerens, J.C.; Kleinhenz, M.D. Sensory quality and mineral and glycoalkaloid concentrations in organically and conventionally grown redskin potatoes (Solanum tuberosum). *J. Sci. Food Agric.* **2005**, *85*, 720–726. [CrossRef]
31. Brown, C.R. Breeding for phytonutrient enhancement of potato. *Am. J. Potato Res.* **2008**, *85*, 298–307. [CrossRef]
32. Gąsiorowska, B.; Płaza, A.; Rzążewska, E.; Cybulska, A.; Górski, R. The potato tuber content of microelements as affected by organic fertilisation and production system. *Environ. Monit. Assess.* **2018**, *190*, 522. [CrossRef]
33. Olsen, N.L.; Hiller, L.K.; Mikitzel, L.J. The dependence of internal brown spot development upon calcium fertility in potato tubers. *Potato Res.* **1996**, *39*, 165–178. [CrossRef]
34. Pedreschi, F.; Mariotti, S.; Granby, K.; Risum, J. Acrylamide reduction in potato chips by using commercial asparaginase in combination with conventional blanching. *LWT Food Sci. Technol.* **2011**, *44*, 1473–1476. [CrossRef]

Publisher's Note: MDPI stays neutral with regard to jurisdictional claims in published maps and institutional affiliations.

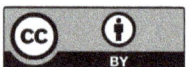

© 2020 by the authors. Licensee MDPI, Basel, Switzerland. This article is an open access article distributed under the terms and conditions of the Creative Commons Attribution (CC BY) license (http://creativecommons.org/licenses/by/4.0/).

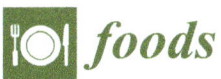

Article

Aglaomorpha quercifolia (L.) Hovenkamp & S. Linds a Wild Fern Used in Timorese Cuisine [†]

Hermenegildo R. Costa [1,2,3], Inês Simão [2], Helena Silva [2], Paulo Silveira [2], Artur M. S. Silva [1] and Diana C. G. A. Pinto [1,*]

[1] LAQV-REQUIMTE & Department of Chemistry, Campus de Santiago, University of Aveiro, 3810-193 Aveiro, Portugal; hrcosta@ua.pt (H.R.C.); artur.silva@ua.pt (A.M.S.S.)
[2] CESAM—Centre for Environmental and Marine Studies & Department of Biology, Campus de Santiago, University of Aveiro, 3810-193 Aveiro, Portugal; ines.simao@ua.pt (I.S.); hsilva@ua.pt (H.S.); psilveira@ua.pt (P.S.)
[3] Faculty of Education, Arts and Humanities, National University Timor Lorosa'e (UNTL), Avenida Cidade de Lisboa, Dili, East Timor
* Correspondence: diana@ua.pt
[†] We dedicate this article to the memory of the prestigious pteridologist Peter Hans Hovenkamp (1953–2019), member of the Naturalis Biodiversity Center (Leiden, The Netherlands), chief editor of Blumea, among other merits. He gave a significant contribution to help H.R.Costa in his efforts towards elaborating a checklist of Timor's ferns, which paved the way to the present article.

Abstract: *Aglaomorpha quercifolia* (L.) Hovenkamp & S. Linds is an extensively used species in traditional medicinal systems in several areas of the world due to some important medicinal properties such as antioxidant, antibacterial, analgesic, and anti-inflammatory activities. In East Timor, different parts of this fern are used either as remedies or as food. The ingestion of a broth made from its rhizome improves lactation, and young fronds of this fern are boiled and eaten with rice by the locals. Nevertheless, its chemical profile is far from being established. The present work aims to establish the chemical profile of both rhizomes and leaves *n*-hexane extracts by Gas Chromatography- Mass Spectrometry (GC-MS). The results showed the leaves richness in fatty acids with interesting nutritional values ($\omega-6/\omega-3 = 0.68$, AI = 0.59, TI = 0.30), being linolenic acid (253.71 ± 0.93 mg/g dry leaves) and palmitic acid (237.27 ± 0.59 mg/g dry leaves) the significant compounds in the extract. Whereas the rhizome extract is mostly rich in terpenoids, such as steroid, cycloartane, and hopanoid derivatives, being hop-16-ene (166.45 ± 0.53 mg/g dry rhizome) and β-sitosterol (50.76 ± 0.11 mg/g dry rhizome) the major compounds. Several compounds are reported for the first time in the species, and the data herein reported contributes to confirming the species nutritional value.

Keywords: *Aglaomorpha quercifolia*; GC-MS profile; rhizome; leaves; *n*-hexane extract; fatty acids; terpenoids; linolenic acid; hop-16-ene

Citation: Costa, H.R.; Simão, I.; Silva, H.; Silveira, P.; Silva, A.M.S.; Pinto, D.C.G.A. *Aglaomorpha quercifolia* (L.) Hovenkamp & S. Linds a Wild Fern Used in Timorese Cuisine . *Foods* **2021**, *10*, 87. https://doi.org/10.3390/foods10010087

Received: 20 November 2020
Accepted: 30 December 2020
Published: 4 January 2021

Publisher's Note: MDPI stays neutral with regard to jurisdictional claims in published maps and institutional affiliations.

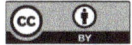

Copyright: © 2021 by the authors. Licensee MDPI, Basel, Switzerland. This article is an open access article distributed under the terms and conditions of the Creative Commons Attribution (CC BY) license (https://creativecommons.org/licenses/by/4.0/).

1. Introduction

Aglaomorpha quercifolia (L.) Hovenkamp & S. Linds., [syn. (*Drynaria quercifolia* (L.) J.Sm., J. Bot. (Hooker)] [1] is an epiphytic, occasionally epilithic medicinal pteridophyte with a short-creeping rhizome, dimorphic fronds, and pinnatifid lamina. It belongs to the Polypodiaceae family, which includes 65 genus and 165 species worldwide [2]. *A. quercifolia* occurs in primary and secondary forests, savannas, and plantations (such as rubber and coconut), but it can also be found along sideroads [3].

Aglaomorpha quercifolia is an extensively used species in traditional medicinal systems in several areas of the world. For example, in India, it is used by tribal communities to cure several different conditions. The juice produced from the rhizome and fronds is taken for body pain [4] and intestinal worms [5]. This fern is also used to treat throat infections, tuberculosis [6], jaundice, dysentery, and typhoid fever [7]. In Bangladesh, several parts of this fern have been used to treat jaundice [8], gonorrhea [9], diabetes [10], and malaria [11].

In East Timor, this fern rhizome is used either as a remedy to treat stomach pain or as food. It is believed that the ingestion of a broth made from its rhizome helps young moms producing more milk [12]. The rhizome is also consumed as a tea, and the young fronds of this fern are boiled and eaten with rice by the locals [12]. A paste made from the rhizome is massaged onto people with malaria [13].

The above-mentioned vast range of traditional uses concerning *A. quercifolia* are most certainly related to its many medicinal properties, such as antioxidant [14], antibacterial [15], analgesic [16], anti-inflammatory [17], anthelmintic [18], antipyretic [19], and antirheumatic [20]. These medicinal properties must be directly related to the secondary metabolites produced by the plant. Although these metabolites are not essential to the plant's life, they contribute directly to its fitness [21] and the interactions between the organism and the environment [22]. It is known that several classes of secondary metabolites with different functions in the plant are responsible for the plant's traditional medicine applications.

In terms of its secondary metabolites, *A. quercifolia* is not an extensively studied species. Studies involving methanolic or ethanolic extracts of the whole plant or the rhizome revealed the identification of several compounds [23–25]. Due to the use of polar solvents in the extraction, several reported compounds are polyphenolic, and others seemed not to be secondary metabolites. So, concerning the use of *A. quercifolia* in traditional medicine and nutrition, further studies focused on the plant's lipophilic constituents are needed to support its traditional use and possible medicinal properties.

Thus, this study aimed to establish the GC-MS profile of both *A. quercifolia* rhizomes and leaves *n*-hexane extract and simultaneously confirm the species' nutritional and medicinal value.

2. Materials and Methods

2.1. Plant Collection

Specimens of *Aglaomorpha quercifolia* (L.) Hovenkamp & S. Linds. were collected from Dare (Vera Cruz, Dili, East Timor) in July 2016. A voucher specimen was identified by the plant taxonomist Paulo Silveira and deposited in the Herbarium of the Department of Biology, University of Aveiro, Portugal (AVE), under the reference number AVE7891 (Costa HR 87).

Several plants were collected (around 100 plants), the plant rhizome and leaves were separated, washed, and dried at room temperature for 7 days. Six samples having ten plant parts were powdered using an electrical blender.

2.2. Extracts Preparation

For the extraction in *n*-hexane, the amount of plant was determined on a precision scale, RADWAG WLC 6/A2, with a precision of 0.1 g. In the process, 100 mL of *n*-hexane for each 10 g of the plant was used. In Table 1, the weights of plant powder and the amount of *n*-hexane are listed. The plant parts were put into an Erlenmeyer flask, a magnetic stirrer was added, and the flasks were placed on a stirring plate. The *n*-hexane was added, see volume in Table 1, and the stirring was started at a speed of 600 rpm. Because some compounds can decompose under the light influence, the flasks were covered with aluminum foil in advance.

Table 1. Dry weight of *A. quercifolia* and added volume of the solvent.

Part of Plant	DW (g)	V (mL)	HeW (g)	PyHe (%)
Leaves	10.01 ± 0.05	300.0 ± 0.1	0.58 ± 0.03	5.79 ± 0.09
Rhizomes	10.03 ± 0.05	300.0 ± 0.1	0.37 ± 0.01	3.69 ± 0.05

DW = Dry weight of the plant part used; V = Volume of *n*-hexane added; HeW = Hexane extract weight; PyHe = Percentage yield of the hexane extract.

One extraction ran for 48 h, and the solvent was changed at least twice until no intensive color and increase of extraction weight of the solvent occurred. After an extraction cycle, the solvent was filtered and evaporated. After the three extraction cycles, the extracts were dried until mass consistency before further usage. The procedure was repeated for two more samples, and the average weights of *n*-hexane dried extracts (after constant mass) are shown in Table 1.

2.3. Standards and Reagents

Several pure compounds were used as standards to ensure the identification of the phytochemicals and to perform the calibration curves for quantification purposes. Tetradecane (99%), hexadecane (99.5%), tetracosane (99%), octadecane (99%), 1-monopalmitin (>99%), β-sitosterol (98%), lupeol, 5α-cholestan-3β-ol (99%), D-mannitol (98%), 1-tetradecanol (98%), sorbitol (99%), D-(+)-galactose (>99%), D-(+)-mannose (>99%), D-(+)-xylose (>99%), D-(−)-ribose (>99.5%), D-fructose (99%), sucrose (>99%), maltose (>98%), stigmasterol (97%), cycloartenol (>99%), campesterol (95%), lupeol (99%), ursolic (98%), oleanolic (98%), palmitic (≥99%) and stearic (99%) acids, were purchased from Sigma-Aldrich (St. Louis, MO, USA). Malonic acid (98%), linoleic acid (≥99%), and glycerol (>99%) were purchased from BDH analytical chemicals (London, UK), D-(−)-cellobiose (>98%), α- and β-tocopherol (98%) from Merk (Darmstadt, Germany), and D-(−)-arabinose (>99%) from Fluka (Bucharest, Romania) while, eicosane, docosane, hexatriacontane, and *n*-paraffin mixtures (C5–C8, C7–C10, C10–C16, C18–C24, C24–C36, C25–C35) were supplied by Supelco Inc. (Bellefonte, PA, USA).

For extraction, hexane pro-analysis (p.a) was used while dichloromethane (p.a.) (DCM) was employed to dissolve the extracts. Pyridine p.a., N, O-bis(trimethylsilyl)trifluoroacetamide (BSTFA) (99%) and trimethylsilyl chloride (TMSCl) (99%) (Sigma-Aldrich) were applied in the sample derivatization by silylation.

2.4. Gas Chromatography—Mass Spectrometry Analysis

The GC-MS analysis of the *n*-hexane extracts was done using a Shimadzu GCMS-QP2010 Ultra system equipped with autosampler AOC-20i, ion source: electronic impact high-performance Quadrupole mass filter. Separation of the compounds was carried out in a DB-5J&W capillary column (30.0 m in length × 0.25 mm in diameter × 0.25 μm thickness of the film). The spectroscopic detection from the mass spectrometer utilized 0.1 kV electron ionization. Helium was used as a carrier gas with a column flow of 1.18 mL/min. GC-injection temperature was set to ϑ = 320 °C and split ratio of 50 was applied to an injection volume of 1 μL. The mass spectrometer ion source temperature was set to ϑ = 250 °C and the interface temperature to ϑ = 300 °C.

The extracts were weight with approximately m = 20 mg on an analytical scale into a tube. DCM was used as a solvent and *n*-tetracosane as an internal standard, added to the tube with 1 mL in total. The extracts were then dissolved in an ultra-sonic bath. For the silylation, 250 μL pyridine, 250 μL BSTFA, and 50 μL TMSCl were added. The mixture was maintained in a water bath at ϑ = 70 °C for 45 min being the hydroxy and the carboxy groups present in each secondary metabolite converted to trimethylsilyl (TMS) ethers and esters, respectively. Afterwards were injected twice in the GC-MS apparatus. The silylation reagents quantity, the water bath temperature and the reaction time were previously optimized to ensure a total conversion of all compounds with hydroxy groups into the correspondent TMS derivatives.

The chromatographic conditions were as follows: start time of record at 6.5 min; initial temperature ϑ = 90 °C, hold for 4.00 min; temperature rate, 16 °C/min up to ϑ = 180 °C; temperature rate, 6 °C/min up to ϑ = 250 °C; followed by temperature rate, 3 °C/min up to ϑ = 300 °C and then hold for 5.00 min.

From the total ion chromatogram, the peaks were identified by comparing their mass spectra with the mass spectra libraries NIST 2014, NIST 2008, and WILEY 2007, and with mass spectra fragmentation published in the literature [26–30]. If possible, it was also compared with the retention time and mass spectra of standard compounds injected in the same chromatographic conditions. Furthermore, identification of some compounds was done using the retention index relative to n-alkanes (C5–C36) injected in the same chromatographic conditions and using the Equation (1). Where z is the number of carbon atoms in the alkane before the unknown compound and Z the number of the longer alkane. The retention time is t_r [31]:

$$I = 100 \cdot \left[z + (Z - z) \cdot \frac{t_{r(unknown)} - t_{r(z)}}{t_{r(Z)} - t_{r(z)}} \right]. \quad (1)$$

For quantification purposes, four independent replicates of each sample were submitted to silylation procedure and each one injected in duplicate. The internal standard method was applied and the amount of metabolites present was achieved from the calibration curves obtained with the most closed pure standard compounds available or its TMS derivatives (if they have hydroxy groups). All the injected samples and standards solutions contain a fixed quantity of internal standard (tetracosane). The calibration curves were obtained by injection of at least six different concentrations (5 µg mL^{-1} to 1.5 mg mL^{-1}) and the detection and quantification limits (LOD and LOQ, respectively) were determined from the parameters of the calibration curves represented in Table 2 (LOD = 3 standard deviation/slope and LOQ = 10 standard deviation/slope). Values of correlation coefficients confirmed linearity of the calibration plots (Table 2). The concentrations of the standards were chosen in order to guarantee the quantification of each compound in the samples by intrapolation in the calibration curve. The results were expressed in mg of compound/g of extract, as mean values ± standard deviation (MV ± SD) of four independent analyses.

Table 2. Linearity (y = mx + b, where y corresponds to the standard peak area/internal standard peak area ratio and x corresponds to the mass of standard/mass of internal standard ratio), LOD and LOQ of pure compounds used as reference.

Standard Compound	Slope (m) [§]	Intercept (b) [§]	R^2	LOD [§§]	LOQ [§§]
Palmitic acid	0.2143	0	0.9944	15	50
1-Monopalmitin	7.2283	−0.0009	0.9975	3	10
Glycerol	7.2366	−0.0037	0.9937	3	10
Triacontane	2.0154	−0.0311	0.9991	10	33
Maltose	4.1401	−0.0801	0.9998	3	10
Mannose	4.1380	−0.1126	0.9999	5	17
β-Sitosterol	2.5254	−0.0033	0.9983	12	40
α-Tocopherol	2.4738	−0.0028	0.9993	5	17

[§] in area counts mg^{-1}; [§§] in µg/mL.

2.5. Statistics

Independent replicates of each sample were analyzed and each aliquot was injected twice. The presented results are the average of four concordant values obtained for each sample (less than 5% variation between injections of the same aliquot and between aliquots of the same sample) and expressed as mean values ± standard deviation (MV ± SD). One-way analysis of variance (ANOVA) followed by Duncan's multiple-range test were performed using the GraphPad Prism version 7 for Windows (Graphpad Software, Inc.) to compare the results of each independent replicates. A p-value lower than 0.0001 was considered statistically significant in all analyses.

3. Results and Discussion

Although the known use of *A. quercifolia* in traditional medicine [12,13] and a few studies involving GC-MS analysis were reported [23–25], this species still is, from the chemical profile point of view, underexplored. So, both rhizome and leaves were extracted with n-hexane at room temperature, aiming to obtain the lipophilic profile. Although this type of extraction was not reported for this species, our experience indicates that low extraction yields, such as the ones herein reported (Table 3), are typical in plants growing in warm environments [32]. Nevertheless, it was possible the identification and quantification, using GC-MS, of the major compounds present in both rhizome and leaves extracts, whose chromatograms demonstrate the richness in lipophilic compounds, although some only in traces (Figure 1). This analysis allowed identifying a total of 59 compounds, 31 in rhizome extract, and 34 in leaves extract. These were distributed through several chemical families, explicitly amid fatty acids, short-chain carboxylic acids, carbohydrates, terpenoids, alkanes, and alcohols. The retention time, identification, and content of each compound in mg/g of dried rhizome or leaves ± standard deviation of each species are presented in Table 3.

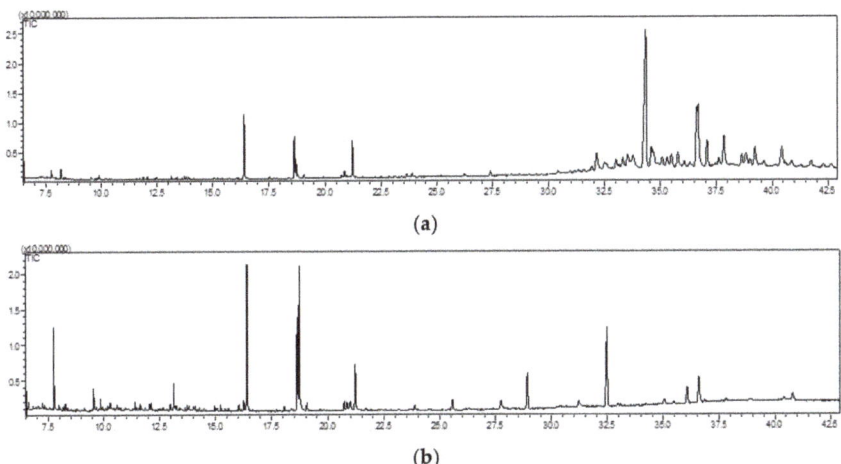

Figure 1. Total ion chromatogram (TIC) of *A. quercifolia* rhizomes (**a**) and leaves (**b**) *n*-hexane extracts with time in minutes.

Table 3. Identified compounds on the *n*-hexane extract of *A. quercifolia* rhizome and leaves.

Identification *	Rt (min)	RI_{NIST}	RI_{cal}	Rhizome **	Leaves **
Carboxylic acids and derivatives					
Butanedioic acid [b,c,d]	8.26	1170	1171	-	tr
Undecanoic acid [b,c,d]	9.55	1704	1704	-	21.78 ± 0.19
Malic acid [a,b,c]	9.86	1390	1392	-	tr
L-Glutamic acid [a,b,c]	10.30	-	-	-	9.87 ± 0.23
Shikimic acid [a,b,c]	13.14	1904	1904	-	28.58 ± 0.08
Citric acid [a,b,c]	13.26	1944	1945	-	tr
Quininic acid [a,b,c]	13.66	-	-	-	tr
Myristic acid	13.83	1788	1787	-	tr
3,4-Dihydroxyhydrocinnamic acid [a,b,c]	14.96	1964	1962	-	tr
Dodecanedioic acid [b,c,d]	15.42	1965	1966	-	tr
Glucaric acid [a,b,c]	15.58	2249	2250	-	tr
Oct-3-enoic acid [b,c,d]	16.26	1200	1202	-	15.67 ± 0.09
Palmitic acid [a,b,c]	16.40	1987	1987	107.65 ± 0.12	237.27 ± 0.59
Linoleic acid [a,b,c]	18.63	2202	2202	60.97 ± 0.08	153.81 ± 0.11
Linolenic acid [a,b,c]	18.73	2210	2211	-	253.71 ± 0.93
Oleic acid [a,b,c]	18.80	2194	2192	12.33±0.05	14.48 ± 0.24
Stearic acid [a,b,c]	19.05	2186	2184	17.00 ± 0.02	15.49 ± 0.08
Arachidonic acid [a,b,c]	20.72	2417	2415	-	19.13 ± 0.04
Oleoamide (9-Octadecenamide) [a,b,c]	20.84	2228	2230	-	13.12 ± 0.03
Monopalmitin [a,b,c]	23.63	2581	2583	0.50 ± 0.01	-
Lignoceric acid [a,b,c]	27.75	2782	2783	-	tr

Table 3. Cont.

Identification *	Rt (min)	RI$_{NIST}$	RI$_{cal}$	Rhizome **	Leaves **
		Terpenoids			
Neophytadiene [b,c,d]	13.76	-	1832	-	tr
Squalene [b,c,d]	27.39	2914	2910	2.59 ± 0.01	-
Cycloeucalenol acetate derivative [b,c,d]	32.13	-	2909	14.61 ± 0.02	-
Stigmastan-3,5-diene [c,d,e]	32.47	2525	2526	tr	-
α-Tocopherol [a,b,c]	32.99	3226	3227	6.89 ± 0.01	-
Cycloeucalenol acetate [b,c,d,§]	33.29	2900	2901	tr	tr
Serratene [b,c,d]	33.53	2744	2745	tr	-
Lupeol [a,b,c]	33.76	2848	2845	tr	-
Hop-16-ene [b,c,d]	34.34	3420	3421	166.45 ± 0.53	-
Cycloartenol acetate [b,c,d]	34.58	2907	2906	9.49 ± 0.01	-
9,19-Cycloergost-24-en-3-ol acetate [b,c,d]	34.70	2956	2957	14.58 ± 0.03	-
Cholest-5-en-3(α)-ol [b,c,d]	35.07	2954	2955	16.49 ± 0.02	-
Lupenone [b,c,d]	35.28	3483	3481	7.22 ± 0.01	-
Stigmasterol [a,b,c]	35.48	2797	2796	9.44 ± 0.01	-
4,14-Dimethyl-9,19-cyclolanost-24(28)-en-3-ol [b,c,d]	35.76	2760	2761	10.75 ± 0.01	-
γ-Sitosterol [a,b,c]	36.05	2731	2731	12.11 ± 0.05	-
β-Sitosterol [a,b,c]	36.60	2789	2789	50.76 ± 0.11	-
Hop-21-ene [b,c,d]	36.67	2659	2659	6.23 ± 0.01	-
Diploptene [Hop-22(29)-ene] [b,c,d]	37.06	-	2667	48.01 ± 0.13	-
Cycloeucalenone [b,c,d]	37.81	-	2981	26.75 ± 0.02	-
9,19-Cyclolanost-23-ene-3,25-diol 3-acetate [b,c,d,§]	38.62	3071	3070	12.99 ± 0.01	-
Hop-17(21)-ene [b,c,d]	38.80	-	2672	14.99 ± 0.01	-
3-O-Acetyl-6-methoxycycloartenol [b,c,d]	39.01	3093	3091	5.94 ± 0.02	-
Cyclolaudenol [b,c,d]	39.21	2834	2834	19.32 ± 0.06	-
Campesterol [a,b,c]	39.62	2689	2685	25.64 ± 0.12	tr
31-Norcyclolaudenone [b,c,d,§§]	40.43	-	3095	21.05 ± 0.06	-
		Alcohols			
Glycerol [a,b,c]	7.74	-	-	-	0.39 ± 0.01
Pentitol [b,c,d]	12.13	-	-	-	0.95 ± 0.01
Phytol [b,c,d]	18.07	2086	2086	-	16.43 ± 0.05
		Alkanes			
n-Docosane [e]	25.56	-	-	-	5.02 ± 0.02
n-Octacosane [e]	28.91	-	-	-	38.05 ± 0.03
n-Tritetracontane [b,c,d]	32.48	-	-	-	131.35 ± 0.64
n-Hentriacontane [b,c,d]	36.06	-	-	-	13.04 ± 0.05
		Carbohydrates			
D-Psicofuranose [b,c,d]	12.99	2029	2029	-	1.73 ± 0.02
D-Tagatose [b,c,d]	14.03	1982	1980	-	tr
D-Galactose [a,b,c]	14.11	1970	1973	-	tr
D-Glucose [a,b,c]	15.23	2037	2035	-	5.76 ± 0.04
Sucrose [a,b,c]	23.86	3552	3551	1.97 ± 0.01	-

RT = retention time; RI$_{NIST}$ = NIST14 mass spectral data retention index; RI$_{cal}$ = retention index relative to n-alkanes (C$_5$–C$_{36}$); MV = mean value; SD = standard deviation; - = not found; tr = traces; * all compounds possessing hydroxy groups are identified as the correspondent TMS derivatives. Compounds were identified by: [a] comparison with pure silylated standards, [b] comparison with the GC-MS spectral libraries NIST14.lib and WILEY229.lib, [c] comparison with spectra found in the literature, [d] interpretation of MS spectrum fragmentation pattern; [e] comparison with pure standards; ** Values in MV ± SD; [§] (3β,4α,5α,9β)-4,14-dimethyl-9,19-cycloergost-24(28)-en-3-yl acetate; [§§] 4-Monomethylcycloartane.

It is evident that the rhizomes and leaves lipophilic profiles are not very rich in secondary metabolites (Figure 1). Different results were observed regarding the mass of compounds identified in each extract, 70.3% in rhizomes and 99.6% in leaves. However, the percentage of compounds not identified by GC-MS was, therefore, approximately 30% for rhizome and less than 1% for leaves.

Regarding rhizomes extract, the most abundant chemical family present is terpenoids (50.2%), which included diterpenes, triterpenes, and steroids (Table 3, Figure 2). The rhizome chemical profile was dominated by hop-16-ene (166.45 ± 0.53 mg/g dry rhizome) and β-sitosterol (50.76 ± 0.11 mg/g dry rhizome). The second major chemical family identified in this plant part lipophilic extract was carboxylic acids and derivatives, summing a total of 19.8% of the identified compounds (Figure 2). The fatty acids palmitic and linoleic dominated the family with 107.65 ± 0.12 mg/g dry rhizome and 60.97 ± 0.08 mg/g dry rhizome, respectively (Table 3).

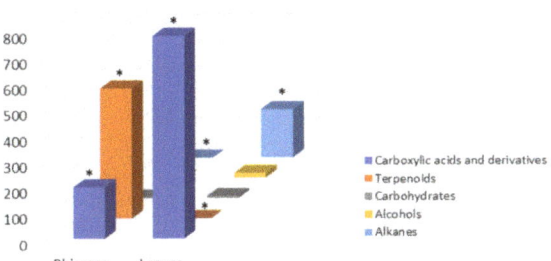

Figure 2. Graphical presentation of the total amount of each class of compounds for the two studied plant parts. * Statistically different (Tukey's test) $p < 0.001$.

Leaves extract showed more diversity in the chemical families present and their representativity (Figure 2). The major chemical family in its lipophilic extract, representing 78.3% of the identified compounds, was the carboxylic acids and derivatives. In addition, among the identified compounds, palmitic, linolenic, and linoleic acids were the ones found in the highest amount, respectively 237.27 ± 0.59 mg/g dry leaves, 253.71 ± 0.93 mg/g dry leaves, and 153.81 ± 0.11 mg/g dry leaves (Table 3). Alkanes were the second major class observed, representing 18.7% of the identified compounds (Figure 2), being the n-tritetracontane found in significant quantities (131.3 ± 0.64 mg/g dry leaves). The remaining chemical families represent 0.2% and 2.5% of the rhizome and leaves' identified compounds, respectively (Figure 2).

Alkanes represent more than 70% of the wax cuticle constitution, which is indispensable to prevent water loss [33], so their detection in *A. quercifolia* leaves seems quite normal. n-Alkanes are easily distinguishable by their mass spectrum due to the first fragment ion peak, represented by $[M - 29]^+$ ion (loss of a $^\bullet CH_2CH_3$), the base peak occurs at 43 or 57 m/z, and peaks differing by 14 m/z units (e.g., 43, 57, 71, 85, etc.) are present [34]. Nevertheless, their identification was possible mainly using pure standards and comparing with GC-MS databases.

A detailed analysis of Table 3 shows that *A. quercifolia* leaves are incredibly rich in fatty acids, both saturated fatty acids (SFA) and polyunsaturated fatty acids (PUFA), from which, respectively, palmitic acid (237.27 ± 0.59 mg/g dry leaves) and linolenic acid (253.71 ± 0.93 mg/g dry leaves) can be highlighted (Table 3). The plant rhizome also presents a high quantity of palmitic acid (107.65 ± 0.12 mg/g dry rhizome), contributing to a higher amount of SFA compared to PUFA (Table 3). However, it should be emphasized that recent evidence points out that SFA in the human diet may not have such an adverse health effect [35]. In the case of leaves, it is evident that some nutritional indexes, such as $\omega-6/\omega-3$ (total of omega-6 acids/total of omega-3 acids ratio), atherogenicity index (AI), and thrombogenicity index (TI), present values ($\omega-6/\omega-3 = 0.68$; AI = 0.59; TI = 0.30) that suggest nutritional and health-promoting values [36,37].

Concerning the rhizome, it is evident its richness in terpenoid derivatives (Figure 2), from which cycloartane, hopanoid, and phytosterol derivatives can be highlighted and being the major compounds hop-16-ene (166.45 ± 0.53 mg/g dry rhizome), β-sitosterol (50.76 ± 0.11 mg/g dry rhizome), diploptene (48.01 ± 0.13 mg/g dry rhizome), cycloeucalenone (26.75 ± 0.02 mg/g dry rhizome), campesterol (25.64 ± 0.12 mg/g dry rhizome), and 31-norcyclolaudenone (21.05 ± 0.06 mg/g dry rhizome) (Table 3 and Figure 3).

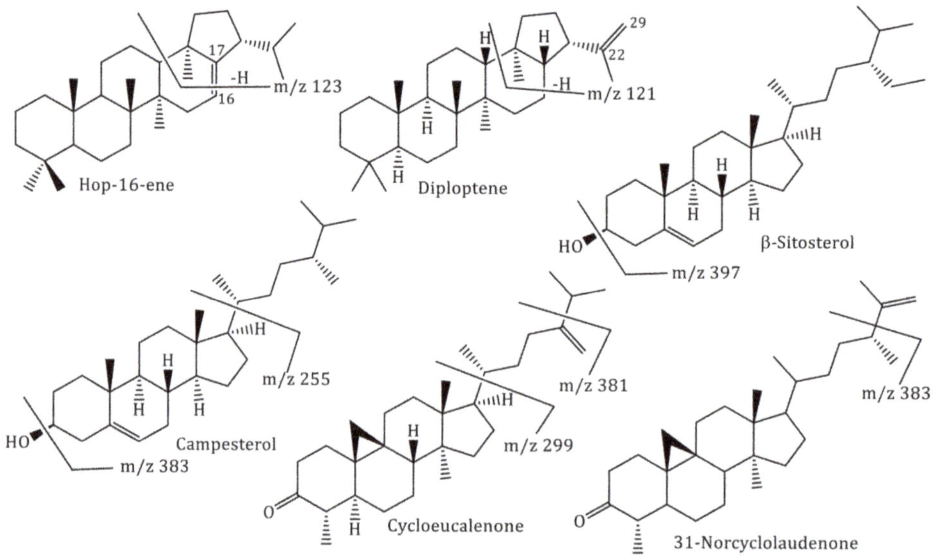

Figure 3. Chemical structure of some of the identified terpenoids and some of the most significant fragments.

Some of the terpenoids found in *A. quercifolia* rhizomes are commonly found in plants, including some phytosterols found in our previous works [32,38]. Cycloartane triterpenoids' natural occurrence is also vast through the plant kingdom [39], being cycloartenol the most recognized due to its rule in the phytosterols biosynthesis [40] and consequently in the regulation of important plant functions [41]. The occurrence of this type of triterpenoids in *A. quercifolia* rhizomes (Table 3) may explain the effect that the rhizome intake promotes on young moms. Actually, there are references to the use of several plants to improve breastfeeding [42–44] and evidence that terpenoids are also involved [42,43].

Lastly, it seems imperative to mention the hopanoids triterpenes, which are the major class found in *A. quercifolia* rhizomes, mainly due to the presence of hop-16-ene (Table 3 and Figure 3). This type of triterpenes frequently occurs in ferns and was described for the first time by John Hope, a British botanist [45,46]. Several hopanoids, including hop-16-ene and diploptene (Figure 3), were found in *Davallia mariesii* rhizomes, and our results are identical to those previously reported [47]. The mass fragments confirm, in particular, the position of the double bond at C16 = C17 in hop-16-ene and C22 = C29 in diploptene (Figure 3). Moreover, the NMR data showed a proton sign at δ 5.28 ppm correlated with a carbon sign at δ 115.6 ppm characteristics of the hop-16-ene vinylic proton and carbon. Whereas in the case of diploptene, it is possible to detect the vinylic proton and carbon, respectively, at δ 4.78 and δ 109.9 ppm, data that are similar to the ones previously reported [47]. It is also important to highlight that the hop-16-ene DEPT 90 and DEPT 135 spectra confirm the presence of 6 methine, 10 methylene, and 8 methyl carbons, data that also ensure the proposed structure (Figure 3).

4. Conclusions

The *A. quercifolia* rhizomes and leaves GC-MS profiles were established and revealed the plant nutritional value. Almost all the compounds herein reported were found for the first time in the species. The leaves richness in PUFA should be highlighted not only because it attests to their nutritional value but also will incentive its use in Timorese cuisine. The rhizomes richness in terpenoids should also be emphasized, particularly the cycloartane derivatives, compounds involved in phytosterols' biosynthesis, which validate this plant's use of rhizome to incentive the production of milk by young moms. The hopanoid derivatives herein revealed for the first time in this species, although common in ferns, may differentiate the species.

Author Contributions: Conceptualization, D.C.G.A.P. and A.M.S.S.; methodology, H.R.C. and D.C.G.A.P.; formal analysis, D.C.G.A.P. and A.M.S.S.; writing—original draft preparation, I.S. and D.C.G.A.P.; writing—review and editing, D.C.G.A.P., I.S., H.S., P.S. and A.M.S.S.; supervision, D.C.G.A.P.; funding acquisition, H.S. and A.M.S.S. All authors have read and agreed to the published version of the manuscript.

Funding: This research was funded by FCT/MCT, which gives the financial support to LAQV-REQUIMTE (UIDB/50006/2020 + UIDP/50006/2020) and to FCT/MCTES for the financial support to CESAM (UIDP/50017/2020+UIDB/50017/2020), through national funds.

Institutional Review Board Statement: Not applicable.

Informed Consent Statement: Not applicable.

Data Availability Statement: Not applicable.

Acknowledgments: Thanks are due to the University of Aveiro, FCT/MCT and FEDER, within the PT2020 Partnership Agreement, and to the Portuguese NMR Network, for their support. Thanks, are also due to U.N.T.L. (Dili, East Timor) for a grant attributed to H.R. Costa.

Conflicts of Interest: The authors declare no conflict of interest.

References

1. Lindsay, S.; Hovenkamp, P.H.; Middleton, D.J. New combinations and typifications in Aglaomorpha (Polypodiaceae). *Gard. Bull. Singapore* **2017**, *69*, 149–155. [CrossRef]
2. Hovenkamp, P.H. Polypodiaceae. In *Flora Malesiana, Seri II—Pteridophyta*; Kalkman, C., Kirkup, D.W., Nooteboon, H.P., Saw, L.G., Stevens, P.F., Wilde, W.J.J., Eds.; New York Botanical Garden: New York, NY, USA, 1998; Volume 3, pp. 1–234.
3. PPG. A community-derived classification for extant lycophytes and ferns. *J. Systemat. Evolut.* **2016**, *54*, 563–603. [CrossRef]
4. Kalaiselvan, M.; Gopalan, R. Ethnobotanical studies on selected wild medicinal plants used by Irula tribes of Bolampatty Valley, Nilgiri Biosphere Reserve (NBR), Southern Western Ghats, India. *Asian J. Pharm. Clin. Res.* **2014**, *7*, 22–26.
5. Das, H.B.; Majumdar, K.; Datta, B.K.; Ray, D. Ethnobotanical uses of some plants by Tripuri and Reang tribes of Tripura. *Nat. Prod. Rad.* **2009**, *8*, 172–180.
6. Sen, A.; Ghosh, P.D. A note on the ethnobotanical studies of some pteriddophytes in Assam. *Indian J. Tradit. Knowl.* **2011**, *10*, 292–295.
7. Ramanathan, R.; Bhuvaneswari, R.; Indhu, M.; Subramanian, G.; Dhandapani, R. Survey of ethnobotanical observation on wild tuberous medicinal plants of Kollihills, Namakkal district, Tamilnadu. *J. Med. Plants Stud.* **2014**, *2*, 50–58.
8. Rahmatullah, M.; Jahan, R.; Seraj, S.; Islam, F.; Jahan, F.I.; Khatun, Z.; Sanam, S.; Monalisa, M.N.; Khan, T.; Biswas, K.R. Medicinal Plants Used by Folk and Tribal Medicinal Practitioners of Bangladesh for Treatment of Gonorrhea. *Am Eurasian J. Sustain. Agric.* **2011**, *5*, 276–281.
9. Rahmatullah, M.; Mukti, I.J.; Haque, A.; Mollik, M.D.; Parvin, K.; Jahan, R.; Chowdhury, M.H.; Rahman, T. An Ethnobotanical Survey and Pharmacological Evaluation of Medicinal Plants used by the Garo Tribal Community living in Netrakona district, Bangladesh. *Adv. Nat. App. Sci.* **2009**, *3*, 402–418.
10. Rahmatullah, M.; Azam, M.D.; Khatun, Z.; Seraj, S.; Islam, F.; Rahman, M.D.; Jahan, S.; Aziz, M.D.S. Medicinal plants used for treatment of diabetes by the Marakh sect of the Garo tribe living in Mymensingh district, Bangladesh. *Afr. J. Tradit. Complement. Alternat. Med.* **2012**, *9*, 380–385. [CrossRef]
11. Mollik, A.; Hasan, N.; Hossan, S.; Jahan, R.; Rahmatullah, M. Medicinal plants used against malaria in several regions of Bogra district, Bangladesh. *Planta Med.* **2009**, *75*, PD39. [CrossRef]
12. Costa, H.R. The Pteridophytes of Timor, with Special Focus on Timor-Leste. Ph.D. Thesis, University of Aveiro, Aveiro, Portugal, 2021.
13. Taek, M.M.; Prajogo, B.E.W.; Agil, M. Plants used in traditional medicine for the treatment of malaria by the Tetun ethnic people in West Timor Indonesia. *Asian Pac. J. Trop. Med.* **2018**, *11*, 630–637. [CrossRef]
14. Prasanna, G.; Anuradha, R. Evaluation of in vitro antioxidant activity of rhizome extract of *Drynaria quercifolia* L. *Int. J. Chem. Tech. Res.* **2015**, *8*, 183–187.

15. Mithraja, M.J.; Irudayaraj, V.; Kiruba, S.; Jeeva, S. Antibacterial efficacy of *Drynaria quercifolia* (L.) J. Smith (Polypodiaceae) against clinically isolated urinary tract pathogens. *Asian Pac. J. Trop. Biomed.* **2012**, *2*, S131–S135. [CrossRef]
16. Anuja, G.I.; Latha, P.G.; Shine, V.J.; Suja, S.R.; Shikha, P.; Kumar, K.S.; Rajasekharan, S. Antioedematous and Analgesic Properties of Fertile Fronds of *Drynaria quercifolia*. *ISRN Inflammation* **2014**, *2014*, 1–8. [CrossRef]
17. Anuja, G.I.; Latha, P.G.; Suja, S.R.; Shyamal, S.; Shine, V.J.; Sini, S.; Pradeep, S.; Shikha, P.; Rajasekharan, S. Anti-inflammatory and analgesic properties of *Drynaria quercifolia* (L.) J. Smith. *J. Ethnopharmacol.* **2010**, *132*, 456–460. [CrossRef]
18. Kulkarni, G.K.; Kadolkar, R.V.; Maisale, A.B. Anthelmintic activity of *Drynaria quercifolia* (L.) J. Smith. *J. Pharm. Res.* **2010**, *3*, 975–977.
19. Khan, A.; Haque, E.; Mukhlesur, R.M.; Mosaddik, A.; Rahman, M.; Sultana, N. Isolation of antibacterial constituent from rhizome of *Drynaria quercifolia* and its sub-acute toxicological studies. *DARU J. Fac. Pharm.* **2007**, *15*, 205–211.
20. Saravanan, S.; Mutheeswaran, S.; Saravanan, M.; Chellappandian, M.; Paulraj, M.G.; Raj, M.K.; Ignacimuthua, S.; Duraipandiyanac, V. Ameliorative effect of *Drynaria quercifolia* (L.) J. Sm., an ethnomedicinal plant, in arthritic animals. *Food Chem. Toxicol.* **2013**, *51*, 356–363. [CrossRef]
21. Pagare, S.; Bhatia, M.; Tripathi, N.; Pagare, S.; Bansal, Y.K. Secondary Metabolites of Plants and their Role: Overview. *Curr. Trends Biotechnol. Pharm.* **2015**, *9*, 293–304.
22. Erb, M.; Kliebenstein, D.J. Plant secondary metabolites as defenses, regulators, and primary metabolites: The blurred functional trichotomy. *Inaugural Trop. Rev. Plant Physiol.* **2020**, *184*, 39–52. [CrossRef]
23. Prasanna, G.; Chitra, M. Phytochemical screening and GC-MS analysis of *Drynaria quercifolia* rhizome. *Am. J. Adv. Drug Deliv.* **2014**, *3*, 72–78.
24. Rajesh, K.D.; Subramanian, V.; Panneerselvam, A.; Rajesh, N.V.; Jeyathilakan, N. GC-MS analysis of secondary metabolites from the whole plant methanolic extract of *Drynaria quercifolia* (L.) J. Smith (Polypodiaceae). *J. Adv. Appl. Scientif. Res.* **2016**, *1*, 84–89.
25. Nithin, M.K.; Veeramani, G.; Sivakrishnan, S. Phytochemical screening and GC-MS analysis of rhizome of *Drynaria quercifolia*. *Res. J. Pharm. Tech.* **2020**, *13*, 2266–2268. [CrossRef]
26. Füzfai, Z.; Boldizsár, I.; Molnar-Perl, I. Characteristic fragmentation patterns of the trimethylsilyl and trimethylsilyl-oxime derivatives of various saccharides as obtained by gas chromatography coupled to ion-trap mass spectrometry. *J. Chromatogr. A* **2008**, *1177*, 183–189. [CrossRef]
27. Razboršek, M.I.; Vončina, D.B.; Doleček, V.; Vončina, E. Determination of oleanolic, betulinic and ursolic acid in lamiaceae and mass spectral fragmentation of their trimethylsilylated derivatives. *Chromatographia* **2008**, *67*, 433–440. [CrossRef]
28. Suttiarporn, P.; Chumpolsri, W.; Mahatheeranont, S.; Luangkamin, S.; Teepsawang, S.; Leardkamolkarn, V. Structures of phytosterols and triperrnoids with potential anti-cancer activity in bran of black non-glutinous rice. *Nutrients* **2015**, *7*, 1672–1687. [CrossRef]
29. AOCS Lipid Library, Lipid Chemistry, Biology, Technology & Analysis. Available online: http://lipidlibrary.aocs.org/index.html (accessed on 15 November 2020).
30. Golm Metabolome Database (GMD). Available online: http://gmd.mpimp-golm.mpg.de/ (accessed on 15 November 2020).
31. Nič, M.; Jirát, J.; Košata, B.; Jenkins, A.; McNaught, A. *Compendium of Chemical Terminology*; IUPAC: Research Triangle Park, NC, USA, 2009.
32. Rahmouni, N.; Pinto, D.C.G.A.; Santos, S.A.O.; Beghidja, N.; Silva, A.M.S. Lipophilic composition of *Scabiosa stellata* L.: An underexploited plant from Batna (Algeria). *Chem. Pap.* **2018**, *72*, 753–762. [CrossRef]
33. Bourdenx, B.; Bernard, A.; Domergue, F.; Pascal, S.; Léger, A.; Roby, D.; Pervent, M.; Vile, D.; Haslam, R.P.; Napier, J.A.; et al. Overexpression of Arabidopsis ECERIFERUM1 promotes wax very-long-chain alkane biosynthesis and influences plant response to biotic and abiotic stresses. *Plant Physiol.* **2011**, *156*, 29–45. [CrossRef]
34. Sparkman, O.D.; Penton, Z.E.; Kitson, F.G. Hydrocarbons. In *Gas Chromatography and Mass Spectrometry: A Practical Guide*; Sparkman, O.D., Penton, Z.E., Kitson, F.G., Eds.; Elsevier: Burlington, MA, USA, 2011; pp. 331–339.
35. Agostoni, C.; Moreno, L.; Shamir, R. Palmitic acid and health: Introduction. *Crit. Rev. Food Sci. Nutr.* **2016**, *56*, 1941–1942. [CrossRef]
36. Ulbricht, T.L.V.; Southgate, D.A.T. Coronary heart disease: Seven dietary factors. *Lancet* **1991**, *338*, 985–992. [CrossRef]
37. Simopoulos, A.P. The importance of the omega-6/omega-3 fatty axid ratio in cardiovascular disease and other chronic diseases. *Exp. Biol. Med.* **2008**, *233*, 674–678. [CrossRef]
38. Faustino, M.V.; Faustino, M.A.F.; Silva, H.; Silva, A.M.S.; Pinto, D.C.G.A. Lipophilic metabolites of *Spartina maritima* and *Puccinellia maritima* involved in their tolerance to salty environments. *Chem. Biodiversity* **2020**, *17*, e2000316. [CrossRef]
39. Boar, R.B.; Roner, C.R. Cycloartane triterpenoids. *Phytochemistry* **1975**, *14*, 1143–1146. [CrossRef]
40. Myant, N.B. The Biosynthesis of Sterols. In *The Biology of Cholesterol and Related Steroids*; Elsevier Ltd.: Amsterdam, The Netherlands, 1981; Chapter 4; pp. 161–225.
41. Clouse, S.D. Brassinosteroids. *Ref. Module Biomed. Sci.* **2019**. [CrossRef]
42. Kuswaningrum, O.; Suwandono, A.; Ariyanti, I.; Hadisaputro, S.; Suharttono, S. The impact of consuming *Amaranthus spinosus* L. extract on prolactin level and breast milk production in postpartum mothers. *Belitung Nurs. J.* **2017**, *3*, 541–547. [CrossRef]
43. Bekoe, E.O.; Kitcher, C.; Gyima, N.A.M.; Schwingee, G.; Frempong, M. Medicinal plants used as galactagogues. In *Pharmacognosy—Medicinal Plants*; IntechOpen: London, UK, 2018. [CrossRef]

44. Jendras, G.; Monizi, M.; Neinhuis, C.; Lautenschläger, T. Plants, food and treatments used by BaKongo tribes in Uíge (northern Angola) to affect the quality and quantity of human breast milk. *Int. Breastfeeding J.* **2020**, *15*, 88. [CrossRef]
45. Poralla, K. Cycloartenol and other triterpene cyclases. *Compr. Nat. Prod. Chem.* **1999**, *2*, 299–319.
46. Kushiro, T.; Ebizuka, Y. Triterpenes. In *Comprehensive Natural Products II: Chemistry and Biology*; Elsevier Ltd.: London, UK, 2010; pp. 673–708.
47. Shiojima, K.; Ageta, H. Fern constituents: Two new triterpenoid hydrocarbons, hop-16-ene and isohop-22(29)-ene, isolated from *Davallia mariesii*. *Chem. Pharm. Bull.* **1999**, *38*, 347–349. [CrossRef]

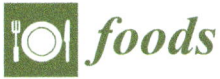

Review

Natural Compounds for the Prevention and Treatment of Cardiovascular and Neurodegenerative Diseases

Rosalba Leuci [†], Leonardo Brunetti [†], Viviana Poliseno, Antonio Laghezza, Fulvio Loiodice, Paolo Tortorella and Luca Piemontese *

Dipartimento di Farmacia-Scienze del Farmaco-University of Bari "Aldo Moro", Via E. Orabona 4, 70125 Bari, Italy; r.leuci6@studenti.uniba.it (R.L.); leonardo.brunetti@uniba.it (L.B.); v.poliseno1@studenti.uniba.it (V.P.); antonio.laghezza@uniba.it (A.L.); fulvio.loiodice@uniba.it (F.L.); paolo.tortorella@uniba.it (P.T.)
* Correspondence: luca.piemontese@uniba.it
† The two authors contributed equally to this work.

Abstract: Secondary metabolites from plants and fungi are stimulating growing interest in consumers and, consequently, in the food and supplement industries. The beneficial effects of these natural compounds are being thoroughly studied and there are frequent updates about the biological activities of old and new molecules isolated from plants and fungi. In this article, we present a review of the most recent literature regarding the recent discovery of secondary metabolites through isolation and structural elucidation, as well as the in vitro and/or in vivo evaluation of their biological effects. In particular, the possibility of using these bioactive molecules in the prevention and/or treatment of widely spread pathologies such as cardiovascular and neurodegenerative diseases is discussed.

Keywords: secondary metabolites; plants; fungi; food supplements; cardiovascular diseases; neurodegenerative diseases; Alzheimer's disease; metabolic syndrome

Citation: Leuci, R.; Brunetti, L.; Poliseno, V.; Laghezza, A.; Loiodice, F.; Tortorella, P.; Piemontese, L. Natural Compounds for the Prevention and Treatment of Cardiovascular and Neurodegenerative Diseases. *Foods* **2021**, *10*, 29. https://dx.doi.org/10.3390/foods10010029

Received: 24 November 2020
Accepted: 22 December 2020
Published: 24 December 2020

Publisher's Note: MDPI stays neutral with regard to jurisdictional claims in published maps and institutional affiliations.

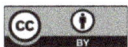

Copyright: © 2020 by the authors. Licensee MDPI, Basel, Switzerland. This article is an open access article distributed under the terms and conditions of the Creative Commons Attribution (CC BY) license (https://creativecommons.org/licenses/by/4.0/).

1. Introduction

Fungi and plants represent an important source of numerous bioactive compounds and have historically been used for medicinal purposes by virtually all human cultures [1].

Plants produce various secondary metabolites (SMs) in order to defend themselves from external attacks and as signals. These SMs show interesting biological and pharmacological activities: for this reason, they are often isolated and used for therapeutic purposes [2]. Plant-derived compounds are currently used in oncology therapy worldwide because they are considered less toxic and thus better accepted by patients [3], even if this consideration cannot be extended to all natural compounds and can be dangerous. Taxanes, used for the treatment of patients with breast cancer, are an excellent example of a valuable drug: paclitaxel is isolated from the bark of *Taxus brevifolia* (Pacific yew tree), while docetaxel is extracted from the needles of *Taxus baccata* (European yew tree) [4]. Other anticancer treatments obtained from plants are the vinca alkaloids vincristine and vinblastine, derived from the periwinkle plant *Catharanthus roseus* [5].

Polyphenols are another remarkable class of plant-derived SM, endowed with protective effects against pathologies such as cancer, cardiovascular diseases, diabetes, and neurodegenerative disorders [6]. These are classified into phenolic acids, flavonoids, stilbenes, coumarins, lignins, and tannins. Coumarins are found in a variety of plants such as tonka bean (*Dipteryx odorata*), sweet woodruff (*Galium odoratum*), sweet grass (*Hierochloe odorata*), deer-tongue (*Dichanthelium clandestinum*), vanilla grass (*Anthoxanthum odoratum*), mullein (*Verbascum* spp.), and sweet-clover (*Melilotus* sp.) [7]. Resveratrol, a stilbenoid present in many fresh fruits and plants such as *Polygonum cuspidatum*, *Arachis hypogea*, *Cassia* sp., *Eucalyptus*, *Morus rubra*, and *Vitis vinifera*, has been reported to have numerous biological properties, such as antioxidant, anti-inflammatory, anti-cancer, anti-aging, anti-obesity, anti-diabetes, cardioprotective and neuroprotective effects [8].

In recent years, the interest on the medicinal properties of compounds from *Cannabis* species has been steadily growing. More than 100 phyto-cannabinoids have been identified from *C. sativa*; among them, the most potent psychoactive activity is displayed by trans-Δ^9-tetrahydrocannabinol (THC). According to several studies, cannabis derivatives can be useful in conditions such as pain, anorexia-cachexia, skin pathologies, neurodegenerative diseases, epilepsy, sleep disorders and infections. However, legislation regarding these compounds is still ambiguous, insufficient, and plagued by controversies linked to their adverse effects and their consumption as recreational drugs [9,10].

Fungi also produce bioactive natural products that are exploited for pharmaceutical purposes. Fungal metabolites with clinical use include beta lactams, e.g., penicillins G and V, statins, cholesterol-lowering blockbuster drugs, the immunosuppressant cyclosporin and the anti-migraine ergotamine [11]. Beta-lactams are the most widely used class of antibiotics that, with the discovery of penicillin, produced by the fungus *Penicillium notatum*, early in the twentieth century, marked a new era for the treatment of bacterial infections [12]. Cyclosporin is employed for the treatment of autoimmune diseases such as psoriasis; it is a peptide isolated from *Tolypocladium inflatum* [13].

Many natural compounds from fungi and plants are extensively used as food supplements for the treatment and prevention of neurodegenerative and cardiovascular diseases [14], showing the growing interest in this field of research. Among the best-selling products, monacolin K, a component of red yeast rice fermented with several patented *Monascus purpureus* strains, is a widely discussed case. Considering its chemical structure and biological activity [15], the use of the food supplement containing this bioactive compound should be more strictly regulated. This review focuses on another important aspect of research regarding natural compounds: the isolation of secondary metabolites of fungi and plants and their biological evaluation as potential useful compounds for neurodegenerative and cardiovascular disorders.

2. Natural Compounds and Neurodegenerative Diseases

The prevention and treatment of neurodegenerative diseases (NDs), such as Parkinson's disease (PD) and Alzheimer's disease (AD), is an important avenue of research due to the increasing occurrence of these pathologies in the rapidly aging world population. Their multifactorial nature complicates their diagnostic and therapeutic profile and only few drugs are available [16–18]. Lifestyle factors, including dietary habits, influence the development of NDs, further cementing the role of food-derived compounds such as plant SMs in the long-term physiological balance of the nervous system [19]. Table 1 summarizes the body of literature regarding plant and fungal SMs with potential activity toward NDs.

Table 1. Natural compounds and neurodegenerative diseases.

Source	Bioactive Compounds	Effects	Main Activities	Ref.
Cetraria islandica L. Ach	Furmarprotocetraric acid	Neuroprotective and antioxidant activities	Oxygen radical absorbance capacity (ORAC) 5.07 ± 0.43 μmol TE/mg	[20]
Spongionella sp.	Gracilin A, H, K, J, L, and tetrahydroaplysulphurin-1	Neuroprotective activity	(Caspase 3 inh.) $3.88\text{–}4.04 \times 10^3$ RFU	[21]
Lepidium meyenii	N-(3-methoxybenzyl)oleamide, (N-(3-methoxybenzyl)linolenamide, N-(3-methoxybenzyl)linolenamide	Neuroprotective activity, peroxisome proliferator-activated receptor (PPAR) γ interaction, inhibition of fatty acid amide hydrolase (FAAH)	(PPARγ act., EC$_{50}$) 20.4–22.6 μM	[22]

Table 1. Cont.

Source	Bioactive Compounds	Effects	Main Activities	Ref.
Aspergillus terreus Y10	Asperteretal F, G_1, G_2, H and others	Inhibition of Tumor Necrosis Factor α (TNFα)	(TNFα inh., IC_{50}) 7.6–9.9 μM	[23]
Sarcophyton glaucum	Sarcophytolide	Antimicrobic and cytoprotective activities	(MIC) 0.13–0.22 μg/mL	[24]
Hericius erinaceus and Hericius flagellum	Erinacine A, B, C, E, F, and others	Neurotrophic activity	(increased NGF expression) 0.8–12 μg/mL	[25]
Narcissus tazetta L.	(−)-9-O-methylpseudolycorine, (−)-narcissidine, (−)-pancratinine-C, (+)-9-O-demethyl-2-a-hydroxyhomolycorine	Inhibition of acetylcholine esterase AChE and butyrylcholine esterase (BChE)	(AChE inh, IC_{50}) 0.67–32.51 μM	[26]
Embelia ribes and others	Embelin and others	Inhibition of AChE, BChE and Beta-secretase 1 (BACE-1); induction of P-glycoprotein 1 (P-gp)	(AChE inh, IC_{50}) 2.50–6.98 μM	[27]
Rumex abyssinicus	Helminthosporin, emodin, chryso-phanol, physcion	Inhibition of AChE and BChE	(AChE inh, IC_{50}) 2.63–33.7 μM	[28]
Oxalis corniculate L.	Flavonoids 1-9	Inhibition of AChE, BChE and carbonic anhydrases II (CA-II)	(AChE inh, IC_{50}) 49.52–109.55 μg/mL	[29]
Lichens	Atranorin, perlatolic acid, physodic acid, usnic acid and others	Neurotrophic activity and AChE inhibition	(AChE inh, IC_{50}) 6.8–27.1 μM	[30]
Fungi and plants	Tenuazonic acid, epi-racidinol, mycophenolic acid, radicinin, visoltricin, 6-methoxymellein	Inhibition of AChE, BChE and Aβ-aggregation; antioxidant activity, metal chelation	(AChE inh, IC_{50}) 6.86–11.4 μM	[31]
S. flavescens	(−)-maackian and others	Inhibition of monoamine oxidases (MAOs)	(MAO-B inh, IC_{50}) 0.68–52.3 μM	[32]
Renealmia Alpinia	Desmethoxyangonin and others	Inhibition of MAOs	(MAO-B inh, Ki) 31–110 nM	[33]
Ginkgo biloba	Ginkgolic acid and anacardic acid	Decreased accumulation of α-synuclein (αSN) aggregates	(αSN aggr inh) 10–100 μM	[34]
Ampelopsis grossedentata	Dihydromyricetin	Neuroprotective activity and inhibition of αSN fibril formation	(αSN aggr inh) 50–100 μM	[35]

Oxidative stress and neuroinflammation are considered two of the causes of NDs [19,36]. For this reason, neuroprotective agents targeting these pathological factors can be useful for the prevention and treatment of these disorders [36]. In recent years, several natural compounds have been explored for their neuroprotective and antioxidant activity. For example, polyphenols, which are secondary metabolites of plants present in various food and drinks, have shown important antioxidant properties [37]. However, numerous studies in the recent past have been focused on different and more original matrices.

Cetraria islandica L. Ach (or Iceland moss), as an example, is the most famous cetrarioid lichen species. It has been used for the treatment of various inflammatory diseases, and recently the neuroprotective properties of its major metabolite, fumarprotocetraric acid (FUM) were evaluated on neuron-like SH-SY5Y cells and glial U373-MG cells. FUM revealed different activities, acting as a scavenger of peroxyl radicals, decreasing reactive oxygen species (ROS) production, reducing GSH depletion and increasing the ratio of reduced glutathioneto oxidized glutathione (GSH/GSSG ratio). Moreover, FUM decreased mitochondrial Ca^{2+} levels, protected the mitochondrial membrane against H_2O_2-induced damage, suppressed H_2O_2-induced expression of protease caspase-3, decreased pro-apoptotic factor Bax levels and increased the anti-apoptotic Bcl-2 levels [20].

Another interesting research is the in vitro screening of the antioxidant action of six diterpene derivatives, named Gracilin A, H, K, J, L, and tetrahydroaplysulphurin-1, isolated from *Spongionella* sp., a marine sponge. The two parameters for the evaluation of antioxidant activity were MTT (3-(4,5-dimethylthiazol-2-yl)-2,5-diphenyltetrazolium bromide) assay and LDH levels: the first is correlated with mitochondrial function, the second is a cytoplasmic enzyme released in the culture medium following cell membrane damage. The tested compounds showed significant neuroprotective activity, interacting with targets such as mitochondrial oxidative phosphorylation and kinases involved in apoptosis [21].

Looking at innovative targets, a recent paper describes Macamides, a group of secondary metabolites isolated from the plant *Lepidium meyenii* (Maca). These compounds are benzylamides of fatty acids, active as analogues of the endocannabinoid anandamide (AEA) and studies have demonstrated that they inhibit fatty acid amide hydrolase (FAAH), blocking AEA hydrolysis. Gugnani et al. demonstrated a neuroprotective role of macamides in vitro and in vivo. Macamides reduced Mn-induced mitochondrial toxicity in glioblastoma U-87 MG cells, probably by binding the CB_1 receptor, and it could thus be useful in the treatment of neurodegenerative diseases, especially Alzheimer's Disease. Like AEA, macamides can interact with PPARγ, regulating inflammation, energetic metabolism and glucose homeostasis, all important factors for the prevention of AD [22,38].

Other interesting bioactive secondary metabolites are butenolides, from the fungus *Aspergillus terreus*. The chemical structures of these compounds were recently elucidated and their effects against the expression of TNFα in lipopolysaccharide (LPS)-activated BV2 microglia cells were tested. The most promising compound was asperteretal F, which inhibited the expression of TNFα in a dose-dependent mode, making it an anti-neuroinflammatory candidate for the treatment of NDs [23].

Sarcophytolide, instead, is a lacton cembrane diterpene derived from soft coral *Sarcophyton glaucum* that was recently shown to possess antimicrobic activity towards *Staphylococcus aureus*, *Pseudomonas aeruginosa*, and *Saccharomyces cerevisiae*. Moreover, pretreatment of primary cortical cells with sarcophytolide had a strong cytoprotective effect against glutamate-induced neurotoxicity and increased the expression of Bcl-2. This mechanism confirmed by evidence that sarcophytolide showed a cytoprotective activity only if added before and not after the exposure of neuronal cells to glutamate [24].

Meanwhile, Rupcic et al. discovered two new metabolites of the medicinal mushrooms *Hericius erinaceus* and *Hericius flagellum* (a rare species). They determined the chemical structures of these new compounds and of other metabolites previously isolated from the two species through Nuclear Magnetic Resonance (NMR) and High-Resolution Mass Spectroscopy (HRMS), identifying them as cyathane diterpenes. All these compounds were tested in vitro on PC12 cells for their neurotrophic activity, showing that, although none of them was endowed with intrinsic neurotrophic properties, all of them promoted the production of neurotrophins NGF (Nerve Growth Factor) and BDNF (Brain-Derived Neurotrophic Factor) in astrocytic cells [25].

2.1. Alzheimer's Disease

Alzheimer's disease (AD) is the most common neurodegenerative disorder, characterized by several cognitive and behavioral disfunctions, and it affects mainly old people, although rare early onset of this disease is also known [39,40]. Several hypotheses have been formulated regarding its pathogenesis, including deposition of amyloid β (Aβ), damaged cholinergic transmission, oxidative stress and hyperphosphorylated Tau aggregation [41,42].

According to the so-called "cholinergic hypothesis", AD is linked to decreased levels of acetylcholine (ACh) accompanied by a loss of cholinergic neurons in the central nervous system. In order to raise the concentration of this neurotransmitter, inhibitors of acetylcholine esterase (AChE), the main enzyme responsible for the degradation of ACh, have found use in clinical practice, improving functional autonomy and cognitive functions in AD patients [43]. Among these drugs are natural compounds such as galantamine, the most important *Amaryllidaceae* alkaloid [44]. For this reason, the potential use in AD of other *Amaryllidaceae* alkaloids, isolated from *Narcissus tazetta* L., was recently evaluated. Their structures were determined by NMR and mass spectroscopy, while in vitro AChE and butyrylcholinesterase (BChE) inhibitory activity was evaluated using Ellman's colorimetric method, with galantamine as reference. (+)-11-Hydroxygalanthine had the highest selective inhibitory activity on AChE, and narcissidine also inhibited AChE rather than BChE; while (−)-pancratinine-C was a selective BChE inhibitor. Docking studies confirmed bioactivity results [26].

The screening of libraries of natural compounds has also proven to be a promising strategy to identify multi-target compounds for the treatment of AD. Embelin, a 1,4-benzoquinone isolated from *Embelia ribes* fruits, recently emerged from one such screening, showing inhibitory activity towards AChE, BChE and beta-secretase 1 (BACE-1, involved in the deposition of Aβ). Another two natural products present in the library, L-tetrahydropalmatine and papaverine, exhibited a good inhibition of AChE. Moreover, embelin, in LS-180 cells, acted as an inductor of P-gp, an ATP-dependent efflux pump situated in the blood-brain barrier (BBB) whose decreased levels can lead to the accumulation of Aβ plaques [27].

Anti-AChE activity was exhibited also by four secondary metabolites (helminthosporin, emodin, chrysophanol, and physcion) of the African medicinal plant *Rumex Abyssinias*. These compounds, sharing an anthraquinone structure, were isolated and showed significant AChE inhibitory activity. Helminthosporin also displayed activity as a non-competitive BChE inhibitor, while the other compounds were only weakly active against this target. Moreover, the tricyclic flat structure makes helminthosporin lipophilic enough to cross the BBB, balancing its low LogP value [28].

Biologically active secondary metabolites such as phenols, alkaloids flavonoids, terpenes, sterols, and tannins from the ethanolic extract of *Oxalis corniculata* L. are endowed with carbonic anhydrase and cholinesterase inhibitory activity, with potential uses against epilepsy and Alzheimer's disease, respectively. Moreover, nine flavonoids were isolated from chloroform and ethyl acetate fractions, displaying ChEs and carbonic anhydrase II (CA-II) inhibitory activity [29].

Lichens have also been used as a source of natural compounds for the treatment of AD. During a recent study conducted on murine neuroblastoma Neuro2A cells, lichen-derived secondary metabolites (atranorin, perlatolic acid, physodic acid and usnic acid) displayed an important increase in neurite outgrowth, with perlatolic acid achieving better results than reference compound resveratrol. MTT assays revealed that only usnic acid showed cytotoxicity at neurotrophic doses. The molecular mediators of these effects are NGF, which is upregulated by atranorin, perlatolic acid and physodic acid, and BDNF, which is upregulated by atranorin and physodic acid. Only perlatolic acid had a potential inhibitory activity on AChE, at a concentration that was comparable with galantamine and lower than biroquinone, another lichen metabolite reported as AChE inhibitor [30].

Detailed knowledge of the structure of plant and fungal secondary metabolites has also proven useful directing screening activities. Due to their similarity to existing nuclei used in AChE inhibitors and metal chelators, fungal secondary metabolites tenuazonic acid (TA), *epi*-radicinol (ROH), mycophenolic acid (MA), radicinin (RAD), visoltricin/fungerin (FU) and plant metabolite 6-methoxymellein (6-MM) were screened for various activities such as inhibition of AChE, BChE and Aβ-aggregation, antioxidant effect and Cu and Zn interaction. A preliminary UV spectrophotometry test for metal chelation of Cu (II) and Zn (II) at physiological pH revealed that TA, MA and 6-MM probably interacted with Cu (II). TA and ROH exhibited a significant selective AChE inhibitory activity, while FU was the only compound that inhibited BChE. 2,2-diphenyl-1-picrylhydrazyl (DPPH) radical scavenging activity assay suggested that TA and MA behaved as antioxidants. Moreover, all molecules were inhibitors of $A\beta_{1-40}$ aggregation, as demonstrated by spectrofluorimetric assays, with ROH being the most active compound [31].

2.2. Parkinson's Disease

Parkinson's disease (PD) is a very common neurodegenerative disease characterized by motor symptoms, such as rigidity, bradykinesia and tremor, and non-motor symptoms, including sleep disorders and cognitive abnormalities [45]. The principal causes of this pathology are the depletion of dopamine in nerve terminals to the striatum and the progressive degeneration of dopaminergic neurons in the substantia nigra [46]. The therapy involves the use of levodopa associated with an inhibitor of the peripheral metabolism of levodopa, for example carbidopa. Additionally, other drugs can be administered, such as dopaminergic agonists, monoamine oxidase-B inhibitors and catechol *O*-methyltransferase inhibitors [47].

Monoamine oxidases (MAOs) are enzymes responsible for the oxidative deamination of both xenobiotic and endogenous neurotransmitters. Both MAO isoforms (MAO-A and MAO-B) are involved in the degradation of dopamine; however, MAO-B is the predominant isoform in the human brain. For this reason, MAO-B selective inhibitors, like selegiline and rasagiline, are used for the treatment of PD, raising striatal dopaminergic activity through the inhibition of dopamine metabolism [48–50].

In recent years, many natural inhibitors of MAO-B have been discovered and characterized, representing a powerful source of inspiration for further drug development [51].

MAO-A and MAO-B inhibitory activities of seven compounds isolated from the extract of *S.flavescens* were recently investigated, highlighting (−)-maackian as a potent inhibitor of MAO-B and as a candidate for the development of drugs for Parkinson's disease. The structurally related compound (−)-4-hydroxy-3-methoxy-8,9-methylenedioxypterocarpan was a non-selective inhibitor of both isoforms, as well as formononetin and genistein. Sophora-flavanone B weakly inhibited MAO-A, but not MAO-B, while kushenol F showed a good inhibitory activity on MAO-A and a weak one on MAO-B [32].

A dichloromethane extract of *Renealmia Alpinia*, was recently shown to possess a potent inhibitory activity towards both MAO-A and MAO-B. From this extract, desmethoxyangonin, a kavalactone, was isolated. It exhibited a potent, selective and competitive inhibition of MAO-B rather than MAO-A, confirmed by molecular modeling studies, leading to its selection as a candidate for further drug development. Other isolated molecules from the extract displayed moderate inhibition of both isoforms [33].

The aggregation of α-synuclein (αSN) in cytoplasmic inclusions called Lewy bodies is another important pathogenetic mechanism involved in PD. The formation of αSN fibrils leads to the disruption of synaptic homeostasis and neurodegeneration. While the exact mechanism is not clear, αSN is an interesting target for natural and synthetic drugs alike [52,53].

A natural compound extracted from *Ginkgo biloba* leaves, ginkgolic acid (GA), and its related molecule anacardic acid (AA) were screened for their influence on αSN aggregates. The treatment of KCl-depolarized SH-SY5Y neuroblastoma cells with GA and AA led to a progressive and relevant decrease in αSN-positive aggregates, probably also due to increased activation of macro-autophagy, that resulted in increased survival of the neural cells [34]. It should be noted that extracts from this plant, containing as low as 5 mg/kg GA, still showed potential to improve cognitive function in mild dementia patients after >24 weeks administration at a dosage of 240 mg/day [54]. Dihydromyricetin (DHM) is a flavonoid isolated from *Ampelopsis grossedentata*, a herb used in traditional Chinese medicine. Previous studies demonstrated that this compound played a neuroprotective role, and DHM, as proved by MTT assays on PC12 cells, blocked αSN fibrillo-genesis and its cytotoxicity. Moreover, DHM also disassembled preformed αSN fibrils, making it a potential molecule for the therapy of PD [35].

3. Metabolic Syndrome and Cardiovascular Risk

Metabolic syndrome (MS) is an increasingly prevalent condition that comprises a variety of pathological states, ranging from type 2 diabetes mellitus (T2DM) to obesity, hyperlipidemia and hypertension [55]. Obesity and hyperlipidemia are known causes of hyperinflammatory states, leading to the expression of pro-inflammatory cytokines and to reduced levels of nitric oxide (NO, which regulates endothelial homeostasis). Moreover, insulin-resistance leads to a blocking of the vasodilating effects of insulin itself, causing endothelial dysfunction. All these factors increase cardiovascular risk [56] and contribute significantly to the morbidity and mortality of cardiovascular diseases (CVD), the most prevalent cause of death worldwide.

Unfortunately, available drugs for the treatment of metabolic disorders are few and sometimes expensive: for this reason, researchers are focusing on the discovery of new and effective drugs [57,58]. In the last decade, it has become clear that an approach covering all underlying pathological conditions is required for the therapy of metabolic syndrome. Although the first step in such a therapeutic regime consists of increased physical exercise and dietary intervention, in many cases pharmacological action is necessary [59].

Over the years, the different aspects of metabolic syndrome have been thoroughly studied, and a number of potential molecular targets have been identified and characterized. Peroxisome Proliferator-Activated Receptors (PPARs), a family of nuclear receptors involved in all aspects of energetic metabolism, have attracted much interest as targets for therapy, considering their important role in the recent past in the treatment of both dyslipidemic and glucose-related pathologies [60,61]. Three PPAR receptor subtypes have been identified to date, respectively PPARα, PPARγ and PPARδ, each of which binds different endogenous ligands and is selectively expressed in different organs and tissues [62–64]. Their differential expression and ligand specificity mirror their different physiological roles: PPARα and PPARδ are mostly responsible for catabolic functions such as lipid oxygenation and glucose consumption, while PPARγ regulates glucose uptake and anabolic functions, particularly lipid storage and adipose tissue formation [65].

An enhanced understanding of the pharmacological profile of PPAR agonists has led to increased interest in their development, focusing particularly on obtaining a selective modulation of their subtypes, in order to maximize their beneficial effects and to minimize adverse reactions [66–69]. This focus on PPAR agonists is, however, not exclusive to medicinal chemists, and PPAR agonism or related activities have been reported for various secondary metabolites derived from plant and fungal extracts.

Table 2 summarizes the body of literature regarding plant and fungal SMs with potential activity toward MS and CVD.

Table 2. Natural compounds with potential use in the therapy of metabolic syndrome and/or with additional effects for the reduction of cardiovascular risk.

Source	Bioactive Compounds	Effects	Main Activities	Ref.
Acalypha fluticosa	2-methyl-5,7-dihydroxychromone 5-*O*-b-D-glucopyranosid, acalyphin, apigenin, and Kaempferol 3-*O*-rutinoside and an acetylated derivate of chromone glucoside	Agonism of PPARα and PPARγ; anti-inflammatory properties	(PPARα act., FI) 1.16–2.25 at 50 µM	[70]
Talisia nervosa Radlk	(−)-catechin, methyl gallate, ethyl gallate, and β-D-glucopyranose,1,4,6-tris(3,4,5-trihydroxybenzoate)	Agonism of PPARα, PPARγ and liver X receptor (LXR); reduction of NO production	(PPARγ act., FI) 1.85–3.02 at 50 µM	[71]
Penicillium chrysogenum J08NF-4	A new bile acid trifluoroacetate	Agonism of PPARγ, anti-inflammatory properties	(PPARγ act., FI) 2.0 at 50 µM	[72]
Cyanobium sp. LEGE 07,175 and *Nodosilinea* sp. LEGE 06001	13^2-hydroxy-pheopytin a and 13^2-hydroxy-pheofarnesin a	Increase of PPARγ mRNA expression	(Lipid-reducing Activity, EC_{50}) 8.9–15.5 µM	[73]
Penicillium expansum Y32	Communesin A, B, I, fumiquinazoline Q, protuboxepin A, B, E, and others	Mitigation of bradycardia, vasculo-genetic effect	(Acid sphingomyelinase mitigation) 20–100 µM	[58]
Lichens	Thirty-seven secondary metabolites and semisynthetic derivates	Anti-AGE activity, vasodilation	(Pentosidine-like AGEs formation, IC_{50}) 0.08–0.70 mM	[74]
Schisandra chinensis	Acidic polysaccharide (SCAP)	Anti-diabetic and anti-apoptotic role	(H_2O_2-induced apoptosis inh) 15.6–62.5 µM	[75]
Sesbania grandiflora	Quercetin, kaempferol, vomifoliol, loliolide and others	Inhibition of α-amylase and α-glucosidase; antioxidant activity	(α-Glucosidase inh, IC_{50}) 17.45–388.48 µM	[76]
Cassia bakeriana craib	Kaempeferol-3-*O*-rhamnoside and kaempferol	Inhibition of α-amylase and antioxidant activity	(α-Glucosidase inh, IC_{50}) 0.36–0.61 mg/mL	[77]
Ocimum campechianum Mill.	Methyl rosmarinate, rosmarinic acid, 5-demethyl nobiletin, 5-demethyl sinensetin, luteolin	Inhibition of α-glucosidase, antihyperglycemic action	(α-Glucosidase inh) 12.86–82.77% at 0.75 mM	[78]
Aspergillus terreus MC751	Butyrolactone I and II, three acetylated derivates of butyrolactone I	Inhibition of α-glucosidase, antioxidant activity	(α-Glucosidase inh, IC_{50}) 52.17–175.18 µM	[79]
Ganoderma australe	Stella-steroid	Inhibition of α-glucosidase and Dipeptidyl peptidase 4 (DPP-4)	(α-Glucosidase inh, IC_{50}) 314.54 µM	[80]

Table 2. Cont.

Source	Bioactive Compounds	Effects	Main Activities	Ref.
Aspergillus sydowii	Asperentin B	Inhibition of Protein-tyrosine phosphatase 1B (PTP1B)	(PTP1B inh, IC$_{50}$) 2.05 µM	[81]
Moringa oleifera	Two sulfur-contained compounds	Anti-adipogenic activity	(Lipid accumulation, inh, IC$_{50}$) 29.6 µM	[82]
Allium sativum L.	Three eugenol diglycosides and three β-carboline alkaloids	Inhibition of adipogenesis and lipid accumulation	(Lipid accumulation, inh) active at 20 µM	[83]
Curcuma amada	Two natural labdane diterpenes and one drimane sesquiterpene	Inhibition of lipase and α-glucosidase	(Lipase inh, IC$_{50}$) 6.1–665.9 µM	[84]
Magnolia spp.	Honokiol	Inhibition of Histone deacetylase (HDAC)-mediated cystathionine γ-lyase degradation	(HDAC6 inh) active at 5 µM	[85]
Panax spp. (Ginseng)	Ginsenoside K	Promotion of macrophage and foam cell apoptosis	(Reduction of foam cell formation) 1.25 µg/mL	[86]
Unspecified	Lupeol	Promotion of macrophage development into the M2 anti-inflammatory phenotype	(Proinflammatory cytokine secretion, inh) active at 50 µM	[87]
Tripterygium Wilfordi	Cerastrol	Action as leptin sensitizer	(Leptin sensitization) active at 150 µg/kg	[88]

Acalypha fluticosa extracts were recently screened for PPAR agonism and anti-inflammatory properties. Following a preliminary screening, four compounds were isolated from the methanol extract, namely 2-methyl-5,7-dihydroxychromone-5-O-b-D-glucopyranosid, acalyphin, apigenin, and kaempferol-3-O-rutinoside. Moreover, an acetylated derivate of chromone glucoside was synthesized and tested. In vitro on human hepatoma (HepG2) cells, acalyphin exhibited a specific PPARγ agonist activity, while apigenin revealed a weak PPARα agonism. Chromone glucoside displayed activity as a dual PPARα/γ agonist, while its acetylated derivative showed increased activity towards PPARα. These molecules, in particular acalyphin, also had anti-inflammatory properties, probably due to the inhibition of NF-κB and/or iNOS. Importantly, tested extracts and compounds were not found to be cytotoxic in vitro against human cells [70].

The ethanolic extract of stems of the Panamanian plant *Talisia nervosa* was also studied, along with its isolated components, for potential use in metabolic disorders. The extract displayed dual PPARα/γ agonism and also increased liver X receptor (LXR) activation. Therefore, four secondary metabolites, namely (−)-catechin, methyl gallate, ethyl gallate, and β-D-glucopyranose-1,4,6-tris(3,4,5-trihydroxybenzoate) were isolated and characterized. In vitro assays on HepG2 revealed that while (−)-catechin activated only PPARγ and not PPARα, the other three compounds activated PPARα, PPARγ and LXR, with methyl gallate being more potent than ethyl gallate on all three targets. The two gallates also reduced nitric oxide (NO) production in mouse macrophages (RAW 264.7) cells [71].

Aside from five known bile acids, a new bile acid trifluoroacetate was isolated from jellyfish-derived fungus *Penicillium chrysogenum* J08NF-4. Its chemical structure and mechanism of action were similar to those of synthetic steroid mifepristone, which is clinically used for the treatment of hypercholesterolemia and recently turned out to be a PPARγ agonist. Docking studies confirmed that this new bile acid, like mifepristone, is capable of binding the ligand binding domain (LBD) of PPARγ, thus suppressing the NF-kB pathway and downregulating the pro-inflammatory mediators iNOS, TNF-α, and NO, with generalized anti-inflammatory effects, as confirmed by in vitro assay on LPS-induced RAW 264.7 macrophages [72].

Other than plants and fungi, marine cyanobacteria have been a promising source of secondary metabolites with potential medicinal use. As an example, chlorophyll derivatives 13^2-hydroxy-pheopytin-a and the novel 13^2-hydroxy-pheofarnesin-a were recently isolated from *Cyanobium* sp. LEGE 07,175 -and *Nodosilinea* sp. LEGE 06001, respectively. The zebrafish Nile red fat metabolism assay confirmed a neutral lipid-reducing activity of both compounds after 48 h of exposure, with no toxic effects. In order to explain the biological mechanism behind this activity profile, 13^2-hydroxy-pheopytin-a was found to increase PPARγ mRNA expression. In light of these data, the presence of this compound in several foods, such as spinach, cabbage, *Spirulina* and *Chlorella*, makes it an important nutraceutical agent [73].

3.1. Diabetes

Type 2 diabetes (T2DM, or non-insulin dependent diabetes mellitus) is the most common form of diabetes. It is characterized by peripheral insulin resistance and hyperglycemia, leading to a loss of pancreatic β-cells which further exacerbates the pathology. No cure is currently available for this disease, however, various drugs capable of ameliorating the patients' quality of life and useful to control the disease have been approved [89]. Studies confirmed that natural products can also be used for the prevention and/or treatment of type 2 diabetes [90].

The therapy of T2DM usually focuses on reducing postprandial glycemia, restoring peripheral insulin sensitivity and improving β-cell survival. Other than the previously discussed PPARγ, molecular targets for the therapy of T2DM include intestinal α-glucosidase and pancreatic α-amylase [91], which catalyze the hydrolysis of dietary carbohydrates and whose inhibition leads to decrease of postprandial blood glucose levels, thanks to a decreased digestion and uptake of carbohydrates [86]. Dipeptidyl peptidase-4 (DPP-4) is another target for the treatment of this pathology: this enzyme metabolizes glucagon-like peptide-1 (GLP-1), an incretin hormone which stimulates insulin secretion, inhibits glucagon secretion and delays gastric emptying [92]. Moreover, recent studies have proven the role of enzyme protein tyrosine phosphatase 1B (PTP1B) in the negative regulation of insulin signaling, making it a novel target for the treatment of T2DM [93].

An acidic polysaccharide from *Schisandra chinensis* (SCAP) was recently evaluated as a potential therapeutic agent in the streptozotocin-induced mouse model of diabetes. SCAP led to increased levels of fasting blood insulin and superoxide dismutase and to decreased levels of fasting blood glucose and malondialdehyde. This polysaccharide also prevented apoptosis of pancreatic β-cells through the up-regulation of factors such as BAX and Bcl-2, suggesting a possible mechanism for its antidiabetic activity. [75].

In another recent study, fourteen known compounds were isolated from *S. grandiflora* crude extract and tested against α-amylase and α-glucosidase in vitro. Two flavonoids (quercetin and kaempferol) and two terpenoids (vomifoliol and loliolide) showed inhibitory activity toward these enzymes, which was justified through docking studies. Finally, all bioactive molecules acted as antioxidants in the ABTS (2,2′-azino-bis(3-ethylbenzothiazoline-6-sulfonic acid) radical scavenging assay. Quantitative analysis highlighted high concentrations of the most active compounds in the plant extract, suggesting a potential use of the edible *S. grandiflora* for the control of postprandial blood glucose in diabetic patients [76].

Similarly, flavonoids kaempferol-3-O-rhamnoside and kaempferol, isolated from *Cassia bakeriana* (pink cassia) extracts, were also recently studied for their antidiabetic activities. While kaempferol was unambiguously able to inhibit α-amylase, the evaluation of the antioxidant activities of these compounds led to somewhat contrasting results, with both being active when tested via oxygen radical absorbance capacity (ORAC) method, and only kaempferol-3-O-rhamnoside being active in DPPH assay. It is worth noting that the isolated compounds are less active than the whole extract, suggesting the importance of synergic effects between the various components of the extract [77].

The leaf infusion of *Ocimum campechianum* (or wild basil) was reported to play an antidiabetic role through α-glucosidase inhibition. Five poly-methoxylated flavones were isolated and their structures were elucidated, with two of these compounds (methyl rosmarinate and rosmarinic acid) displaying strong inhibition of α-glucosidase in vitro and a marked decrease of blood glucose in vivo [78].

Natural compound stella-steroid was instead isolated from fungal plant pathogen *Ganoderma australe*, and its structure was elucidated via NMR spectroscopy. This compound showed inhibitory activity towards DPP-4 and α-glucosidase in silico and in vitro, with higher activity toward the latter target [80].

Two natural compounds from *Aspergillus terreus*, known as butyrolactone I and II, along with three synthetic acetylated derivatives of butyrolactone I, were also screened in a different study for their activity as α-glucosidase inhibitors and as antioxidants. Butyrolactone I showed both α-glucosidase inhibitory and antioxidant activities, while butyrolactone II was the most potent antioxidant compound, but had a lower inhibitory activity toward α-glucosidase. Synthetic derivatives were less active, probably because of the acetylation of the hydroxyl groups of butyrolactone I [79].

Another fungus from the *Aspergillus* genus, *Aspergillus sydowii*, was found to produce a compound with significant antidiabetic potential, asperentin B. In vitro, this compound inhibited PTP1B six times more strongly than the positive control suramin. Interestingly, the structurally related compound asperentin did not display any inhibitory activity towards PTP1B. Future studies on structure-activity relationships and chemical modifications will be necessary to explain and enhance the antidiabetic activity of asperentin B [81].

3.2. Obesity

Obesity and overweight, defined as excess body weight, affect a growing number of adults, children and adolescents. Obesity in particular is often associated with the development of other disorders such as T2DM, cardiovascular disease and nonalcoholic fatty liver disease. Behavioral interventions, including dietary changes and increased physical exercise, are important to prevent obesity and to induce weight loss, however pharmacological treatment is often necessary in obese patients [94–96].

A viable strategy for the treatment of metabolic disorders like obesity is decreasing the absorption of dietary components such as fats and carbohydrates through the inhibition of metabolic enzymes, including lipase and, again, α-glucosidase [97]. On the other hand, it is also necessary to act on signaling pathways that might be dysregulated as a result of obesity. Leptin is a protein involved in one such pathway; it is expressed in the adipocytes and it controls body weight and the mass of adipose tissue through the inhibition of food intake and the stimulation of energy expenditure. Defects in leptin production cause severe obesity [98].

A growing body of literature demonstrates the potential anti-obesity action of natural bioactive compounds, mostly derived from plants [99]. As an example, extracts from seeds and leaves *Moringa oleifera* were recently tested for various properties such as antioxidant, anti-inflammatory and anti-hyperlipidemic effects. Two sulfur-containing compounds were isolated from these extracts and were evaluated for their anti-adipogenic activity on pre-adipocyte 3T3-L1 cell line. One compound had no significant anti-adipogenic activity, while the other one showed a significant inhibition of intracellular lipid accumulation, probably due to the presence of an isothiocyanate group (ITC) in its structure. For this reason, a series of ITC derivatives were prepared, and most of them also showed anti-adipogenic activity [82]. Similarly, three eugenol diglycosides and three β-carboline alkaloids isolated from Garlic (*Allium sativum* L.) were screened on 3T3-L1 cells for their effects on adipogenesis and lipid metabolism. Among them, one β-carboline alkaloid inhibited adipogenesis and lipid accumulation through the regulation of adipogenic, lipogenic and lipolytic genes [83].

In another recent study, two natural labdane diterpenes and a drimane sesquiterpene were isolated from the hexane extract of *Curcuma amada* and they were tested for their inhibitory activity against rat intestinal α-glucosidase and porcine pancreatic lipase. One of the two diterpenes showed relevant inhibitory activity toward both enzymes. Therefore, some semi-synthetic derivatives of this molecule were prepared and screened: a reduced derivative maintained α-glucosidase inhibitory activity, while it lost lipase inhibition. At the opposite end of the spectrum, oxidized and acetate derivatives acted as good lipase inhibitors but had a weak α-glucosidase inhibitory activity [84].

Another terpene, specifically a pentacyclic triterpene from the roots of *Tripterygium Wilfordi*, was recently discovered to be a leptin sensitizer. In hyperleptinemic diet-induced obese (DIO) mice it led to effects such as a significant decrease of food intake, increased hypothalamic leptin sensitivity, and weight loss, a promising profile for the treatment of obesity [88].

3.3. Hypertension and Hyperinflammation-Managing Cardiovascular Risk in Metabolic Syndrome

Hypertension and hyperinflammation are another important component of MS which, along with hypercholesterolemia, cause atherosclerosis and therefore significantly raise the cardiovascular risk linked to this syndrome [55].

In this case, too, secondary metabolites of plants and fungi have shown promise as preventative or therapeutic agents. As an example, honokiol, a natural compound from magnolia plants, was very recently shown to ameliorate Angiotensin II-induced hypertension and endothelial dysfunction via inhibition of histone deacetylase 6 (HDAC6) [85].

A very promising way to prevent cardiovascular risk related to hyperinflammation and atherosclerosis is to target the macrophages that accumulate in the site of the atherogenic lesion and bind low density lipoprotein (LDL), transforming in foam cells and driving inflammation further [100]. An aqueous bark extract from the plant *Terminalia Arjuna*, containing a number of polyphenols including gallic acid, epigallocatechin gallate and ellagic acid, displayed significant activity in stimulating apoptosis in macrophages and foam cells during the early stages of atherogenesis, thereby driving back inflammation and potentially reducing cardiovascular risk [101]. Similar effects were shown by ginseng-derived compound ginsenoside K [86], while lupeol, a pentacyclic terpene which can be found in a variety of fruits and vegetables, including mango, red grapes and tomato, was shown to be capable of shunting macrophage development towards the anti-inflammatory, reparative M2 phenotype (as opposed to the pro-inflammatory M1 phenotype) [87].

The formation of advanced-end glycation products (AGEs) is involved in several pathologies such as atherosclerosis, arterial stiffness, but also Parkinson's disease and Alzheimer's disease. In a recent study, a group of lichen secondary metabolites and one semisynthetic derivative were shown to possess relevant inhibitory activity towards AGE formation. Although some of these compounds were endowed with antioxidant activity, it was not necessarily linked to the inhibition of AGE formation. Moreover, the tested compounds proved to have vasodilative effects, potentially useful in alleviating hypertension linked to atherosclerosis [74].

Finally, three new alkaloids (communesin I, fumoquinazoline Q and protuboxepin E) and nine known alkaloids (communesin A and B, cottoquinazoline A, prelapatin B, glyantrypine, protuboxepin A and B, chaetoglobosin C and penochalasin E) were recently isolated from the marine-derived fungus *Penicillium expansum* Y32. All molecules were screened in vivo on a zebrafish model for their cardiovascular effects. All of them exhibited a mitigative activity on bradycardia induced by astemizole; moreover, all compounds, except for communesin B, showed vasculo-genetic effects [58].

4. Conclusions

The research reviewed in this paper confirms the rising importance of natural compounds in the inspiration of new therapeutic protocols for the prevention and/or treatment of chronic diseases.

However, the use of secondary metabolites requires in many cases a specific formulation, when we consider that they are often insoluble in water, and the problems related to the abuse of supplements containing bioactive molecules, while outside the scope of this review, must still be carefully considered, taking into account the side effects of the active ingredients themselves and the possibility of external contamination [102]. The already mentioned case of Monacolin K, a blockbuster product which presents the same problems as statins (being a statin itself) and a high possibility of contamination with citrinin (fermented red rice with *Monascus Purpureus* strains is the only regulated matrix in EU for this mycotoxin [103]), must be a wake-up call to the food supplement industry. Therefore, future research must definitely focus on the analysis of natural contaminants such as ochratoxin A [104] and other mycotoxins, as well as residues of pesticides and heavy metals, if these bioactive compounds are to be included in plant food supplements [105].

The design of new potential drugs starting from the structures of natural compounds and the preparation of these molecules with a semi-synthetic or a total-synthetic approach will be another significant challenge in future years. Several research groups are working on this fascinating, though not always linear, route [72,82,106], and important results are expected.

Author Contributions: L.P. performed the bibliographic research and wrote the manuscript along with L.B., V.P. and R.L. L.B., A.L., F.L., P.T. and L.P. provided helpful discussions and revised the manuscript. All authors have read and agreed to the published version of the manuscript.

Funding: This research received no external funding.

Acknowledgments: The authors would like to thank Nicoletta Gadaleta for providing the picture in the graphical abstract.

Conflicts of Interest: The authors declare no conflict of interest.

References

1. Salem, M.A.; De Souza, L.P.; Serag, A.; Fernie, A.R.; Farag, M.A.; Ezzat, S.M.; Alseekh, S. Metabolomics in the context of plant natural products research: From sample preparation to metabolite analysis. *Metabolites* **2020**, *10*, 37. [CrossRef] [PubMed]
2. Wink, M. Modes of Action of Herbal Medicines and Plant Secondary Metabolites. *Medicines* **2015**, *2*, 251–286. [CrossRef] [PubMed]
3. Seca, A.; Pinto, D. Plant Secondary Metabolites as Anticancer Agents: Successes in Clinical Trials and Therapeutic Application. *Int. J. Mol. Sci.* **2018**, *19*, 263. [CrossRef] [PubMed]
4. Saloustros, E.; Mavroudis, D.; Georgoulias, V. Paclitaxel and docetaxel in the treatment of breast cancer. *Expert Opin. Pharmacother.* **2008**, *9*, 2603–2616. [CrossRef]
5. Kumar, A. Vincristine and vinblastine: A review. *Int. J. Med. Pharm. Sci.* **2016**, *6*, 23–30.
6. Vacca, R.A.; Valenti, D.; Caccamese, S.; Daglia, M.; Braidy, N.; Nabavi, S.M. Plant polyphenols as natural drugs for the management of Down syndrome and related disorders. *Neurosci. Biobehav. Rev.* **2016**, *71*, 865–877. [CrossRef]
7. Shahidi, F.; Yeo, J.D. Bioactivities of phenolics by focusing on suppression of chronic diseases: A review. *Int. J. Mol. Sci.* **2018**, *19*, 1573. [CrossRef]
8. Huang, X.-T.; Li, X.; Xie, M.-L.; Huang, Z.; Huang, Y.-X.; Wu, G.-X.; Peng, Z.-R.; Sun, Y.-N.; Ming, Q.-L.; Liu, Y.-X.; et al. Resveratrol: Review on its discovery, anti-leukemia effects and pharmacokinetics. *Chem. Biol. Interactions* **2019**, *306*, 29–38. [CrossRef]
9. Gonçalves, J.; Rosado, T.; Soares, S.; Simão, A.; Caramelo, D.; Luís, Â.; Fernández, N.; Barroso, M.; Gallardo, E.; Duarte, A. Cannabis and Its Secondary Metabolites: Their Use as Therapeutic Drugs, Toxicological Aspects, and Analytical Determination. *Medicines* **2019**, *6*, 31. [CrossRef]
10. Bonini, S.A.; Premoli, M.; Tambaro, S.; Kumar, A.; Maccarinelli, G.; Memo, M.; Mastinu, A. Cannabis sativa: A comprehensive ethnopharmacological review of a medicinal plant with a long history. *J. Ethnopharmacol.* **2018**, *227*, 300–315. [CrossRef]
11. Misiek, M.; Hoffmeister, D. Fungal genetics, genomics, and secondary metabolites in pharmaceutical sciences. *Planta Med.* **2007**, *73*, 103–115. [CrossRef] [PubMed]
12. Tahlan, K.; Jensen, S.E. Origins of the β-lactam rings in natural products. *J. Antibiot.* **2013**, *66*, 401–410. [CrossRef] [PubMed]
13. Ho, V.C. The use of ciclosporin in psoriasis: A clinical review. *Br. J. Dermatol. Suppl.* **2004**, *150*, 1–10. [CrossRef] [PubMed]

14. Leuci, R.; Brunetti, L.; Laghezza, A.; Tortorella, P.; Loiodice, F.; Piemontese, L. A Review of Recent Patents (2016-2019) on Plant Food Supplements with Potential Application in the Treatment of Neurodegenerative and Metabolic Disorders. *Recent Pat. Food. Nutr. Agric.* **2020**, *11*, 145–153. [CrossRef]
15. Journoud, M.; Jones, P.J.H. Red yeast rice: A new hypolipidemic drug. *Life Sci.* **2004**, *74*, 2675–2683. [CrossRef]
16. Brunetti, L.; Laghezza, A.; Loiodice, F.; Tortorella, P.; Piemontese, L. Combining fatty acid amide hydrolase (FAAH) inhibition with peroxisome proliferator-activated receptor (PPAR) activation: A new potential multi-target therapeutic strategy for the treatment of Alzheimer's disease. *Neural Regen. Res.* **2020**, *15*, 67–68. [CrossRef]
17. Fancellu, G.; Chand, K.; Tomás, D.; Orlandini, E.; Piemontese, L.; Silva, D.F.; Cardoso, S.M.; Chaves, S.; Santos, M.A. Novel tacrine–benzofuran hybrids as potential multi-target drug candidates for the treatment of Alzheimer's Disease. *J. Enzym. Inhib. Med. Chem.* **2020**, *35*, 211–226. [CrossRef]
18. Piemontese, L.; Loiodice, F.; Chaves, S.; Santos, M.A. The Therapy of Alzheimer's Disease: Towards a New Generation of Drugs. *Front. Clin. Drug Res. Alzheimer Disord.* **2019**, *8*, 33–80. [CrossRef]
19. Popa-Wagner, A.; Dumitrascu, D.; Capitanescu, B.; Petcu, E.; Surugiu, R.; Fang, W.-H.; Dumbrava, D.-A. Dietary habits, lifestyle factors and neurodegenerative diseases. *Neural Regen. Res.* **2020**, *15*, 394–400. [CrossRef]
20. Fernández-Moriano, C.; Divakar, P.K.; Crespo, A.; Gómez-Serranillos, M.P. In vitro neuroprotective potential of lichen metabolite fumarprotocetraric acid via intracellular redox modulation. *Toxicol. Appl. Pharmacol.* **2017**, *316*, 83–94. [CrossRef]
21. Leirós, M.; Sánchez, J.A.; Alonso, E.; Rateb, M.E.; Houssen, W.E.; Ebel, R.; Jaspars, M.; Alfonso, A.; Botana, L.M. Spongionella secondary metabolites protect mitochondrial function in cortical neurons against oxidative stress. *Mar. Drugs* **2014**, *12*, 700–718. [CrossRef] [PubMed]
22. Gugnani, K.S.; Vu, N.; Rondón-Ortiz, A.N.; Böhlke, M.; Maher, T.J.; Pino-Figueroa, A.J. Neuroprotective activity of macamides on manganese-induced mitochondrial disruption in U-87 MG glioblastoma cells. *Toxicol. Appl. Pharmacol.* **2018**, *340*, 67–76. [CrossRef] [PubMed]
23. Yang, L.H.; Ou-Yang, H.; Yan, X.; Tang, B.W.; Fang, M.J.; Wu, Z.; Chen, J.W.; Qiu, Y.K. Open-ring butenolides from a marine-derived anti-neuroinflammatory fungus aspergillus terreus Y10. *Mar. Drugs* **2018**, *16*, 428. [CrossRef] [PubMed]
24. Badria, F.A.; Guirguis, A.N.; Perovic, S.; Steffen, R.; Müller, W.E.G.; Schröder, H.C. Sarcophytolide: A new neuroprotective compound from the soft coral Sarcophyton glaucum. *Toxicology* **1998**, *131*, 133–143. [CrossRef]
25. Rupcic, Z.; Rascher, M.; Kanaki, S.; Köster, R.W.; Stadler, M.; Wittstein, K. Two new cyathane diterpenoids from mycelial cultures of the medicinal mushroom hericium erinaceus and the rare species, hericium flagellum. *Int. J. Mol. Sci.* **2018**, *19*, 740. [CrossRef] [PubMed]
26. Karakoyun, Ç.; Bozkurt, B.; Çoban, G.; Masi, M.; Cimmino, A.; Evidente, A.; Somer, N.U. A comprehensive study on narcissus tazetta subsp. tazetta L.: Chemo-profiling, isolation, anticholinesterase activity and molecular docking of amaryllidaceae alkaloids. *S. Afr. J. Bot.* **2020**, *130*, 148–154. [CrossRef]
27. Nuthakki, V.K.; Sharma, A.; Kumar, A.; Bharate, S.B. Identification of embelin, a 3-undecyl-1,4-benzoquinone from Embelia ribes as a multitargeted anti-Alzheimer agent. *Drug Dev. Res.* **2019**, *80*, ddr.21544. [CrossRef]
28. Augustin, N.; Nuthakki, V.K.; Abdullaha, M.; Hassan, Q.P.; Gandhi, S.G.; Bharate, S.B. Discovery of Helminthosporin, an Anthraquinone Isolated from Rumex abyssinicus Jacq as a Dual Cholinesterase Inhibitor. *ACS Omega* **2020**, *5*, 1616–1624. [CrossRef]
29. Imran, M.; Irfan, A.; Ibrahim, M.; Assiri, M.A.; Khalid, N.; Ullah, S.; Al-Sehemi, A.G. Carbonic anhydrase and cholinesterase inhibitory activities of isolated flavonoids from Oxalis corniculata L. and their first-principles investigations. *Ind. Crops Prod.* **2020**, *148*, 112285. [CrossRef]
30. Reddy, R.G.; Veeraval, L.; Maitra, S.; Chollet-Krugler, M.; Tomasi, S.; Dévéhat, F.L.L.; Boustie, J.; Chakravarty, S. Lichen-derived compounds show potential for central nervous system therapeutics. *Phytomedicine* **2016**, *23*, 1527–1534. [CrossRef]
31. Piemontese, L.; Vitucci, G.; Catto, M.; Laghezza, A.; Perna, F.M.; Rullo, M.; Loiodice, F.; Capriati, V.; Solfrizzo, M. Natural scaffolds with multi-target activity for the potential treatment of Alzheimer's disease. *Molecules* **2018**, *23*, 2182. [CrossRef] [PubMed]
32. Lee, H.W.; Ryu, H.W.; Kang, M.G.; Park, D.; Oh, S.R.; Kim, H. Potent selective monoamine oxidase B inhibition by maackiain, a pterocarpan from the roots of Sophora flavescens. *Bioorganic Med. Chem. Lett.* **2016**, *26*, 4714–4719. [CrossRef] [PubMed]
33. Chaurasiya, N.D.; León, F.; Ding, Y.; Gómez-Betancur, I.; Benjumea, D.; Walker, L.A.; Cutler, S.J.; Tekwani, B.L. Interactions of Desmethoxyyangonin, a Secondary Metabolite from Renealmia alpinia, with Human Monoamine Oxidase-A and Oxidase-B. *Evid. Based Complement. Altern. Med.* **2017**, *2017*, 4018724. [CrossRef] [PubMed]
34. Vijayakumaran, S.; Nakamura, Y.; Henley, J.M.; Pountney, D.L. Ginkgolic acid promotes autophagy-dependent clearance of intracellular alpha-synuclein aggregates. *Mol. Cell. Neurosci.* **2019**, *101*, 103416. [CrossRef]
35. Jia, L.; Wang, Y.; Sang, J.; Cui, W.; Zhao, W.; Wei, W.; Chen, B.; Lu, F.; Liu, F. Dihydromyricetin Inhibits α-Synuclein Aggregation, Disrupts Preformed Fibrils, and Protects Neuronal Cells in Culture against Amyloid-Induced Cytotoxicity. *J. Agric. Food Chem.* **2019**, *67*, 3946–3955. [CrossRef] [PubMed]
36. Hsieh, H.L.; Yang, C.M. Role of redox signaling in neuroinflammation and neurodegenerative diseases. *Biomed Res. Int.* **2013**, *2013*, 484613. [CrossRef] [PubMed]
37. Albarracin, S.L.; Stab, B.; Casas, Z.; Sutachan, J.J.; Samudio, I.; Gonzalez, J.; Gonzalo, L.; Capani, F.; Morales, L.; Barreto, G.E. Effects of natural antioxidants in neurodegenerative disease. *Nutr. Neurosci.* **2012**, *15*, 1–9. [CrossRef] [PubMed]

38. Basavarajappa, B.S.; Shivakumar, M.; Joshi, V.; Subbanna, S. Endocannabinoid system in neurodegenerative disorders. *J. Neurochem.* **2017**, *142*, 624–648. [CrossRef]
39. González, J.F.; Alcántara, A.R.; Doadrio, A.L.; Sánchez-Montero, J.M. Developments with multi-target drugs for Alzheimer's disease: An overview of the current discovery approaches. *Expert Opin. Drug Discov.* **2019**, *14*, 879–891. [CrossRef]
40. Mendez, M.F. Early-onset Alzheimer disease and its variants. *Continuum* **2019**, *25*, 34–51. [CrossRef]
41. Du, X.; Wang, X.; Geng, M. Alzheimer's disease hypothesis and related therapies. *Transl. Neurodegener.* **2018**, *7*, 2. [CrossRef] [PubMed]
42. Baig, M.H.; Ahmad, K.; Rabbani, G.; Choi, I. Use of Peptides for the Management of Alzheimer's Disease: Diagnosis and Inhibition. *Front. Aging Neurosci.* **2018**, *10*, 21. [CrossRef] [PubMed]
43. Martorana, A.; Esposito, Z.; Koch, G. Beyond the Cholinergic Hypothesis: Do Current Drugs Work in Alzheimer's Disease? *CNS Neurosci. Ther.* **2010**, *16*, 235–245. [CrossRef] [PubMed]
44. Harvey, A.L. The pharmacology of galanthamine and its analogues. *Pharmacol. Ther.* **1995**, *68*, 113–128. [CrossRef]
45. Jankovic, J. Parkinson's disease: Clinical features and diagnosis. *J. Neurol. Neurosurg. Psychiatry* **2008**, *79*, 368–376. [CrossRef]
46. Park, J.S.; Leem, Y.H.; Park, J.E.; Kim, D.Y.; Kim, H.S. Neuroprotective effect of β-lapachone in MPTP-induced parkinson's disease mouse model: Involvement of astroglial p-AMPK/Nrf2/HO-1 signaling pathways. *Biomol. Ther.* **2019**, *27*, 178–184. [CrossRef]
47. Gazewood, J.D.; Richards, D.R.; Clebak, K. Parkinson Disease: An Update. *Am. Fam. Physician* **2013**, *87*, 267–273.
48. Kumar, B.; Sheetal, S.; Mantha, A.K.; Kumar, V. Recent developments on the structure-activity relationship studies of MAO inhibitors and their role in different neurological disorders. *RSC Adv.* **2016**, *6*, 42660–42683. [CrossRef]
49. Fernandez, H.H.; Chen, J.J. Monoamine oxidase-B inhibition in the treatment of Parkinson's disease. *Pharmacotherapy* **2007**, *27*, 174S–185S. [CrossRef]
50. Finberg, J.P.M. Update on the pharmacology of selective inhibitors of MAO-A and MAO-B: Focus on modulation of CNS monoamine neurotransmitter release. *Pharmacol. Ther.* **2014**, *143*, 133–152. [CrossRef]
51. Carradori, S.; Gidaro, M.C.; Petzer, A.; Costa, G.; Guglielmi, P.; Chimenti, P.; Alcaro, S.; Petzer, J.P. Inhibition of Human Monoamine Oxidase: Biological and Molecular Modeling Studies on Selected Natural Flavonoids. *J. Agric. Food Chem.* **2016**, *64*, 9004–9011. [CrossRef] [PubMed]
52. Stefanis, L. α-Synuclein in Parkinson's disease. *Cold Spring Harb. Perspect. Med.* **2012**, *2*, a009399. [CrossRef] [PubMed]
53. Recchia, A.; Debetto, P.; Negro, A.; Guidolin, D.; Skaper, S.D.; Giusti, P. α-Synuclein and Parkinson's disease. *FASEB J.* **2004**, *18*, 617–626. [CrossRef]
54. Liu, H.; Ye, M.; Guo, H. An Updated Review of Randomized Clinical Trials Testing the Improvement of Cognitive Function of Ginkgo biloba Extract in Healthy People and Alzheimer's Patients. *Front Pharmacol.* **2019**, *10*, 1688. [CrossRef] [PubMed]
55. Eckel, R.H.; Grundy, S.M.; Zimmet, P.Z. The metabolic syndrome. *Lancet* **2005**, *365*, 1415–1428. [CrossRef]
56. Ritchie, S.A.; Connell, J.M.C. The link between abdominal obesity, metabolic syndrome and cardiovascular disease. *Nutr. Metab. Cardiovasc. Dis.* **2007**, *17*, 319–326. [CrossRef]
57. Luna-Vázquez, F.J.; Ibarra-Alvarado, C.; Rojas-Molina, A.; Rojas-Molina, I.; Zavala-Sánchez, M.Á. Vasodilator compounds derived from plants and their mechanisms of action. *Molecules* **2013**, *18*, 5814–5857. [CrossRef]
58. Fan, Y.Q.; Li, P.H.; Chao, Y.X.; Chen, H.; Du, N.; He, Q.X.; Liu, K.C. Alkaloids with cardiovascular effects from the marine-derived fungus Penicillium expansum Y32. *Mar. Drugs* **2015**, *13*, 6489–6504. [CrossRef]
59. Saklayen, M.G. The Global Epidemic of the Metabolic Syndrome. *Curr. Hypertens. Rep.* **2018**, *20*, 12. [CrossRef]
60. Carrieri, A.; Giudici, M.; Parente, M.; De Rosas, M.; Piemontese, L.; Fracchiolla, G.; Laghezza, A.; Tortorella, P.; Carbonara, G.; Lavecchia, A.; et al. Molecular determinants for nuclear receptors selectivity: Chemometric analysis, dockings and site-directed mutagenesis of dual peroxisome proliferator-activated receptors α/γ agonists. *Eur. J. Med. Chem.* **2013**, *63*, 321–332. [CrossRef]
61. Laghezza, A.; Piemontese, L.; Cerchia, C.; Montanari, R.; Capelli, D.; Giudici, M.; Crestani, M.; Tortorella, P.; Peiretti, F.; Pochetti, G.; et al. Identification of the First PPARα/γ Dual Agonist Able to Bind to Canonical and Alternative Sites of PPARγ and to Inhibit Its Cdk5-Mediated Phosphorylation. *J. Med. Chem.* **2018**, *61*, 8282–8298. [CrossRef]
62. Schoonjans, K.; Staels, B.; Auwerx, J. Role of the peroxisome proliferator-activated receptor (PPAR) in mediating the effects of fibrates and fatty acids on gene expression. *J. Lipid Res.* **1996**, *37*, 907–925. [PubMed]
63. Michalik, L.; Wahli, W. Peroxisome proliferator-activated receptors: Three isotypes for a multitude of functions. *Curr. Opin. Biotechnol.* **1999**, *10*, 564–570. [CrossRef]
64. Piemontese, L.; Fracchiolla, G.; Carrieri, A.; Parente, M.; Laghezza, A.; Carbonara, G.; Sblano, S.; Tauro, M.; Gilardi, F.; Tortorella, P.; et al. Design, synthesis and biological evaluation of a class of bioisosteric oximes of the novel dual peroxisome proliferator-activated receptor α/γ ligand LT175. *Eur. J. Med. Chem.* **2015**, *90*, 583–594. [CrossRef]
65. Lamichane, S.; Dahal Lamichane, B.; Kwon, S.-M. Pivotal Roles of Peroxisome Proliferator-Activated Receptors (PPARs) and Their Signal Cascade for Cellular and Whole-Body Energy Homeostasis. *Int. J. Mol. Sci.* **2018**, *19*, 949. [CrossRef]
66. Penumetcha, M.; Santanam, N. Nutraceuticals as ligands of PPARγ. *PPAR Res.* **2012**, *2012*, 858352. [CrossRef] [PubMed]
67. Fracchiolla, G.; Lavecchia, A.; Laghezza, A.; Piemontese, L.; Trisolini, R.; Carbonara, G.; Tortorella, P.; Novellino, E.; Loiodice, F. Synthesis, biological evaluation, and molecular modeling investigation of chiral 2-(4-chloro-phenoxy)-3-phenyl-propanoic acid derivatives with PPARα and PPARγ agonist activity. *Bioorganic Med. Chem.* **2008**, *16*, 9498–9510. [CrossRef]

68. Fracchiolla, G.; Laghezza, A.; Piemontese, L.; Parente, M.; Lavecchia, A.; Pochetti, G.; Montanari, R.; Di Giovanni, C.; Carbonara, G.; Tortorella, P.; et al. Synthesis, biological evaluation and molecular investigation of fluorinated peroxisome proliferator-activated receptors α/γ dual agonists. *Bioorganic Med. Chem.* **2012**, *20*, 2141–2151. [CrossRef]
69. Laghezza, A.; Montanari, R.; Lavecchia, A.; Piemontese, L.; Pochetti, G.; Iacobazzi, V.; Infantino, V.; Capelli, D.; DeBellis, M.; Liantonio, A.; et al. On the Metabolically Active Form of Metaglidasen: Improved Synthesis and Investigation of Its Peculiar Activity on Peroxisome Proliferator-Activated Receptors and Skeletal Muscles. *ChemMedChem* **2015**, *10*, 555–565. [CrossRef]
70. Fawzy, G.A.; Al-Taweel, A.M.; Perveen, S.; Khan, S.I.; Al-Omary, F.A. Bioactivity and chemical characterization of Acalypha fruticosa Forssk. growing in Saudi Arabia. *Saudi Pharm. J.* **2017**, *25*, 104–109. [CrossRef]
71. Vásquez, Y.; Zhao, J.; Khana, S.I.; Gupta, M.P.; Khana, I.A. Constituents of talisia nervosa with potential utility against metabolic syndrome. *Nat. Prod. Commun.* **2019**, *14*, 51–54. [CrossRef]
72. Liu, S.; Wang, Y.; Su, M.; Song, S.J.; Hong, J.; Kim, S.; Im, D.S.; Jung, J.H. A bile acid derivative with PPARγ-mediated anti-inflammatory activity. *Steroids* **2018**, *137*, 40–46. [CrossRef] [PubMed]
73. Freitas, S.; Silva, N.G.; Sousa, M.L.; Ribeiro, T.; Rosa, F.; Leão, P.N.; Vasconcelos, V.; Reis, M.A.; Urbatzka, R. Chlorophyll derivatives from marine cyanobacteria with lipid-reducing activities. *Mar. Drugs* **2019**, *17*, 229. [CrossRef] [PubMed]
74. Schinkovitz, A.; Le Pogam, P.; Derbré, S.; Roy-Vessieres, E.; Blanchard, P.; Thirumaran, S.L.; Breard, D.; Aumond, M.C.; Zehl, M.; Urban, E.; et al. Secondary metabolites from lichen as potent inhibitors of advanced glycation end products and vasodilative agents. *Fitoterapia* **2018**, *131*, 182–188. [CrossRef] [PubMed]
75. Tao, X.; Liang, S.; Che, J.Y.; Li, H.; Sun, H.X.; Chen, J.G.; Du, X.X.; Wang, C.M. Antidiabetic activity of acidic polysaccharide from schisandra chinensis in STZ-induced diabetic mice. *Nat. Prod. Commun.* **2019**, *14*, 1–9. [CrossRef]
76. Thissera, B.; Visvanathan, R.; Khanfar, M.A.; Qader, M.M.; Hassan, M.H.A.; Hassan, H.M.; Bawazeer, M.; Behery, F.A.; Yaseen, M.; Liyanage, R.; et al. Sesbania grandiflora L. Poir leaves: A dietary supplement to alleviate type 2 diabetes through metabolic enzymes inhibition. *S. Afr. J. Bot.* **2020**, *130*, 282–299. [CrossRef]
77. Silva, T.D.C.; Justino, A.B.; Prado, D.G.; Koch, G.A.; Martins, M.M.; Santos, P.D.S.; De Morais, S.A.L.; Goulart, L.R.; Cunha, L.C.S.; Sousa, R.M.F.; et al. Chemical composition, antioxidant activity and inhibitory capacity of α-amylase, α-glucosidase, lipase and non-enzymatic glycation, in vitro, of the leaves of Cassia bakeriana Craib. *Ind. Crops Prod.* **2019**, *140*, 111641. [CrossRef]
78. Ruiz-Vargas, J.A.; Morales-Ferra, D.L.; Ramírez-Ávila, G.; Zamilpa, A.; Negrete-León, E.; Acevedo-Fernández, J.J.; Peña-Rodríguez, L.M. α-Glucosidase inhibitory activity and in vivo antihyperglycemic effect of secondary metabolites from the leaf infusion of Ocimum campechianum mill. *J. Ethnopharmacol.* **2019**, *243*, 112081. [CrossRef]
79. Dewi, R.T.; Tachibana, S.; Darmawan, A. Effect on α-glucosidase inhibition and antioxidant activities of butyrolactone derivatives from Aspergillus terreus MC751. *Med. Chem. Res.* **2014**, *23*, 454–460. [CrossRef]
80. Budipramana, K.; Junaidin, J.; Wirasutisna, K.R.; Pramana, Y.B.; Sukrasno, S. An integrated in silico and in vitro assays of dipeptidyl peptidase-4 and α-glucosidase inhibition by stellasterol from Ganoderma australe. *Sci. Pharm.* **2019**, *87*, 21. [CrossRef]
81. Wiese, J.; Aldemir, H.; Schmaljohann, R.; Gulder, T.A.M.; Imhoff, J.F.; Kerr, R. Asperentin B, a new inhibitor of the protein tyrosine phosphatase 1B. *Mar. Drugs* **2017**, *15*, 191. [CrossRef] [PubMed]
82. Huang, L.; Yuan, C.; Wang, Y. Bioactivity-guided identification of anti-adipogenic isothiocyanates in the moringa (Moringa oleifera) seed and investigation of the structure-activity relationship. *Molecules* **2020**, *25*, 2504. [CrossRef] [PubMed]
83. Baek, S.C.; Nam, K.H.; Yi, S.A.; Jo, M.S.; Lee, K.H.; Lee, Y.H.; Lee, J.; Kim, K.H. Anti-adipogenic Effect of β-Carboline Alkaloids from Garlic (Allium sativum). *Foods* **2019**, *8*, 673. [CrossRef]
84. Yoshioka, Y.; Yoshimura, N.; Matsumura, S.; Wada, H.; Hoshino, M.; Makino, S.; Morimoto, M. α-Glucosidase and pancreatic lipase inhibitory activities of diterpenes from indian mango ginger (curcuma amada roxb.) and its derivatives. *Molecules* **2019**, *24*, 4071. [CrossRef]
85. Chi, Z.; Le, T.P.H.; Lee, S.K.; Guo, E.; Kim, D.; Lee, S.; Seo, S.Y.; Lee, S.Y.; Kim, J.H.; Lee, S.Y. Honokiol ameliorates angiotensin II-induced hypertension and endothelial dysfunction by inhibiting HDAC6-mediated cystathionine γ-lyase degradation. *J. Cell Mol. Med.* **2020**, *24*, 10663–10676. [CrossRef]
86. Lu, S.; Luo, Y.; Sun, G.B.; Sun, X.B. Ginsenoside Compound K Attenuates Ox-LDL-Mediated Macrophage Inflammation and Foam Cell Formation via Autophagy Induction and Modulating NF-κB, p38, and JNK MAPK Signaling. *Front. Pharmacol.* **2020**, *11*, 567238. [CrossRef]
87. Saha, S.; Profumo, E.; Togna, A.R.; Riganò, R.; Saso, L.; Buttari, B. Lupeol Counteracts the Proinflammatory Signalling Triggered in Macrophages by 7-Keto-Cholesterol: New Perspectives in the Therapy of Atherosclerosis. *Oxid. Med. Cell. Longev.* **2020**, *2020*, 1–12. [CrossRef]
88. Liu, J.; Lee, J.; Hernandez, M.A.S.; Mazitschek, R.; Ozcan, U. Treatment of obesity with celastrol. *Cell* **2015**, *161*, 999–1011. [CrossRef]
89. Olokoba, A.B.; Obateru, O.A.; Olokoba, L.B. Type 2 diabetes mellitus: A review of current trends. *Oman Med. J.* **2012**, *27*, 269–273. [CrossRef]
90. Hays, N.P.; Galassetti, P.R.; Coker, R.H. Prevention and treatment of type 2 diabetes: Current role of lifestyle, natural product, and pharmacological interventions. *Pharmacol. Ther.* **2008**, *118*, 181–191. [CrossRef]
91. Salehi, P.; Asghari, B.; Esmaeili, M.A.; Dehghan, H.; Ghazi, I. -Glucosidase and -amylase inhibitory effect and antioxidant activity of ten plant extracts traditionally used in Iran for diabetes. *J. Med. Plants Res.* **2013**, *7*, 257–266. [CrossRef]

92. Ahrén, B.; Schmitz, O. GLP-1 receptor agonists and DPP-4 inhibitors in the treatment of type 2 diabetes. *Horm. Metab. Res.* **2004**, *36*, 867–876. [CrossRef] [PubMed]
93. Montalibet, J.; Kennedy, B.P. Therapeutic strategies for targeting PTP1B in diabetes. *Drug Discov. Today Ther. Strateg.* **2005**, *2*, 129–135. [CrossRef]
94. Kopelman, P.G. Obesity as a medical problem. *Nature* **2000**, *404*, 635–643. [CrossRef] [PubMed]
95. Ogden, C.L.; Yanovski, S.Z.; Carroll, M.D.; Flegal, K.M. The Epidemiology of Obesity. *Gastroenterology* **2007**, *132*, 2087–2102. [CrossRef] [PubMed]
96. Hussain, S.S.; Bloom, S.R. The pharmacological treatment and management of obesity. *Postgrad. Med.* **2011**, *123*, 34–44. [CrossRef] [PubMed]
97. Mohapatra, S.; Prasad, A.; Haque, F.; Ray, S.; De, B.; Ray, S.S. In silico investigation of black tea components on α-amylase, α-glucosidase and lipase. *J. Appl. Pharm. Sci.* **2015**, *5*, 42–47. [CrossRef]
98. Paracchini, V.; Pedotti, P.; Taioli, E. Genetics of leptin and obesity: A HuGE review. *Am. J. Epidemiol.* **2005**, *162*, 101–114. [CrossRef]
99. Torres-Fuentes, C.; Schellekens, H.; Dinan, T.G.; Cryan, J.F. A natural solution for obesity: Bioactives for the prevention and treatment of weight gain. A review. *Nutr. Neurosci.* **2015**, *18*, 49–65. [CrossRef]
100. Libby, P.; Buring, J.E.; Badimon, L.; Hansson, G.K.; Deanfield, J.; Bittencourt, M.S.; Tokgözoğlu, L.; Lewis, E.F. Atherosclerosis. *Nat. Rev. Dis. Prim.* **2019**, *5*, 56. [CrossRef]
101. Bhansali, S.; Khatri, S.; Dhawan, V. Terminalia Arjuna bark extract impedes foam cell formation and promotes apoptosis in ox-LDL-stimulated macrophages by enhancing UPR-CHOP pathway. *Lipids Health Dis.* **2019**, *18*, 195. [CrossRef] [PubMed]
102. Piemontese, L. Plant Food Supplements with Antioxidant Properties for the Treatment of Chronic and Neurodegenerative Diseases: Benefits or Risks? *J. Diet Suppl.* **2017**, *14*, 478–484. [CrossRef] [PubMed]
103. Commission Regulation (EU) No 212/2014 of 6 March 2014. *Amending Regulation (EC) No 1881/2006 as Regards Maximum Levels of the Contaminant Citrinin in Food Supplements based on Rice Fermented with Red Yeast Monascus purpureus (Text with EEA relevance)*; European Union: Brussels, Belgium, 2014.
104. Piemontese, L.; Perna, F.M.; Logrieco, A.; Capriati, V.; Solfrizzo, M. Deep eutectic solvents as novel and effective extraction media for quantitative determination of Ochratoxin A in wheat and derived products. *Molecules* **2017**, *22*, 121. [CrossRef] [PubMed]
105. Moncalvo, A.; Marinoni, L.; Dordoni, R.; Garrido, G.D.; Lavelli, V.; Spigno, G. Waste grape skins: Evaluation of safety aspects for the production of functional powders and extracts for the food sector. *Food Addit. Contam. Part A Chem. Anal. Control. Exp. Risk Assess.* **2016**, *33*, 1116–1126. [CrossRef] [PubMed]
106. Poliseno, V.; Chaves, S.; Brunetti, L.; Loiodice, F.; Carrieri, A.; Laghezza, A.; Tortorella, P.; Magalhaes, J.D.; Cardoso, S.M.; Santos, M.A.; et al. Derivatives of Tenuazonic Acid as Potential New Multi-Target Anti-Alzheimer's Disease Agents. *Biomolecules* **2021**, *11*, 111. [CrossRef]

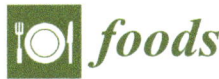

Review

Bioactive Compounds from Plant-Based Functional Foods: A Promising Choice for the Prevention and Management of Hyperuricemia

Lin-Lin Jiang [1], Xue Gong [2], Ming-Yue Ji [2], Cong-Cong Wang [2], Jian-Hua Wang [1,*] and Min-Hui Li [1,2,3,4,5,*]

1. Department of Pharmacy, Inner Mongolia Medical University, Hohhot 010110, China; jianglinlin27@163.com
2. Department of Pharmacy, Baotou Medical College, Baotou 014060, China; gongxue_2017@yeah.net (X.G.); Jimingyue9@163.com (M.-Y.J.); WangCongCong0@163.com (C.-C.W.)
3. Department of Pharmacy, Qiqihar Medical University, Qiqihar 161006, China
4. Pharmaceutical Laboratory, Inner Mongolia Institute of Traditional Chinese Medicine, Hohhot 010020, China
5. Inner Mongolia Key Laboratory of Characteristic Geoherbs Resources Protection and Utilization, Baotou Medical College, Baotou 014060, China
* Correspondence: ny_wjh513@163.com (J.-H.W.); prof_liminhui@yeah.net (M.-H.L.); Tel.: +86-472-716-7795 (M.-H.L.)

Received: 7 June 2020; Accepted: 20 July 2020; Published: 23 July 2020

Abstract: Hyperuricemia is a common metabolic disease that is caused by high serum uric acid levels. It is considered to be closely associated with the development of many chronic diseases, such as obesity, hypertension, hyperlipemia, diabetes, and cardiovascular disorders. While pharmaceutical drugs have been shown to exhibit serious side effects, and bioactive compounds from plant-based functional foods have been demonstrated to be active in the treatment of hyperuricemia with only minimal side effects. Indeed, previous reports have revealed the significant impact of bioactive compounds from plant-based functional foods on hyperuricemia. This review focuses on plant-based functional foods that exhibit a hypouricemic function and discusses the different bioactive compounds and their pharmacological effects. More specifically, the bioactive compounds of plant-based functional foods are divided into six categories, namely flavonoids, phenolic acids, alkaloids, saponins, polysaccharides, and others. In addition, the mechanism by which these bioactive compounds exhibit a hypouricemic effect is summarized into three classes, namely the inhibition of uric acid production, improved renal uric acid elimination, and improved intestinal uric acid secretion. Overall, this current and comprehensive review examines the use of bioactive compounds from plant-based functional foods as natural remedies for the management of hyperuricemia.

Keywords: hyperuricemia; plant-based functional food; xanthine oxidase; adenosine deaminase; uric acid transporter; bioactive compound

1. Introduction

Hyperuricemia (HUA) is a common metabolic disease caused by an imbalance between endogenous production and excretion of urate [1]. Recently, considerable evidence has indicated that uric acid (UA), an endogenous antioxidant present in low concentrations in the human plasma, plays an active role in life processes [2,3]. However, the over-production of UA easily results in the formation of monosodium urate crystals, which increases inflammation and causes gout [4]. In recent years, the incidence of HUA has been increasing every year worldwide, and the prevalence of HUA is particularly high in China and the United States [5–7]. HUA is considered to be a major risk factor of metabolic disorders after hypertension, hyperlipidemia, and hyperglycemia [8], and is considered to be the major pathological basis of gout, whereby approximately 5–12% of HUA patients have the possibility of developing gout [9]. Moreover, a large number of epidemiological studies have reported that HUA is closely related to diabetes, hypertension, obesity, cardiovascular disease, and kidney disease [10–13], which suggests that complications associated with HUA may increase in the coming years.

As mentioned above, HUA can be caused by either an increase in UA production or a decrease in UA metabolism in the body, with reduced urate excretion being the most common mechanism, accounting for about 90% of cases [9]. As a result, a means to reduce the body UA levels could be considered an effective treatment. However, the production and metabolism of UA are complex physiological processes. Endogenous UA is derived from the metabolism of nucleic acids within the body, and accounts for 80–90% of the body's total UA content [14,15]. Xanthine oxidase (XOD) and adenosine deaminase (ADA) are key enzymes that catalyze the production of UA. XOD is known to catalyze the oxidation of hypoxanthine to xanthine and xanthine to UA [16], while also converting purines from protein-rich foods into UA. In addition, ADA catalyzes the conversion of adenosine to inosine, which in turn is catalyzed to hypoxanthine and xanthine. Therefore, ADA plays a key role in indirectly catalyzing the formation of UA [17]. The catalytic process for UA production is presented in Figure 1. In contrast, exogenous UA is derived from the intake of purine-containing foods. As previously reported, the consumption of seafood, animal giblets, eggs, soy products, wheat, sugary beverages, and high-fructose foods will increase UA production, which is associated with a high risk of gout and HUA [18–20]. During UA metabolism, approximately 70% of UA is eliminated through kidneys and the other 30% by the intestinal pathway [21]. In humans, UA metabolism in the body mainly takes place in the kidneys, involving processes such as reabsorption and secretion (Figure 2). UA relies on the cooperative excretion of multiple transporters to complete metabolism, whereby the urate transporter 1 (URAT1), the organic anion transporters 4 (OAT4), and the glucose transporter 9 (GLUT9) mainly regulate UA reabsorption, while the organic anion transporters 1 (OAT1) and 3 (OAT3) are responsible for regulating renal UA excretion [22–25]. Therefore, lowering UA levels can be achieved by inhibiting UA synthesis and promoting UA metabolism, as well as encouraging high-risk people to change their dietary structure can prevent and control HUA. Currently, the clinical drugs available for HUA can be categorized into UA synthesis inhibitors (allopurinol, febuxostat, etc.) and UA excretion promoters (probenecid, benzbromarone, etc.) [26]. Although these drugs aid in reducing UA levels, many exhibit serious side effects, such as gastrointestinal reactions, skin rashes, liver and kidney dysfunction, and hepatotoxicity [27]. It is therefore necessary to discover alternative effective agents for the treatment of HUA.

Plant-based functional foods are derived from natural or unprocessed plant foods, or plant foods modified via biotechnological means [28]. They are products that have a relevant effect on well-being and health or reduce the risk of disease [29]. Interestingly, many such functional foods have been links with lowered incidences of various health disorders, such as cardiovascular disease, diabetes, cancers, and gout, and so there is growing interest in the research and development of plant-based functional foods [30–33]. In recent years, with the increase in numbers of HUA patients, studies into the treatment of HUA using plant-based functional foods have received increasing attention. For example, sea buckthorn was found to exhibit high antioxidant capacity and XOD inhibition capacity, while lemon water extract can directly promote the metabolism of excess UA, thereby indicating a potential to treat HUA [34–36]. Previous studies have found that these functions are associated with the presence of large quantities of phytochemicals, which are chemical compounds originating from plants [37]. Furthermore, bioactive components from plant-based functional foods have been extensively screened for their potential anti-HUA activities both in vivo and in vitro [32,38]. Table 1 briefly summarizes the animal models of HUA. The identified constituents can be divided into six categories, namely flavonoids, phenolic acids, saponins, alkaloids, polysaccharides, and others. This review highlights the biological components of plant-based functional foods towards the treatment of HUA, as well as the mechanisms by which these components exhibit hypouricemic effects. We expect that the contents of this review will aid in the understanding of potential applications for plant-based functional foods in the treatment of HUA.

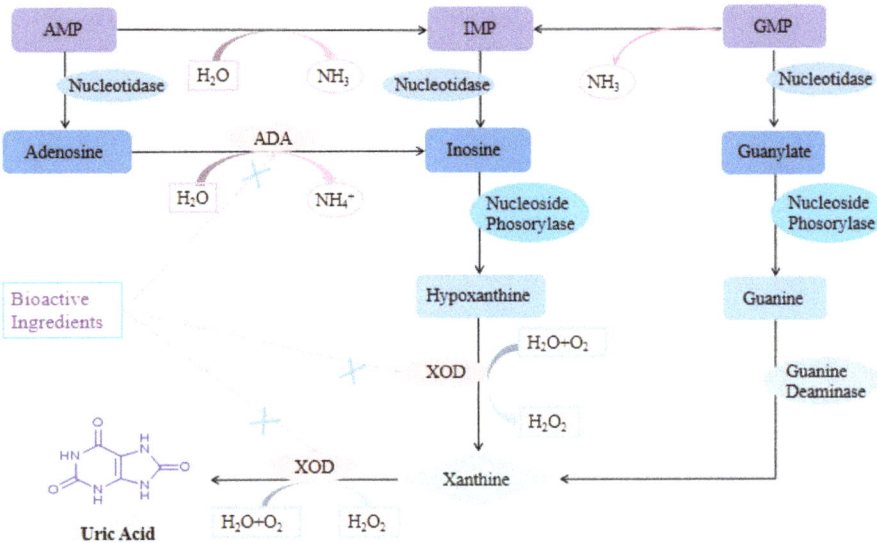

Figure 1. Xanthine oxidase (XOD) and adenosine deaminase (ADA) inhibitory mechanisms of bioactive ingredients.

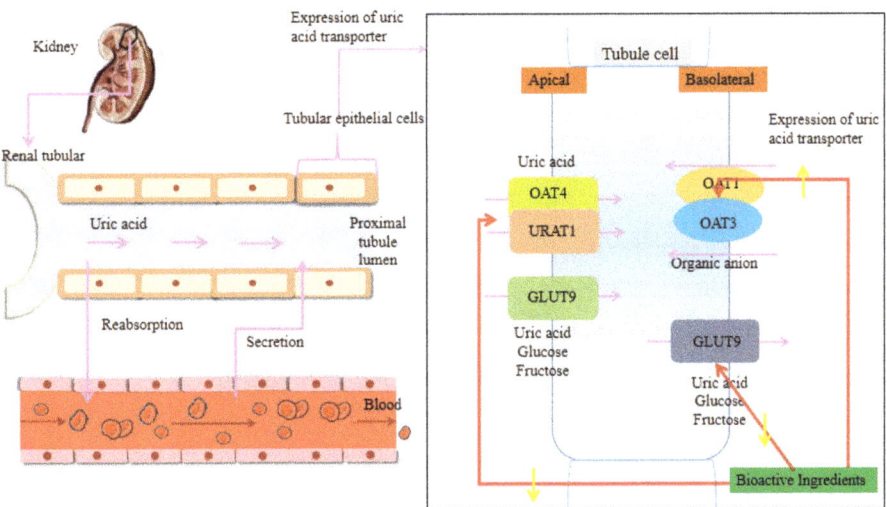

Figure 2. Effect of bioactive components of plant-based functional foods on renal transporters.

Table 1. Establishment of an animal model of Hyperuricemia (HUA) by drugs.

No.	Drug	Animal	Dosage (mg/kg)	Mode of Administration
A	Potassium oxonate	Mice	-	Intragastric administration
B	Potassium oxonate	Rats	200	Intragastric administration
C	Potassium oxonate	Mice	250	Oral gavage
D	Potassium oxonate	Mice	250	Intragastric administration
E	Potassium oxonate	Mice	270	Intragastric administration
F	Potassium oxonate	Mice	300	Intragastric administration
G	Potassium oxonate	Mice	500	Intragastric administration
H	Adenine	Mice	75	Intragastric administration
I	Adenine + potassium oxonate	Mice	100 + 250	Intragastric administration
J	Adenine + ethylamine butanol	Rats	-	Intragastric administration
K	Inosine + potassium oxonate	Rats	400 + 280	Intragastric administration
L	Yeast + potassium oxonate	Rats	1500 + 200	Intragastric administration
M	Purine	Mice	300	Intragastric administration
N	Uric acid	Rats	150	Intragastric administration
O	Uric acid	Rats	180	Intragastric administration
P	High purine diet	Rats	-	Oral gavage
Q	Yeast	Quails	6 mL	Oral gavage
R	High purine diet	Quails	-	Oral gavage

2. Bioactive Components of Plant-Based Functional Foods

Flavonoids are polyphenols with a basic 2-phenyl-chromone structure [39], and they are found widely in plants. Hence, flavonoids are introduced to the human diet through vegetables, fruits, grains, tea, and other plant-derived foods [40]. Previous studies have demonstrated that they are also known to be potent inhibitors of XOD and ADA, and they could significantly reduce the production of UA [41]. Indeed, molecular docking results indicate that the hydrophobic action of flavonoids plays an important role in the binding of such compounds to XOD, and various tested flavonoids are competitive inhibitors. More specifically, the hydroxyl groups at the C-7 and C-5 positions, in addition to the carbonyl group at the C-4 position, interact with a large number of XOD amino acid residues, which promotes hydrogen bonding and electrostatic interactions with XOD [42,43]. Upon increasing the affinity between flavonoids and XOD, a stronger XOD inhibition ability was achieved, whereby substitution at the C-7 position of the basic flavonoid structure was particularly effective [40]. In addition, flavonoids have also been found to promote UA excretion through regulation of the UA transporters in the kidneys, such as URAT1. The molecular virtual docking study has revealed that the hydroxyl group of morusin can combine with the oxygen in the structure of URAT1 to form a hydrogen bond, resulting in an inhibitory effect on the expression of URAT1, which is superior to that of the known drug benzbromarone [44].

At present, only a few clinical studies have shown that flavonoids from plant-based functional foods can effectively lower UA levels. For example, following the isolation of puerarin from *Pueraria lobata* (Willd.) Ohwi and Wang et al. randomly divided 120 HUA patients into a control group, a myricetin group, and a puerarin group. After injection with 5 mL/d puerarin injection and 5 mL/d myricetin, the changes in the UA levels in patients with HUA were observed. The obtained results showed that the serum uric acid (SUA) levels of the myricetin and puerarin groups decreased significantly ($p < 0.05$), indicating that myricetin and puerarin present obvious therapeutic effects on HUA [45].

Quercetin, one of the major flavonols mainly found in onions and sophora japonica (*Sophora japonica* L.), exhibits a variety of biological activities. In their study into the effect of quercetin on HUA rats, whereby a rat model of HUA was induced via the administration of potassium oxonate. Xie et al. found that after three weeks of administration, quercetin (10 mg/kg/d) significantly reduced the levels of SUA and inhibited the activities of XOD and ADA in both serum and the liver ($p < 0.05$) [46]. In addition, one clinical trial investigated the effect of oral quercetin over four weeks on the SUA levels in 22 healthy male volunteers with high baseline SUA. It was found that the oral administration of 500 mg/d quercetin significantly lowered plasma UA levels 26.5 µM, while the extraction of UA and the patient blood pressure were not affected [47]. Furthermore, molecular docking studies confirmed that quercetin could bind to the XOD active center, which prevents xanthine from entering the XOD active center and thereby inhibits XOD activity [48]. Quercetin is therefore able to inhibit the catalytic activities of both XOD and ADA to reduce the production of UA.

Ipomoea batatas L. possesses a high content of anthocyanins (ACNs) [49]. In one study, ACNs were administered to potassium oxonate, inosine, and yeast-induced HUA mice model for three weeks, and it was found that the groups treated with 400 and 800 mg/kg of ACNs exhibited significant reductions in their SUA levels by 30.2% and 37.9%, respectively ($p < 0.01$), in addition to effective decreases in the serum and liver XOD activities in mice ($p < 0.05$). Furthermore, treatment with high doses of ACNs significantly down-regulated the mRNA expression levels of the URAT1 and GLUT9 ($p < 0.001$), while up-regulating the mRNA expression levels of OAT1, OAT3, and ATP-binding cassette subfamily G member 2 (ABCG2) ($p < 0.05$) in the kidney. Moreover, ACNs treatment lowered blood urea nitrogen (BUN) and serum creatinine (Scr) levels, while up-regulating the mRNA expression levels of organic cation transporters (OCT1 and OCT2) and organic carnitine transporter (OCTN1 and OCTN2) compared with the model group ($p < 0.01$). It has also been suggested that ACNs exhibit hepatoprotective activities and nephroprotective effects, thereby suggesting overall that ACNs are potential treatments for HUA [50].

The hypouricemic effect of flavonoids has been studied in particular detail compared to other natural products. Although the majority of previous studies have focused on the inhibition of XOD, the number of studies on UA transporters are gradually increasing. Besides, studies on monomeric compounds remain scarce, and in general, there is a lack of high-quality clinical research. For example, it has been shown that stevia residue extract can reduce SUA levels in HUA mice, and this was attributed to the presence of flavonoids [51], thereby indicating that the effects of flavonoids in the treatment of HUA require further study. The established hypouricemic effects and mechanisms of action of the bioactive components of flavonoids in plant-based functional foods are summarized in Tables 2 and 3, and the structures of flavonoids obtained from these plant-based functional foods are illustrated in Figure 3.

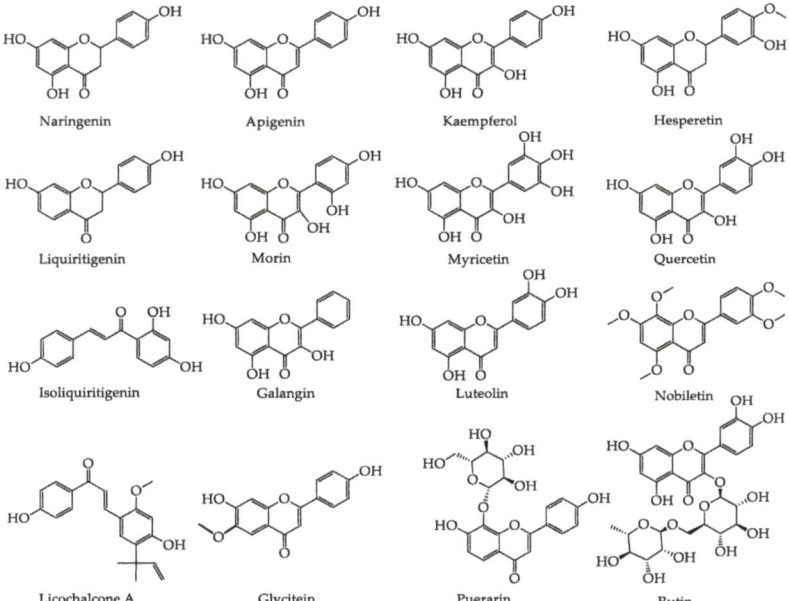

Figure 3. The basic structure of hypouricemic effects from flavonoids bioactive components in plant-based functional foods.

Table 2. Experiment and mechanism of flavonoids bioactive components from plant-based functional foods on hyperuricemia.

Source	Bioactive Compound	Model	Dose	Effects	Mechanisms	Ref.
Apium graveolens L./Celery	Apigenin	C	40 and 80 mg/kg	SUA, urinary UA and the protein expression of URAT1 levels were significantly decreased, while 24 h urinary creatinine were significantly increased	This is associated with promoting renal excretion of UA by down-regulating the expression of URAT1	[52]
Apium graveolens L./Celery	Kaempferol	E	150 and 300 mg/kg	Significantly decreased SUA	Inhibit UA production by inhibiting XOD	[53]
Camellia sinensis var. Assamica/Pu-erh tea	Myricetin	D	4 mg/kg	Significantly lowered SUA level, it also markedly inhibited liver XOD and ADA activities	It is mainly involved in inhibiting UA production by inhibiting XOD and ADA activities	[54]
Glycyrrhiza uralensis Fisch/Liquorice Root	Liquiritigenin	G	10 mg/kg	SUA level significantly reduced, fractional excretion of UA was increased	This is related to promoting renal excretion of UA by down-regulating the transport expression of URAT1	[55]
Glycyrrhiza uralensis Fisch/Liquorice Root	Isoliquiritigenin	G	10 mg/kg	SUA level significantly reduced, fractional excretion of UA was increased	This is related to inhibiting UA reabsorption by down-regulating the transport of OAT4	[55]
Glycyrrhiza uralensis Fisch/Liquorice Root	Licochalcone A	G	10 mg/kg	SUA level significantly reduced, fractional excretion of UA was increased	This is related to inhibiting UA reabsorption by down-regulating the transport of OAT4	[55]
Vaccinium vitisidaea L./Lingonberry	Flavonoids from fruit residues of lingonberry	B	100 and 200 mg/kg	SUA was significantly reduced at 100 mg/kg, while 200 mg/kg inhibited the activity of XOD in liver	It is mainly involved in inhibiting XOD activity	[56]
Smilax china L./Rhizome Glabrous Greenbrier	Astilbin	B	10 and 20 mg/kg	SUA, Scr and BUN were significantly reduced, and urinary UA and renal UA excretion effectively increased	It is related to promoting renal excretion of UA by suppressing role in GLUT9 and URAT1 expression and up-regulating the expression of ABCG2, OAT1, OAT3	[57]
Pueraria lobata (Willd.) Ohwi/Puerraria	Puerarin	L	200 mg/kg	SUA, and BUN were significantly reduced	It is mainly involved in inhibiting XOD activity to inhibit UA production	[58]
Glycyrrhiza uralensis Fisch/Liquorice Root	3,5,2′,4′-tetrahydroxychalcone	N	4 mg/kg	SUA and the content of Hepatic XOD were significantly reduced	It is mainly involved in inhibiting XOD activity to inhibit UA production and down-regulating the protein expression of GLUT9 to inhibit UA re-absorption	[59]
Morus alba L./Mori Cortex	Flavonoids of Mori Cortex	H	1 mg/kg	URAT1 was significantly decreased, the content of OAT1 mRNA was significantly increased	It may be related to the down-regulation of URAT1 and the up-regulation OAT1 to promote renal excretion of UA	[60]
Morus alba L./Mulberry Leaf	Morusin	J	40 and 80 mg/kg	Increased urinary UA/creatinine ratio and resulting in reduction of SUA level	Down-regulated of renal mGLUT9 and mURAT1, and increased urate secretion via up-regulating of renal mOAT1 to promote renal excretion of UA	[44]

Table 2. Cont.

Source	Bioactive Compound	Model	Dose	Effects	Mechanisms	Ref.
Morus alba L./Mulberry Leaf	Mulberry leaf flavonoids	H	50, 100, and 200 mg/kg	SUA and urea nitrogen were effectively lowered, XOD was inhibited	It is related to inhibiting the activity of XOD to inhibit UA production	[61]
Morus alba L./Mulberry	Mulberry flavonoids	H	200 mg/kg	SUA were effectively lower	It is related to inhibiting the activity of XOD to inhibit UA production	[56]
Crataegus pinnatifida Bge./Hawthorn	Flavonoids of hawthorn leaves	J	3, 6, and 9 mg/kg	SUA was effectively lowered, XOD was inhibited	It is related to inhibiting the activity of XOD to inhibit UA production	[62]
Sophora japonica L./Sophora Japonica	Rutin	D	50 and 100 mg/kg	Significantly decreased SUA, BUN, and Scr, and increased urine creatinine excretion	It is related to promoting renal excretion of UA by down-regulating mRNA and protein levels of URAT1 and GLUT9, and up-regulating mRNA and protein levels of OAT1	[63,64]
Hippophae rhamnoides L./Seabuckthorn	Isorhamnetin	M	300 mg/kg	Significantly reduced plasma and hepatic UA level, also decreased hepatic XOD activity	It is related to inhibiting the activity of XOD to inhibit UA production	[65]

Table 3. In vitro experiment and mechanism of flavonoids bioactive components from plant-based functional foods on hyperuricemia.

Source	Bioactive Compound	Model	Dose	IC_{50}	Effects	Mechanisms	Ref.
Pueraria lobata (Willd.) Ohwi/Pueraria	Puerarin	Human renal proximal tubular epithelial cells (HK2 cells)	100 mg/L	16.48 µM	Effectively promoted ABCG2 protein expression in HK2 cells	It is related to up-regulating of ABCG2 to promote renal excretion of UA	[66]
Citrus aurantium L./Fructus Aurantii	Hesperetin	XOD inhibitor screening model in vitro	20 µM	16.48 µM	Significantly inhibited XOD activity	This is related to inhibit XOD to inhibit UA production	[67]
Citrus aurantium L./Fructus Aurantii	Nobiletin	XOD inhibitor screening model in vitro	20 µM	16.48 µM	Significantly inhibited XOD activity	This is related to inhibit XOD to inhibit UA production	[67]
Citrus reticulata Blanco/Citrus	Acacatechin	XOD model in vitro	100 µg/mL	27 ± 1.16 µg/mL	Significantly inhibited XOD activity	It showed competitive type of XOD inhibition to inhibit UA production	[68]
Citrus reticulata Blanco/Citrus	Glycitein	XOD model in vitro	100 µg/mL	12 ± 0.86 µg/mL	Significantly inhibited XOD activity	It showed competitive type of XOD inhibition to inhibit UA production	[68]
Citrus reticulata Blanco/Citrus	Myricetin	XOD model in vitro	100 µg/mL	26 ± 0.72 µg/mL	Significantly inhibited XOD activity	It showed competitive type of XOD inhibition to inhibit UA production	[68]
Carthamus tinctorius L./Carthami Flos	Galuteolin	XOD inhibitor screening model in vitro	100 µg/mL	12 ± 0.86 µg/mL	Significantly inhibited XOD activity	This is related to inhibiting XOD to inhibit UA production	[68]
Citrus reticulata Blanco/Citrus	Naringenin	XOD model in vitro	100 µg/mL	22 ± 0.64 µg/mL	Significantly inhibited XOD activity	It showed competitive type of XOD inhibition to inhibit UA production	[68]
Carthamus tinctorius L./Carthami Flos	Kaemperfol	XOD inhibitor screening model in vitro	100 µg/mL	12 ± 0.86 µg/mL	Significantly inhibited XOD activity	This is related to inhibiting XOD to inhibit UA production	[69]

2.1. Phenolic Acids

Phenolic acids, which are secondary metabolites, are non-flavonoid phenolic compounds. They represent a substantial part of the human diet [70]. In recent years, phytochemicals such as phenolic acids have been found to exhibit XOD and ADA inhibitory activities, and are thought to be applicable in the prevention and treatment of HUA. For example, compounds such as chicory acid, caffeic acid, and chlorogenic acid, inhibit the activity of XOD [71].

In the context of chicory acid, which was isolated from *Cichorium intybus* L., Zhu et al. established a quail HUA model to elucidate the active ingredients and mechanism of *C. intybus* L. in combating HUA. After 21 days of administration, chicory acid (150 mg/kg/d) significantly reduced the quail SUA ($p < 0.05$). Moreover, the quail serum ADA and XOD levels were also significantly reduced ($p < 0.05$), which may be related to inhibition of the XOD and ADA activities. Overall, chicory acid significantly reduced quail SUA levels by inhibiting the XOD and ADA activities [72,73].

Phenolic antioxidants, including phenolic acids, have been isolated from Adlay (*Coix lachryma-jobi* L.) [74]. Upon the administration of various doses of caffeic acid (i.e., 25, 50, and 100 mg/kg) to potassium oxonate-induced HUA rats, the UA levels were reduced in the high-dose group ($p < 0.05$). Moreover, the BUN and Scr levels were significantly reduced compared with the model control group, and caffeic acid was found to reduce BUN to the normal range. Besides, an in vivo study showed that caffeic acid regulated the transcription levels in a dose-dependent manner by up-regulating the expression of UA secretory transporters OAT1 and ABCG2 mRNA, and down-regulating UA reabsorption transporters URAT1 and GLUT9 mRNA. Furthermore, an in vitro study showed that caffeic acid can inhibit XOD by competitively binding to xanthine, with an IC_{50} value of 53.45 μM being recorded [75]. Therefore, it is believed that caffeic acid presents a dual effect in lowering UA levels, and so presents a potential application for the treatment of HUA.

However, to date, despite extensive research into phenolic acids, few studies exist regarding the regulation of UA transporters. In addition, there is a lack of anti-HUA clinical data, and few reports have been published on the role of phenolic acids in regulating transport proteins. These issues must, therefore, be solved to enhance the applicability of phenolic acids for the treatment of HUA. The hypouricemic effects and mechanisms of action of the various bioactive phenolic acids found in plant-based functional foods are listed in Table 4, and their structures are illustrated in Figure 4.

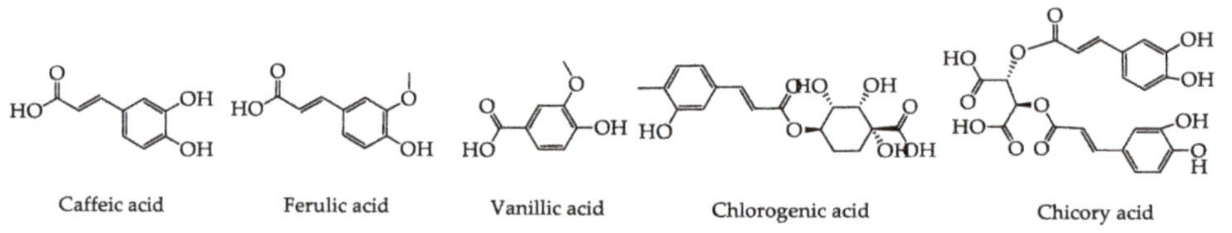

Figure 4. The basic structure of hypouricemic effects from phenolic acid bioactive components in plant-based functional foods.

Table 4. Experiment and mechanism of phenolic acid bioactive components from plant-based functional foods on hyperuricemia.

Source	Bioactive Compound	Model	Dose	Effects	Mechanisms	Ref.
Cichorium intybus L./Chicory	Chlorogenic acid	R	50 and 150 mg/kg	SUA level significantly was reduced, XOD and ADA levels showed different degrees of inhibition	This is related to promoting UA excretion by down-regulating the expression of mURAT1 and inhibiting XOD and ADA	[76]
Glycyrrhiza uralensis Fisch/Liquorice Root	Protocatechuic acid	F	10 mg/kg	SUA level significantly reduced, fractional excretion of uric acid was increased	This is related to down-regulation the transport activity of URAT1 by inhibiting UA re-absorption	[55]
Coix lachryma-jobi L/Adlay	Vanillic acid	B	166 mg/kg	SUA level significantly reduced, XOD was inhibited	This is related to inhibiting the activity of XOD	[74]
Coix lachryma-jobi L/Adlay	Ferulic acid	B	166 mg/kg	SUA level significantly reduced, XOD was inhibited	This is related to inhibiting the activity of XOD	[74]

2.2. Alkaloids

Alkaloids are a class of nitrogen-containing organic compounds that exist in many organisms [77]. Due to their complex structures and strong biological activities, their role in lowering UA should not be ignored. Recently, it has been reported that alkaloids can not only inhibit XOD and ADA activities, but also play a role in promoting UA excretion and inhibiting UA reabsorption [78].

Recently, Sang et al. evaluated the effective components present in a total alkaloid extract from *Nelumbinis folium* (lotus leaf) for the lowering of the UA levels. UHPLC-Q-TOF-MS and 3D docking analysis were employed to show that roemerine was a potentially active component. More specifically, roemerine bound with XOD through hydrophobic interactions, inhibited the activity of XOD, and reduced the production of UA [78,79]. Furthermore, nuciferine, a major aporphine alkaloid of the lotus leaf, was found to decrease SUA levels and improve kidney function in potassium oxonate-induced HUA mice. After seven days of treatment, the SUA, BUN, and Scr levels were dramatically reduced ($p < 0.05$), and the excretion of UA increased significantly ($p < 0.05$) for the high-dose nuciferine group (40 mg/kg). It has since been reported that the mechanism of lowering UA is related to down-regulation of the expression of URAT1, GLUT9, and up-regulation of the expression of OAT1 and ABCG2 in HUA mice [80].

Evodiamine is the main active component of *Evodia rutaecarpa* (Juss.) Benth, and has been shown to exhibit an obvious effect on lowering SUA levels. Tao et al. established animal models of HUA in rats and chickens to observe the effect of evodiamine on lowering SUA after 7 and 14 days of administration. Compared with the model group, the low and high dosage groups (9 and 18 mg/kg) reduced SUA values in rats, while the low dose group showed significantly reduced SUA values in HUA chicken [81]. Similarly, Song et al. studied the effects and mechanisms of evodiamine dispersing tablets (5 mg/kg) on SUA in HUA chickens. Their results showed that after 14 days of the administration, UA levels were significantly reduced, as were the activities of XOD and ADA. This experiment suggested that evodiamine dispersible tablets could apply to the treatment of HUA by lowering UA levels in clinical applications [82].

Although alkaloids have been shown to prevent and control HUA through a variety of mechanisms, exhibiting a significant effect on lowering UA levels, due to a lack of clinical data, larger numbers of studies must be conducted in the context of clinical trials and toxic doses. The hypouricemic effects of alkaloid bioactive components in plant-based functional foods and their mechanisms of action are summarized in Table 5, while their structures are illustrated in Figure 5.

Table 5. Experiment and mechanism of alkaloids bioactive components from plant-based functional foods on hypouricemia.

Source	Bioactive Compound	Model	Dose	Effects	Mechanisms	Ref.
Evodia rutaecarpa (Juss.) Benth./Euodiae Fructus	Evodiamine	Q	8 mg/kg	SUA and XOD could be significantly reduced	This is related to inhibiting the activity of XOD to inhibit of UA production	[83]
Lycium barbarum L./Lycii Fructus	Betaine	D	10, 20, and 40 mg/kg	SUA, BUN, and Scr levels significantly reduced, fractional excretion of uric acid was increased	This is related to down-regulating mRNA and protein levels of URAT1 and GLUT9, and up-regulating mRNA and protein levels of OAT1 to promote uric acid excretion	[84,85]

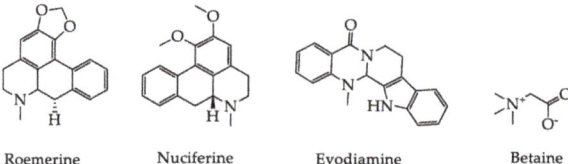

Roemerine   Nuciferine   Evodiamine   Betaine

Figure 5. The basic structure of hypouricemic effects from alkaloids bioactive components in plant-based functional foods.

2.3. Saponins

Saponins are mainly distributed in terrestrial plants, and small amounts are also found in marine life. Based on their different aglycones, saponins can be divided into steroidal saponins and triterpenoid saponins. In recent years, studies have shown that saponins can reduce UA production by inhibiting the activity of XOD and ADA, and that they can also increase UA excretion by regulating the expression of UA transporters [86].

As an example, the anti-HUA mechanism dioscin, which is mainly distributed in *Dioscorea opposita* L. [87], was investigated in HUA mice. More specifically, HUA mice were induced with potassium oxonate (250 mg/kg), and dioscin was orally administered to HUA mice at dosages of 319.22, 638.43, 1276.86 mg/kg/d for 10 days. Following treatment, the SUA levels were significantly reduced, and the Scr levels were lower than those found in the model group ($p < 0.05$). In addition, dioscin significantly increased the 24 h cumulative urinary excretion of creatinine ($p < 0.05$), the protein level of renal mOAT1 in HUA mice treated by dioscin increased significantly at high dosages (1276.86 mg/kg/d), and the protein level of renal mURAT1 decreased. Thus, the mechanism by which dioscin lowers UA levels involves transporter regulation [88].

HUA rats were also treated with saponins from *Gynostemma pentaphyllum* (Thunb.) Makino (GPS). Compared with the model group, the low (15 mg/kg) and high dosage groups (60 mg/kg) exhibited dramatically reduced SUA levels ($p < 0.01$, $p < 0.05$). Moreover, after being treated with a high dosage of GPS, the UA level was close to normal ($p < 0.01$), and the levels of XOD and ADA in the serum and liver decreased ($p < 0.05$). Treatment with GPS also increased the kidney index, downregulated URAT1 and GLUT9 expression, and upregulated OAT1 expression in the kidney. GPS may, therefore, be an effective treatment for HUA through the inhibition of XOD and ADA, and an increase in UA excretion by regulation of the URAT1, GLUT9, and OAT1 transporters [89,90].

Overall, saponin extracts act by inhibiting UA generation, promoting UA excretion, and protecting the kidneys. At present, research into the anti-HUA activities of saponin extracts are in their initial stages, and the identification of additional pharmaceutically active monomer components is necessary. Moreover, investigations into the pharmacological mechanisms of any monomeric species are desirable, as is the development of safe and effective new drugs demonstrating anti-HUA properties.

2.4. Polysaccharides

Significant attention has been paid to the extraction and bioactivity of biomacromolecules, such as polysaccharides. Polysaccharides obtained from natural sources tend to exhibit a low toxicity in addition to various bioactivities, such as anti-bacterial, anti-inflammatory activities [91,92]. In recent years, studies reporting their inhibition of UA production and enhancement of UA elimination have been published, indicating that polysaccharides may be a candidate for the development of new natural anti-HUA agents.

Lonicera japonica (Thunb) is recognized as a medicine food homology species. The *L. japonica* polysaccharides have been studied for their hypouricemic effect in potassium oxonate-induced HUA mice. Interestingly, with an increase in the polysaccharide dose, the level of UA was significantly lowered, demonstrating that the oral administration of polysaccharides could treat HUA in a dose-dependent manner. In particular, in the high-dose group, the level of SUA was reduced, and compared with the model group, SUA levels in the middle and low dose groups decreased by 47.93% and 43.41%, respectively ($p < 0.01$). The low, middle, and high dose groups (100, 200, and 300 mg/kg) showed the capability to inhibit the activity of XOD (28.71%, 46.31%, and 54.69%, respectively), thereby indicating that *L. japonica* (Thunb) polysaccharides could significantly attenuate HUA in rats [93].

To further study the effect of pachman (polysaccharides of Poria Cocos, PPC) on HUA, Wang et al. fed rats with potassium oxonate and ethambutol to establish an animal model for HUA, and then treated with PPC. The high-dose PPC group (2.0 g/kg/d) exhibited an increase in the fractional excretion of UA, while the level of SUA and any pathological changes in renal tubules were reduced compared with the model group ($p < 0.05$). The protein expression results showed that the expression of URAT1 was significantly down-regulated compared with the model group, while the expression of OAT1 was significantly increased. These results revealed that PPC increased the reabsorption of UA by down-regulating the expression of URAT1, while up-regulating the expression of OAT1 to reduce the re-secretion of UA [94].

Some polysaccharides have also been shown to play an important role in reducing UA. However, previous studies have shown that a high fructose intake was associated with a higher risk of gout and HUA. For example, Lecoultre et al. evaluated 16 healthy adults who were induced by a high fructose, which found UA clearance rate was decreased and SUA was increased [95]. Moreover, an increase in SUA induced by fructose metabolism could have some effects on kidney injury [96]. Cirillo et al. showed that fructose can induce proximal tubular injury in vitro by fructokinase to generate oxidants and UA [97]. As a result, further studies into the pharmacological effects of polysaccharides are required, as are the corresponding clinical trials.

2.5. Others

In addition to the above bioactive ingredients, other components (e.g., terpenoids, stilbene glycosides, and coumarin) have also been found to exhibit UA-lowering effects. For example, gardenoside and acteoside have been reported to present significant hypouricemic effects [98,99]. Moreover, Moriwaki et al. studied changes in SUA concentration after intake of oligonol in six healthy subjects. Subjects were treated with 2 g/d oligonol, 1h UA excretion, and partial UA clearance were significantly reduced, with decreased SUA concentration [100]. The UA-lowering effects and mechanisms of action of these other components are summarized in Table 6, and their basic structures are shown in Figure 6. Moreover, compounds-targets network diagrams for the plant-based functional foods exhibiting hypouricemic effects were established using Cytoscape 3.7.1 software, as shown in Figure 7. In Figure 7, the bioactive compounds of plant-based functional foods for hyperuricemia are divided into six categories, namely flavonoids, phenolic acids, alkaloids, saponins, polysaccharides, and others. The compounds-targets results show that XOD is a major target for UA reduction of plant-based functional foods active ingredients. Besides, except for polysaccharides, other plant-based functional foods active ingredients of plants act on CLUT9 targets and all but saponins on URAT1. Moreover, flavonoids, saponins, and phenolic acids can inhibit the activity of ADA to inhibit the production of UA. In addition, saponins, phenolic acids, and polysaccharides can act on OAT1 targets. Furthermore, among these components, only flavonoids could down-regulate OAT4 and up-regulate OAT3 expression.

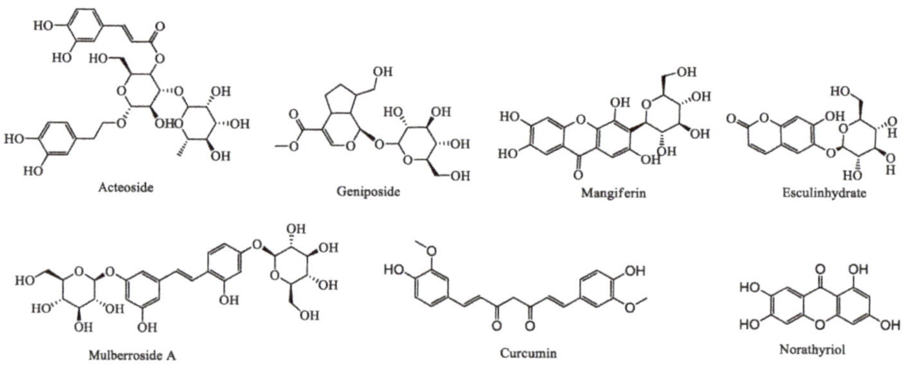

Figure 6. The basic structure of hypouricemic effects from other bioactive components in plant-based functional foods.

Table 6. Experiment and mechanism of other bioactive components from plant-based functional foods on Hyperuricemia.

Source	Bioactive Compound	Model	Dose	Effects	Mechanisms	Ref.
Camellia sinensis L./Green tea	Green tea polyphenols	P	600 mg/kg	Decreased SUA and increased excretion of exceeding UA significantly	It can inhibit XOD activities	[101]
Plantago asiatica L./Plantaginis Semen	Acteoside	D	200 mg/kg	UA and creatinine levels were obviously reduced and the activity of hepatic XOD was inhibited. Furthermore, the mRNA expression of URAT1 and GLUT9 were obviously down-regulated	The mechanism of lowering SUA level can inhibit XOD activity and down-regulate the mRNA expression of URAT1 and GLUT9	[99, 102]
Morus alba L./Mori Cortex	Mulberroside A	C	10, 20 and 40 mg/kg	Decreased SUA level and increased urinary UA excretion and fractional excretion of UA. Furthermore, down-regulated mRNA and protein levels of mGLUT9 and mURAT1, and upregulating mRNA and protein levels of mOAT1, mOCT1, mOCT2, mOCTN1, and mOCTN2	Hypouricemic effect is achieved by down-regulating mRNA and protein levels of mGLUT9 and mURAT1, and upregulating mRNA and protein levels of mOAT1 to promote UA excretion	[103]
Cichorium intybus L./Chicory	Esculinhydrate	M	50 and 150 mg/kg	SUA level significantly increased, XOD and ADA levels showed different degrees of inhibition	This is related to down-regulation the expression of mURAT1 to promote UA excretion	[76]
Gardenia jasminoides Ellis/Cape Jasmine	Geniposide	B	50 and 100 mg/kg	The protein and mRNA expression of URAT1 and GLUT9 and serum UA significantly decreased, while 24 h urinary, the protein and mRNA expression of OAT1 were significantly increased	Down-regulated URAT1 and GLUT9, and up-regulated OAT1 to promote UA excretion	[98]
Mangifera indica L./Mango	Mangiferin	B	6 mg/kg	SUA and the protein expression of URAT1, and GLUT9 were significantly decreased, while 24 h urinary creatinine, the expression of mABCG2 were significantly increased	This is related to down-regulation the protein expression of URAT1, GLUT9 and up-regulation the expression of ABCG2 to promote UA excretion	[104, 105]
Mangifera indica L./Mango	Norathyriol	O	4 mg/kg	Decreased SUA and markedly increased the fractional excretion of UA	The mechanism of lowering SUA can inhibit XOD activity and up-regulated OAT1.	[106]
Curcuma longa L./Turmeric	Curcumin	G	20 and 40 mg/kg	Decreased SUA markedly increased	The mechanism of lowering SUA can inhibit XOD activity	[107, 108]

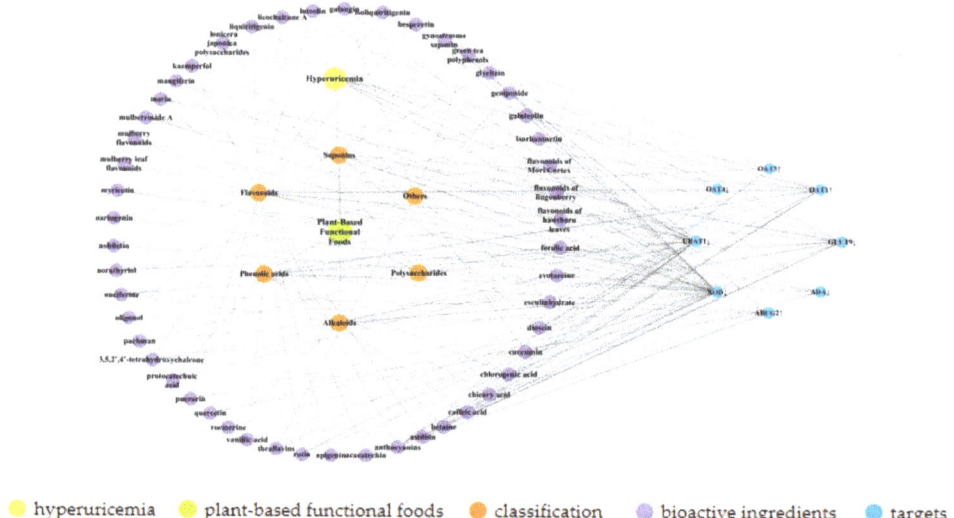

Figure 7. The hypouricemic effects on the compounds–targets network from the plant-based functional foods.

3. Uric Acid Reduction Effects of Plant-Based Functional Foods

As mentioned above, the bioactive components of plant-based functional foods prevent UA disorders by inhibiting the enzyme responsible for UA production, by enhancing the excretion of UA, and by preventing its reabsorption. These mechanisms of action are summarized as follows.

3.1. Inhibition of Uric Acid Production

XOD and ADA are key enzymes that catalyze the production of UA. XOD catalyzes the oxidation of hypoxanthine to xanthine and xanthine to UA [16]. ADA plays a key role in indirectly catalyzing the formation of UA [17]. Thus, inhibiting UA synthesis through XOD and ADA inhibition can be considered a therapeutic target to reduce the level of UA in the body. Indeed, in vitro and animal studies have indicated that bioactive components of plant-based functional foods could inhibit XOD and ADA. Notably, increasing molecular docking studies have revealed that polyphenols could bind to an amino acid of XOD and enter the molybdopterin center to form a complex, effectively inhibiting XOD [109]. Further studies have shown that flavonoids and phenolic acids not only exhibit good XOD inhibitory activities, but also present a certain ability to scavenge oxygen free radicals, which can alleviate the damage caused to the body by peroxides generated by XOD [110].

Luteolin is mainly present in *L. japonica* Thunb. and *Dendranthema morifolium* (Ramat.) Tzvel., and exhibits its anti-HUA effect by inhibiting the excess production of UA [111]. Hao et al. showed that the intragastric administration of luteolin (20, 40, and 80 mg/kg) to potassium oxonate-induced HUA mice for seven days reduced the levels of UA and XOD in a dose-dependent manner. Compared with the model group, the high-dose group showed significantly reduced levels of SUA, XOD, BUN, and Scr ($p < 0.01$) [53]. In another study, Yan et al. found that luteolin presents a competitive inhibitory effect on XOD. They postulated that the mechanism of this activity involves luteolin binding to amino acids in the active site of XOD at a single binding site, which is mainly driven by hydrophobic interactions. Molecular docking results revealed that a combination of luteolin and XOD changed the conformation of XOD, and inhibited the synthesis of UA [112], thereby confirming the XOD inhibition activity and hypouricemic effects of luteolin.

Lipid emulsion-induced HUA rats have been used to study the effects of GPS on lowering UA levels. In this study, the low (15 mg/kg) and high dosage groups (60 mg/kg) presented dramatically reduced SUA levels ($p < 0.01$, $p < 0.05$), whereby the UA level was close to normal for the high dosage group ($p < 0.01$). Moreover, the serum and liver levels of XOD and ADA also decreased ($p < 0.05$). These results confirmed that GPS significantly reduced the production of UA through inhibition of the XOD and ADA activities [90].

Galangin extracted from *Rhizoma Alpiniae* was used to treat HUA mice, with high and medium dose groups (300 and 150 mg/kg) resulting in lower UA levels than for the model group ($p < 0.05$), and a significantly decreased XOD activity for the high dose group ($p < 0.05$) [113]. Recently, Zhang et al. reported the XO inhibitory mechanism of galangin, predicting that galangin could enter the Mo center and occupy the catalytic center of XOD to inhibit the activity of XOD, thereby preventing xanthine from entering the active center to block the generation of UA [114].

3.2. Regulation of the Renal Uric Acid Transporter

Physiologically, UA production and excretion are in a dynamic balance. However, when UA excretion is reduced and excess UA is produced, thereby leading to HUA [98]. As a result, promoting the excretion of UA could be an effective means to treat HUA. In the process of promoting excretion, UA relies on the cooperative excretion of multiple transporters on the proximal tubular epithelial cells of the apical and basolateral membranes [22]. In addition, various studies have confirmed that the reabsorption of UA can be categorized into two steps, namely UA uptake into renal tubular epithelial cells through the anion transporters *SLC22A12* (URAT1) and *SLC22A11* (OAT4), and release into the blood through the anion transporter SLC2A9 (GLUT9) from the renal tubular epithelial basolateral membrane [23–25]. GLUT9 has two splice variants, which are GLUT9a and GLUT9b. GLUT9a of the renal tubular epithelial cell basolateral membranes is responsible for UA reabsorption, while URAT1 and OAT4, localized in the apical membrane of proximal tubules, also control renal urate reabsorption. In contrast, organic anion transporters on the basolateral membrane of renal proximal tubules (e.g., *SLC22A6* (OAT1) and *SLC22A8* (OAT3)), in addition to GLUT9b on the apical membrane of proximal tubules, play an important role in the secretion of UA [22].

Numerous studies have demonstrated that the bioactive components of plant-based functional foods increase UA elimination by up-regulating (OAT1, OAT3) and down-regulating (URAT1, OAT4, and GLUT9) UA transporters in the kidneys [33]. They also improve renal function by regulating the transport and excretion of organic cations (OCTs) and carnitine transporters (OCTNs) in the kidneys [115,116], and so are likely to be important agents in the treatment of HUA.

Theaflavins are important functional ingredients in black tea. Among them, studies have shown that the three theaflavin monomer, namely theaflavin (TF), theaflavin-3-gallate (TF-3-G), and theaflavin-3-3′-gallate (TFDG) exhibit significant hypouricemic effects on HUA mice. Compared with the model group, the TF (20, 50, and 100 mg/kg), TFDG (50 and 100 mg/kg), and TF-3-G (100 mg/kg) groups notably decreased SUA levels ($p < 0.01$), while TFDG (20 mg/kg) and TF-3-G (50 mg/kg) also clearly reduced the SUA levels ($p < 0.05$). These results indicated that the hypouricemic effect of TF was superior to those of TFDG and TF-3-G at the same dosage. With the exceptions of TFDG (20 mg/kg) and TF-3-G (20 mg/kg), BUN was also reduced in other treatment dose groups ($p < 0.01$), while TF(20 mg/kg), TFDG (20 and 50 mg/kg), and TF-3-G (20, 50, and 100 mg/kg) also decreased Scr ($p < 0.001$). These components could, therefore, treat renal damage in HUA mice by decreasing BUN and Scr levels. In addition, they down-regulated the expression of the genes and proteins of GLUT9 and URAT1, while up-regulating the gene and protein expression of OCTN1, OCT1, OCT2, OAT1, and OAT2 [117]. These findings indicated that TF, TFDG, and TF-3-G could exhibit potential application prospects in the prevention and therapy of HUA.

The effects of licochalcone A from the *Glycyrrhiza uralensis* Fisch were also investigated in a 60 mice model of HUA induced by potassium oxonate and xanthine. The results indicated that licochalcone A can significantly reduce the level of SUA of HUA mice, increase the excretion of UA, and reduce the level of Scr and BUN. Besides, licochalcone A can notably inhibit the transport activity of OAT4 [55]. Besides, a further study has also investigated the effect of green tea polyphenols (GTP) on potassium oxonate-induced HUA mice, and explored the underlying mechanisms of action. It was reported that GTP significantly decreased the SUA levels of HUA mice in a dose-dependent manner ($p < 0.05$), while GTP dosages of 300 and 600 mg/kg markedly reduced the XOD activities in the serum and liver of HUA mice ($p < 0.05$). Furthermore, these dosages reduced the expression of URAT1 ($p < 0.05$), as well as increasing the expression of OAT1 and OAT3 in the kidneys ($p < 0.01$). Overall, the results suggested that GTP reduced UA levels by inhibiting UA production and increasing its excretion [101].

Furthermore, to examine the lowering UA effects of rutin from Sophora japonica (*Sophora japonica* L.), a potassium oxonate-induced HUA model was established in mice. HUA mice were randomly divided into six groups. Compared to that in control mice, treatment with rutin (50, and 100 mg/kg) caused significant reduction SUA, Scr, and BUN, serum and kidney uromodulin levels, while elevating UA excretion in HUA mice. Further, rutin was administered orally 1 h, significantly downregulated mRNA and protein levels of mice GLUT9 and URAT1, and upregulated mRNA and protein levels of OAT1 and OCTs in the kidney of HUA mice. In conclusion, rutin exerted its hypouricemic and renal function improvement by the regulation of renal organic ion transporters [64].

In addition, the SLC2A9 and SLC22A12 are mentioned as genes that have been found to play a role in regulating SUA concentrations through urate reabsorption. However, genetic variants in SLC22A12 and SLC2A9 can result in hereditary renal hypouricemia 1 and 2, leading to severe hypouricemia [118]. In the study, hypouricemia reflected excessive UA excretion, which may lead to UA stones and acute renal failure. In everyday life, people with hypouricemia should eat more foods rich in antioxidants, such as glutathione, vitamin E, vitamin C, etc. At present, vitamin C and E have been isolated in plant-based functional foods. For example, Vitamin C is found in blueberries. Moreover, sea buckthorn berry is rich in vitamins C and E [119–121]. Therefore, these plant functional foods may also have the potential to prevent hypouricemia.

3.3. Enhancement in Intestinal UA Secretion

Similar to the kidneys, the intestines also play an important role in the excretion of UA. To maintain normal daily body UA levels, approximately two-thirds of UA is eliminated through the kidneys while the other third is eliminated by the intestinal pathway [122]. Urate transport is a complex process involving several transmembrane proteins that promote reabsorption (e.g., URAT1, GLUT9) and secretion (ABCG2). ABCG2 plays a significant role in regulating UA transport in the gastrointestinal tract and is a high-capacity urate transporter that is most active in the jejunum and the ileum [123]. It plays a crucial role in renal urate overload and extra-renal urate underexcretion. ABCG2 dysfunction leads to the blockade of renal and intestinal urate excretion, thereby inducing HUA due to a renal urate overload and its overflow into the kidney. The ABCG2 population-attributable percentage risk for HUA has been reported to be 29.2%, which is significantly higher than those with more typical environmental risks [124]. Stiburkova et al. studied 58 patients with primary HUA and 176 patients with gout in the Czech Republic, among whom 17 patients with HUA and 14 patients with gout were pediatric-onset patients. At the same time, 115 cases of normal anemia control group were compared. Fifteen ABCG2 exons were amplified and sequenced. The chi-square fitting test was used to compare the small allele frequencies, and the logarithmic rank test was employed to compare the empirical distribution functions. The obtained results suggested that genetic factors affecting the ABCG2 function should be considered routinely in the diagnosis of hyperuricemia/gout, especially in pediatric patients [123].

However, the mechanisms involved in the elimination of UA from the intestine remain unclear. To date, only a few studies have shown that ABCG2 is the main UA transporter to maintain serum UA levels, with its most active expression being in the jejunum and the ileum [125].

In addition, Morimoto et al. found that the expression of ABCG2 in an HUA rat group was up-regulated in the intestinal villi and crypt. They confirmed that ABCG2 is involved in the intestinal excretion of UA in humans and rats as an extrarenal excretion pathway, thereby providing some clarification regarding UA metabolism along the intestine by focusing on a novel UA exporter, ABCG2 [126]. Furthermore, Wang et al. [127] confirmed that chicory extract ameliorates intestinal UA elimination by modulating the ABCG2 transporter. In 10% fructose-induced HUA rats, the administration of chicory water extract (6.6 g/kg) significantly reduced SUA levels, and significantly increased intestinal UA excretion ($p < 0.05$). Compared with the model group, ABCG2 was up-regulated on the jejunum and the ileum. Further research showed that chicory can significantly increase ABCG2 mRNA expression to reduce UA levels in the jejunum and ileum.

4. Conclusions and Future Perspectives

HUA can lead to life-threatening disorders that are rapidly increasing in frequency worldwide, and so the consumption of functional foods could be considered an alternative to medication to prevent or treat HUA. In this context, plant-based functional foods are of particular interest since they contain thousands of naturally beneficial phytochemicals. Numerous in vitro and in vivo experiments have therefore been conducted to elucidate the mechanism by which these plant-based foods lower UA levels, whereby active ingredients such as flavonoids, phenolic acids, and alkaloids reduce the production of UA or promote its excretion. Indeed, it was confirmed that plant-based functional foods are very helpful for the management of UA disorders; however, these studies have their limitations. For example, although animal models can fully reflect the pharmacological actions and metabolic processes of active ingredients, rapid and simple screening is challenging due to the long cycle, and current animal models are limited due to differences in the UA metabolism in humans and animals. In addition, the majority of in vitro experiments carried out to date mainly screen for XOD inhibition, and there is a lack of comprehensive animal model base studies. Furthermore, the anti-HUA effects of many plants have been examined without the determination of the bioactive compounds responsible for their activities, and there is a lack of substantial clinical data and dose-toxicity data to support the applicability of bioactive ingredients in humans. Moreover, there is a lack of relevant research data on intestinal UA elimination by bioactive compounds, and studies focusing on the mechanisms by which such active ingredients act are scarce and vague.

Novel approaches are therefore required to identify bioactive ingredients from plant-based functional foods, evaluate their efficacy in human and animal models, and develop a sustainable and natural means of treating or preventing HUA. In this context, molecular docking technology has been used to elucidate the mechanism and structural characteristics of polyphenols inhibiting XOD, which is of great significance for the development and synthesis of XOD inhibitors for the treatment of HUA. Since the function of the UA transporter is essential for the maintenance of normal UA levels, further studies into the function of the UA transporter will provide a new strategy for the treatment of HUA and related diseases. In addition, the intestinal tract should be investigated in further detail as a new route to UA secretion, providing a potential new target for the development of natural drugs against HUA. In combination with clinical trials, a comprehensive study into the bioactive ingredients present in plant-based functional foods is necessary, and the diets of patients at high risk from suffering high UA levels should be altered. In conclusion, a large number of studies have confirmed that many biologically active compounds from plant-based functional foods possess anti-HUA activities, which therefore provides a theoretical basis for the synthesis of novel anti-HUA drugs, and suggests the potential of plant-based functional foods for the future prevention and management of HUA.

Author Contributions: Conceptualization, M.-H.L., J.-H.W., and L.-L.J. Writing—original draft preparation, L.-L.J., X.G., M.-Y.J., and C.-C.W. Writing—review and editing, L.-L.J. Supervision, M.-H.L. and J.-H.W. All authors have read and agreed to the published version of the manuscript.

Funding: This research was funded by the National Natural Science Foundation of China (No. 81874336).

Conflicts of Interest: The authors declare no conflict of interest.

References

1. Wang, Y.N.; Zhao, M.; Xin, Y.; Liu, J.J.; Wang, M.; Zhao, C.J. ^{1}H-NMR and MS based metabolomics study of the therapeutic effect of Cortex Fraxini on hyperuricemic rats. *J. Ethnopharmacol.* **2016**, *185*, 272–281. [CrossRef] [PubMed]
2. Zhang, Y.L.; Su, H.; Zhang, J.; Kong, J. The effects of ginsenosides and anserine on the up-regulation of renal aquaporins 1–4 in hyperuricemic mice. *Am. J. Chin. Med.* **2019**, *47*, 1–15. [CrossRef]
3. Corey-Bloom, J.; Haque, A.; Aboufadel, S.; Snell, C.; Fischer, R.S.; Granger, S.W.; Granger, D.A.; Thomas, E.A. Uric acid as a potential peripheral biomarker for disease features in huntington's patients. *Front. Neurosci.* **2020**, *14*, 73. [CrossRef] [PubMed]
4. Brook, R.A.; Forsythe, A.; Smeeding, J.E.; Lawrence Edwards, N. Chronic gout: Epidemiology, disease progression, treatment and disease burden. *Curr. Med. Res. Opin.* **2010**, *26*, 2813–2821. [CrossRef] [PubMed]
5. Xia, Y.; Wu, Q.J.; Wang, H.Y.; Zhang, S.; Jiang, Y.T.; Gong, T.T.; Xu, X.; Chang, Q.; Niu, K.J.; Zhao, Y. Global, regional and national burden of gout, 1990–2017: A systematic analysis of the Global Burden of Disease Study. *Rheumatology* **2019**, *59*, 1529–1538. [CrossRef]
6. Michael, C.X.; Yokose, C.; Rai, S.K.; Pillinger, M.H.; Choi, H.K. Contemporary prevalence of gout and hyperuricemia in the united states and decadal trends: The national health and nutrition examination survey 2007–2016. *Arthritis Rheumatol.* **2019**, *71*, 991–999. [CrossRef]
7. Mu, Z.P.; Wang, W.; Wang, J.; Lv, W.S.; Chen, Y.; Wang, F.; Yu, X.L.; Wang, Y.G.; Cheng, B.F.; Wang, Z.C. Predictors of poor response to urate-lowering therapy in patients with gout and hyperuricemia: A post-hoc analysis of a multicenter randomized trial. *Clin. Rheumatol.* **2019**, *38*, 3511–3519. [CrossRef]
8. Chen, S.; Guo, X.F.; Dong, S.Y.; Yu, S.S.; Chen, Y.T.; Zhang, N.J.; Sun, Y.X. Association between the hypertriglyceridemic waist phenotype and hyperuricemia: A cross-sectional study. *Clin. Rheumatol.* **2017**, *36*, 1111–1119. [CrossRef]
9. Ragab, G.; Elshahaly, M.; Bardin, T. Gout: An old disease in new perspective—A review. *J. Adv. Res.* **2017**, *8*, 495–511. [CrossRef]
10. Li, C.G.; Hsieh, M.C.; Chang, S.J. Metabolic syndrome, diabetes, and hyperuricemia. *Curr. Opin. Rheumatol.* **2013**, *25*, 210–216. [CrossRef]
11. Petreski, T.; Ekart, R.; Hojs, R.; Bevc, S. Asymptomatic hyperuricemia and cardiovascular mortality in patients with chronic kidney disease who progress to hemodialysis. *Int. Urol. Nephrol.* **2019**, *51*, 1013–1018. [CrossRef] [PubMed]
12. Liu, F.; Du, G.L.; Song, N.; Ma, Y.T.; Li, X.M.; Gao, X.M.; Yang, Y.N. Hyperuricemia and its association with adiposity and dyslipidemia in Northwest China: Results from cardiovascular risk survey in Xinjiang (CRS 2008–2012). *Lipids Health Dis.* **2019**, *19*, 58. [CrossRef] [PubMed]
13. Jeon, H.J.; Oh, J.; Shin, D.H. Urate-lowering agents for asymptomatic hyperuricemia in stage 3–4 chronic kidney disease: Controversial role of kidney function. *PLoS ONE* **2019**, *14*, e0218510. [CrossRef] [PubMed]
14. Guo, L.F.; Chen, X.; Lei, S.S.; Li, B.; Zhang, N.Y.; Ge, H.Z.; Yang, K.; Lv, G.Y.; Chen, S.H. Effects and mechanisms of Dendrobium officinalis six nostrum for treatment of hyperuricemia with hyperlipidemia. *Evid. Based Complement. Altern. Med.* **2020**, *2020*, 2914019. [CrossRef] [PubMed]
15. Maiuolo, J.; Oppedisano, F.; Gratteri, S.; Muscoli, C.; Mollace, V. Regulation of uric acid metabolism and excretion. *Int. J. Cardiol.* **2016**, *213*, 8–14. [CrossRef] [PubMed]
16. Chen, C.Y.; Lv, J.M.; Yao, Q. Hyperuricemia-related diseases and xanthine oxidoreductase (XOR) inhibitors: An overview. *Med. Sci. Monit.* **2016**, *22*, 2501–2512. [CrossRef]
17. Han, S.; Wei, R.H.; Han, D.; Zhu, J.X.; Luo, W.Z.; Ao, W.; Zhong, G.Y. Hypouricemic effects of extracts from Urtica *hyperborea* Jacq. ex Wedd. in hyperuricemia mice through XOD, URAT1, and OAT1. *BioMed Res. Int.* **2020**, *2020*, 1–8. [CrossRef]
18. Liu, X.R.; Huang, S.S.; Xu, W.D.; Zhou, A.J.; Li, H.; Zhang, R.; Liu, Y.; Yang, Y.; Jia, H. Association of dietary patterns and hyperuricemia: A cross-sectional study of the Yi ethnic group in China. *Food Nutr. Res.* **2018**, *62*, 1380. [CrossRef]
19. Li, R.R.; Yu, K.; Li, C.W. Dietary factors and risk of gout and hyperuricemia: A meta-analysis and systematic review. *Asia. Pac. J. Clin. Nutr.* **2018**, *27*, 1344–1356. [CrossRef]

20. Büsing, F.; Hägele, F.A.; Nas, A.; Döbert, L.V.; Fricker, A.; Dörner, E.; Podlesny, D.; Aschoff, J.; Pöhnl, T.; Schweiggert, R.; et al. High intake of orange juice and cola differently affects metabolic risk in healthy subjects. *Clin. Nutr.* **2018**, *38*, 812–819. [CrossRef]
21. Perez-Ruiz, F.; Dalbeth, N.; Bardin, T. A review of uric acid, crystal deposition disease, and gout. *Adv. Ther.* **2015**, *32*, 31–41. [CrossRef] [PubMed]
22. Ristic, B.; Sikder, M.O.F.; Bhutia, Y.D.; Ganapathy, V. Pharmacologic inducers of the uric acid exporter ABCG2 as potential drugs for treatment of gouty arthritis. *Asian J. Pharm. Sci.* **2020**, *15*, 173–180. [CrossRef] [PubMed]
23. Xu, L.Q.; Shi, Y.F.; Zhuang, S.G.; Liu, N. Recent advances on uric acid transporters. *Oncotarget* **2017**, *8*, 100852–100862. [CrossRef] [PubMed]
24. Tan, P.K.; Liu, S.; Gunic, E.; Miner, J.N. Discovery and characterization of verinurad, a potent and specific inhibitor of URAT1 for the treatment of hyperuricemia and gout. *Sci. Rep.* **2017**, *7*, 665. [CrossRef] [PubMed]
25. DeBosch, B.J.; Kluth, O.; Fujiwara, H.; Schürmann, A.; Moley, K. Early-onset metabolic syndrome in mice lacking the intestinal uric acid transporter SLC2A9. *Nat. Commun.* **2014**, *5*, 4642. [CrossRef] [PubMed]
26. Liu, N.X.; Wang, Y.; Yang, M.F.; Bian, W.X.; Zeng, L.; Yin, S.G.; Xiong, Z.Q.; Hu, Y.; Wang, S.Y.; Meng, B.L.; et al. New rice-derived short peptide potently alleviated hyperuricemia induced by potassium oxonate in rats. *J. Agric. Food Chem.* **2018**, *67*, 220–228. [CrossRef]
27. Gliozzi, M.; Malara, N.; Muscoli, S.; Mollace, V. The treatment of hyperuricemia. *Int. J. Cardiol.* **2016**, *213*, 23–27. [CrossRef]
28. Pinela, J.; Carocho, M.; Dias, M.I.; Caleja, C.; Barros, L.; Ferreira, I.C.F.R. Wild plant-based functional foods, drugs, and nutraceuticals. *Wild Plants Mushrooms Nuts.* **2016**, 315–351. [CrossRef]
29. Kumar, A.; Mosa, K.A.; Ji, L.Y.; Kage, U.; Dhokane, D.; Karre, S.; Madalageri, D.; Pathania, N. Metabolomics assisted biotechnological interventions for developing plant-based functional foods and nutraceuticals. *Crit. Rev. Food. Sci. Nutr.* **2018**, *58*, 1791–1807. [CrossRef]
30. Ji, M.Y.; Bo, A.; Yang, M.; Xu, J.F.; Jiang, L.L.; Zhou, B.C.; Li, M.H. The pharmacological effects and health benefits of *Platycodon grandiflorus*-A medicine food homology species. *Foods* **2020**, *9*, 142. [CrossRef]
31. Gong, X.; Ji, M.Y.; Xu, J.P.; Zhang, C.H.; Li, M.H. Hypoglycemic effects of bioactive ingredients from medicine food homology and medicinal health food species used in China. *Crit. Rev. Food Sci. Nutr.* **2019**, 1–24. [CrossRef] [PubMed]
32. Badimon, L.; Vilahur, G.; Padro, T. Nutraceuticals and atherosclerosis: Human trials. *Cardiovasc. Ther.* **2010**, *28*, 202–215. [CrossRef] [PubMed]
33. Mehmood, A.; Zhao, L.; Wang, C.T.; Nadeem, M.; Raza, A.; Ali, N.; Shah, A.A. Management of hyperuricemia through dietary polyphenols as a natural medicament: A comprehensive review. *Crit. Rev. Food Sci.* **2019**, *59*, 1433–1455. [CrossRef]
34. Arimboor, R.; Arumughan, C. Effect of polymerization on antioxidant and xanthine oxidase inhibitory potential of sea buckthorn (*H. rhamnoides*) proanthocyanidins. *J. Food Sci.* **2012**, *77*, C1036–C1041. [CrossRef] [PubMed]
35. Ji, M.Y.; Gong, X.; Li, X.; Wang, C.C.; Li, M.H. Advanced research on the antioxidant activity and mechanism of polyphenols from *Hippophae* Species—A Review. *Molecules* **2020**, *25*, 917. [CrossRef]
36. Chen, L.; Li, M.; Wu, J.L.; Li, J.X.; Ma, Z.C. Effect of lemon water soluble extract on hyperuricemia in mouse model. *Food Funct.* **2019**, *10*, 6000–6008. [CrossRef]
37. Kapinova, A.; Stefanicka, P.; Kubatka, P.; Zubor, P.; Uramova, S.; Kello, M.; Mojzis, J.; Blahutova, D.; Qaradakhi, T.; Zulli, A.; et al. Are plant-based functional foods better choice against cancer than single phytochemicals? A critical review of current breast cancer research. *Biomed. Pharmacother.* **2017**, *96*, 1465–1477. [CrossRef]
38. Lin, S.Y.; Zhang, G.W.; Liao, Y.J.; Pan, J.H. Inhibition of chrysin on xanthine oxidase activity and its inhibition mechanism. *Int. J. Biol. Macromol.* **2015**, *81*, 274–282. [CrossRef]
39. Patra, J.C.; Chua, B.H. Artificial neural network-based drug design for diabetes mellitus using flavonoids. *J. Comput. Chem.* **2011**, *32*, 555–567. [CrossRef]
40. Lin, S.Y.; Zhang, G.W.; Liao, Y.J.; Pan, J.H. Dietary flavonoids as xanthine oxidase inhibitors: Structure-Affinity and Structure-Activity relationships. *J. Agric. Food Chem.* **2015**, *63*, 7784–7794. [CrossRef]
41. Lin, C.M.; Chen, C.S.; Chen, C.T.; Liang, Y.C.; Lin, J.K. Molecular modeling of flavonoids that inhibits xanthine oxidase. *Biochem. Biophys. Res. Commun.* **2002**, *294*, 167–172. [CrossRef]

42. Cheng, L.C.; Murugaiyah, V.; Chan, K.L. Flavonoids and phenylethanoid glycosides from Lippia nodiflora as promising antihyperuricemic agents and elucidation of their mechanism of action. *J. Ethnopharmacol.* **2015**, *176*, 485–493. [CrossRef] [PubMed]
43. Montoro, P.; Braca, A.; Pizza, C.; De Tommasi, N. Structure-antioxidant activity relationships of flavonoids isolated from different plant species. *Food Chem.* **2005**, *92*, 349–355. [CrossRef]
44. Wang, C.P.; Wang, X.; Zhang, X.; Shi, Y.W.; Liu, L.; Kong, L.D. Morin improves urate excretion and kidney function through regulation of renal organic ion transporters in hyperuricemic mice. *J. Pharm. Pharm. Sci.* **2010**, *13*, 411–427. [CrossRef] [PubMed]
45. Xing, Z.H.; Ma, Y.C.; Li, X.P.; Zhang, B.; Zhang, M.D.; Wan, S.M.; Yang, X.; Yang, T.F.; Jiang, J.W.; Bao, R. Research progress of puerarin and its derivatives on anti-inflammatory and anti-gout activities. *China J. Chin. Mater. Med.* **2017**, *42*, 3703–3708. [CrossRef]
46. Xie, K.L.; Li, Z.H.; Dong, X.Z.; Gong, M.X. Research progress of quercetin on inhibiting the activity of xanthine oxidase. *Lishizhen Med. Mater. Med. Res.* **2019**, *30*, 2223–2225. [CrossRef]
47. Shi, Y.L.; Williamson, G. Quercetin lowers plasma uric acid in pre-hyperuricaemic males: A randomised, double-blinded, placebo-controlled, cross-over trial. *Brit. J. Nutr.* **2016**, *115*, 800–806. [CrossRef]
48. Zhang, C.; Wang, R.; Zhang, G.W.; Gong, D.M. Mechanistic insights into the inhibition of quercetin on xanthine oxidase. *Int. J. Biol. Macromol.* **2018**, *112*, 405–412. [CrossRef] [PubMed]
49. Zhang, Z.C.; Su, G.H.; Luo, C.L.; Pang, Y.L.; Wang, L.; Li, X.; Zhang, J.L. Effects of anthocyanins from purple sweet potato (Ipomoea batatas L. cultivar Eshu No. 8) on the serum uric acid level and xanthine oxidase activity in hyperuricemic mice. *Food Funct.* **2015**, *6*, 3045–3055. [CrossRef]
50. Qian, X.Y.; Wang, X.; Luo, J.; Liu, Y.; Pang, J.; Zhang, H.Y.; Xu, Z.L.; Xie, J.W.; Jiang, X.W.; Ling, W. Hypouricemic and nephroprotective roles of anthocyanins in hyperuricemic mice. *Food Funct.* **2019**, *10*, 867–878. [CrossRef]
51. Meehmood, A.; Zhao, L.; Chengtao, W.; Hossen, I.; Raka, R.N.; Zhang, H. Stevia residue extract increases intestinal uric acid excretion via interacting with intestinal urate transporters in hyperuricemic mice. *Food Funct.* **2019**, *10*, 7900–7912. [CrossRef]
52. Miao, M.X.; Wang, X.; Lu, Y.; Wang, X. Mechanism Study on effects of apigenin on reducing uric acid and renal protection in oteracil potassium-induced hyperuricemia mice. *China Pharm.* **2016**, *27*, 4794–4796. [CrossRef]
53. Hao, Y.; Jiao, A.N.; Yu, M.; Gao, J.Z.; He, X.; Zhang, M.H.; Jiao, L.Q.; Zhang, J. Activity screening of thirty flavonoids on the inhibition of xanthine oxidase. *Chin. Tradit. Pat. Med.* **2019**, *41*, 55–59. [CrossRef]
54. Zhao, R.; Chen, D.; Wu, H.L. Pu-erh ripened tea resists to hyperuricemia through xanthine oxidase and renal urate transporters in hyperuricemic mice. *J. Funct. Foods.* **2017**, *29*, 201–207. [CrossRef]
55. Wang, Z.; Ci, X.Y.; Cui, T.; Wei, Z.H.; Zhang, H.B.; Liu, R.; Li, Y.Z.; Yi, X.L.; Zhang, T.J.; Gu, Y.; et al. Effects of Chinese herb ingredients with different properties on OAT4, URAT1 and serum uric acid level in acute hyperuricemia mice. *Chin. Trad. Herb. Drugs* **2019**, *50*, 1157–1163. [CrossRef]
56. Wang, H.Q.; Zhan, J.; Wang, X.B.; Zou, L. Research progress in treatment of hyperuricemia with active ingredients of traditional Chinese medicine. *Chin. J. Pharmacol. Toxicol.* **2015**, *29*, 471–476. [CrossRef]
57. Wang, M.; Zhao, J.; Zhang, N.; Chen, J.H. Astilbin improves potassium oxonate-induced hyperuricemia and kidney injury through regulating oxidative stress and inflammation response in mice. *Biomed. Pharm.* **2016**, *83*, 975–988. [CrossRef] [PubMed]
58. Shi, K.; Zhang, R.T.; Shang, X.Y.; Wang, N.; Li, S.; Zhang, Z.S. Effect of puerarin on serum uric acid in hyperuricemic rat. *Food Sci. Technol.* **2014**, *39*, 216–220. [CrossRef]
59. Pu, J.Y.; Niu, Y.F.; Gao, L.H.; Lin, H.; Tu, C.X.; Li, L. Effects of 3,5,2′,4′-tetrahydroxychalcone on urate excretion in hyperuricemic mice. *Chin. Pharmacol. Bull.* **2015**, *31*, 1091–1095. [CrossRef]
60. Dang, Y.X.; Liang, D.L.; Zhou, X.X.; Qin, Y.; Gao, Y.; Li, W.M. Protective effect of Mori Cortex on kidney in rats with hyperlipidemia and hyperuricemia based on molecular docking technique. *Chin. Trad. Herb. Drugs* **2019**, *50*, 1175–1181. [CrossRef]
61. Zhang, H.C.; Zhang, Y.; Lv, G.F.; Wang, E.P.; Chen, X. The puerarin impact on the expression of ABCG2 in human renal proximal tubule epithelial cells. *SH J. TCM Mar.* **2016**, *50*, 74–77. [CrossRef]
62. Wang, K.; Wang, R.P.; Li, J.; Zhao, D.; Wang, J.Q.; Ran, X.; Qu, W.J. The preventive and therapeutic effects of mulberry leaf flavonoids on adenine induced hyperuricemia and kidney injury in rats. *Nat. Prod. Res. Dev.* **2012**, *24*, 172–175, 202. [CrossRef]

63. Zhang, Z.G.; Yang, H. Effects of total flavone of hawthorn leaf on serum uric acid and vascular endothelial cell function in hyperuricemia rats. *Chin. J. Exp. Trad. Med. Formulae* **2012**, *18*, 259–261. [CrossRef]
64. Liu, J.L.; Li, L.Y.; He, G.H.; Zhang, X.; Song, X.H.; Cui, G.L.; Liao, S.Q. Quality evaluation of Flos Sophorae Immaturus from different habitats by HPLC coupled with chemometrics and anti-oxidant ability. *Chin. Trad. Herb. Drugs* **2018**, *49*, 4644–4652. [CrossRef]
65. Chen, Y.S.; Hu, Q.H.; Zhang, X.; Zhu, Q.; Kong, L.D. Beneficial effect of rutin on oxonate-induced hyperuricemia and renal dysfunction in mice. *Pharmacology* **2013**, *92*, 75–83. [CrossRef] [PubMed]
66. Adachi, S.I.; Kondo, S.; Sato, Y.; Yoshizawa, F.; Yagasaki, K. Anti-hyperuricemic effect of isorhamnetin in cultured hepatocytes and model mice: Structure-activity relationships of methylquercetins as inhibitors of uric acid production. *Cytotechnology* **2019**, *71*, 181–192. [CrossRef] [PubMed]
67. Liu, K.; Wang, W.; Guo, B.H.; Gao, H.; Liu, Y.; Liu, X.H.; Yao, H.L.; Cheng, K. Chemical evidence for potent xanthine oxidase inhibitory activity of ethyl acetate extract of *Citrus aurantium* L. dried immature fruits. *Molecules* **2016**, *21*, 302. [CrossRef] [PubMed]
68. Umamaheswari, M.; Madeswaran, A.; Asokkumar, K. Virtual screening analysis and in-vitro xanthine oxidase inhibitory activity of some commercially available flavonoids. *Iran. J. Pharm. Res.* **2013**, *12*, 317–323. [CrossRef]
69. Yu, S.H.; Song, H.P.; Gao, W.; Zhang, H. Study on the inhibitory activity of flavonoids in *Carthami Flos* on xanthine oxidase. *Chin. J. Ethnomed. Ethnopharm.* **2017**, *26*, 23–26.
70. González-Castejón, M.; Rodriguez-Casado, A. Dietary phytochemicals and their potential effects on obesity: A review. *Pharmacol. Res.* **2011**, *64*, 438–455. [CrossRef]
71. Irondi, E.A.; Agboola, S.O.; Oboh, G.; Boligon, A.A.; Athayde, M.L.; Shode, F.O. Guava leaves polyphenolics-rich extract inhibits vital enzymes implicated in gout and hypertension in vitro. *J. Intercult. Ethnopharm.* **2016**, *5*, 122–130. [CrossRef] [PubMed]
72. Zhu, C.S.; Zhang, B.; Lin, Z.J.; Bai, Y.F. Pharmacodynamics authentication research on uric acid-lowering active ingredients of *Cichorium intybus* L. *China J. Trad. Chin. Med. Pharm.* **2018**, *33*, 4933–4936.
73. Zhu, C.S.; Lin, Z.J.; Zhang, B.; Wang, H.B.; Wang, X.J.; Niu, H.J.; Wang, Y.; Niu, A.Z. Spectrum-effect relationships on uric acid lowering effect of *Cichorium intybus*. *Chin. Trad. Herb. Drugs* **2015**, *46*, 3386–3389. [CrossRef]
74. Zhao, M.M.; Zhu, D.S.; Sun-Waterhouse, D.X.; Su, G.W.; Lin, L.Z.; Wang, X.; Dong, Y. In vitro and in vivo studies on adlay-derived seed extracts: Phenolic profiles, antioxidant activities, serum uric acid suppression, and xanthine oxidase inhibitory effects. *J. Agric. Food Chem.* **2014**, *62*, 7771–7778. [CrossRef] [PubMed]
75. Wan, Y.; Wang, F.; Zou, B.; Shen, Y.F.; Li, Y.Z.; Zhang, A.X.; Fu, G.M. Molecular mechanism underlying the ability of caffeic acid to decrease uric acid levels in hyperuricemia rats. *J. Funct. Foods.* **2019**, *57*, 150–156. [CrossRef]
76. Zhu, C.S.; Lin, Z.J.; Zhang, B.; Bai, Y.F. Uric acid-lowering active ingredients and mechanism of *Cichorium intybus*. *Chin. Trad. Herb. Drugs* **2017**, *48*, 957–961. [CrossRef]
77. Qiu, S.; Sun, H.; Zhang, A.H.; Xu, H.Y.; Yan, G.L.; Han, Y.; Wang, X.J. Natural alkaloids: Basic aspects, biological roles, and future perspectives. *Chin. J. Nat. Med.* **2014**, *12*, 401–406. [CrossRef]
78. Zou, L.; Feng, F.Q. Research progress of uric acid-lowering bioactive compounds in food and their mechanisms. *Sci. Technol. Food Ind.* **2019**, *40*, 352–357, 364. [CrossRef]
79. Sang, M.M.; Du, G.Y.; Hao, J.; Wang, L.L.; Liu, E.W.; Zhang, Y.; Wang, T.; Gao, X.M.; Han, L. Modeling and optimizing inhibitory activities of Nelumbinis folium extract on xanthine oxidase using response surface methodology. *J. Pharm. Biomed.* **2017**, *139*, 37–43. [CrossRef]
80. Wang, M.X.; Liu, Y.L.; Yang, Y.; Zhang, D.M.; Kong, L.D. Nuciferine restores potassium oxonate-induced hyperuricemia and kidney inflammation in mice. *Eur. J. Pharmacol.* **2015**, *747*, 59–70. [CrossRef]
81. Tao, Z.Y.; Cheng, Y.; Tang, Y.; Tan, Y.M.; Li, J. Effect of evodiamine on the animal model of Hyperuricemia. *Pharm. Clin. Chin. Mater. Med.* **2014**, *5*, 69–71.
82. Song, Y.; Li, J.; Cheng, Y.; Lin, Z.; He, B.Y.; Wang, C.Y. Lowering effect of evodiamine dispersible tablets on uric acid in chickens. *Chin. J. New Drugs* **2015**, *24*, 1057–1060.
83. Hu, M.; Liu, J.W.; Song, Y.; Zeng, N. Effect and mechanism study of evodiamine on hyperuricemia model quail. *Pharmacol. Clin. Chin. Mater. Med.* **2014**, *30*, 38–40. [CrossRef]
84. Tan, L.; Ji, T.; Cao, J.Y.; Hu, F.Z. Determination of betaine contents in Fructus Lycii from different origins by dual wavelength TLC scanning. *Nat. Prod. Res. Dev.* **2014**, *26*, 388–391, 397. [CrossRef]

85. Liu, Y.L.; Pan, Y.; Wang, X.; Fan, C.Y.; Zhu, Q.; Li, J.M.; Wang, S.J.; Kong, L.D. Betaine Reduces Serum Uric Acid Levels and Improves Kidney Function in Hyperuricemic Mice. *Planta Med.* **2013**, *80*, 39–47. [CrossRef] [PubMed]
86. Li, P.; Song, Z.B.; Chen, M.M.; Song, J.; Cui, H.X. Research progress of therapeutic drug of hyperuricemia and its action target. *China Mod. Med.* **2018**, *25*, 16–19.
87. Gong, L.X.; Chi, J.W.; Wang, J.; Ren, Y.Q.; Sun, B.G. Research progress on main functional component and action mechanism of *Dioscorea opposita*. *Sci. Technol. Food Ind.* **2019**, *40*, 312–319. [CrossRef]
88. Su, J.X.; Wei, Y.H.; Liu, M.L.; Liu, T.X.; Li, J.H.; Ji, Y.C.; Liang, J.P. Anti-hyperuricemic and nephroprotective effects of *Rhizoma Dioscoreae* septemlobae extracts and its main component dioscin via regulation of mOAT1, mURAT1 and mOCT2 in hypertensive mice. *Arch. Pharm. Res.* **2014**, *37*, 1336–1344. [CrossRef]
89. Shi, S.; Wang, N.; Shang, X.Y.; Zhang, R.T.; Li, S.; Zhang, Z.S. Effect of gypenoside on serum uric acid of hyperuricemic rats. *Nat. Prod. Res. Dev.* **2014**, *26*, 1285–1289, 1315. [CrossRef]
90. Pang, M.X.; Fang, Y.Y.; Chen, S.H.; Zhu, X.X.; Shan, C.W.; Su, J.; Yu, J.J.; Li, B.; Yang, Y.; Chen, B.; et al. Gypenosides inhibits xanthine oxidoreductase and ameliorates urate excretion in hyperuricemic rats induced by high cholesterol and high fat food (Lipid Emulsion). *Med. Sci. Monit.* **2017**, *23*, 1129–1140. [CrossRef]
91. Meng, F.C.; Li, Q.; Qi, Y.M.; He, C.W.; Wang, C.M.; Zhang, Q.W. Characterization and immunoregulatory activity of two polysaccharides from the root of *Ilex asprella*. *Carbohydr. Polym.* **2018**, *197*, 9–16. [CrossRef] [PubMed]
92. Liu, M.; Li, S.S.; Wang, X.X.; Zhu, Y.F.; Zhang, J.J.; Liu, H.; Jia, L. Characterization, anti-oxidation and anti-inflammation of polysaccharides by *Hypsizygus marmoreus* against LPS-induced toxicity on lung. *Int. J. Biol. Macromol.* **2018**, *111*, 121–128. [CrossRef] [PubMed]
93. Yang, Q.X.; Wang, Q.L.; Deng, W.W.; Sun, C.Y.; Wei, Q.Y.; Adu-Frimpong, M.; Shi, J.X.; Yu, J.N.; Xu, X.M. Anti-hyperuricemic and anti-gouty arthritis activities of polysaccharide purified from *Lonicera japonica* in model rats. *Int. J. Biol. Macromol.* **2019**, *123*, 801–809. [CrossRef] [PubMed]
94. Deng, L.J.; Yan, J.X.; Wang, P.; Zhou, Y.; Wu, X.A. Effects of pachman on the expression of renal tubular transporters rURAT1, rOAT1 and rOCT2 of the rats with hyperuricemia. *West. J. Tradit. Chin. Med.* **2019**, *32*, 10–14. [CrossRef]
95. Lanaspa, M.A.; Ishimoto, T.; Cicerchi, C.; Tamura, Y.; Roncal-Jimenez, C.A.; Chen, W.; Johnson, R.J. Endogenous fructose production and fructokinase activation mediate renal injury in diabetic nephropathy. *J. Am. Soc. Nephrol.* **2014**, *25*, 2526–2538. [CrossRef]
96. Lecoultre, V.; Egli, L.; Theytaz, F.; Despland, C.; Schneiter, P.; Tappy, L. Fructose-induced hyperuricemia is associated with a decreased renal uric acid excretion in humans. *Diabetes Care* **2013**, *36*, e149–e150. [CrossRef]
97. Cirillo, P.; Gersch, M.S.; Mu, W.; Scherer, P.M.; Kim, K.M.; Gesualdo, L.; Henderson, G.N.; Johnson, R.J.; Sautin, Y.Y. Ketohexokinase-dependent metabolism of fructose induces proinflammatory mediators in proximal tubular cells. *J. Am. Soc. Nephrol.* **2009**, *20*, 545–553. [CrossRef]
98. Zhou, J.; Sun, C.; Li, F. Research advances in mechanism of active components of traditional Chinese medicine for reducing uric acid. *Chin. Pharmacol. Bull.* **2018**, *34*, 19–22. [CrossRef]
99. Zeng, J.X.; Xu, B.B.; Wang, J.; Bi, Y.; Wang, X.Y.; Zhong, G.Y.; Ren, G.; Zhu, J.X.; Li, M.; Zhu, Y.Y. Hypouricemic effects of acteoside and isoacteoside from *Plantaginis Semen* on mice with acute hyperuricemia and their possible mechanisms. *Chin. Tradit. Pat. Med.* **2016**, *38*, 1449–1454. [CrossRef]
100. Moriwaki, Y.J.; Okuda, C.; Yamamoto, A.; Ka, T.; Tsutsumi, Z.; Takahashi, S.; Yamamoto, T.; Kitadate, K.; Wakame, K. Effects of oligonol, an oligomerized polyphenol formulated from lychee fruit, on serum concentration and urinary excretion of uric acid. *J. Func. Foods* **2011**, *3*, 13–16. [CrossRef]
101. Nugraheni, P.W.; Rahmawati, F.; Mahdi, C.; Prasetyawan, S. Green tea extract (*Camellia sinensis* L.) effects on uric acid levels on hyperuricemia rats (*Rattus norvegicus*). *J. Pure App. Chem. Res.* **2017**, *6*, 246–254. [CrossRef]
102. Huang, C.G.; Shang, Y.J.; Zhang, J.; Zhang, J.R.; Li, W.J.; Jiao, B.H. Hypouricemic effects of phenylpropanoid glycosides acteoside of scrophularia ningpoensis on serum uric acid levels in potassium oxonate-pretreated mice. *Am. J. Chin. Med.* **2008**, *36*, 149–157. [CrossRef] [PubMed]
103. Wang, C.P.; Wang, Y.; Wang, X.; Zhang, X.; Ye, J.F.; Hu, L.S.; Kong, L.D. Mulberroside A possesses potent uricosuric and nephroprotective effects in hyperuricemic mice. *Planta Med.* **2011**, *77*, 786–794. [CrossRef] [PubMed]
104. Xu, X.W.; Niu, Y.F.; Gao, L.H.; Li, L.; Lin, H. Analysis of hypouricemic mechanism of mangiferin based on intestinal urate transporter ABCG2. *Chin. J. Exp. Tradit. Med. Formulae* **2018**, *24*, 145–149. [CrossRef]

105. Yang, H.; Gao, L.H.; Niu, Y.F.; Zhou, Y.F.; Lin, H.; Jiang, J.; Kong, X.F.; Liu, X.; Li, L. Mangiferin inhibits renal urate reabsorption by modulating urate transporters in experimental hyperuricemia. *Biol. Pharm. Bull.* **2015**, *38*, 1591–1598. [CrossRef]
106. Lin, H.; Tu, C.X.; Niu, Y.F.; Li, F.S.; Yuan, L.X.; Li, N.; Xu, A.P.; Gao, L.H.; Li, L. Dual actions of norathyriol as a new candidate hypouricaemic agent: Uricosuric effects and xanthine oxidase inhibition. *Eur. J. Pharmacol.* **2019**, *853*, 371–380. [CrossRef]
107. Chen, Y.E.; Li, C.T.; Duan, S.N.; Yuan, X.; Liang, J.; Hou, S.Z. Curcumin attenuates potassium oxonate-induced hyperuricemia and kidney inflammation in mice. *Biomed. Pharmacother.* **2019**, *118*, 109195. [CrossRef]
108. Ao, G.Z.; Zhou, M.Z.; Li, Y.Y.; Li, S.N.; Wang, H.N.; Wan, Q.W.; Li, H.Q.; Hu, Q.H. Discovery of novel curcumin derivatives targeting xanthine oxidase and urate transporter 1 as anti-hyperuricemic agents. *Bioorg. Med. Chem.* **2017**, *25*, 166–174. [CrossRef]
109. Li, X.Z.; Zheng, L.L.; Ai, B.L.; Zheng, X.Y.; Yang, Y.; Yang, J.S.; Sheng, Z.W. The inhibitory kinetics and mechanism of xanthine oxidase by screened polyphenols. *Food Res. Dev.* **2020**, *41*, 12–19, 97. [CrossRef]
110. Lin, L.; Yang, Q.; Zhao, K.; Zhao, M. Identification of the free phenolic profile of Adlay bran by UPLC-QTOF-MS/MS and inhibitory mechanisms of phenolic acids against xanthine oxidase. *Food Chem.* **2018**, *253*, 108–118. [CrossRef]
111. Lin, L.C.; Pai, Y.F.; Tsai, T.H. Isolation of luteolin and luteolin-7-O-glucoside from *Dendranthema morifolium* Ramat Tzvel and their pharmacokinetics in rats. *J. Agric. Food Chem.* **2015**, *63*, 7700–7706. [CrossRef] [PubMed]
112. Yan, J.; Zhang, G.; Hu, Y.; Ma, Y. Effect of luteolin on xanthine oxidase: Inhibition kinetics and interaction mechanism merging with docking simulation. *Food Chem.* **2013**, *141*, 3766–3773. [CrossRef] [PubMed]
113. Pu, Z.Q.; Wang, Q.L.; Xu, X.M.; Yu, J.N. Separation, purification of galangin and its effect on reducing uric acid. *J. Jiangsu Univ.* **2017**, *27*, 338–343. [CrossRef]
114. Zhang, C.; Zhang, G.W.; Pan, J.H.; Gong, D.M. Galangin competitively inhibits xanthine oxidase by a ping-pong mechanism. *Food Res. Int.* **2016**, *89*, 152–160. [CrossRef]
115. Komazawa, H.; Yamaguchi, H.; Hidaka, K.; Ogura, J.; Kobayashi, M.; Iseki, K. Renal Uptake of substrates for organic anion transporters Oat1 and Oat3 and organic cation transporters Oct1 and Oct2 is altered in rats with adenine-induced chronic renal failure. *J. Pharm. Sci.* **2013**, *102*, 1086–1094. [CrossRef]
116. Nakanishi, T.; Fukushi, A.; Sato, M.; Yoshifuji, M.; Gose, T.; Shirasaka, Y.; Ohe, K.; Kobayashi, M.; Kawai, K.; Tamai, I. Functional characterization of apical transporters expressed in rat proximal tubular cells (PTCs) in primary culture. *Mol. Pharm.* **2011**, *8*, 2142–2150. [CrossRef]
117. Tai, L.L.; Liu, Z.H.; Sun, M.H.; Xie, Q.J.; Cai, X.Q.; Wang, Y.; Dong, X.; Xu, Y. Anti-hyperuricemic effects of three theaflavins isolated from black tea in hyperuricemic mice. *J. Funct. Foods.* **2020**, *66*, 103803. [CrossRef]
118. Yin, Y.C.; Ma, C.C.; Wu, J.; Yu, S.L.; Guo, X.Z.; Hou, L.A.; You, T.T.; Wang, D.C.; Li, H.L.; Xu, T.; et al. Association of SLC22A12 and SLC2A9 genetic polymorphisms with hypouricemia in Ningxia populatio. *Basic Clin. Med.* **2018**, *38*, 638–642. [CrossRef]
119. Liu, D.P. Hypouricemia. *Chin. J. Cardiovasc. Med.* **2016**, *21*, 104–107. [CrossRef]
120. Dong, S.T.; Chen, Y.; Gao, Q.Y. Research progress on bioactive compounds and function of sea buckthorn berry. *Chin. Brew.* **2020**, *39*, 26–32. [CrossRef]
121. Pei, J.B.; Li, X.Y.; Wang, J.H. Study on variation of sugar, acid, vitamin C and pigments contents during fruit development of blueberries. *J. Northeast Agric. Univ.* **2011**, *42*, 76–79. [CrossRef]
122. Mandal, A.K.; Mount, D.B. The molecular physiology of uric acid homeostasis. *Annu. Rev. Physiol.* **2015**, *77*, 323–345. [CrossRef] [PubMed]
123. Stiburkova, B.; Pavelcova, K.; Pavlikova, M.; Ješina, P.; Pavelka, K. The impact of dysfunctional variants of ABCG2 on hyperuricemia and gout in pediatric-onset patients. *Arthritis Res. Ther.* **2019**, *21*. [CrossRef] [PubMed]
124. Nakayama, A.; Matsuo, H.; Nakaoka, H.; Nakamura, T.; Nakashima, H.; Takada, Y.; Oikawa, Y.; Takada, T.; Sakiyama1, M.; Shimizu1, S.; et al. Common dysfunctional variants of ABCG2 have stronger impact on hyperuricemia progression than typical environmental risk factors. *Sci. Rep.* **2014**, *4*, 5227. [CrossRef]
125. Matsuo, H.; Yamamoto, K.; Nakaoka, H.; Nakayama, A.; Sakiyama, M.; Chiba, T. Genome-wide association study of clinically defined gout identifies multiple risk loci and its association with clinical subtypes. *Ann. Rheum. Dis.* **2015**, *75*, 652–659. [CrossRef]

126. Morimoto, C.; Tamura, Y.; Asakawa, S.; Kuribayashi-Okuma, E.; Nemoto, Y.; Li, J.P.; Murase, T.; Nakamura, T.; Hosoyamada, M.; Uchida, S.; et al. ABCG2 expression and uric acid metabolism of the intestine in hyperuricemia model rat. *Nucleosides Nucleotides Nucleic Acids* **2020**, *39*, 744–759. [CrossRef]
127. Wang, Y.; Lin, Z.; Zhang, B.; Nie, A.Z.; Bian, M. *Cichorium intybus* L. promotes intestinal uric acid excretion by modulating ABCG2 in experimental hyperuricemia. *Nut. Metab.* **2017**, *14*, 1–11. [CrossRef]

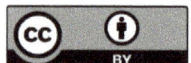

© 2020 by the authors. Licensee MDPI, Basel, Switzerland. This article is an open access article distributed under the terms and conditions of the Creative Commons Attribution (CC BY) license (http://creativecommons.org/licenses/by/4.0/).

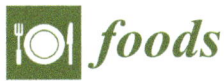

Review

Research Advances on Health Effects of Edible *Artemisia* Species and Some Sesquiterpene Lactones Constituents

Antoaneta Trendafilova [1,*], Laila M. Moujir [2], Pedro M. C. Sousa [3] and Ana M. L. Seca [4,5,*]

1. Institute of Organic Chemistry with Centre of Phytochemistry, Bulgarian Academy of Sciences, Acad. G. Bonchev Str., bl. 9, 1113 Sofia, Bulgaria
2. Department of Biochemistry, Microbiology, Genetics and Cell Biology, Facultad de Farmacia, Universidad de La Laguna, 38206 La Laguna, Tenerife, Spain; lmoujir@ull.edu.es
3. Faculty of Sciences and Technology, University of Azores, 9500-321 Ponta Delgada, Portugal; sdoffich@gmail.com
4. cE3c—Centre for Ecology, Evolution and Environmental Changes/Azorean Biodiversity Group & Faculty of Sciences and Technology, University of Azores, Rua Mãe de Deus, 9500-321 Ponta Delgada, Portugal
5. LAQV-REQUIMTE, University of Aveiro, 3810-193 Aveiro, Portugal
* Correspondence: trendaf@orgchm.bas.bg (A.T.); ana.ml.seca@uac.pt (A.M.L.S.); Tel.: +359-2-960-6144 (A.T.); +351-296-650-174 (A.M.L.S.)

Citation: Trendafilova, A.; Moujir, L.M.; Sousa, P.M.C.; Seca, A.M.L. Research Advances on Health Effects of Edible *Artemisia* Species and Some Sesquiterpene Lactones Constituents. *Foods* 2021, *10*, 65. https://doi.org/10.3390/foods10010065

Received: 27 November 2020
Accepted: 25 December 2020
Published: 30 December 2020

Publisher's Note: MDPI stays neutral with regard to jurisdictional claims in published maps and institutional affiliations.

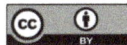

Copyright: © 2020 by the authors. Licensee MDPI, Basel, Switzerland. This article is an open access article distributed under the terms and conditions of the Creative Commons Attribution (CC BY) license (https://creativecommons.org/licenses/by/4.0/).

Abstract: The genus *Artemisia*, often known collectively as "wormwood", has aroused great interest in the scientific community, pharmaceutical and food industries, generating many studies on the most varied aspects of these plants. In this review, the most recent evidence on health effects of edible *Artemisia* species and some of its constituents are presented and discussed, based on studies published until 2020, available in the Scopus, Web of Sciences and PubMed databases, related to food applications, nutritional and sesquiterpene lactones composition, and their therapeutic effects supported by in vivo and clinical studies. The analysis of more than 300 selected articles highlights the beneficial effect on health and the high clinical relevance of several *Artemisia* species besides some sesquiterpene lactones constituents and their derivatives. From an integrated perspective, as it includes therapeutic and nutritional properties, without ignoring some adverse effects described in the literature, this review shows the great potential of *Artemisia* plants and some of their constituents as dietary supplements, functional foods and as the source of new, more efficient, and safe medicines. Despite all the benefits demonstrated, some gaps need to be filled, mainly related to the use of raw *Artemisia* extracts, such as its standardization and clinical trials on adverse effects and its health care efficacy.

Keywords: *Artemisia*; clinical trials; health effects; adverse effects; anticancer; antiparasitic; artemisinin; santonin; achillin; tehranolide

1. Introduction

Artemisia genus (Asteraceae family) comprise more than 2290 plant name records in the "The Plant List" database, being only 530 of these taxa with accepted Latin botanical name [1], which shows how challenging the taxonomy of this genus is. In this review, the complete accepted Latin botanical name, according to the "The Plant List" database, is presented in the first species citation, with an indication of any synonym when the latter is the one mentioned in the original publication. In the remaining citations, the genre name is abbreviated to *A.* and omitted the authority name. The *Artemisia* species are herbs and shrubs, which could be perennial, biennial and annual plants, distributed on all continents except Antarctica, mainly on Northern Hemisphere, with only 25 species on the Southern Hemisphere [2], being the Asian the zone where higher species diversity is concentrated [3,4]. They exhibit a great ability to grow on different ecosystems from the sea level to the mountains and from arid areas to wet regions, but the majority of the species live on temperate zones [2]. This ability contributed very significantly to the fact that some species of *Artemisia*, although originating in a specific zone, are now widely distributed. For example, *Artemisia vulgaris* L. is native to Europe and Asia but has now a large distribution in natural habitats worldwide, can be found in abundance in very distant areas ranging from Africa, North America to the Himalayas and Australia [5]. Some *Artemisia* species exhibit so high ability to adapt to new habitats that they become invasive species in these environments, posing a significant threat to biodiversity. This is the case of *Artemisia princeps* L. which, being native to Japan, China and Korea, is currently classified as an invasive species in Belgium and Netherlands [6] while *Artemisia verlotiorum* Lamotte is an alien invasive species in Croatia [7].

The use of *Artemisia* species in traditional medicine is well-documented [5,8–17] and demonstrates the great ethnopharmacological value of this genus. *Artemisia annua* L. and *Artemisia absinthium* L. are the best known for their uses in traditional medicine around of the World. For example, *A. annua* is cited in several ancient books as being suitable for the treatment of consumptive fever, jaundice, summer heat wounds, tuberculosis, lice, scabies, dysentery, and hemorrhoids in addition to pain relievers, while in Iran is used as antispasmodic, carminative, or sedative remedy for children [9,16,18]. In turn, *A. absinthium* has been traditionally used to treat mainly gastrointestinal diseases and as anthelmintic although for example in Italy it is also used as an antiparasitic, antihypertensive and anti-inflammatory, while in France it is also used to stimulate appetite, as an antipyretic, and emmenagogue [17,19]. However, many other species are used on each continent. For example, *Artemisia afra* Jacq. ex Willd. is one of the most widely used herbal remedies in South Africa to treat inflammation and pain [20]. It is also used to treat various ailments including coughs, colds, asthma, fever, influenza, diabetes and malaria [20], and by certain South African traditional healers to treat rhinitis [21]. *Artemisia dracunculus* L. is widely used in North America, for example by the Chippewa and Costanoan Indians as abortifacient and medicine to treat chronic dysentery, heart palpitations, wounds, colic in babies, and also to strengthen hair and make it grow [22]. In the Iranian Traditional Medicine *A. vulgaris* is used to treat cervicitis [23], while this species is reported in the ethnobotany of Karok, Kiowa, Miwok Paiute, Pomo and Tlingit areas, as a drug with several applications such as in childbirth, steam bath for pleurisy, gonorrheal sore, cold, rheumatism, headache, a 'worm' medicine, pains of afterbirth [24]. The traditional use of *Artemisia* species in Europe is mainly as food, spices and beverages (discussed in more detail in Section 2). However, *Artemisia* species are also used in the treatment of various diseases, as for example *Artemisia umbelliformis* Lam. and *Artemisia genipi* Weber ex Stechm. also known as Alpine wormwoods and génépis species, that are used traditionally to fight cold fever, fatigue, dyspepsia and respiratory infections, as wound-healing agents and to treat bruises, while wines aromatized with these species stimulate appetite, promote digestion, and fight the mountain sickness [10].

Even some *Artemisia* species less scientifically known such as *Artemisia ordosica* Krasch, have significant ethnomedicinal applications. This species was recorded on the traditional Mongolian and Chinese medicine books, as having a beneficial effect on the nasal bleeding, rheumatoid arthritis, headache, sore throat and carbuncle [25] and was used by Mongolian "barefoot" doctors for nasosinusitis treatment [26]. *Artemisia tripartita* (Nutt.) Rydb. was reported on Native American Ethnobotany database [27] as diaphoretic and remedy to treat cold and sore throats, while *Artemisia verlotiorum* Lamotte, distributed in all northern hemisphere, is used in Tuscany folk medicine to treat hypertension [28], and to alleviate stomach problems in Gilgit-Baltistan, Pakistan [29].

Artemisia species, as well as other herbal medicines, with proven pharmacological effects has been incorporated into conventional medicine. This incorporation is supported by the world health organization, which considers that traditional and complementary medicine can make a significant contribution to the goal of achieving universal health coverage by being included in the provision of essential health services [30]. Nevertheless, international research into traditional herbal medicines should be subject to the same ethical and methodological requirements as all research involving humans. Therefore, criteria to promote the safety, quality and effectiveness of the plants used in traditional medicine have been discussed and established [31,32].

Encouraged by this wide application in traditional medicine, the scientific community has dedicated itself to investigating in each *Artemisia* species evidence to support these applications. In the laboratory, the properties of the plant and extracts are tested using different models (in vitro, in vivo, clinical trial), and the active principles present in these species are wanted.

The result of this vast investigation showed the *Artemisia* species (extracts and essential oils) as exhibiting antiparasitic, anticancer and anti-inflammatory action in addition to antioxidant, wound healing, antinociceptive, immunoregulation, hepatoprotective, neuroprotective, anti-asthmatic, antidiabetic, antihypertensive, anti-adipogenic, anti-ulcerogenic, antiviral, antibacterial, antifungal, and anti-osteoporotic activities [10–13,18,19,33–39].

The search for bioactive compounds responsible for these biological activities has led to *Artemisia* species are privileged sources of compounds with highly diversified structures that exhibit a high level and diversity of biological activities, providing the basis for the development of new drugs, some of which are already used in clinical therapeutics [4,8,10,13,40–47].

The *Artemisia* secondary metabolites belong to the several organic compounds families [44,47–49] such as terpenoids [14,44], mostly monoterpenes in essential oils [31,44] and sesquiterpene lactones [40,41,50], flavonoids [14,46,51,52], lignans [52–55], alkaloids [56], steroids [14,57], phenolic acids [37,47,58] and coumarins [14,53,59], all of them well known for their large range of biological activities.

Given the large number of papers published on the theme of health effects of products related to *Artemisia* species (plant, extracts, pure compounds, studies in vitro, in vivo and clinical trials), all publications related to in vitro studies were excluded from this review. In fact, although these studies are essential for a first assessment of the species' potential, they are the ones that are farthest from the final objective, which is, the application in patients. Thus, the results of these studies are those that weigh less in the realistic assessment of the therapeutic effects of the plant and/or its constituents.

This review is intended to gather and discuss the most impactful research concerning the health effects of edible *Artemisia* species, based on their applications as food, their nutritional composition and therapeutic applications supported by clinical studies. It is also discussed the therapeutic relevance of some sesquiterpene lactones constituents of *Artemisia* species and its derivatives.

The method consisted of searching the Scopus, Web of Science, PubMed and Google Scholar databases for original and review articles in English language, published from 2015 to 2020, while ClinicalTrials.gov was used to find registered clinical trials. For a systematic search, "Artemisia" as the primary keyword, associated with other keywords such as "chemical composition", "nutritional", "food", "adverse effects" and "covid-19" for Sections 2–4 and 7; "Artemisia" and "clinical trial" for Section 5; For Section 6 are used the name of each sesquiterpene lactone and terms like "biological activity", "cancer", "malaria". The in vitro studies were excluded (NOT "in vitro"). More than 300 references were considered, and the most significant results discussed and presented here.

2. Use of *Artemisia* Species as Food, Spices, Condiments and Beverages

In addition to the traditional medicine applications, *Artemisia* species exhibit high food value since many of them are species used in culinary.

The most extensive use of *Artemisia* species as food is found in the countries of Europe, Asia (Japan, Korea, China and India) as well as in North America. The literature data describing the utilization of *Artemisia* species as a food, spices, condiments and beverages are summarized in Table 1.

Table 1. Application of *Artemisia* species as food, spices, condiments and beverages.

Species	Common Name	Distribution *	Edible Part	Use	Ref.
Artemisia abrotanum L.	Southernwood	S. Europe	Young shoots	Flavoring cakes, salads and vinegars; herb tea	[60–65]
A. absinthium	Mugwort, common wormwood, absinthe	Europe, Asia	Herb	Spice; flavoring beer, wine, vermouth, absinthe, liquors and aperitifs; pelinkovac	[60–62,65–72]
A. afra	African wormwood	Africa	Herb	Flavoring; preparation of vermouth; as a tea	[60–67]
Artemisia alba Turra (syn. *A. camphorata* Vill.)	Camphor absinthe	S. Europe, C. Europe, N.W. Africa	Herb	Spice and flavoring	[60]
A. annua	Qing Hao, Sweet sagewort	S.E. Europe to W. Asia.	Leaves	Essential oil in the leaves is used as a flavoring in spirits such as vermouth; as a vegetable	[67]
Artemisia arborescens (Vaill.) L.	Silver wormwood	N. Africa, S. Europe	Herb	Spice added to the green tea prepared by Moroccans	[60,65,67]
Artemisia argyi H. Lév. & Vaniot	Aicao, Gaiyou, Seomae mugwort	N. Asia, N. Europe, N. America	Leaves, buds, herb	As a tea or other forms of food supplements; dried leaves as a flavoring and colorant for the Chinese dish Qingtua	[46,73]
Artemisia balchanorum Krasch.		Turkmenia	Herb	Spice; potherb	[60]
Artemisia capillaris Thunb.	Yin Chen Hao	E. Asia—China, Japan, Korea	Leaves, stems, shoots	Soaked and boiled eaten as food supplements in times of famine	[67,74]
Artemisia carvifolia Buch.-Ham. ex Roxb.		E. Asia—China, Japan, Himalayas	Leaves	Flavoring for tea and coffee; Young plants—cooked in the spring	[67]
Artemisia dracunculoides Pursh.	Russian Tarragon, Tarragon, French Tarragon	N. America. N. Europe. N. Asia—Siberia	Leaves, seeds	Leaves—raw in salads; The N. American Indians bake the leaves between hot stones and then eat them with salt water; Seed—raw or cooked as an oily texture.	[62,67,68,75]

Table 1. *Cont.*

Species	Common Name	Distribution *	Edible Part	Use	Ref.
A. dracunculus	Tarragon, French Tarragon	S. Europe to W. Asia.	Leaves, young shoots	Leaves—raw or used as a flavoring in soups, oily foods, salads, vinegar, etc.; The young shoots can also be cooked and used as a potherb	[60,62,63,66,67,70,76]
Artemisia frigida Willd.	Fringed Wormwood, Prairie sagewort	N. America, N. Asia.	Leaves	The leaves are used by the Hopi Indians as a flavoring for sweet corn	[68,76]
A. genipi.	Genepi, black wormwart, black wormwood, génépi noir	S. Europe	Leaves, flower heads	Spice, flavoring for liqueurs	[10,60,61,66,67]
Artemisia glacialis L.	Glacier wormwood	C. Europe	Herb, flower heads	Flavoring in vermouth and liqueurs	[10,60,61,67]
Artemisia granatensis Boiss.		Spain	Herb	Herb tea	[77]
Artemisia herba-alba Asso		Africa, Mediterranean area	Herb	Herb tea; Flavoring tea and coffee	[78]
Artemisia indica Willd.		E. Asia—China, Japan, India.	Leaves	Young leaves—cooked and eaten with barley; the leaves pounded with steamed rice dumplings to give a flavor and coloring	[60,70]
Artemisia japonica Thunb.		E. Asia—China, Japan, Korea.	Young leaves	Raw as a vegetable or cooked	[70]
Artemisia keiskeana Miq.		E. Asia—China, Japan, Korea, E. Russia.	Leaves, shoot tips	Cooked	[67]
Artemisia ludoviciana Nutt.	White Sage, Louisiana Sage, Prairie Sage, Western Mugwort	N. America	Leaves, flowering heads	Flavoring or garnish for sauces, gravies, etc.; Used like absinthe; herb tea	[60,61,67,75,76]
Artemisia maritima L.	Sea Wormwood	Europe, E. Asia, C. Asia.	Leaves	Spice; flavoring in some Danish schnapps, beer and liqueurs	[60,61,67]
Artemisia montana (Nakai.) Pamp.		E. Asia—China, Japan.	Leaves	Young leaves—cooked; herb tea	[79]
Artemisia pallens Wall. ex DC.	Davana	N.E. India, Thailand	Herb	Spice; flavoring for cakes, pastries, candy, chewing gum, ice cream, beverages, tobacco; for production of essential oil (davana oil)	[60,61,67]

Table 1. Cont.

Species	Common Name	Distribution *	Edible Part	Use	Ref.
Artemisia pontica L.	Roman wormwood; Small absinthe	S.E. Europe to Siberia, C. Asia	Leaves, herb	Spice, flavoring, like A. absinthium	[60,61,66,67]
A. princeps	Mugwort mochi, Yomogi	E. Asia—China, Japan, Korea.	Leaves, young seedlings	Raw or cooked in salads and soups; for flavoring and coloring of rice dumplings ('mochi')	[60,67,80]
Artemisia schmidtiana Maxim.	Sagebrush, Silvermound, Wormwood, Mugwort	E. Asia—Japan.	Stems	Cooked; for flavoring and coloring of rice dumplings ('mochi')	[78,80]
Artemisia sphaerocephala Krasch.		China	Seed	Seed powder added to noodles and other traditional Chinese foods to improve sensory qualities such as elasticity and chewing quality	[81]
Artemisia tilesii Ledeb.	Wormwood, Tilesius' wormwood	E. Asia, N.W. America.	Leaves, shoots	The fresh shoots are peeled and eaten, usually with oil; Flavoring rice dumplings	[67]
Artemisia tridentata Nutt.	Sage Brush, Big sagebrush, Bonneville big sagebrush	N. America	Leaves, seeds	Leaves—cooked, as a condiment and to make a tea with sage-like flavor; Seed—can be roasted then ground into a powder and mixed with water or eaten raw	[61,75,76]
A. umbelliformis (syn. A. mutellina Vill.)	Alpine Wormwood	Europe—Alps, N. Apennines	Herb, leaves, flower heads	As a condiment; preparation of a tea and a liqueur, often with the addition of absinthe	[10,60,66,67,82]
Artemisia vallesiaca All.	Alpine Wormwood, Valais wormwood	Europe—N. Italy, Switzerland, S. E. France	Herb	Flavoring for liqueurs; product of santonin	[10,60,66]
A. vulgaris	Mugwort, Common wormwood, Felon Herb, Chrysanthemum Weed, Wild Wormwood	Temperate regions of Europe and Asia	Leaves, young shoots, flowering tops	Flavoring fatty foods; to give color and flavor to rice dumplings ('mochi'); as a potherb; flavoring in beer and liqueurs	[60,61,66,67,70,71,80]
Artemisia wrightii A. Gray.		N. America	Leaves, seeds	Raw or cooked—an oily texture; Seed—ground with water, made into balls and steamed	[75]

* S.—south; E.—east; C.—central; N.—north; W—west; S. E.—south-east; N.W.—north-west; N. E.—north-east.

Taxa of the *A. vulgaris* is collected and cultivated for different alimentary purposes [60,67,80]. Their leaves are one of the ingredients of kusa-mochi and hishi-mochi, two kinds of rice cakes or dumplings, one variant of which is called yomogi-mochi, yomogi being the Japanese name of these *Artemisia* species [80]. A type of soba, Japanese noodles used in soups and similar dishes, made with wheat and buckwheat also contains *A. princeps*, which gives it a green color. The young plants (leaves, stems, or shoot tips) of *A. dracunculus*, *A. dracunculoides*, *A. vulgaris*, *A. japonica*, *A. capillaris*, *A. carvifolia*, *A. indica*, *A. keiskeana*, *A. montana*, *A. schmidtiana*, *A. tilesii*, *A. tridentata*, *A. wrightii*, etc. (Table 1) can be eaten fresh in salads or cooked in soups and food supplements. *Sabzi khordan* is an Iranian (Persian) mixture of fresh herbs (served with lunch and dinner) that typically includes tarragon (*A. dracunculus*) [83]. Although the seeds of *A. dracunculoides* and *A. tridentata* are very small, they can be roasted, ground into a powder, and mixed with water or eaten raw [75]. Similarly, the seed of *A. wrightii* is crushed with water, made into balls and steamed [75].

On the other hand, the flavoring use of an *Artemisia* species is worldwide and especially of *A. dracunculus* (French tarragon, German tarragon, true tarragon or estragon) and closely related *A. dracunculoides* (Russian tarragon). The early culinary history is obscure, but the name "tarragon" is derived from *tarkhūn*, the Arabic name [83]. Tarragon became popular as a flavoring agent in the 16th century and is one of the most sought after herbs amongst gourmet chefs because of its delicate anise flavor, reminiscent of licorice. *Herbes vénitiennes* are a mixture of aromatic herbs (tarragon, chervil, parsley and sorrel) traditionally used in France to flavor butter. Tarragon vinegar is made by steeping a few fresh leafy twigs in a bottle of white wine vinegar. It is an essential ingredient of famous sauces such as béarnaise, hollandaise and tartare that classically accompany asparagus, green beans, peas and other vegetables (as tarragon cream) or chicken, meat and eggs. Leaves (preferably fresh) are used to flavor meat dishes, stews, fish dishes, salads, pickles and mustard sauces. Russian tarragon (*A. dracunculoides*) is very similar but more robust (and less aromatic). Tarragon is largely cultivated and commercialized as living plants in pots. Dried leaves of *A. argyi* are utilized as flavoring and colorant for the Chinese dish Qingtua [46], and *A. ludoviciana*—for sauces, gravies and as a garnish for pork and game [60,67]. Dried leaves of *A. vulgaris* (mugwort) make a bitter seasoning for poultry stuffing, especially for goose, and soups, and fresh leaves can be rubbed on fatty meats before roasting [61]. Some gourmands like cheese use seasoning with a mixture of wormwood (*A. absinthium*), thyme, and rosemary (at ratio 4:2:1) [84]. Small farmers in Lithuania are using a mix of wormwood and tansy (*Tanacetum vulgare*) for preservative purposes (to protect smoked meats from flies blow, other pests, and spoilage) as well as for flavoring (it gives a specific pleasant smell to the meat) [84]. The leaves of *A. frigida* are used by the Hopi Indians as a flavoring for sweet corn [68,76]. *A. abrotanum* is the sweetest *Artemisia* with slight lemon scent is a natural choice for seasoning cakes, pastries and vinegars [61]. Similarly, the leaves of *A. pallens* are delicately scented and the flowers yield a balsamic essential oil (davana) with application in baked goods, candy, chewing gum, and ice cream [61].

Many *Artemisia* species are applied in the preparation of different non-alcoholic beverages, giving them a bitter taste and alleged tonic properties. Thus, *A. absinthium*, *A. abrotanum*, *A. agryi*, *A. ludoviciana*, *A. montana*, *A. tridentata*, *A. granatensis*, etc. are consumed as herbal tea with digestive properties (Table 1). Silver wormwood (*A. arborescens*) and *A. herba-alba* are added to the green tea or the coffee in North Africa [67,78] and *A. carvifolia* has the same use in Asia [67]. Tarragon (*A. dracunculus*) is an ingredient of Georgian carbonated soft drink called *Tarkhuna* [75]. *A. maritima*, *A. abrotanum*, *A. absinthium*, *A. vulgaris*, etc. (Table 1) have been applied as a flavoring ingredient in beer production before the common application of hops.

Undoubtedly, the most famous *Artemisia* species employed in alcoholic drinks is *A. absinthium*, among which two are most noteworthy: vermouth and absinthe. Vermouth is a low alcoholic drink prepared from wine and a cocktail of botanical ingredients with *A. absinthium* as a principal component [85]. There are similar drinks in some countries of the Balkan Peninsula—pelin in Bulgaria [86] and vin pelin in Romania [87]. The spirit drink absinthe was created in French-speaking Switzerland in the late eighteenth century [88] and is produced by macerating *A. absinthium* leaves, anise and fennel seeds in alcohol (85 vol%) [84,89]. Wormwood (*A. absinthium*) is also used for the preparation of a bitter liqueur with lower content of alcohol (28–35 vol%) called pelinkovac (pelinkovec, pelinovec, pelen or pelin) and popular in Croatia, Serbia, Montenegro, Bosnia-Herzegovina, North Macedonia as well as in Slovenia [71].

Another popular herbal liqueurs in which *Artemisia* species present are genepy or génépi (*A. genipi* and related taxa such as *A. glacialis* and *A. umbelliformis*) [10] and ratafia (*A. abrotanum, A. absinthium, A. arborescens* and *Artemisia chamaemelifolia* Vill. [65]).

3. Nutritional Value of *Artemisia* Species

As demonstrated above *Artemisia* species are widely consumed by human as a traditional food, a tea and dietary supplements, owing to the fact that they are rich in fatty acids, carbohydrates, dietary fiber, protein, essential amino acids, vitamins and minerals as demonstrated in Table 2.

Table 2. Nutritional composition of some edible *Artemisia* species.

Plant Species	Plant Part	Nutrient Composition *	Ref.
A. absinthium	Oil cake **	Sugars (9.4%)	[90]
	Leaves	Protein (27.1%); TAA (27.6%), EAA (16.1%), NEAA (11.5%); Crude fat (8.34%); Minerals: K (26.3 mg/g DM), Ca (11.5 mg/g DM), Mg (7.1 mg/g DM), P (7.1 mg/g DM), S (3.9 mg/g DM), Fe (0.2 mg/g DM), Mn (0.2 mg/g DM), Zn (0.06 mg/g DM); Vitamin A (<0.3 µg/100 g DM); Vitamin E (22.63 mg/kg)	[91]
	Inflorescence	Protein (18.4%); Crude fat (10.5%); TAA (18.3%), EAA (10.14%), NEAA (8.11%); Minerals: K (24.6 mg/g DM), Ca (4.4 mg/g DM), Mg (2.3 mg/g DM), P (3.4 mg/g DM), S (4.6 mg/g DM), Fe (0.2 mg/g DM), Mn (0.3 mg/g DM), Zn (0.06 mg/g DM); Vitamin A (<0.3 µg/100 g DM); Vitamin E (19.38 mg/kg)	
A. annua	Stems	Protein (10.7%); Crude fat (2.60%); TAA (10.3%), EAA (5.91%), NEAA (4.38%); Minerals: K (13.3 mg/g DM), Ca (0.9 mg/g DM), Mg (0.9 mg/g DM), P (0.7 mg/g DM), S (0.5 mg/g DM), Fe (0.7 mg/g DM), Mn (0.02 mg/g DM), Zn (0.08 mg/g DM); Vitamin A (<0.3 µg/100 g DM); Vitamin E (1.19 mg/kg)	
	Roots	Protein (8.23%); Crude fat (2.13%); TAA (8.01%), EAA (4.34%), NEAA (3.66%); Minerals: K (11.1 mg/g DM), Ca (11.5 mg/g DM), Mg (7.1 mg/g DM), P (7.1 mg/g DM), S (3.9 mg/g DM), Fe (0.2 mg/g DM), Mn (0.2 mg/g DM), Zn (0.06 mg/g DM); Vitamin A (<0.3 µg/100 g DM); Vitamin E (1.36 mg/kg)	
	Leaves	Protein (24.37 mg/100 g); Crude fat (6.07%); TFA (4.19 mg/g FW), SFA (22.9%) UFA (77.1%), MUFA (8.4%), PUFA (68.7%) Carbohydrates (8%); Fibre (14.2%); Vitamins: Tocopherol (2.74%)	[92,93]
	Achene	Lipids: SFA (29.21%), UFA (70.87%), MUFA (13.99%), PUFA (56.88%)	[94]
A. arborescens	Leaves	Lipids: TFA (3.31 mg/g FW), SFA (47.4%), UFA (52.6%), MUFA (16.3%), PUFA (36.3%)	[92]

Table 2. Cont.

Plant Species	Plant Part	Nutrient Composition *	Ref.
A. argyi	Leaves	Protein (22.0 mg/g FW); Free amino acids: EAA (3.71 mg/g DW), NEAA (2.42 mg/g DW), FAA (6.13 mg/g DW); Total lipid (24.7 mg/g FW); SFA (40.8%), MUFA (7.1%), PUFA (52.1%); Total carbohydrates (52.3 mg/g FW); Dietary fiber (39.9 mg/g FW); Minerals: K (74.22 mg/100 g FW), Ca (14.74 mg/100 g FW), Mg (36.64 mg/100 g FW), Zn (0.89 mg/100 g FW), Cu (0.13 mg/100 g FW), Mn (0.76 mg/100 g FW), Fe (3.15 mg/100 g FW); Vitamin C (total ascorbic acid) 2.09 mg/g DW	[46,73]
A. austriaca Jacq.	Achene	Lipids: SFA (47.43%), UFA (49.02%), MUFA (9.65%), PUFA (39.37%)	[94]
A. campestris L.	Leaves	Lipids: TFA (10.22 mg/g FW), SFA (21.0%), UFA (79.0%), MUFA (3.6%), PUFA (75.3%)	[92]
A. camphorata Vill.	Aerial	Crude protein (115 mg/g DM)	[95]
A. capilaris	Leaves	Lipids: TFA (14.82 mg/g FW), SFA (37.4%), UFA (62.6%), MUFA (8.3%), PUFA (54.3%)	[92]
A. frigida	Leaves	Lipids: TFA (6.01 mg/g FW), SFA (16.0%), UFA (84.0%), MUFA (4.7%), PUFA (79.4%)	[92]
	Aerial	Crude protein (17.9%); Minerals: K (18.34 mg/g DM), Ca (7.46 mg/g DM), P (2.54 mg/g DM), Mg (2.17 mg/g DM), Cu (1.1 mg/100 g DM), Mn (24 mg/100 g DM), Fe (20.0 mg/100 g DM) Zn (1.9 mg/100 g DM); Na (5 mg/100 g DM)	[96]
A. glacialis	Leaves	Lipids: TFA (8.95 mg/g FW), SFA (21.6%), UFA (78.4%), MUFA (6.8%), PUFA (71.6%)	[92]
A. gmellini Weber ex Stechm.	Leaves	Lipids: TFA (14.11 mg/g FW), SFA (25.5%), UFA (74.5%), MUFA (4.5%), PUFA (70.0%)	[92]
A. herba-alba	Aerial	Crude protein (103.4–153.6 mg/g DM); Crude fibre (407.9 mg/g DM)	[95,97,98]
A. jacutica Drobow	Leaves	Lipids: SFA (61.21–68.12%), UFA (31.88–38.79%)	[99]
A. ludoviciana	Leaves	Lipids: TFA (14.28 mg/g FW), SFA (19.6%), UFA (80.4%), MUFA (5.3%), PUFA (75.1%)	[92]
A. macrocephala Jaq. ex Bess	Leaves	Lipids: UFA (50.80–65.22%), SFA (34.78–49.20%).	[99]
A. oleandica (Besser) Krasch	Leaves	Lipids: TFA (9.84 mg/g FW), SFA (17.6%), UFA (82.4%), MUFA (4.7%), PUFA (77.7%)	[92]
A. princeps	Leaves	Lipids: TFA (6.49 mg/g FW), SFA (20.2%), UFA (79.8%), MUFA (5.7%), PUFA (74.1%)	[92]
	Leaves	Lipids: SFA (27.5%), MUFA (35.1%), PUFA (37.4%); Free amino acids: EAA (3.19 mg/g DW), NEAA (2.42 mg/g DW), FAA (5.61 mg/g DW); Vitamin C (total ascorbic acid) 1.01 mg/g DW;	[73]
A. santolinifolia Turcz. ex Bess	Leaves	Lipids: SFA (51.8–65.02%), PFA (9.74–44.14%), MFA (4.06–30.85%)	[100]

Table 2. Cont.

Plant Species	Plant Part	Nutrient Composition *	Ref.
A. santonicum L.	Achene	Lipids: SFA (43.70%), UFA (56.33%), MUFA (8.26%), PUFA (48.07%)	[94]
A. sieberi Besser	Aerial	Crude protein (55 mg/g DM); Crude fiber (484 mg/g DM); Minerals: K (13.1 mg/g DM), Ca (15.9 mg/g DM), P (2.5 mg/g DM), Mg (1.8 mg/g DM), Cu (1.37 mg/100 g DM), Mn (2.26 mg/100 g DM), Fe (20.0 mg/100 g DM) Zn (21.2 mg/100 g DM)	[101]
A. sieversiana Ehrh. ex Willd	Leaves	Lipids: UFA (64.11–73.23%), SFA (26.77–35.89%)	[99]
A. sphaerocephala	Seed	Carbohydrate (73%)	[102]
A. stelleriana Bess	Leaves	Lipids: TFA (17.78 mg/g FW), SFA (70.2%), UFA (29.8%), MUFA (1.3%), PUFA (28.4%)	[92]
A. tridentata subsp. wyomingensis Beetle & A.L. Young	Leaves	Crude protein (15.7%)	[103]
A. vallesiaca	Leaves	Lipids: TFA (5.27 mg/g FW), SFA (17.1%), UFA (82.9%), MUFA (9.3%), PUFA (73.6%)	[92]
A. vulgaris	Leaves	Lipids: TFA (13.32 mg/g FW), SFA (15.2%), UFA (84.8%), MUFA (3.7%), PUFA (81.1%)	[92]

* Free (FAA), essential (EAA) and non-essential (NEAA) amino acids; total (TFA), saturated (SFA), unsaturated (UFA), monounsaturated (MUFA) and polyunsaturated (PUFA) fatty acids; DW—dry weight; FW—fresh weight; DM—dry matter. ** Oil cake remaining after the extraction of essential oil.

Fatty acids (FA) have chemo-preventive effects and are pharmacologically active in chronic or degenerative diseases. Research has proved that diets rich in saturated fatty acids (SFA) are a risk factor for cardiovascular diseases unlike diets rich in monounsaturated fatty acids (MUFA) and polyunsaturated fatty acids (PUFA), which reduce or inhibit such cardiovascular disease [104]. Linoleic and linolenic acids are essential for human health growth health promotion and disease prevention [104–108]. They could not be synthesized endogenously in the human body and therefore they need to be supplied by food. The studies on the fatty acid profile of *Artemisia* species (Table 2) showed a very variable fatty acid content, ranging from 3.31 mg/g FW in *A. arborescens* [92] to 24.7 mg/g FW in *A. argyi* [46]. With exception of *A. jacutica* [99], *A. santolinifolia* [100] and *A. stelleriana* [92], unsaturated fatty acids (UFA) predominated in all investigated species, followed by polyunsaturated fatty acids (PUFA) and saturated fatty acids (SFA) (Table 2). Among individual compounds, linolenic and linoleic acids are the major fatty acids. These results determine *Artemisia* plants as a valuable source of unsaturated fatty acids with significance from both dietary and nutritional point of view. Palmitic acid was found to be the most abundant component in *A. stelleriana* (70%) [92], *A. princeps* (34.9%) [73] and *A. jacutica* (20.6–21.8%) [99].

Carbohydrates are important for keeping the body supply with energy and stamina. Recently, *A. sphaerocephala* carbohydrates have been the subject of a bibliographic review [109], showing their high nutritional value and versatility in terms of applications. For instance, the total amount of carbohydrates in *A. sphaerocephala* seed oil is 73% [83,110] while in *A. annua* is only 8% [93]. Recently, it has been found that the oil cake remaining after the extraction of essential oils from *A. absinthium* contains 9.4% of sugars [90]. The authors propose an application of the aqueous extracts of oil cake for the formulations of gelled desserts.

Dietary fiber possesses an ability to prevent or relieve constipation and foods containing fiber can provide other health benefits as well, such as helping to maintain a healthy weight and lowering your risk of diabetes, heart disease and some types of cancer [111]. Few *Artemisia* species have been studied for the content of dietary fiber (Table 2). The amount of crude fiber in the fresh *A. argyi* leaves, *A. annua*, *A. herba-alba* leaves and *A. sibieri* is 39.9 mg/g, 142 mg/g, 407.9 mg/g and 484 mg/g, respectively (Table 2).

Proteins play critical roles in cellular functions, structure and regulations of metabolic activities in all living organisms and have primary importance in the daily diets of consumers. Crude protein content was assessed in *A. argyi* and *A. princeps* [73], *A. herba-alba* [95–97], *A. campestris* [97], *A. sieberi* [101], *A. frigida* [96], *A. tridentata* ssp. *wyomingensis* [103] and *A. annua* [93]. It has been found that leaves and inflorescence of *A. annua* are rich in protein (27.1 and 18.4%, respectively) when compared to stems and roots (10.7 and 8.23%, respectively) [91]. The comparative study of the nutritional constituents of *A. princeps* and *A. argyi* showed significant difference in the content of free amino acids [73]. The content of the essential amino acids valine and phenylalanine is significantly higher in *A. argyi* (by approximately 63% and 41%, respectively) than in *A. princeps*. The amount of total essential amino acids is approximately 57% in *A. princeps* and 61% in *A. argyi*. γ-Aminobutyric acid is the main component in *A. argyi*. This acid is a natural non-protein amino acid with great therapeutic potential in neurological disorders and mental illnesses, because it acts as the major inhibitory neurotransmitter in the central nervous system [112]. Reflective of the protein content in the various tissues of *A. annua*, the highest concentration of amino acids was registered in the leaves and inflorescence and leucine was the most abundant one [91].

As can be seen in Table 2, few *Artemisia* species have been investigated for the presence of vitamins and minerals. Thus, the content of vitamin C (measured as ascorbic acid) in *A. argyi* was found to be twice higher than in *A. princeps* [73]. The content of vitamin E varies in the different plant parts of *A. annua*, from 1.19 mg/kg (stems) to 22.63 mg/kg (leaves) [91] and is significantly lower from that reported by Iqbal et al. [93]. The different values of vitamin E are probably due to the different methods used for the quantitative determination. The measured concentration of vitamin A in the different parts of *A. annua* was under detection limit level (<0.3 μg/100 g) [91]. Among minerals, potassium was detected in the highest concentration in all studied *Artemisia* species so far (Table 2) followed by calcium and magnesium (Table 2). Potassium is important in a balance for cellular metabolism and regulating transfer of nutrients to cells, maintaining blood pressure and electrolyte balance, transmitting electrochemical impulses and for the correct functioning of blood, endocrine/digestive and nervous systems, heart, kidneys, muscles and skin [113]. High levels of phosphorous were found in aerial parts of *A. frigida* [96] and *A. sieberi* [101], in *A. annua* leaves and inflorescence [91]. Phosphorous is an essential component to maintain electrolyte balance, correct functioning of brain cells, circulatory and digestive systems, eyes, liver, muscles, nerves and teeth/bones. A balance of magnesium, calcium and phosphorus is required for these minerals to be used effectively [113]. Regarding the microelements, iron, manganese and zinc in different amounts dominated all studied samples (Table 2). Probably, the functions of all these macro- and microelements in the body to maintain water balance and to stimulate normal movement in the intestinal tract can explain the traditional use of the *Artemisia* plants as an herbal tonic.

4. Adverse Effects Reported to *Artemisia* Species and Some Constituents

Pollen from the various *Artemisia* species is one of the most frequent and serious pollinosis causes in many parts of the world [114–118]. It has been verified as an allergen by nasal challenge and bronchial provocation tests, and these allergens have been shown to occur not only in its pollen but also in its leaves and stems. Studies on the immunological changes from *Artemisia* pollen allergic subjects revealed that *Artemisia* pollen can trigger not only allergic rhinitis but also asthma alone or both [118,119]. Almost half of the patients with autumnal pollen allergic rhinitis developed seasonal allergic asthma within 9 years [118]. The immunoelectrophoretic comparison of the allergen extracts from pollen of six *Artemisia* species and morphological studies on the pollen grains showed an extensive degree of similarity and cross-reactivity between the studied species [120]. Screening of both Korean and Norwegian patient sera against extracts from *A. vulgaris* and *A. princeps* showed that both groups of patients had the same pattern of reactivity towards both extracts [120]. The mugwort (*A. vulgaris*) pollen contained allergenic substances with IgE reactivity [121], which can cause immediate Type I allergic reactions such as anaphylactic shock [122]. Another study on the pollen collected from plants across Europe has shown that the highest levels of endotoxin were detected on *A. vulgaris* pollen [123]. The investigation on *Artemisia* pollen allergenicity revealed significant daily, seasonal and species-specific variability [124]. The analysis of *Artemisia* pollen concentrations evidenced the presence of a bimodal curve with two peaks. The first peak was attributed to *A. vulgaris* (early flowering species) and the second one—to late flowering species (*A. campestris, A. annua, A. verlotiorum*, etc.) [115,124]. The authors supposed that the spread of these species could affect human health, increasing the length and severity of allergenic pollen exposure in autumn.

Skin contact with some members of the genus *Artemisia* can cause dermatitis or other allergic reactions in some people [125–128]. Several cases of contact dermatitis are described in the literature [129–132]. Mugwort (*A. vulgaris*) has demonstrated a medium sensitizing capacity in guinea pigs [133]. According to Park [134], nearly 43% of patients with allergic rhinitis and asthma have positive reactions to mugwort on skin prick testing. Wormwood tea (*A. absinthium*) induced positive patch test reactions in 13 of 19 Compositae-allergic patients [135]. Erythema multiforme, is probably an expression of a delayed hypersensitivity reaction and appears clinically as acute or chronic dermatitis of exposed sites [127,128]. Skin contact dermatitis caused by *Artemisia* species is attributed to the presence of sesquiterpene lactones [129,136,137].

Absinthe and the use of wormwood extracts (*A. absinthium*) for food purposes were prohibited around the years 1910–1920 in many countries as their consumption was associated with a range of severe adverse symptoms called absinthism, including convulsions, blindness, hallucinations and mental deterioration [89,138–140]. Padosch et al. [139] reviewed the available data concerning medical and toxicological aspects experienced and discovered before the prohibition of absinthe. Numerous studies did not give a clear answer whether the toxicity is due to thujone alone, to a combination of the alcohol and thujone or whether it can be traced back to toxic components used in the manufacture of absinthe liqueur [89,140]. Nowadays, *A. absinthium* is permitted in foods and alcoholic beverages according to the regulation of the European Parliament and Council [141]. In addition, European Food Safety Authority (EFSA) states that thujone content in alcoholic beverages, including absinthe, must not exceed 10 mg/kg [142], while the European Medicines Agency (EMA) also proposed a daily maximum intake of thujone in *Absinthii herba*, which was set at 3.0 mg thujone/day/person as acceptable for a maximum duration of 2 weeks in the wormwood monograph [143].

Some *Artemisia* species such as *A. vulgaris* [144], *A. herba-alba* [145], *A. annua* [146,147], *A. arborescens* and *A. douglasiana* Besser ex Besser [67] are used in regulating fertility and should be avoided in pregnancy. Thus, the consumption of *A. herba-alba* during pregnancy of mice offspring significantly decreased the fertility ratio and increased the weight and body size of preweaning offspring mice [148]. In addition, administration of *A. herba-alba* prolonged the time of completing the reflex response of surface righting, negative geotaxis, cliff avoidance and jumping test of mice offspring. In another study, treatment of pregnant rats with *A. kopetdaghensis* "Krasch, Popov & Lincz. ex Poljakov" hydroalcoholic extract (200 and 400 mg/kg) from the 2nd to 8th day of pregnancy led to 30 and 44% abortion in animals but had no significant effect on duration of pregnancy, average number of neonates, and weight of neonates [149]. The abortifacient effect of *A. kopetdaghensis* was attributed to the high content of camphor, for which is known that can crosses the placenta [150]. Gomes et al. [151] reviewed the results of non-clinical and clinical studies with artemisinin derivatives, their mechanisms of embryotoxicity and discussed the safety of their use during pregnancy. The mechanisms of embryotoxicity are not completely understood, but might not be so relevant for humans, considering the short time of treatment (3–7 days) compared with the longer period of target cell formation in the human embryo (~3 weeks).

The sesquiterpene lactone artemisinin isolated from the herb *A. annua* and its derivatives (artemether, arteether, and sodium artesunate) are successively applied in the malaria chemotherapy [152]. Extensive studies and meta-analyses of thousands of patients did not show serious side effects [152–156], although proper monitoring of adverse side effects in developing countries might not be a trivial task [155]. Common side effects were nausea, vomiting, and diarrhea, which are also symptoms of malaria itself. Efferth and Kaina [157] have summarized the available data on toxicity studies (neurotoxicity, embryotoxicity, genotoxicity, hemato- and immunotoxicity, cardiotoxicity, nephrotoxicity, and allergic reactions) in cell culture, animals (mice, rats, rabbits, dogs, monkeys) and in human clinical trials of artemisinin and its derivatives and concluded that artemisinin did not cause toxicity if are taken in appropriate doses for short periods.

5. Therapeutic Uses of *Artemisia* Species Based on Clinical Trials

Encouraged by long traditional use of many *Artemisia* species for treatment of various ailments, research into their pharmacological effects has been carried out and seem to support the traditional applications [5,12,15–17]. In this regard, *Artemisia* species and their biologically active compounds have already been introduced as antimalarial, antioxidant, cytotoxic, antispasmodic, anthelmintic, antinociceptive, neuroprotective, anti-inflammatory, and antimicrobial agents, among others [16,44]. It is noteworthy that although *Artemisia* species have been intensively studied in vitro as cytotoxic agents, there are no reports on their clinical evaluation for cancer therapy in humans [4]. However, one report by Saeed et al. showed that supplementing pet food with an *A. annua* formulation (Luparte®) clearly improved survival prognosis in veterinary treatment of small tumors [158].

Nevertheless, clinical evaluations of *Artemisia* species for a range of other diseases have been carried out [4]. The effect of *A. annua* in traditional medicine in China for treating fever, inflammation and malaria [9] have been evaluated in clinical trials for stiffness and functional limitation associated with osteoarthritis of the hip and knee, pain management, experimental heterophyid infection and treatment of malaria [159–161].

Artemisia dracunculus has been used for glycemic control, insulin sensitivity, and insulin secretion [162] and likewise, *A. princeps* was evaluated for the same effects in subjects with impaired fasting glucose and mild-type 2 diabetes [163] and *A. absinthium* in the control of diabetes type 2 [164].

Ointments and liniments of *A. absinthium* can be effective in the treatment of knee osteoarthritis [165]. Based on the suppressor activity of *A. absinthium* compounds on tumor necrosis factor alpha (TNF-α) and other interleukins [166], Krebs et al. [167] established the curative effect of this *Artemisia* species in patients with Crohn's disease. There was improvement in symptoms after treatment with dried powder of the plant together with a conventional therapy, and a cardamonin present in the plant was considered responsible for the anti-inflammatory activity.

In addition to being widely used clinically to treat itching in icteric and dialytic patients, owing to its anti-histaminic and anti-allergenic effects, *A. vulgaris* (mugwort) lotion has also provided good results in patients with post-burn hypertrophic scars [168].

Recently, the preventive effect on hepatitis B cirrhosis of *A. capillaris* decoction combined with the entecavir has been evaluate by a randomized, double-blind and placebo controlled clinical trial (Chinese Clinical Trial Registry: ChiCTR1900021521), to assess its efficacy and safety [169].

Artemisia annua and *A. vulgaris* are the species of the genus that produce the highest levels of allergens in their pollen, being one of the main causes of seasonal allergic rhinitis ("hayfever"). Lou et al. [170] carried out a phase III clinical trial (ClinicalTrials.gov identifier: NCT03990272) from March 2017 (approximately 4 months before the local natural *Artemisia* pollen season) to October 2017, involving patients from 13 centres across Northern China. The aim was to test the efficacy and safety of sublingual immunotherapy (SLI) with drops of *A. annua* for allergic rhinitis related to this plant. Results indicated that *A. annua* was a safe and significantly effective therapy. However, longer term follow-up is required, particularly to determine the mechanism of action.

Based in previous study where Xiao et al. [25] demonstrated using in vivo models, the ability of *A. ordosica* Krasch. extracts to control the allergic inflammatory response in rhinitis, clinical trials using nasal spray preparations of *A. abrotanum* containing its essential oils and flavonols have been performed with good results [171].

Munyangi et al. [172] published a randomized controlled clinical trial reporting far superior cure rates of *A. afra* and *A. annua* infusions than with artemisinin combination therapy (artesunate—amodiaquine), in the treatment of malaria. Contrastingly, a recent review by Toit and van der Kooy [15] concluded that tea infusions do not have in vitro activity, and in fact contain no artemisinin. Another randomized large-scale double-blind controlled trial on *A. annua* and *A. afra* tea vs. praziquantel for the treatment of schistosomiasis was documented by Munyangi et al. [173]. Controversially, Gillibert found scientific and ethical issues such as the article on schistosomiasis referring to the same ethics committee registration number as the malaria article [174].

Sensitive skin was initially believed to be an unusual reaction occurring in only a small subset of individuals. However, during recent decades, it has been shown to affect half the population of the world [175]. Accordingly, extensive in vitro, preclinical, and clinical research with artemisinin and its derivatives has been undertaken, notably into their anti-inflammatory, immunomodulatory and antioxidant properties [176]. Yu et al. [177] tested the effectiveness of cosmetics containing *A. annua* extract in repairing sensitive skin. In this study, the xylene-induced ear swelling and human clinical efficacy tests were used, and the authors found that applications containing *A. annua* extract can inhibit inflammation, repair the skin barrier, improve damaged skin, and reduce redness and other sensitive skin symptoms. Aside from this, its leaves are eaten in salads in some Asian countries and in the United States, and several companies currently sell ground leaves and their extracts as dietary supplements [178].

6. Some Sesquiterpene Lactones Constituents of *Artemisia* Species with High Clinical Relevance

The pharmaceutical industry has always been interested in the secondary metabolites produced by plants, for the treatment of diseases, in cosmetics, dyes, fragrances and flavorings [179]. The *Artemisia* species are well known by its content of sesquiterpene lactones [40,41,43,50]. These family of compounds have been studied and reveal high therapeutic potential [180,181]. Here are presented some of the most studied and promise sesquiterpene lactones constituents of edible *Artemisia* species (does not intent to be an exhaustive list) which, due to its medicinal properties discussed above, could contributes to the benefits effects of the *Artemisia* species. Sesquiterpene lactones such as arglabin parthenolide, cynaropicrin, helenalin, costunolide and thapsigargin identified in species of the genus *Artemisia* [40,41,50,180] and other genera, exhibit high pharmacological potential, including in in vivo studies and clinical trials, as demonstrated and discussed very recently [181]. So, they will not be considered in this work. The most recent and relevant experimental evidence of other sesquiterpene lactones medical potential will be highlighted discussed below. In this selection, was considerate mainly the in vivo and clinical studies, once they are the last steps of new drugs development and their results are the most significant to drug development.

The chemical structures of the selected sesquiterpene lactones discussed below are indicated in the Figure 1.

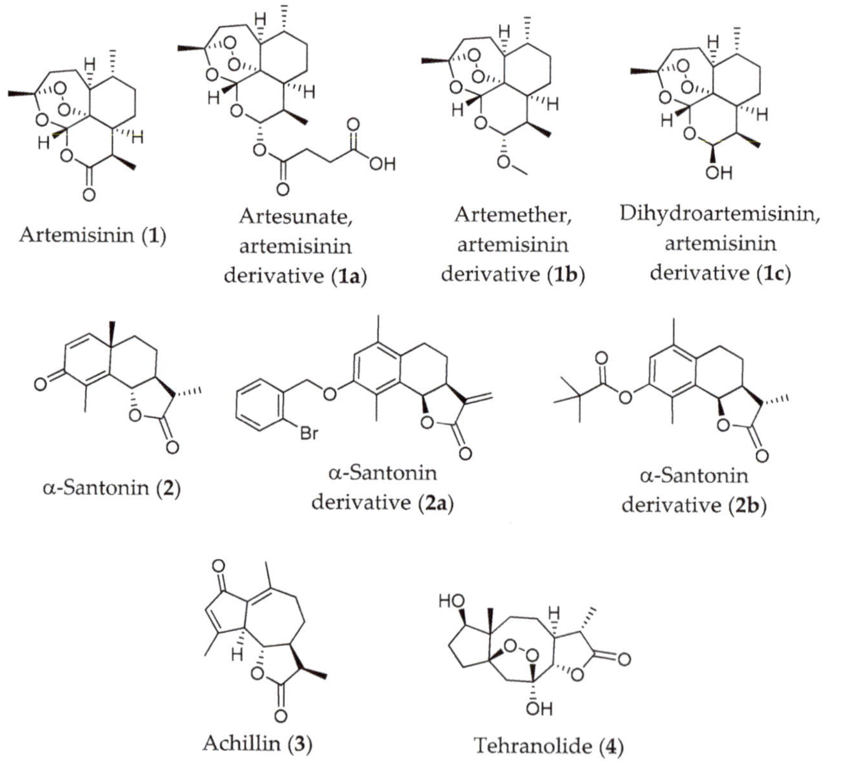

Figure 1. Chemical structures of some sesquiterpene lactones constituents of edible *Artemisia* sp. and derivatives with pharmacological relevance.

6.1. Artemisinin and Its Derivatives

Artemisinin (**1**) is a sesquiterpene lactone with an unusual peroxide bridge (cadinene sub-group), that was discovered and isolated from the Chinese herb *A. annua* by Tu YouYou in the early 1970s [182], who was awarded the Nobel Prize in 2015, for discoveries concerning the novel artemisinin therapy against malaria.

Artemisinin (**1**) has low solubility in both water and oil, resulting in weak erratic absorption after oral administration. It also has a short half-life and high first-passage metabolism [183]. Therefore, preserving its pharmacophore, a series of derivatives were designed. The 5–10 times more potent hemiacetal, dihydroartemisinin (DHA, **1c**), also known as dihydroqinghaosu or artenimol, is produced by reducing the lactone. Alkylation of the hemiacetal yields arteether (artemotil) and artemether, while artesunate is reached by acylation of the hemiacetal with succinic acid [184]. In in vivo systems, artesunate (**1a**) and artemether (**1b**) are converted back to dihydroartemisinin (**1c**). The most clinical widely used derivative is artesunate [185]. These derivatives showed better efficacy, tolerability, and oral bioavailability (all well absorbed by mouth and rapidly eliminated) than artemisinin, as well as minimal adverse effects [186,187]. Artemisinin (**1**) and its derivatives have been highlighted for their potent activity against species of *Plasmodium* genus responsible for malaria, as well as in the treatment of leishmaniasis, schistosomiasis and trypanomiasis [188–190]. They have also shown efficacy on several cancer lines, along with anti-inflammatory activity, modulating the immune response by regulating cell proliferation and cytokine release [191–193]. They also have anti-ulcerous [194], antinociceptive [195], antiviral [196], antifungal [180], and antibacterial [197] activities, besides being effective in other disorders such as respiratory [198], and related to metabolic syndromes, including obesity, diabetes and atherosclerosis [199,200], being many of the effects mentioned evaluated in in vivo models

6.1.1. Antiparasitic Activity In Vivo and Clinical Trials

Malaria is the most common tropical disease and is caused by protozoan parasites of the genus *Plasmodium* (*P. malariae*, quartan fevers; *P. vivax* and *P. ovale*, tertian fevers; *P. falciparum*, malignant tertians and *P. knowlesi*) [201]. Artemisinin (**1**) and its derivatives contain a 1,2,4-trioxane moiety responsible for the drug's action mechanism [193,202], which despite intensive study remains debatable. The compound is believed to act in two phases. Firstly, the haem iron attacks and breaks its endoperoxide linkage to produce oxy and carbon free radicals. In the second step, the latter free radical alkylates specific malarial proteins, killing the parasite. artemisinin (**1**) also has another target, the mitochondria and endoplasmic reticulum, where it inhibits PfATP6, the enzyme responsible for Ca^{++} delivery into vesicles. This is a parasite-encoded sarcoplasmic-endoplasmic reticulum calcium ATPase (SERCA), which is crucial for parasite development [193,201–205]. Furthermore, compound **1** exhibits a direct antiparasitic effect against several *Leishmania* species, by increasing NO production and iNOS expression in uninfected macrophages, and an indirect immunomodulatory effect. In addition, treatment with artemisinin (**1**) in a BALB/c mouse model led to significant reduction in splenic weight, a strong inhibition of parasites, and a restoration of Th1 cytokines such as interferon-γ and interleukin-2 (IL-2) [206].

The 11th World Malaria Report 2018 by the WHO estimated a 2 million increase in global malaria cases with respect to 2017. Examples of growing challenges are urban malaria, the parasite's drug resistance, malaria in pregnancy, resistance towards insecticides, etc. [207]. Artemisinin (**1**) and its analogues **1a**, **1b** and **1c** show marked activity against multidrug resistant strains of *Plasmodium* species and cerebral malaria both in vivo and in vitro. For this reason, the WHO recommends them as first choice treatment as part of artemisinin combination therapy (ACT) [208].

Artesunate (**1a**) is widely used to treat multidrug-resistant malaria [209,210]. The African Quinine Artesunate Malaria Trial multicenter study (AQUAMAT) conducted clinical trials with it in more than 5400 children under 15 years of age with severe malaria.

As a result of these, the WHO revised the guidelines for malaria and recommended intravenous artesunate as a choice to treat severe malaria [211,212].

After a cluster-randomized trial carried out in several African countries, it was concluded that rectal derivative **1a** takes 4–6 h to reduce parasitemia and affect progression of the disease. Consequently, when malaria patients cannot be treated orally, rectal artesunate prior to hospital referral can prevent death and disability. In fact, the WHO recommends this, to reduce the risk of death or permanent disability [213].

In 2019, as part of a double-blind, randomized, placebo-controlled trial in Mozambique by Dobaño et al. [214], monthly chemoprophylaxis with sulfadoxine-pyrimethamine plus artesunate (**1a**) (ASSP) was tested to selectively control timing of malaria exposure during infancy. It was observed that a balanced proinflammatory and regulatory cytokine signature (probably by innate cells), around 2 years of age, is associated with a lower risk of clinical malaria. In addition, excellent results were obtained with ASSP therapy in patients affected with uncomplicated *P. falciparum* in India, obtaining an 84.1% cure rate. The 15% failure was due to an artemisinin-resistant isolate [215].

Recent reports highlight the capacity of iron oxide nanoparticles to enhance the efficacy of artesunate (**1a**). In fact, this combination was efficient to retard growth of *P. falciparum* at a reduced drug concentration, with significant damage to macromolecules mediated by enhanced ROS production. Its efficacy against the artemisinin-resistant strain of *P. falciparum* is noteworthy, which suggests artesunate can be developed into a potent therapeutic agent against multidrug-resistant strains [216]. Despite the success of artemisinin derivative artesunate (**1a**), the two major antimalarial policy options are dihydroartemisinin (**1c**)–piperaquine (DHA–PQP) and artemether (**1b**)–lumefantrine (AL) "first-line treatment of uncomplicated *P. falciparum* malaria worldwide" [217]. The benefits of DHA–PQP in children have been validated in endemic countries [218]. The AL combined therapy exerts its effects against the erythrocytic stages of *Plasmodium* spp. In the body, artemether (**1b**) is rapidly metabolized into the active metabolite dihydroartemisinin (**1c**). It is thought that **1b** derivative provides rapid symptomatic relief by reducing the number of malarial parasites. However, lumefantrine has a much longer half-life and is believed to clear residual parasites. Extensive clinical trials of the combination were carried out against *P. falciparum* in China and elsewhere, the success of which led to marketing the combination worldwide under the name "Coartem". This resulted in many independent comparative drug studies, which further confirmed its efficacy [219,220].

A prospective, open label, non-randomized, interventional clinical trial of artemether (**1b**)–lumefantrine (AL) combined therapy was conducted in Zambia. It involved 152 HIV-infected patients with uncomplicated falciparum malaria, who were on efavirenz-based anti-retro-viral therapy. They received a 3-day directly observed standard AL treatment and were followed up until day 63. The results showed that while AL was well tolerated and efficacious in treating uncomplicated falciparum malaria, 16.4% of the participants had a recurrent malaria episode by day 42. This highlights the need in this sub-population for additional malaria prevention measures after treatment [221].

Furthermore, a systematic review compared the efficacies of artemether (**1b**)–lumefantrine (AL) and dihydroartemisinin (**1c**)–piperaquine (DHA–PQP) with or without primaquine (PQ) on the risk of *P. vivax* recurrence [222]. It revealed that administration of DHA–PQP considerably reduced *P. vivax* recurrence by day 42, compared with AL, although at day 63 the risk of recurrence following DHA–PQP was also reduced substantially by co-administration of PQ.

Malaria causes serious maternal and fetal complications, for this reason control of infection in in pregnancy is very important. Centers for Disease Control and Prevention (CDC) recommended artemether (**1b**)–lumefantrine combined therapy as an additional option for treatment of pregnant women with uncomplicated malaria in the United States during the second and third trimesters of pregnancy, at the same doses recommended for non-pregnant adults [223,224].

6.1.2. Antitumor Activity In Vivo and Clinical Trials

Artemisinin (**1**) and its derivatives (**1a**, **1b** and **1c**) are very potent anticancer compounds, highly selective on cancer cells with almost no side effects on normal cells. This specificity is due to certain tumor cell characteristics, such as increased metabolism and the high concentration of ferrous ion required to assist their rapid proliferation. There is indeed a high concentration of transferrin, an iron transporter protein situated on the surface cell, and also a susceptibility to reactive oxygen species (ROS) [225]. Furthermore, interest in artemisinin (**1**) and its derivatives resides in their minimal toxicity and adverse effects, which suggest the possibility of utilizing them as antineoplastic drugs [186].

Recent studies have shown that compound **1** and derivatives inhibit the growth of numerous types of neoplasm cells, including breast, ovarian, prostate, lung, colon, leukemia, pancreas, melanoma, renal, hepatic, gastric, and CNS cancer cells. Several reviews have been published in the last few years describing the outstanding antitumor activities of artemisinin (**1**) and derivatives upon different pathways in human cancer cells [186,198,226,227]. Therefore, we will only point to the most relevant aspects of the in vivo and clinical trials carried out.

The antitumor mechanism of artemisinin (**1**) is also based on cleavage of its endoperoxide bridge by the ferrous iron in cancer cells and formation of ROS. Such free radicals produce cell alterations such as apoptosis, DNA damage, autophagy and cell cycle arrest G0/G1 [227]. They can also inhibit angiogenesis by inhibiting the secretion of VEGF, VEGFR2, and KDR/flk-1 in tumors [228,229]. They also may affect signaling pathways and transcription factors associated with tumor growth, including the Wnt/β-catenin and AMPK pathways, nitric oxide signaling, NF-κB, CREBP, MYC/MAX, mTOR, and AP-1 [230].

Some derivatives have reached the phase of clinical trials against several cancers such as breast, cervical, hepatocellular carcinoma, non-small cell lung, squamous cell laryngeal [229,231,232]. However, insufficient large-scale clinical studies have been conducted on their applications in cancer therapy.

Artenusate (**1a**) was used in phase I clinical trial to treat metastatic breast cancer (ClinicalTrials.gov identifier: NCT00764036) and concluded that 200 mg per day are recommended for future trials [233]. This compound (**1a**) is also being tested regarding colorectal cancer phase I (ISRCTN registry: ISRCTN05203252) and its safety and efficiency in stage II/III to the same disease (ClinicalTrials.gov identifier: NCT02633098), as treatment in patients with cervical dysplasia (ClinicalTrials.gov identifier: NCT02354534) and as treatment of HPV-associated anal intraepithelial neoplasia (ClinicalTrials.gov identifier: NCT03100045). Recently, Trimble et al. [234] assess for the first time the safety and efficacy of intravaginal artesunate (**1a**) to treat cervical intraepithelial neoplasia 2/3 (CIN2/3) with good results which support continuing phase II clinical (ClinicalTrials.gov identifier: NCT04098744). A phase-one study was also conducted to evaluate its safety and pharmacokinetic properties when administered orally in patients with advanced hepatocellular carcinoma (ClinicalTrials.gov identifier: NCT02304289) [235]. One double-blind placebo-controlled trial consisted of giving human colorectal cancer patients oral compound **1a** prior to surgery. During a median follow-up of 42 months, 1 patient in the artesunate group had a recurrence of colon cancer compared to 6 patients in the placebo group [236].

Artemether (**1b**) has also been included in a phase I/IIa study to assess its potential use in treating subjects with advanced solid tumors (ClinicalTrials.gov identifier: NCT02263950) [235]. Another report describes beneficial improvement in a patient with pituitary macroadenoma treated with it for 12 months [237].

The pilot clinical phase I/II trial of dihydroartemisinin (**1c**) [238] against advanced cervical carcinoma indicates that after three weeks of treatment in ten women, the majority showed improvement in the signs and symptoms. This included the vaginal discharge and pain, with no evidence of severe toxicity. These patients had a lower expression of epidermal growth factor receptor (EGFR) and Ki-67 oncogenes.

Furthermore, with the goal of increasing the antineoplastic effect of these drugs, the combination of the usual chemotherapy with artemisinin or its derivatives has been investigated, showing that their multifactorial action on various pathways may improve overall activity [232]. Interestingly, Wang et al. [239], demonstrated that dihydroartemisinin (**1c**) improves the anticancer effect of gemcitabine, a drug used in pancreatic cancer, which develops resistance over time. They confirmed by in vitro and in vivo analysis that compound **1c** induced increased growth inhibition and apoptosis 4- and 2-fold, using both drugs and alone, respectively.

Tilaoui et al. [240] observed a synergistic effect when they used vincristine and artemisinin (**1**), in combination, against murine mastocytoma (P815) cells. A randomized controlled trial with artesunate (**1a**) combine with a chemotherapy regime using vinorelbine plus cisplatin, in patients with advanced non-small cell lung cancer (NSCLL) shown that this treatment can raise the short-term survival rate and prolong the progression time, without extra side effects [241]. Liu et al. [242] found that a combination of artesunate (**1a**) with lenalinomide, commonly used for the treatment of multiple myeloma, caused an impressive enhancement of antineoplastic activity in polyploid cell lines [243], while Singh and Verna [244] described significant improvement and 70% reduction in tumor size after 2 weeks of treating a patient diagnosed with stage II cancer of the larynx with the same compound **1a** (50 mg). Additionally, the first long-term treatment of two patients with metastatic uveal melanoma with artesunate (**1a**), in combination with standard chemotherapy, was reported [245]. The standard therapy alone was ineffective in stopping tumor growth, while the disease was stabilized after adding compound **1a** to this chemotherapy, followed by objective regressions of spleen and lung metastases [245].

Another characteristic of tumors and cancer cells is their ability to develop resistance to chemotherapy due to their rapid cell-division rate and genetic mutations [246]. In this context, Reungpatthanaphong et al. [247] report that artemisinin (**1**), artesunate, and dihydroartemisinin (**1c**), combined with doxorubicin and pirarubicin, increased the cytotoxic effect induced by pirarubicin or doxorubicin only in MDR cell lines. They proposed that artemisinin and its derivatives reverse the MDR phenomenon at the mitochondrial level.

Currently, another series of derivatives are being explored that present a longer plasma life and are more powerful and effective at lower concentrations. These include artemisinin dimers and trimers, hybrid compounds, and tagging of the compounds to molecules that are involved in the intracellular iron-delivery mechanism. These compounds are promising potent anticancer agents that produce significantly less side effects than conventional chemotherapeutic agents [226].

6.2. α-Santonin and Its Derivatives

Santonin ($C_{15}H_{18}O_3$) (**2**) (Figure 1) is an eudesmanolide sesquiterpene lactone first isolated from A. santonicum by Kahler in 1830 [248], but it is much less known than artemisinin (**1**). Santonin exists in two isomeric forms, α-santonin and β-santonin [249], with α-santonin being the most studied form due to its higher stability [250].

Its isolation and characterization proved an arduous and grueling task for chemists at the time [251]. Its mevalonoid biosynthesis pathways has long been studied, revealing that it is formed by a methylene reduction, C-1 hydroxylation and C-3 oxidation of the precursor costunolide, sharing an identical initial pathway [252,253]. The synthesis of santonin (**2**) was first described by Marshall and Wuts in 1978 [250] and involved the reduction-alkylation of m-toluic acid with lithium in ammonia.

Santonin is the most abundant sesquiterpene lactone in *Artemisia cina* Berg ex Poljakov and was isolated from several *Artemisia* species [254–256], including some edible species such as *A. absinthium*, *A. frigida*, *A. tridentata* [34,255]. *Artemisia santonicum* is commonly referred to as "wormseed", a name historically attributed to the plants' anthelmintic ("worms") activity [251]. Indeed, santonin was one of the most frequently used treatments for intestinal nematode infections up until the 1970s [257]. Nowadays santonin has fallen out of use due to a wealth of better anthelmintic therapeutics [258]. Nevertheless, santonin has been revealed to have many other bioactivities worthy of investigating. In a recent publication [259] santonin proved to have potent insect growth inhibitory effect on the cotton bollworm, *Helicoverpa armigera*, a widespread pest of significant agricultural and economic impact. In this work, the researchers showed that a 2 mg/mL dose of santonin in wet feed would cause a significant (~80%) decrease in larval weight compared to the control. This is explained by the results obtained from the excised midguts, which revealed that trehalase activity had decreased to 32% of the control in treated larva. Trehalase is an important enzyme in the metabolism of trehalose, an abundant simple sugar in plants. This enzyme inhibitory activity could also be allied with santonin's effect of rupturing insect midgut cell lining [260]. Overall, this shows there is clear signs of a potential value for the compound in possible environmentally friendly pesticidal formulations, as well as a continued interest in the compound. We would also like to note the high quality of this publication, particularly in its clarity of language and presentation of data, something which is sorely missed in similar publications.

In modern times attention has mostly been devoted to α-santonin derivatives as opposed to the actual compound. This is because α-santonin's chemical structure lends itself very well to modifications, the compound a cheap and easy to use platform for drug synthesis [261]. Indeed, two reviews were recently published [256,261] about α-santonin derivatives and how different structural changes affect their bioactivities. In vitro results are much more abundant for santonin derivatives, mainly detailing the synthesis of novel cancer therapeutic agents. Santonin tumor inhibitory derivatives have included a diacetoxy acetal form [262]; spiro-isoxazoline and spiro-isoxazolidine derivatives [263,264]; cinnamic acid derivatives [265], immunosuppressants [266]; anti-inflammatory bromoketone [267–269]. Given the scope of the previously cited reviews, here it will be highlighting the main recently published derivatives showing potent in vivo effects.

Regarding in vivo effects, a recently published work [270] presents an α-santonin derivative (a benzyl ether derivative containing *o*-bromine named (3a*S*,9b*R*)-8-((2-bromobenzyl)oxy)-6,9-dimethyl-3-methylene3a,4,5,9b-tetrahydronaphtho[1,2-b]furan-2(3*H*)-one) (compound **2a**, Figure 1) with potent anti-inflammatory bioactivity. In this work [270], the α-santonin derivative **2a** was synthesized and screened for in vitro activity where it was the most potent one and selected for further in vivo assays. This compound was administered orally to an arthritis rat model with very similar characteristics to rheumatoid arthritis human patients. Rats were treated with doses of 5 and 20 mg/kg (*w*/*w*) per day of the selected derivative **2a** and monitored for arthritic disease progression. Results showed a significant improvement of arthritis symptomatology in the treated rats, with ~40% lower clinical disease scores (associated with the degree of limb swelling) and significant reduction of hind paw volume. It is also worth noting that the response seems to not be dose-dependent, since both doses tested revealed almost identical activity. After mechanistic studies, the authors attribute this effect to the selective bonding of the derivative with the active site of UbcH5c, a key enzyme for ubiquitination during TNF-α-triggered activation of the NF-κB inflammatory pathway. These results seem to indicate the potent anti-inflammatory bioactivity of this novel derivative **2a**, with potential future applications in the development of a new anti-rheumatoid arthritis (RA) drug.

However, some criticism can be levelled at the work of Chen et al. [270], primarily for the way the researchers measure disease progression; their score system seems simplistic and overly reliant on somewhat subjective and qualitative observation (swelling vs. no swelling), rather than more quantitative records and measures, rendering it quite unwieldy and difficult to understand. Another addition to this work we consider beneficial would have been to include a positive control. By including a known and widely used anti-rheumatic in this in vivo assay, we could assess the bioactivity of this novel compound by comparison with a known therapeutic. We believe more studies are required in order to better understand this new agent, and hope to see clinical trials in the near future.

Novel immunosuppressant drugs are currently in very high demand due to the high cost and serious side effects of currently used therapeutics [271]. A very interesting research was published in 2017 [272], exhibiting a novel α-santonin derivative with in vivo immunosuppressant properties. In this paper [272] the authors describe the synthesis of several O-aryl/aliphatic ether, ester and amide α-santonin derivatives and the in vitro assay for immunosuppressant bioactivity, showed one particular compound exhibiting ~75–80% proliferation suppression rates for B and T lymphocytes. This derivative, a trimethyl acetate ester α-santonin analogue (compound **2b**, Figure 1), was used for in vivo immunosuppression testing using BALB/c mice. Rats were injected with 6.25 mg/kg (*w/w*), 12.5 mg/kg (*w/w*) and 25 mg/kg (*w/w*). Rat humoral immune response was assessed by quantification of post-challenge antibody production and cell mediated immune response was assayed by post-challenge left hind footpad thickness measurement. Results were impressive: humoral response was suppressed by 28% with the lowest dose (6.25 mg/kg (*w/w*)), and 41% at the highest dose (25 mg/kg (*w/w*)); and cell mediated immune response was suppressed by ~30% in the medium and highest doses. These results were comparable to the positive control cyclophosphamide regarding humoral response but fell considerably shorter of the positive control in the cell mediated response assay. Nevertheless, these results show that the novel derivative synthesized is capable of both humoral and cell mediated immune suppression, with reasonable potency, making it a prime candidate for future drug development. More tests with this compound, particularly exploring the mode of action, which was not presented by Dangroo et al. [272] and future clinical trials are expected.

From these studies and cited reviews, it is concluded that santonin and its derivatives are highly interesting, with new papers and bioactivities being constantly researched and published. It is expected to see some of these compounds enter pre-clinical testing soon.

6.3. Achillin

Achillin (**3**) (Figure 1) a sesquiterpene lactone ($C_{15}H_{18}O_3$) of the guaianolide class, first identified in *Achillea millefolium* L. (syn *Achillea lanulosa* Nutt.) in 1963 by White and Winter [273] and synthesized in 1967 [274].

Although achillin (**3**, Figure 1) is mainly extracted from plants of the *Achillea* genus, it has also been identified in edible *Artemisia* species such as *A. capillaris* [275], *A. frigida* [276], *Artemisia feddei* H. Lév. & Vaniot [277] and *A. ludoviciana* [278]. It has also been identified in plants of other species, such as *Taraxacum platycarpum* [279] and *Anthemis scrobicularis* [280]. Achillin biosynthesis pathway starts with the eudesmane skeleton of α-santonin, and involves the hydrolysis of an acetate precursor, followed by epimerization at C-11 and finishing with an allylic oxidation [281].

The first bioactivity for achillin (**3**) described it as a strong antifeedant agent against two grasshopper species [282]. This study showed that a concentration of only 0.5% (% dry weight) of compound **3** was enough to repel *Melanoplus sanguinipes* from feeding. This antifeedant effect was measured qualitatively rather than quantitatively, so it is difficult to accurately assess the full extent of the antifeedant bioactivity. Nevertheless, the rather limited preliminary study [282] was enough to show there was potential application to achillin (**3**). Subsequent in vitro assays followed, showing it had anti-allergic effect (IC_{50} = 100 μM) [279]; increasing chemosensitivity to paclitaxel, with potency comparable to known therapeutics at 100 μM concentration [283]; and antitumor against endocervical cell lines (IC_{50} = 160.3 μg/mL after 72 h [48].

Achillin (**3**) has proven to possess interesting and potent bioactivities tested in vivo. Firstly, the work of Rivero-Cruz et al. [278] showed compound **3** had potent antinociceptive effect in mice assessed using the formalin test. This work started by focusing on the effects of *A. ludoviciana* (edible species), showing it had strong in vivo analgesic and anti-inflammatory effects. Subsequent analysis by HPLC attributed the bioactivity to the presence of two sesquiterpene lactones being one of them achillin and the other dehydroleucodin. Regarding achillin (**3**), it was individually tested using the formalin assay and showed significant activity causing near 50% reduction in formalin wound time with a dose of 17.7 mg/kg (*w/w*). Researchers did not specify a mode of action for this activity but cited a previous work [284] attributing the effect to the NF-κB inhibition by sesquiterpene lactones. Another point of critique to the work of Rivero-Cruz et al. [278] would be the heavy emphasis on assaying the plant extract as opposed to the isolated compounds. More extensive testing with the purified compounds would be desirable, producing far more relevant and compelling results. Nevertheless, this work proved achillin possesses interesting antinociceptive bioactivity, which should be studied further, particularly in finding out its mode of action.

Another highly relevant study with achillin (**3**) in animal model was its effect as an inhibitor of meiosis in toad (*Rhinella arenarum*) oocytes was carried out by Zapata-Martínez et al. [285], where denuded toad oocytes were exposed to different concentrations of achillin prior to the necessary hormonal stimulus necessary for meiotic resumption. Results showed a marked overall decrease of germinal vesicle breakdown (GVBD) in occytes with exposure to **3**. It is also worth noting that the response was dose-dependent; a 6 μM concentration of achillin (**3**) showed a ~10% reduction of GVBD compared the control, whereas a 36 μM concentration reduced GVBD by ~35% more than control oocytes. So, it appears achillin (**3**) has meiosis inhibiting potential, which the authors [285] attribute to the covalent bonds formed between achillin's partially electrophilic center and the nucleophilic center of target molecules. The meiotic inhibitors have been shown to improve human embryonic development in in-vitro fertilization procedures by allowing the embryo to have enough time to finish cytoplasmic maturation [286].

Finally, we present a very recent 2020 paper by Arias-Durán et al. [287] showing achillin's potential as a smooth muscle cell relaxant. The authors used an ex vivo rat trachea model, where the relaxing effects of increasing concentrations of achillin (**3**) were measured in the rat trachea rings. The results showed achillin (**3**) exhibited almost identical activity to theophylline, a widely used medicine for asthma and chronic obstructive pulmonary disease. The effect seems to be mainly due to a release of nitric oxide and calcium channel blockade influx into the smooth muscle cells of the tracheal rings [286]. This result indicates the great potential as a smooth cell muscle relaxant, with possible applications in the treatment of asthma, bronchospasm and chronic bronchitis.

In conclusion, achillin (**3**) exhibits very interesting bioactivities, mainly anti-inflammatory, meiotic inhibitor, and tracheal relaxant. It is also worth noting that this compound has also been identified as the possible bioactive agent behind interesting *Artemisia* extracts bioactivities, such as allelopathic [276] and anticarcinogenic [275]. It would be very interesting to follow-up on these results with more assays involving the purified compound, although such would possibly require biosynthetic methods, since it is reportedly very difficult to obtain large quantities of purified achillin (**3**) [275]. Nevertheless, there is great potential for its future drug development, but further research is needed.

6.4. Tehranolide

Tehranolide ($C_{15}H_{22}O_6$) (**4**) (Figure 1), also sometimes referred to as artediffusin, is a sesquiterpene lactone first isolated from the aerial parts of *Artemisia diffusa* Krasch. ex Poljakov (edible) [288]. Currently, based on The Plant List database, *A. diffusa* name is a synonym of *Seriphidium diffusum* (Krasch. ex Poljak.) Y.R. Ling.

A biosynthesis pathway has been suggested by [289], involving the oxidative cleavage of the Δ^4 bond of a eudesmanolide derivative, followed by an internal aldol condensation, rearrangement by hydroxy addition and ending with acetal formation. Chemical synthesis has not been described for compound (**4**) which explains why work done with this compound is predominantly centered in a certain few labs and research groups geographically close to the relatively narrow *A. diffusa* natural distribution. There is continued interest in the eudesmanolide chemical synthesis and its derivatives [290,291].

Structurally, tehranolide (**4**) exhibits great similarity to artemisinin (**1**), including the presence of an endoperoxide (C-O-O-C) bridge common to both compounds. This is very noteworthy, since the endoperoxide group is reported to be vital to artemisinin antimalarial activity [202]. This established connection between structure and function lead to the hypothesis that compound **4** could have antimalarial activity, which was investigated by Rustaiyan et al. [292–294], with in vivo results using the purified compound. In this work, the authors use NMRI infected with *Plasmodium berghei*, a widely used malaria animal model organism. The mice were injected daily with doses ranging from 1.7 g to 17 mg (total dose) of HPLC purified tehranolide (**4**). Results showed the lowest dose (17 mg) significantly reduced *P. berghei* parasitemia by ~10% (compared to negative control) 2 days after infection while the highest dose (1.7 g) significantly reduced it by ~14%. It is important to note that, even though dosages varied by a factor of 100, differences between doses were relatively small, and became almost imperceptible 10 days after infection (while still maintaining ~10% difference to negative control after 10 days). We can then conclude that although some dose-dependence effect was exhibited, it was relatively small, and that over time all doses showed almost identical effect when compared between each other.

Some criticism can be made to this work, particularly the fact that total doses were uniformly used instead of doses adjusted to mouse weight. This means that mouse weight fluctuations translated into differing compound systemic concentrations (i.e., "lighter" mice will exhibit higher compound concentrations than "heavier" mice, which could result in exacerbated effect). This ended up not being very relevant, since the results showed relatively small difference between doses, but could have definitely cast doubt upon the results if compound dose-dependency was more exuberant and should be avoided in future assays. Other points open to criticism could be the use of a relatively small sample size (n = 5, in triplicate), and the lack of usage of a positive control, in order to compare compound **4**'s efficacy against known used therapeutics. Nevertheless, the work serves to prove that the in vivo anti-malarial bioactivity.

The mode of action for this compound has not been specifically described but, it is thought to be very similar to artemisinin's (**1**), due to the similar structure [288]. Mechanistically, the antimalarial bioactivity results from the presence of haem or Fe^{2+} resulting from the *P. falciparum* hemolysis. The Fe^{2+} functions as a catalyst to the opening of the peroxide bridge of the compound, which leads to the formation of free radicals, alkylating *P. falciparum* proteins and eventually causing parasite death.

The bioactivity presented above exhibited by tehranolide (**4**) is very interesting and relevant to current society when consider the ever-increasing *Plasmodium falciparum* antimalarial drug resistance [295]. There is indeed an urgent need for novel antimalarial compounds which exhibit potential as a possible therapeutic and the compound **4** was considered a very promise antimalaria agent [296]. Given these facts, it would be expected to see more work done with this compound, hopefully aiming at pre-clinical testing.

Tehranolide (**4**) has also proven to be a very promising anticancer agent, with several recent publications supporting in vivo effect. Much like before, the initial hypothesis was derived from the structural similarity between compound **4** and artemisinin (**1**), whose anticancer activity is discussed above. The earliest account of **4** anticancer bioactivity was described by Noori et al. [297,298]. These papers are arguably some of the most important works on this subject, due to the in vivo nature of the assays and the immunomodulatory insights provided. In summary, a total dose of 5.64 µg of tehranolide (**4**) per mouse was injected intratumor in Balb/c breast cancer mouse models. Results showed this dose significantly inhibited tumor growth by ~75% compared to negative control. Treated animals also exhibited ~2.5× increase in lymphocyte proliferation, as well as ~12% decrease in $CD4^+CD25^+Foxp3^+$ regulatory T cells, an important factor in tumor tolerance [299], when compared with negative control. These results showed compound **4** had potent in vivo anticancer activity and great potential as an immunotherapeutic regulator. Subsequent follow-up work by the same research group [300] with similarly mice treated (same dose and conditions) revealed a ~80% increase in apoptosis index of tumor cells compared to untreated mice. This result confirms compound **4** indeed possesses in vivo antitumor activity by apoptosis induction (attributed to a tumor cell selective G0/G1 cycle arrest. Finally, Noori et al. [301] describe in detail the mechanism behind compound **4** anticancer activity as being linked to calmodulin and phosphodiesterase type 1 inhibition, as well as cAMP-dependent protein kinase A activity. These processes allow tehranolide (**4**) to selectively inhibit tumor proliferation and induce tumor cell apoptosis.

In conclusion, compound **4** has proven to have great potential as an antimalarial but mainly as anticancer therapeutic. Both of these bioactivities are extremely relevant and important in the modern medical/scientific paradigm, because of the need for novel antimalarials as previously mentioned, as well as rising cancer rates [302]. We hope to see tehranolide (**4**) progress into pre-clinical stages of research with regards to both of these activities.

7. Hotpoint Research: *Artemisia* Species and Its Constituents as Strategy to Treat COVID-19 Infection

Caused by a member of the Coronavirus family (CoV), SARS-CoV-2 (COVID-19) has recently posed a potential threat to the survival of human beings on Earth and was declared a global health emergency by the WHO [303]. The therapeutic strategy to treat infection by this coronavirus has used the knowledge and experience acquired in the previous epidemics caused by SARS-CoV-1 and MERS-CoV. To date, there are no vaccines or specific antiviral agents against coronavirus infections, so it is a great challenge for scientists to find treatments for them. Repositioning of drugs already in clinical use is being studied, as a quick response to provide effective treatments in humans and assess other compounds that may be effective against the virus [304]. The WHO proposed *A. annua* as a possible treatment to be considered for COVID-19 treatment, however its efficacy and side-effects must be determined. Additionally, *A. annua* is one of the of Jinhua Qinggan granule ingredients, one of the Traditional Chinese Patent Medicines recommended in 13 therapeutic regimens of COVID-19 in China [305]. The *A. argyi* it was also mentioned as one of the plants that can be used by aromatherapy method of Traditional Chinese Medicine with effects of contagion prevention [306]. Scientific evidence supporting this proposal is partly based on bioactive compounds present in the plant with antiviral effects against hepatitis B, bovine viral diarrhea, and Epstein–Barr virus [307]. It also contains compounds with antioxidant, anti-inflammatory and immunomodulatory properties [176], which would play an important role in controlling the acute inflammatory process triggered by Covid-19 infection. Another research line requiring further attention in the context of acute Covid-19 is the efficacy of the artesunate to ameliorate bleomycin-induced pulmonary fibrosis pathology in rats, possibly by inhibiting profibrotic molecules [308]. Other promising pointers are that *A. annua* showed significant activity in vitro against SARS-CoV-1-2002 (IC_{50} = 34.5 ± 2.6 µg/mL) [309,310]. Tea infusions of *A. annua* and *A. afra* were found to be highly active against HIV virus, although the role of artemisinin is rather limited [311], as were various *Artemisia* species against Herpes simplex virus type 1 [312] and *A. capillaris* against Hepatitis B [169]. In a recent preliminary in silico study, Rolta et al. [313] evaluated the possibility of binding artemisinin (among other compounds) to the cellular ACE-2 receptors via the spicules of the SARS-CoV-2 membrane, as well as ADMET prediction and toxicity analysis. The results obtained support the possibility that artemisinin can act as an antiviral by means of a predictable binding to the receptor, also being non-carcinogenic, non-cytotoxic and safe to administer.

Clearly, greater scientific attention is placed and needed toward *A. annua* and its bioactive compound/derivatives in addressing the treatment of COVID-19 and they need to be further assessed in clinical trials. Kapepula et al. recently published a review drawing attention to the path to be followed and the errors to avoid [314]. And this assessment already started. The phase II clinical study is currently underway (ClinicalTrials.gov identifier: NCT04530617, recruitment), aiming to evaluate the efficacy of *A. annua* and camostat to inhibit viral entry or replication of SARS-CoV-2 virus and their toxicity, administered immediately after COVID-19 positive testing, in mild to moderate disease patients and with high-risk factors such as diabetes, hypertension and obesity, among others.

8. Conclusions

This review starts to present an overview of *Artemisia* species traditional use as food, spices, condiment and beverage. The plants are mainly used in salads and tea, as well as to flavoring food and beverages. The leaves are the most used edible part, but the aerial parts, mentioned as "herb", is also widely used. The nutritional value of *Artemisia* species is also presented and discussed, based on the fatty acid, proteins, sugars, minerals, and vitamin contents reported in the literature.

Studies already published show that the use of *Artemisia* plants is not risk-free. The allergic reactions, mainly allergic rhinitis caused by pollens and skin dermatitis caused by the presence of sesquiterpene lactones, are the most frequently reported and studied adverse effects. Absinthe drinks are reported as causing some adverse side-effects, so its content is legislated. Some *Artemisia* species cause reduction of fertility, so its use is not recommended during pregnancy.

The evaluation, based on clinical studies, of the *Artemisia* formulations effectiveness remains a hot topic. The application of integral plants or extracts as anti-inflammatory agents is deepened and the spectrum of applications broadened to, for example, the preventive effect on hepatitis B cirrhosis, treatment of malaria, anti-allergenic and glycemic control.

Concerning the *Artemisia* constituents, clinical and in vivo studies involving artemisinin and its derivatives show them as efficient antimalarial and anticancer agents. Additionally, the additive or synergistic interactions of artemisinin and derivatives in combination with a wide array of clinically established drugs to combat different cancer are highlighted. The high therapeutic potential is evident in the WHO proposal to investigate artemisinin and derivatives as well as *A. annua* to the treatment of Covid-19 infection. In addition to artemisinin and its derivatives, other sesquiterpene lactones isolated from different species of *Artemisia*, such as santonin, achillin and tehranolide, have been the target of further studies with a view to the development of new derivatives and their application as medicines. These compounds exhibit very interesting activities, in in vivo models, such as immunosuppressant and anti-inflammatory and potent antinociceptive effect. Achillin acts as a meiotic inhibitor and smooth muscle cell relaxant, properties very relevant to improve human embryonic development in-vitro fertilization procedures and to treat asthma and chronic obstructive pulmonary disease, respectively.

Nevertheless, although this review shows the great potential for *Artemisia* species as dietary supplements, functional foods, source of new and more efficient and safe drugs, further research on action mechanism and involving clinical trials on toxicity, adverse side-effects, efficacy and health care uses continue to be needed.

Author Contributions: Conceptualization, A.M.L.S. and A.T.; writing—original draft preparation, A.M.L.S., A.T., L.M.M., P.M.C.S.; writing—review and editing, A.M.L.S., A.T. and L.M.M. All authors have read and agreed to the published version of the manuscript.

Funding: This research was funded by FCT–Fundação para a Ciência e a Tecnologia, the European Union, QREN, FEDER, COMPETE, by funding the cE3c centre (UIDB/00329/2020) and the LAQV-REQUIMTE (UIDB/50006/2020) research units; Funded by RTI2018-094356-B-C21 Spanish MINECO project, co-funded by European Regional Development Fund (FEDER); And funded by the project EthnoHERBS (H2020-MSCA-RISE-2018, No. 823973).

Data Availability Statement: Not applicable.

Acknowledgments: Thanks are due to the University of Azores, University of La Laguna and Institute of Organic Chemistry with Centre of Phytochemistry, Bulgarian Academy of Sciences.

Conflicts of Interest: The authors declare no conflict of interest.

References

1. The Plant List, a Working List of All Plant Species. Available online: http://www.theplantlist.org/tpl1.1/search?q=Artemisia (accessed on 24 June 2020).

2. Vallès, J.; Garcia, S.; Hidalgo, O.; Martín, J.; Pellicer, J.; Sanz, M.; Garnatje, T. Biology, genome evolution, biotechnological issues and research including applied perspectives in *Artemisia* (Asteraceae). In *Advances in Botanical Research*; Kader, J.-C., Delseny, M., Eds.; Academic Press: Burlington, NJ, USA, 2011; Volume 60, pp. 349–419, ISBN 978-0-12-385851-1.
3. Hussain, A.; Potter, D.; Kim, S.; Hayat, M.Q.; Bokhari, S.A. Molecular phylogeny of Artemisia (Asteraceae-Anthemideae) with emphasis on undescribed taxa from Gilgit-Baltistan (Pakistan) based on nrDNA (ITS and ETS) and cpDNA (psbA-trnH) sequences. *Plant Ecol. Evol.* **2019**, *152*, 507–520. [CrossRef]
4. Taleghani, A.; Emami, S.A.; Tayarani-Najaran, Z. Artemisia: A promising plant for the treatment of cancer. *Bioorg. Med. Chem.* **2020**, *28*, 115180. [CrossRef] [PubMed]
5. Ekiert, H.; Pajor, J.; Klin, P.; Rzepiela, A.; Ślesak, H.; Szopa, A. Significance of *Artemisia vulgaris* L. (Common Mugwort) in the History of Medicine and Its Possible Contemporary Applications Substantiated by Phytochemical and Pharmacological Studies. *Molecules* **2020**, *25*, 4415. [CrossRef] [PubMed]
6. Verloove, F.; Andeweg, R. *Artemisia princeps* L. (Asteraceae), an overlooked invasive Far Eastern weed in Western Europe. *Gorteria* **2020**, *42*, 1–18.
7. Boršić, I.; Milović, M.; Dujmović, I.; Bogdanović, S.; Cigić, P.; Rešetnik, I.; Nikolić, T.; Mitić, B. Preliminary check-list of invasive alien plant species (IAS) in Croatia. *Nat. Croat.* **2008**, *17*, 55–71.
8. Nadeem, M.; Shinwari, Z.K.; Qaiser, M. Screening of folk remedies by genus *Artemisia* based on ethnomedicinal surveys and traditional knowledge of native communities of Pakistan. *Pak. J. Bot.* **2013**, *45*, 111–117.
9. Sadiq, A.; Hayat, M.Q.; Ashraf, M. Ethnopharmacology of *Artemisia annua* L.: A review. In *Artemisia Annua—Pharmacology and Biotechnology*; Aftab, T., Ferreira, J., Khan, M., Naeem, M., Eds.; Springer: Berlin/Heidelberg, Germany, 2014. [CrossRef]
10. Vouillamoz, J.F.; Carlen, C.; Taglialatela-Scafati, O.; Pollastro, F.; Appendino, G. The génépi Artemisia species. Ethnopharmacology, cultivation, phytochemistry, and bioactivity. *Fitoterapia* **2015**, *106*, 231–241. [CrossRef]
11. Dib, I.; Angenot, L.; Mihamou, A.; Ziyyat, A.; Tits, M. Artemisia campestris L.: Ethnomedicinal, phytochemical and pharmacological review. *J. Herb. Med.* **2017**, *7*, 1–10. [CrossRef]
12. Ahuja, A.; Yi, Y.-S.; Kim, M.-Y.; Cho, J.Y. Ethnopharmacological properties of Artemisia asiatica: A comprehensive review. *J. Ethnopharmacol.* **2018**, *220*, 117–128. [CrossRef]
13. Abiri, R.; Silva, A.L.M.; De Mesquita, L.S.S.; De Mesquita, J.W.C.; Atabaki, N.; De Almeida, E.B.; Shaharuddin, N.A.; Malik, S. Towards a better understanding of Artemisia vulgaris: Botany, phytochemistry, pharmacological and biotechnological potential. *Food Res. Int.* **2018**, *109*, 403–415. [CrossRef]
14. Kumar, A.; Aswal, S.; Semwal, R.B.; Chauhan, A.; Semwal, D.K. Insights on the pharmacological, phytochemical and ethnobotanical aspects of Artemisia roxburghiana: A rather less explored but therapeutically important species of lower Himalayas. *Phytochem. Rev.* **2019**, *18*, 199–214. [CrossRef]
15. Du Toit, A.; Van Der Kooy, F. Artemisia afra, a controversial herbal remedy or a treasure trove of new drugs? *J. Ethnopharmacol.* **2019**, *244*, 112127. [CrossRef] [PubMed]
16. Septembre-Malaterre, A.; Rakoto, M.L.; Marodon, C.; Bedoui, Y.; Nakab, J.; Simon, E.; Hoarau, L.; Savriama, S.; Strasberg, D.; Guiraud, P.; et al. Artemisia annua, a Traditional Plant Brought to Light. *Int. J. Mol. Sci.* **2020**, *21*, 4986. [CrossRef] [PubMed]
17. Szopa, A.; Pajor, J.; Klin, P.; Rzepiela, A.; Elansary, H.O.; Al-Mana, F.A.; Mattar, M.A.; Ekiert, H. Artemisia absinthium L.—Importance in the History of Medicine, the Latest Advances in Phytochemistry and Therapeutical, Cosmetological and Culinary Uses. *Plants* **2020**, *9*, 1063. [CrossRef]
18. Feng, X.; Cao, S.; Qiu, F.; Zhang, B.-L. Traditional application and modern pharmacological research of Artemisia annua L. *Pharmacol. Ther.* **2020**, *216*, 107650. [CrossRef]
19. Batiha, G.E.-S.; Olatunde, A.; El-Mleeh, A.; Hetta, H.F.; Al-Rejaie, S.; Alghamdi, S.; Zahoor, M.; Beshbishy, A.M.; Murata, T.; Zaragoza-Bastida, A.; et al. Bioactive Compounds, Pharmacological Actions, and Pharmacokinetics of Wormwood (*Artemisia absinthium*). *Antibiotics* **2020**, *9*, 353. [CrossRef]
20. Liu, N.; Van Der Kooy, F.; Verpoorte, R. Artemisia afra: A potential flagship for African medicinal plants? *S. Afr. J. Bot.* **2009**, *75*, 185–195. [CrossRef]
21. Semenya, S.S.; Maroyi, A. Ethnobotanical study of curative plants used by traditional healers to treat rhinitis in the Limpopo Province, South Africa. *Afr. Health Sci.* **2018**, *18*, 1076–1087. [CrossRef]
22. Native American Ethnobotany. Available online: http://naeb.brit.org/uses/search/?string=Artemisia+dracunculus (accessed on 14 October 2020).
23. Nabimeybodi, R.; Zareshahi, R.; Tansaz, M.; Dastjerdi, M.V.; Hajimehdipoor, H. Scientific Evaluation of Medicinal Plants Used for the Treatment of Cervicitis (Qorohe- Rahem) in Iranian Traditional Medicine. *Iran. J. Pharm. Res.* **2019**, *18*, 1884–1901.
24. Native American Ethnobotany. Available online: http://naeb.brit.org/uses/search/?string=Artemisia+vulgaris (accessed on 14 October 2020).
25. Xiao, B.; Wang, J.-H.; Zhou, C.-Y.; Chen, J.-M.; Zhang, N.; Zhao, N.; Han, X.-Y.; Niu, Y.-X.; Feng, Y.-B.; Du, G.-H. Ethno-medicinal study of *Artemisia* ordosica Krasch. (traditional Chinese/Mongolian medicine) extracts for the treatment of allergic rhinitis and nasosinusitis. *J. Ethnopharmacol.* **2020**, *248*, 112262. [CrossRef]
26. Xiao, B.; Bai, J.J.; Qi, L.; Lu, L.S.; Tian, X.R.; Yin, J.; Su, Y.X. Research progress on resource distribution, chemical components, and pharmacological activities of *Artemisia* ordosica Krasch. *J. Chin. Pharm.* **2016**, *13*, 1862–1864.

27. Native American Ethnobotany. Available online: http://naeb.brit.org/uses/search/?string=Artemisia+tripartita (accessed on 14 October 2020).
28. Calderone, V.; Martinotti, E.; Baragatti, B.; Breschi, M.C.; Morelli, I. Vascular effects of aqueous crude extracts of *Artemisia verlotorum* Lamotte (Compositae): In vivo and in vitro pharmacological studies in rats. *Phytother. Res.* **1999**, *13*, 645–648. [CrossRef]
29. Hussain, A. Distribution and Molecular Phylogeny of *Artemisia* Plants from Gilgit-Baltistan, Pakistan. Ph.D. Thesis, University of International Islamic University Islamabad, Islamabad, Pakistan, March 2019; pp. 69–70, Reg. No. 31-FBAS/PHDBT/F14. Available online: http://prr.hec.gov.pk/jspui/handle/123456789/11070 (accessed on 15 October 2020).
30. World Health Organization. *WHO Global Report on Traditional and Complementary Medicine 2019*; WHO Press: Geneva, Switzerland, 2019; Licence: CC BY-NC-SA 3.0 IGO.
31. Miller, F.G.; Emanuel, E.J.; Rosenstein, D.L.; Straus, S.E. Ethical Issues Concerning Research in Complementary and Alternative Medicine. *JAMA* **2004**, *291*, 599. [CrossRef] [PubMed]
32. Smith, K.; Ernst, E.; Colquhoun, D.; Sampson, W. 'Complementary & Alternative Medicine' (CAM): Ethical and policy issues. *Bioethics* **2016**, *30*, 60–62. [CrossRef] [PubMed]
33. Martinez, M.J.A.; Bedoya, L.M.; Apaza, L.; Bermejo, P. The *Artemisia* L. Genus: A Review of Bioactive Essential Oils. *Molecules* **2012**, *17*, 2542–2566. [CrossRef]
34. Turi, C.E.; Shipley, P.R.; Murch, S.J. North American Artemisia species from the subgenus Tridentatae (Sagebrush): A phytochemical, botanical and pharmacological review. *Phytochemistry* **2014**, *98*, 9–26. [CrossRef]
35. Wan, Y.-J.; Xia, J.-X.; Tang, L. Chemical constituents, biological activities and clinical applications of *Artemisia rupestris*. *Zhongguo Zhongyao Zazhi* **2017**, *42*, 4565–4573.
36. Kefale, A.T.; Dabe, N.E. Antidiabetic effects of artemisia species: A systematic review. *Anc. Sci. Life* **2017**, *36*, 175–181. [CrossRef]
37. Yalçinkaya, E.; Özgüç, S.; Aydinalp, A.; Zeybek, U. The importance of *Artemisia annua* L. in the anticancer activity research. *Ank. Univ. Eczacilik Fak. Derg.* **2017**, *41*, 1–8. [CrossRef]
38. Gondwe, M.; Mpalala, A.; Zongo, L.; Kamadyaapa, D.; Ndebia, E.; Sewani-Rusike, C.; Shauli, M.; Iputo, J. Investigation of anti-inflammatory and antinociceptive effects of aqueous extracts of *Artemisia afra* in wistar rats. *Asian J. Pharm. Clin. Res.* **2018**, *11*, 190–193. [CrossRef]
39. Koyuncu, I. Evaluation of anticancer, antioxidant activity and phenolic compounds of *Artemisia absinthium* L. extract. *Cell. Mol. Biol.* **2018**, *6*, 25–34. [CrossRef] [PubMed]
40. Martínez, M.J.A.; Del Olmo, L.M.B.; Ticona, L.A.; Benito, P.B. The *Artemisia* L. genus: A review of bioactive sesquiterpene lactones. In *Studies in Natural Products Chemistry*; Elsevier B.V.: Amsterdam, The Netherlands, 2012; Volume 37, Chapter 2, pp. 43–65. [CrossRef]
41. Ivanescu, B.; Miron, A.; Corciova, A. Sesquiterpene Lactones from *Artemisia* Genus: Biological Activities and Methods of Analysis. *J. Anal. Methods Chem.* **2015**, *2015*, 1–21. [CrossRef] [PubMed]
42. Mohamed, A.H.H.; El-Sayed, M.A.; Hegazy, M.E.; Helaly, S.E.; Esmail, A.M.; Mohamed, N.S. Chemical constituents and biological activities of *Artemisia herba-alba*. *Rec. Nat. Prod.* **2010**, *4*, 1–25.
43. Bora, K.S.; Sharma, A. The Genus *Artemisia*: A Comprehensive Review. *Pharm. Biol.* **2011**, *49*, 101–109. [CrossRef] [PubMed]
44. Nigam, M.; Atanassova, M.; Mishra, A.P.; Pezzani, R.; Devkota, H.P.; Plygun, S.; Salehi, B.; Setzer, W.N.; Sharifi-Rad, J. Bioactive Compounds and Health Benefits of *Artemisia* Species. *Nat. Prod. Commun.* **2019**, *14*, 1–17. [CrossRef]
45. Gruessner, B.M.; Cornet-Vernet, L.; Desrosiers, M.R.; Lutgen, P.; Towler, M.J.; Weathers, P.J. It is not just artemisinin: *Artemisia* sp. for treating diseases including malaria and schistosomiasis. *Phytochem. Rev.* **2019**, *18*, 1509–1527. [CrossRef]
46. Song, X.; Wen, X.; He, J.; Wang, J.; Li, S.; Wang, M. Phytochemical components and biological activities of *Artemisia* argyi. *J. Funct. Foods* **2019**, *52*, 648–662. [CrossRef]
47. Dib, I.; El Alaoui-Faris, F.E. *Artemisia* campestris L.: Review on taxonomical aspects, cytogeography, biological activities and bioactive compounds. *Biomed. Pharmacother.* **2019**, *109*, 1884–1906. [CrossRef]
48. Liu, S.-J.; Liao, Z.-X.; Tang, Z.-S.; Cui, C.-L.; Liu, H.-B.; Liang, Y.-N.; Zhang, Y.; Shi, H.-X.; Liu, Y.-R. Phytochemicals and biological activities of *Artemisia* sieversiana. *Phytochem. Rev.* **2017**, *16*, 441–460. [CrossRef]
49. Koul, B.; Khatri, T. The *Artemisia* genus: Panacea to several maladies. In *Bioactive Natural Products in Drug Discovery*; Singh, J., Meshram, V., Gupta, M., Eds.; Springer: Singapore, 2020; pp. 3–95. [CrossRef]
50. Zhang, L.; Lv, J. Phytochemistry and bioactivities of sesquiterpenoids from the *Artemisia* species. *J. Chin. Pharm. Sci.* **2017**, *26*, 317–334. [CrossRef]
51. Zhang, W.; Zhao, D.-B.; Li, M.-J.; Liu, X.-H.; Wang, H.-Q. Studies on flavonoid constituents from herbs of *Artemisia ordosica* II. *Zhongguo Zhongyao Zazhi* **2006**, *31*, 1959–1961. [PubMed]
52. Nurbek, S.; Murata, T.; Suganuma, K.; Ishikawa, Y.; Buyankhishig, B.; Kikuchi, T.; Byambajav, T.; Davaapurev, B.-O.; Sasaki, K.; Batkhuu, J. Isolation and evaluation of trypanocidal activity of sesquiterpenoids, flavonoids, and lignans in *Artemisia* sieversiana collected in Mongolia. *J. Nat. Med.* **2020**, *74*, 750–757. [CrossRef] [PubMed]
53. Li, K.-M.; Dong, X.; Ma, Y.-N.; Wu, Z.H.; Yan, Y.-M.; Cheng, Y.-X. Antifungal coumarins and lignans from *Artemisia annua*. *Fitoterapia* **2019**, *134*, 323–328. [CrossRef] [PubMed]
54. Labruzzo, A.; Cantrell, C.L.; Carrubba, A.; Ali, A.; Wedge, D.E.; Duke, S.O. Phytotoxic Lignans from *Artemisia* arborescens. *Nat. Prod. Commun.* **2018**, *13*, 237–240. [CrossRef]

55. Wang, Q.; Gong, J.-H.; Hao, J.-S.; Xu, Y.-H. Structure Elucidation of a New Lignan Glycoside from *Artemisia* ordosica. *Chem. Nat. Compd.* **2019**, *55*, 1007–1009. [CrossRef]
56. Rashid, M.U.; Alamzeb, M.; Ali, S.; Ullah, Z.; Shah, Z.A.; Naz, I.; Khan, M.R. The chemistry and pharmacology of alkaloids and allied nitrogen compounds from *Artemisia* species: A review. *Phytother. Res.* **2019**, *33*, 2661–2684. [CrossRef]
57. Giang, P.M.; Tran, T.T.N.; Phan, T.S.; Otsuka, H.; Matsunami, K. Two new sesquiterpene lactones and other chemical constituents of *Artemisia* roxbughiana. *Biochem. Syst. Ecol.* **2012**, *45*, 115–119. [CrossRef]
58. Megdiche-Ksouri, W.; Trabelsi, N.; Mkadmini, K.; Bourgou, S.; Noumi, A.; Snoussi, M.; Barbria, R.; Tebourbi, O.; Ksouri, R. *Artemisia* campestris phenolic compounds have antioxidant and antimicrobial activity. *Ind. Crop. Prod.* **2015**, *63*, 104–113. [CrossRef]
59. Souhila, T.; Zohra, B.F.; Tahar, H.S. Identification and quantification of phenolic compounds of *Artemisia* herba-alba at three harvest time by HPLC–ESI–Q-TOF–MS. *Int. J. Food Prop.* **2019**, *22*, 843–852. [CrossRef]
60. Seidemann, J. *World Spice Plants: Economic Usage, Botany, Taxonomy*; Springer: Berlin/Heidelberg, Germany, 2005; ISBN 978-3-540-22279-8.
61. Allen, G. *The Herbalist in the Kitchen*; University of Illinois Press: Champaign, IL, USA, 2010; ISBN 025209039X.
62. Vaughan, J.; Geissler, C. *The New Oxford Book of Food Plants*, 2nd ed.; Oxford University Press: Oxford, UK, 2009; ISBN 0191609498.
63. Kains, M.G. *Culinary Herbs: Their Cultivation, Harvesting, Curing and Uses*; Orange Judd Company: New York, NY, USA, 1912.
64. Fern, K. *Plants for a Future: Edible & Useful Plants for a Healthier World*; Permanent Publications: East Meon, UK, 2000; ISBN 9781856230117.
65. Parada, M.; Carrió, E.; Vallès, J. Ethnobotany of food plants in the alt empordà region (Catalonia, Iberian peninsula). *J. Appl. Bot. Food Qual.* **2011**, *84*, 11–25.
66. Wright, C.W. *Artemisia. Medicinal and Aromatic Plants—Industrial Profiles*; Taylor & Francis Ltd.: London, UK, 2003; ISBN 0203303067.
67. Amidon, C.; Barnett, R.; Cathers, J.; Chambers, B.; Hamilton, L.; Kellett, A.; Kennel, E.; Montowski, J.; Thomas, M.A.; Watson, B. *Artemisia: An Essential Guide from The Herb Society of America*; The Herb Society of America: Kirtland, OH, USA, 2014.
68. Densmore, F. *How Indians Use Wild Plants for Food, Medicine, & Crafts*; Dover Publications: Mineola, NY, USA, 1974; ISBN 0486406709.
69. Mladenova, O. *Grapes and Wine in the Balkans: An Ethno-Linguistic Study*; Harrassowitz Verlag: Wiesbaden, Germany, 1998; ISBN 978-3447040372.
70. Koul, B.; Taak, P.; Kumar, A.; Khatri, T.; Sanyal, I. The *Artemisia* Genus: A Review on Traditional Uses, Phytochemical Constituents, Pharmacological Properties and Germplasm Conservation. *J. Glycom. Lipidom.* **2018**, *7*, 1–7. [CrossRef]
71. Pieroni, A.; Quave, C.L. *Ethnobotany and Biocultural Diversities in the Balkans: Perspectives on Sustainable Rural Development and Reconciliation*; Springer: New York, NY, USA, 2014; ISBN 9781493914920.
72. Tonutti, I.; Liddle, P. Aromatic plants in alcoholic beverages: A review. *Flavour Fragr. J.* **2010**, *25*, 341–350. [CrossRef]
73. Kim, J.K.; Shin, E.C.; Lim, H.J.; Choi, S.J.; Kim, C.R.; Suh, S.H.; Kim, C.J.; Park, G.G.; Park, C.S.; Kim, H.K.; et al. Characterization of nutritional composition, antioxidative capacity, and sensory attributes of Seomae Mugwort, a native Korean variety of *Artemisia argyi* H. Lév. & Vaniot. *J. Anal. Methods Chem.* **2015**, *2015*, 916346. [CrossRef] [PubMed]
74. Wang, J.; Seyler, B.C.; Ticktin, T.; Zeng, Y.; Ayu, K. An ethnobotanical survey of wild edible plants used by the Yi people of Liangshan Prefecture, Sichuan Province, China. *J. Ethnobiol. Ethnomedicine* **2020**, *16*, 1–27. [CrossRef] [PubMed]
75. Yanovsky, E. *Food Plants of the North American Indians*; U.S. Dept. of Agriculture: Washington, DC, USA, 1936.
76. Moerman, D.E. *Native American Food Plants: An Ethnobotanical Dictionary*; Timber Press Inc.: Portland, OR, USA, 2010; ISBN 9781604691894.
77. de Santayana, M.P.; Morales, R. Manzanillas ibéricas: Historia y usos tradicionales. *Rev. Fitoter.* **2006**, *6*, 143–153.
78. Bezza, L.; Mannarino, A.; Fattarsi, K.; Mikail, C.; Abou, L.; Hadji-Minaglou, F.; Kaloustian, J. Composition chimique de l'huile essentielle d'*Artemisia* herba-alba provenant de la région de Biskra (Algérie). *Phytothérapie* **2010**, *8*, 277–281. [CrossRef]
79. Kunkel, G. *Plants for Human Consumption: An Annotated Checklist of the Edible Phanerogams and Ferns*; Koeltz Scientific Books: Koenigatein, West Germany, 1984; ISBN 9783874292160.
80. Sanmi, S.; McCabe, S.; Satoko, I. *Chado the Way of Tea: A Japanese Tea Master's Almanac*; Tuttle Publishing: North Clarendon, VT, USA, 2005; ISBN 0804837163.
81. Xing, X.H.; Zhang, Z.M.; Hu, X.Z.; Wu, R.Q.; Xu, C. Antidiabetic effects of *Artemisia* sphaerocephala Krasch. gum, a novel food additive in China, on streptozotocin-induced type 2 diabetic rats. *J. Ethnopharmacol.* **2009**, *125*, 410–416. [CrossRef]
82. Boggia, L.; Pignata, G.; Sgorbini, B.; Colombo, M.L.; Marengo, A.; Casale, M.; Nicola, S.; Bicchi, C.; Rubiolo, P. *Artemisia* umbelliformis Lam. and Génépi Liqueur: Volatile Profile as Diagnostic Marker for Geographic Origin and to Predict Liqueur Safety. *J. Agric. Food Chem.* **2017**, *65*, 2849–2856. [CrossRef]
83. Van Wyk, B.-E. *Culinary Herbs and Spices of the World*; The University of Chicago Press: Chicago, IL, USA, 2013; ISBN 9780226091839.
84. Judžentiene, A. Wormwood (*Artemisia absinthium* L.) oils. In *Essential Oils in Food Preservation, Flavor and Safety*; Elsevier Academic Press: London, UK, 2016; pp. 849–856, ISBN 9780124166448.
85. Morata, A.; Vaquero, C.; Palomero, F.; Loira, I.; Bañuelos, M.A.; Suárez-Lepe, J.A. Technology of vermouth wines. In *Alcoholic Beverages: Volume 7: The Science of Beverages*; Elsevier Woodhead Publishing: Duxford, UK, 2019; pp. 35–63, ISBN 9780128152690.
86. How Prepare Peiln. Available online: https://www.bgfermer.bg/Article/4834261 (accessed on 10 August 2020).

87. Vin de Pelin—Preparare, Administrare, Indicații Terapeutice I LaTAIFAS. Available online: https://lataifas.ro/retete-naturiste/vinuri-medicinale-retete-naturiste/22852/vin-de-pelin-preparare-indicatii-terapeutice/# (accessed on 10 August 2020).
88. Arnold, W.N. Absinthe. *Sci. Am.* **1989**, *260*, 112–117. [CrossRef]
89. Lachenmeier, D.W.; Walch, S.G.; Padosch, S.A.; Kröner, L.U. Absinthe—A Review. *Crit. Rev. Food Sci. Nutr.* **2006**, *46*, 365–377. [CrossRef]
90. Veretnova, O.Y.; Gulenkova, G.S.; Chepeleva, G.G.; Fedchenko, E.A.; Rybakova, G.R. Rationale and methods of the use of *Artemisia absinthium* L., *Ledum palustre* L. and *Tanacetum vulgare* L. for food purposes. In *IOP Conference Series: Earth and Environmental Science*; Institute of Physics Publishing: Bristol, UK, 2020; Volume 421.
91. Brisibe, E.A.; Umoren, U.E.; Brisibe, F.; Magalhäes, P.M.; Ferreira, J.F.; Luthria, D.; Wu, X.; Prior, R.L. Nutritional characterisation and antioxidant capacity of different tissues of *Artemisia annua* L. *Food Chem.* **2009**, *115*, 1240–1246. [CrossRef]
92. Carvalho, I.S.; Teixeira, M.C.; Brodelius, M. Fatty acids profile of selected *Artemisia* spp. plants: Health promotion. *LWT Food Sci. Technol.* **2011**, *44*, 293–298. [CrossRef]
93. Iqbal, S.; Younas, U.; Chan, K.W.; Zia-Ul-Haq, M.; Ismail, M. Chemical Composition of *Artemisia annua* L. Leaves and Antioxidant Potential of Extracts as a Function of Extraction Solvents. *Molecules* **2012**, *17*, 6020–6032. [CrossRef] [PubMed]
94. Ayaz, F.A.; Inceer, H.; Hayirlioglu-Ayaz, S.; Aksu-Kalmuk, N. Achene fatty acid composition in the tribe anthemideae (Asteraceae). *Rom. Biotechnol. Lett.* **2016**, *21*, 11576–11584.
95. Boufennara, S.; Lopez, S.; Bousseboua, H.; Bodas, R.; Bouazza, L. Chemical composition and digestibility of some browse plant species collected from Algerian arid rangelands. *Span. J. Agric. Res.* **2012**, *10*, 88. [CrossRef]
96. Olson, K.A.; Murray, M.G.; Fuller, T.K. Vegetation Composition and Nutritional Quality of Forage for Gazelles in Eastern Mongolia. *Rangel. Ecol. Manag.* **2010**, *63*, 593–598. [CrossRef]
97. Al-Masri, M. Nutritive evaluation of some native range plants and their nutritional and anti-nutritional components. *J. Appl. Anim. Res.* **2013**, *41*, 427–431. [CrossRef]
98. Bouazza, L.; Boufennara, S.; Bensaada, M.; Zeraib, A.; Rahal, K.; Saro, C.; Ranilla, M.J.; López, S. In vitro screening of Algerian steppe browse plants for digestibility, rumen fermentation profile and methane mitigation. *Agrofor. Syst.* **2020**, *94*, 1433–1443. [CrossRef]
99. Randalova, T.E.; Dylenova, E.P.; Renchenbyamba, S.; Zhigzhitzhapova, S.V.; Radnaeva, L.D.; Taraskin, V.V. The composition of fatty acids isolated from plants of Absinthium section of floras of Buryatia and Mongolia. In *IOP Conference Series: Earth and Environmental Science*; Institute of Physics Publishing: Bristol, UK, 2019; Volume 320, p. 012057.
100. Tsybikova, S.Z.; Randalova, T.E.; Radnaeva, L.D. Fatty acid composition of *Artemisia santolinifolia* Turcz. ex Bess. of flora of Buryatia. In *IOP Conference Series: Earth and Environmental Science*; Institute of Physics Publishing: Bristol, UK, 2019; Volume 320, p. 012058.
101. Towhidi, A.; Saberifar, T.; Dirandeh, E. Nutritive value of some herbage for dromedary camels in the central arid zone of Iran. *Trop. Anim. Heal. Prod.* **2011**, *43*, 617–622. [CrossRef]
102. Ren, D.; Zhao, Y.; Nie, Y.; Yang, N.; Yang, X. Hypoglycemic and hepatoprotective effects of polysaccharides from *Artemisia* sphaerocephala Krasch seeds. *Int. J. Biol. Macromol.* **2014**, *69*, 296–306. [CrossRef]
103. Davies, K.G.; Bates, J.D.; Johnson, D.D.; Nafus, A.M. Influence of Mowing *Artemisia tridentata* ssp. wyomingensis on Winter Habitat for Wildlife. *Environ. Manag.* **2009**, *44*, 84–92. [CrossRef] [PubMed]
104. Ros, E.; Mataix, J. Fatty acid composition of nuts—implications for cardiovascular health. *Br. J. Nutr.* **2006**, *96*, S29–S35. [CrossRef] [PubMed]
105. Bourre, J.-M.; Dumont, O. Dietary oleic acid not used during brain development and in adult in rat, in contrast with sciatic nerve. *Neurosci. Lett.* **2003**, *336*, 180–184. [CrossRef]
106. Innis, S.M. Fatty acids and early human development. *Early Hum. Dev.* **2007**, *83*, 761–766. [CrossRef]
107. Innis, S.M. Essential fatty acids in growth and development. *Prog. Lipid Res.* **1991**, *30*, 39–103. [CrossRef]
108. Farvid, M.S.; Ding, M.; Pan, A.; Sun, Q.; Chiuve, S.E.; Steffen, L.M.; Willett, W.C.; Hu, F.B. Dietary Linoleic Acid and Risk of Coronary Heart Disease: A Systematic Review and Meta-Analysis of Prospective Cohort Studies. *Circulation* **2014**, *130*, 1568–1578. [CrossRef]
109. Kakar, M.U.; Kakar, I.U.; Mehboob, M.Z.; Zada, S.; Soomro, H.; Umair, M.; Iqbal, I.; Umer, M.; Shaheen, S.; Syed, S.F.; et al. A review on polysaccharides from *Artemisia* sphaerocephala Krasch seeds, their extraction, modification, structure, and applications. *Carbohydr. Polym.* **2021**, *252*, 117113. [CrossRef]
110. Zhang, L.; Hu, X.; Miao, X.; Chen, X.; Nan, S.; Fu, H. Genome-Scale Transcriptome Analysis of the Desert Shrub *Artemisia* sphaerocephala. *PLoS ONE* **2016**, *11*, e0154300. [CrossRef]
111. Barber, T.M.; Kabisch, S.; Pfeiffer, A.F.H.; Weickert, M.O. The Health Benefits of Dietary Fibre. *Nutrients* **2020**, *12*, 3209. [CrossRef]
112. Zhu, S.; Noviello, C.M.; Teng, J.; Walsh, R.M.; Kim, J.J.; Hibbs, R.E. Structure of a human synaptic GABAA receptor. *Nature* **2018**, *559*, 67–88. [CrossRef]
113. Fellows, P.J. Properties of food and principles of processing. In *Food Processing Technology*; Elsevier: Cambridge, UK, 2017; pp. 3–200.
114. Stach, A.; García-Mozo, H.; Prieto-Baena, J.C.; Czarnecka-Operacz, M.; Jenerowicz, D.; Silny, W.; Galán, C. Prevalence of *Artemisia* species pollinosis in western Poland: Impact of climate change on aerobiological trends, 1995–2004. *J. Investig. Allergol. Clin. Immunol.* **2007**, *17*, 39–47. [PubMed]

115. Cristofori, A.; Bucher, E.; Rossi, M.; Cristofolini, F.; Kofler, V.; Prosser, F.; Gottardini, E. The late flowering of invasive species contributes to the increase of *Artemisia* allergenic pollen in autumn: An analysis of 25 years of aerobiological data (1995–2019) in Trentino-Alto Adige (Northern Italy). *Aerobiologia (Bologna)* **2020**, *36*, 669–682. [CrossRef]
116. D'Amato, G.; Spieksma, F.T.M. Allergenic pollen in europe. *Grana* **1991**, *30*, 67–70. [CrossRef]
117. D'Amato, G.; Spieksma, F.T.M.; Liccardi, G.; Jäger, S.; Russo, M.; Nikkels, H.; Wuthrich, B.; Bonini, S.; Kontou-Fili, K. Pollen-related allergy in Europe. *Allergy* **1998**, *53*, 567–578. [CrossRef] [PubMed]
118. Tang, R.; Sun, J.-L.; Yin, J.; Li, Z. *Artemisia* Allergy Research in China. *BioMed Res. Int.* **2015**, *2015*, 1–9. [CrossRef]
119. Gao, Z.; Fu, W.-Y.; Sun, Y.; Gao, B.; Wang, H.-Y.; Liu, M.; Luo, F.-M.; Zhou, X.; Jin, J.; Zhao, L.; et al. *Artemisia* pollen allergy in China: Component-resolved diagnosis reveals allergic asthma patients have significant multiple allergen sensitization. *Allergy* **2019**, *74*, 284–293. [CrossRef]
120. Brandys, J.; Grimsoen, A.; Nilsen, B.M.; Smestad Paulsen, B.; Park, H.S.; Hong, C.S. Cross-reactivity between pollen extracts from six *Artemisia* species. *Planta Med.* **1993**, *59*, 221–228. [CrossRef]
121. Hirschwehr, R.; Heppner, C.; Spitzauer, S.; Sperr, W.R.; Valent, P.; Bergerd, U.; Horak, F.; Jäger, S.; Kraft, D.; Valenta, R. Identification of common allergenic structures in mugwort and ragweed pollen. *J. Allergy Clin. Immunol.* **1998**, *101*, 196–206. [CrossRef]
122. Ortiz, J.C.G.; Martin, P.C.; Lopez-Asunsolo, A. Allergy to foods in patients monosensitized to *Artemisia* pollen. *Allergy* **1996**, *51*, 927–931. [CrossRef]
123. Oteros, J.; Bartusel, E.; Alessandrini, F.; Núñez, A.; Moreno, D.A.; Behrendt, H.; Schmidt-Weber, C.; Traidl-Hoffmann, C.; Buters, J. *Artemisia* pollen is the main vector for airborne endotoxin. *J. Allergy Clin. Immunol.* **2019**, *143*, 369–377. [CrossRef]
124. Grewling, Ł.; Bogawski, P.; Kostecki, Ł.; Nowak, M.; Szymańska, A.; Frątczak, A. Atmospheric exposure to the major *Artemisia* pollen allergen (Art v 1): Seasonality, impact of weather, and clinical implications. *Sci. Total Environ.* **2020**, *713*, 136611. [CrossRef] [PubMed]
125. Foster, S.; Duke, J.A. *A Field Guide to Medicinal Plants and Herbs of Eastern and Central North America*; Peterson, R.T., Ed.; Houghton Mifflin Harcourt: Boston, MA, USA, 2000; ISBN 0395988144, 9780395988145.
126. Czygan, F.-C. *Herbal Drugs and Phytopharmaceuticals: A Handbook for Practice on a Scientific Basis*; Wichtl, M., Bisset, N.G., Eds.; CRC Press: Boca Raton, FL, USA, 2004; ISBN 0849319617, 9780849319617.
127. Paulsen, E. Systemic allergic dermatitis caused by sesquiterpene lactones. *Contact Derm.* **2017**, *76*, 1–10. [CrossRef] [PubMed]
128. Paulsen, E. Contact sensitization from Compositae-containing herbal remedies and cosmetics. *Contact Derm.* **2002**, *47*, 189–198. [CrossRef] [PubMed]
129. Kurz, G.; Rapaport, M.J. External/internal allergy to plants (*Artemisia*). *Contact Derm.* **1979**, *5*, 407–408. [CrossRef]
130. Wu, P.; He, Y.; Zeng, Z.; Yang, Z.; Li, Y. Allergic contact dermatitis by *Artemisia*: Report of two cases. *Contact Derm.* **2020**, *83*, 31–32. [CrossRef]
131. Mitchell, J.C.; Dupuis, G. Allergic contact dermatitis from sesquiterpenoids of the Compositae family of plants. *Br. J. Dermatol.* **1971**, *84*, 139–150. [CrossRef]
132. Haw, S.; Cho, H.-R.; Lee, M.-H. Allergic contact dermatitis associated with mugwort (*Artemisia vulgaris*). *Contact Derm.* **2010**, *62*, 61–63. [CrossRef]
133. Zeller, W.; de Gols, M.; Hausen, B.M. The sensitizing capacity of Compositae plants—VI: Guinea pig sensitization experiments with ornamental plants and weeds using different methods. *Arch. Dermatol. Res.* **1984**, *277*, 28–35. [CrossRef]
134. Park, Y.M. Relationship between sensitization to outdoor aeroallergen and month of birth. *Pediatr. Allergy Respir. Dis.* **2016**, *15*, 257–262. [CrossRef]
135. Lundh, K.; Hindsén, M.; Gruvberger, B.; Möller, H.; Svensson, Å.; Bruze, M. Contact allergy to herbal teas derived from Asteraceae plants. *Contact Derm.* **2006**, *54*, 196–201. [CrossRef]
136. Amorim, M.H.R.; Gil Da Costa, R.M.; Lopes, C.; Bastos, M.M.S.M. Sesquiterpene lactones: Adverse health effects and toxicity mechanisms. *Crit. Rev. Toxicol.* **2013**, *43*, 559–579. [CrossRef] [PubMed]
137. Denisow-Pietrzyk, M.; Pietrzyk, Ł.; Denisow, B. Asteraceae species as potential environmental factors of allergy. *Environ. Sci. Pollut. Res.* **2019**, *26*, 6290–6300. [CrossRef] [PubMed]
138. Weisbord, S.D.; Soule, J.B.; Kimmel, P.L. Poison on line—Acute renal failure caused by oil of wormwood purchased through the internet. *N. Engl. J. Med.* **1997**, *337*, 825–827. [CrossRef] [PubMed]
139. Padosch, S.A.; Lachenmeier, D.W.; Kröner, L.U. Absinthism: A fictitious 19th century syndrome with present impact. *Subst. Abus. Treat. Prev. Policy* **2006**, *1*, 14. [CrossRef]
140. Lachenmeier, D.W.; Uebelacker, M. Risk assessment of thujone in foods and medicines containing sage and wormwood—Evidence for a need of regulatory changes? *Regul. Toxicol. Pharmacol.* **2010**, *58*, 437–443. [CrossRef]
141. European Parliament and Council. Available online: https://eur-lex.europa.eu/eli/reg/2008/1334/oj (accessed on 12 October 2020).
142. European Commission Health and Consumer Protection Directorate-General. Opinion of the Scientific Committee on Food on Thujone. Available online: https://ec.europa.eu/food/sites/food/files/safety/docs/fs_food-improvement-agents_flavourings-out162.pdf (accessed on 14 October 2020).
143. Community Herbal Monograph on *Artemisia absinthium* L., Herba. EMA/HMPC/234463/2008. 2009. Available online: http://golbid.com/wp-content/uploads/2017/09/artemisia-absinthium.pdf (accessed on 12 October 2020).

144. De Boer, H.J.; Cotingting, C. Medicinal plants for women's healthcare in southeast Asia: A meta-analysis of their traditional use, chemical constituents, and pharmacology. *J. Ethnopharmacol.* **2014**, *151*, 747–767. [CrossRef]
145. Almasad, M.M.; Qazan, W.S.; Daradka, H. Reproductive toxic effects of *Artemisia* herba alba ingestion in female Spague-dawley rats. *Pak. J. Biol. Sci.* **2007**, *10*, 3158–3161. [CrossRef]
146. Abolaji, A.O.; Eteng, M.U.; Ebong, P.E.; Brisibe, E.A.; Dar, A.; Kabir, N.; Choudhary, M.I. A safety assessment of the antimalarial herb *Artemisia annua* during pregnancy in wistar rats. *Phyther. Res.* **2013**, *27*, 647–654. [CrossRef]
147. Abolaji, A.O.; Eteng, M.U.; Ebong, P.E.; Dar, A.; Farombi, E.O.; Choudhary, M.I. *Artemisia annua* as a possible contraceptive agent: A clue from mammalian rat model. *Nat. Prod. Res.* **2014**, *28*, 2342–2346. [CrossRef]
148. Laadraoui, J.; Aboufatima, R.; El Gabbas, Z.; Ferehan, H.; Bezza, K.; Ait Laaradia, M.; Marhoume, F.; Wakrim, E.M.; Chait, A. Effect of *Artemisia herba-alba* consumption during pregnancy on fertility, morphological and behaviors of mice offspring. *J. Ethnopharmacol.* **2018**, *226*, 105–110. [CrossRef]
149. Oliaee, D.; Boroushaki, M.T.; Oliaee, N.; Ghorbani, A. Evaluation of cytotoxicity and antifertility effect of *Artemisia kopetdaghensis*. *Adv. Pharmacol. Sci.* **2014**, *2014*, 745760. [CrossRef] [PubMed]
150. Rabl, W.; Katzgraber, F.; Steinlechner, M. Camphor ingestion for abortion (case report). *Forensic Sci. Int.* **1997**, *89*, 137–140. [CrossRef]
151. Gomes, C.; Boareto, A.C.; Dalsenter, P.R. Clinical and non-clinical safety of artemisinin derivatives in pregnancy. *Reprod. Toxicol.* **2016**, *65*, 194–203. [CrossRef] [PubMed]
152. Meshnick, S.R.; Taylor, T.E.; Kamchonwongpaisan, S. Artemisinin and the antimalarial endoperoxides: From herbal remedy to targeted chemotherapy. *Microbiol. Rev.* **1996**, *60*, 301–315. [CrossRef]
153. Alkadi, H.O. Antimalarial drug toxicity: A review. *Chemotherapy* **2007**, *53*, 385–391. [CrossRef]
154. Adjuik, M.; Babiker, A.; Garner, P.; Olliaro, P.; Taylor, W.; White, N.; International Artemisinin Study Group. Artesunate combinations for treatment of malaria: Meta-analysis. *Lancet* **2004**, *363*, 9–17. [CrossRef]
155. Staedke, S.G.; Jagannathan, P.; Yeka, A.; Bukirwa, H.; Banek, K.; Maiteki-Sebuguzi, C.; Clark, T.D.; Nzarubara, B.; Njama-Meya, D.; Mpimbaza, A.; et al. Monitoring antimalarial safety and tolerability in clinical trials: A case study from Uganda. *Malar. J.* **2008**, *7*, 107. [CrossRef]
156. Ribeiro, I.R.; Olliaro, P. Safety of artemisinin and its derivatives a review of published and unpublished clinical trials. *Med. Trop.* **1998**, *58*, 50–53.
157. Efferth, T.; Kaina, B. Toxicity of the antimalarial artemisinin and its dervatives. *Crit. Rev. Toxicol.* **2010**, *40*, 405–421. [CrossRef]
158. Saeed, M.; Breuer, E.; Hegazi, M.A.; Efferth, T. Retrospective study of small pet tumors treated with *Artemisia annua* and iron. *Int. J. Oncol.* **2020**, *56*, 123–138. [CrossRef]
159. Hunt, S.; Stebbings, S.; McNamara, D. An open-label six-month extension study to investigate the safety and efficacy of an extract of *Artemisia annua* for managing pain, stiffness and functional limitation associated with osteoarthritis of the hip and knee. *N. Z. Med. J.* **2016**, *129*, 97–102. [PubMed]
160. Stebbings, S.; Beattie, E.; McNamara, D.; Hunt, S. A pilot randomized, placebo-controlled clinical trial to investigate the efficacy and safety of an extract of *Artemisia annua* administered over 12 weeks, for managing pain, stiffness, and functional limitation associated with osteoarthritis of the hip and knee. *Clin. Rheumatol.* **2016**, *35*, 1829–1836. [CrossRef] [PubMed]
161. Daddy, N.B.; Kalisya, L.M.; Bagire, P.G.; Watt, R.L.; Towler, M.J.; Weathers, P.J. *Artemisia annua* dried leaf tablets treated malaria resistant to ACT and i.v. artesunate: Case reports. *Phytomedicine* **2017**, *32*, 37–40. [CrossRef] [PubMed]
162. Mendez, V.M.; Puebla-Perez, A.M.; Sanchez-Pena, M.J.; Gonzalez-Ortiz, L.J.; Martinez-Abundis, E.; Gonzalez-Ortiz, M. Effect of *Artemisia dracunculus* administration on glycemic control, insulin sensitivity, and insulin secretion in patients with impaired glucose tolerance. *J. Med. Food.* **2016**, *19*, 481–485. [CrossRef]
163. Choi, J.Y.; Shin, S.K.; Jeon, S.M.; Jeong, T.; Baek, N.I.; Chung, H.G.; Lee, K.T.; Lee, M.K.; Choi, M.S. Dose–response study of sajabalssuk ethanol extract from *Artemisia princeps* Pampanini on blood glucose in subjects with impaired fasting glucose or mild type 2 diabetes. *J. Med. Food.* **2011**, *14*, 101–107. [CrossRef]
164. Li, Y.; Zheng, M.; Zhai, X.; Huang, Y.; Khalid, A.; Malik, A.; Shah, P.; Karim, S.; Azhar, S.; Hou, X. Effect of *Gymnema sylvestre*, *Citrullus colocynthis* and *Artemisia absinthium* on blood glucose and lipid profile in diabetic human. *Acta Pol. Pharm.* **2015**, *72*, 981–985.
165. Basiri, Z.; Zeraati, F.; Esna-Ashari, F.; Mohammadi, F.; Razzaghi, K.; Araghchian, M.; Moradkhani, S. Topical effects of *Artemisia absinthium* ointment and liniment in comparison with piroxicam gel in patients with knee joint osteoarthritis: A randomized double-blind controlled trial. *Iran. J. Med. Sci.* **2017**, *42*, 524–531.
166. Hatziieremia, S.; Gray, A.I.; Ferro, V.A.; Paul, A.; Plein, R. The effects of cardamonin on lipopolysaccharide-induced inflammatory protein production and MAP kinase and NFkappaB signaling pathways in monocytes/macro-phages. *Br. J. Pharmacol.* **2006**, *149*, 188–198. [CrossRef]
167. Krebs, S.; Omer, T.N.; Omer, B. Wormwood (*Artemisia absinthium*) suppresses tumour necrosis factor alpha and accelerates healing in patients with Crohn's disease–A controlled clinical trial. *Phytomedicine* **2010**, *17*, 305–309. [CrossRef]
168. Ogawa, R.; Hyakusoku, H.; Ogawa, N.; Nakao, C. Effectiveness of mugwort lotion for the treatment of post-burn hypertrophic scars. *JPARS* **2008**, *61*, 210–212. [CrossRef]

169. Wu, Q.-J.; Lv, W.-L.; Li, J.-M.; Zhang, T.-T.; Zhou, W.-H.; Zhang, Q.; Wang, J.-C.; Wang, Q.-N.; Zhang, R.X.; Zhao, X.; et al. Efficacy and safety of Yin Qi San Huang antiviral decoction in chronic hepatitis B: Study protocol for a randomized, placebo controlled, double-blinded trial. *Trials* **2020**, *21*, 482. [CrossRef] [PubMed]
170. Lou, H.; Wang, X.; Wei, Q.; Zhao, C.; Xing, Z.; Zhang, Q.; Meng, J.; Zhang, S.; Zhou, H.; Mak, R.; et al. *Artemisia Annua* sublingual immunotherapy for seasonal allergic rhinitis: A multicenter, randomized trial. *WAO J.* **2020**, *13*, 100458. [CrossRef] [PubMed]
171. Remberg, P.; Björk, L.; Hedner, T.; Sterner, O. Characteristics, clinical effect profile and tolerability of a nasal spray preparation of *Artemisia abrotanum* L. for allergic rhinitis. *Phytomedicine* **2004**, *11*, 36–42. [CrossRef] [PubMed]
172. Munyangi, J.; Cornet-Vernet, L.; Idumbo, M.; Lu, C.; Lutgen, P.; Perronne, C.; Ngombe, N.; Bianga, J.; Mupenda, B.; Lalukala, P.; et al. *Artemisia annua* and *Artemisia afra* tea infusions vs. artesunate-amodiaquine (ASAQ) in treating *Plasmodium falciparum* malaria in a large scale, double blind, randomized clinical trial. *Phytomedicine* **2019**, *57*, 49–56. [CrossRef]
173. Munyangi, J.; Cornet-Vernet, L.; Idumbo, M.; Lud, C.; Lutgen, P.; Perronne, C.; Ngombe, N.; Bianga, J.; Mupenda, B.; Lalukala, P.; et al. Effect of *Artemisia annua* and *Artemisia afra* tea infusions on schistosomiasis in a large clinical trial. *Phytomedicine* **2018**, *51*, 233–240. [CrossRef]
174. Gillibert, A.; Stephane, J.; Yves, H.; Xavier, A.; Jordi, L.; Erice, C.; Gaudart Jean, G. TEMPORARY REMOVAL: Comment on *A. annua* and *A. afra* infusions vs. Artesunate-amodiaquine (ASAQ) in treating *Plasmodium falciparum* malaria in a large scale, double blind, randomized clinical trial. *Phytomedicine* **2019**, *59*, 152981. [CrossRef]
175. Farage, M.A. The prevalence of sensitive skin. *Front. Med.* **2019**, *6*, 98. [CrossRef]
176. Zyad, A.; Tilaoui, M.; Jaafari, A.; Oukerrou, M.A.; Mouse, H.A. More insights into the pharmacological effects of artemisinin. *Phytother. Res.* **2017**, *32*, 1–14. [CrossRef]
177. Yu, J.; Wang, G.; Jiang, N. Study on the repairing effect of cosmetics containing *Artemisia annua* on sensitive skin. *J. Cosmet. Dermatol.* **2020**, *10*, 8–19. [CrossRef]
178. El-Askarya, H.I.; Mohamed, S.S.; El-Gohari, H.M.A.; Ezzata, S.M.; Meselhya, M.R. Quinic acid derivatives from *Artemisia annua* L. leaves; biological activities and seasonal variation. *S. Afr. J. Bot.* **2020**, *128*, 200–208. [CrossRef]
179. Guerriero, G.; Berni, R.B.; Muñoz-Sanchez, A.; Apone, F.; Abdel-Salam, E.M.; Qahtan, A.A.; Alatar, A.A.; Cantini, C.; Cai, G.; Hausman, J.-F.; et al. Production of plant secondary metabolites: Examples, tips and suggestions for biotechnologists. *Genes* **2018**, *9*, 309. [CrossRef] [PubMed]
180. Sülsen, V.P.; Martino, V.S. Overview. In *Sesquiterpene Lactones: Advances in their Chemistry and Biological Aspects*; Sülsen, V.P., Martino, V.S., Eds.; Springer International Publishing: Cham, Switzerland, 2018; pp. 3–17. [CrossRef]
181. Moujir, L.M.; Callies, O.; Sousa, P.M.C.; Sharopov, F.; Seca, A.M.L. Applications of sesquiterpene lactones: A review of some potential success cases. *Appl. Sci.* **2020**, *10*, 3001. [CrossRef]
182. Tu, Y. *From Artemisia annua L. to Artemisinins: The Discovery and Development of Artemisinins and Antimalarial Agents*; Academic Press: London, UK, 2017; 468p, ISBN 9780128116562.
183. Letchmanan, K.; Shen, S.; Ng, W.K.; Tan, R.B. Application of transglycosylated stevia and hesperidin as drug carriers to enhance biopharmaceutical properties of poorly-soluble artemisinin. *Colloids Surf. B Biointerfaces* **2018**, *161*, 83–93. [CrossRef] [PubMed]
184. Li, Y. Qinghaosu (artemisinin): Chemistry and pharmacology. *Acta Pharmacol. Sin.* **2012**, *33*, 1141–1146. [CrossRef] [PubMed]
185. White, N.J. Malaria. In *Antibiotics and Chemotherapy*, 9th ed.; Elsevier: Philadelphia, PA, USA, 2010; pp. 809–822. [CrossRef]
186. Konstat-Korzenny, E.; Ascencio-Aragón, J.A.; Niezen-Lugo, S.; Vázquez-López, R. Artemisinin and its synthetic derivatives as a possible therapy for cancer. *Med. Sci.* **2018**, *6*, 19. [CrossRef]
187. Li, Y. Artemisinin and derivatives pharmacodynamics, toxicology, pharmacokinetics, mechanism of action, resistance, and immune regulation. In *Artemisinin-Based and Other Antimalarials*; Li, G., Li, Y., Li, Z., Zeng, M., Eds.; Academic Press: Cambridge, MA, USA, 2018; Chapter 5, pp. 197–351. [CrossRef]
188. Saeed, M.; Krishna, S.; Greten, H.J.; Kremsner, P.G.; Efferth, T. Antischistosomal activity of artemisinin derivatives in vivo and in patients. *Pharmacol. Res.* **2016**, *110*, 216–226. [CrossRef]
189. Pérez del Villar, L.; Burguillo, F.J.; López-Abán, J.; Muro, A. Systematic review and meta-analysis of artemisinin based therapies for the treatment and prevention of schistosomiasis. *PLoS ONE* **2012**, *7*, e45867. [CrossRef]
190. Naß, J.; Efferth, T. The activity of *Artemisia* spp. and their constituents against Trypanosomiasis. *Phytomedicine* **2018**, *47*, 184–191. [CrossRef]
191. Charlie-Silva, I.; Fernandes Fraceto, L.; Ferreira Silva de Melo, N. Progress in nano-drug delivery of artemisinin and its derivatives: Towards to use in immunomodulatory approaches. *Artif. Cells Nanomed. Biotechnol.* **2018**, *4*, S611–S620. [CrossRef]
192. Hou, L.; Huang, H. Immune suppressive properties of artemisinin family drugs. *Pharmacol. Ther.* **2016**, *166*, 123–127. [CrossRef]
193. Wang, J.; Xu, C.; Wong, Y.K.; Li, Y.; Liao, F.; Jiang, T.; Tu, Y.Y. Artemisinin, the magic drug discovered from Traditional Chinese Medicine. *Engineering* **2019**, *5*, 32–39. [CrossRef]
194. Ajeigbe, K.O.; Emikpe, B.O.; Olaleye, S.B. Effects of artemisinin, with or without lumefantrine and amodiaquine on gastric ulcer healing in rat. *J. Basic Clin. Physiol. Pharmacol.* **2018**, *29*, 515–524. [CrossRef] [PubMed]
195. Dehkordi, F.M.; Kaboutari, J.; Zendehdel, M.; Javdani, M. The antinociceptive effect of artemisinin on the inflammatory pain and role of GABAergic and opioidergic systems. *Korean J. Pain* **2019**, *32*, 160–167. [CrossRef] [PubMed]
196. Efferth, T. Beyond malaria: The inhibition of viruses by artemisinin-type compounds. *Biotechnol. Adv.* **2018**, *36*, 1730–1737. [CrossRef] [PubMed]

197. Lin, L.; Mao, X.; Sun, Y.; Cui, H. Antibacterial mechanism of artemisinin/beta-cyclodextrins against methicillin-resistant *Staphylococcus aureus* (MRSA). *Microb. Pathog.* **2018**, *118*, 66–73. [CrossRef] [PubMed]
198. Cheong, D.H.J.; Tan, D.W.S.; Wong, F.W.S.; Tran, T. Anti-malarial drug, artemisinin and its derivatives for the treatment of respiratory diseases. *Pharmacol. Res.* **2020**, *158*, 1049012. [CrossRef] [PubMed]
199. Chen, H.; Du, H.; Chang, C.; Li, X. Artemisinin reduces atherosclerosis in apolipoprotein E deficient mice. *Arterioscler. Thromb. Vasc. Biol.* **2020**, *40* (Suppl. 1), A346. [CrossRef]
200. Jiang, W.; Cen, Y.; Song, Y.; Li, P.; Qin, R.; Liu, C.; Zhao, Y.; Zheng, J.; Zhou, H. Artesunate attenuated progression of atherosclerosis lesion formation alone or combined with rosuvastatin through inhibition of pro-inflammatory cytokines and pro-inflammatory chemokines. *Phytomedicine* **2016**, *23*, 1259–1266. [CrossRef]
201. Karri, S.; Sharma, S.; Kaur, G. Pharmacological and analytical aspects of artemisinin for malaria: Advances and challenges. *Asian Pac. J. Trop. Med.* **2019**, *12*, 339–346. [CrossRef]
202. Rudrapal, M.; Chetia, D. Endoperoxide antimalarials: Development, structural diversity and pharmacodynamic aspects with reference to 1,2,4-trioxane-based structural scaffold. *Drug Des. Devel. Ther.* **2016**, *10*, 3575–3590. [CrossRef]
203. Krishna, S.; Bustamante, L.; Haynes, R.K.; Staines, H.M. Artemisinins: Their growing importance in medicine. *Trends Pharmacol. Sci.* **2008**, *29*, 520–527. [CrossRef] [PubMed]
204. Chaturvedi, D.; Goswami, A.; Saikia, P.P.; Barua, N.C.; Rao, P.G. Artemisinin and its derivatives: A novel class of anti-malarial and anti-cancer agents. *Chem. Soc. Rev.* **2010**, *39*, 435–454. [CrossRef] [PubMed]
205. O'Neill, P.M.; Barton, V.E.; Ward, S.A. The molecular mechanism of action of artemisinin—The debate continues. *Molecules* **2010**, *15*, 1705–1721. [CrossRef] [PubMed]
206. Sen, R.; Ganguly, S.; Saha, P.; Chatterjee, M. Efficacy of artemisinin in experimental visceral leishmaniasis. *Int. J. Antimicrob. Agents* **2010**, *36*, 43–49. [CrossRef]
207. WHO. *The World Malaria Report 2018*; WHO: Geneva, Switzerland, 2018. Available online: https://www.who.int/malaria/publications/world-malaria-report-2018/en/ (accessed on 26 October 2020).
208. Muangphrom, P.; Seki, H.; Fukushima, E.O.; Muranaka, T. Artemisinin-based antimalarial research: Application of biotechnology to the production of artemisinin, its mode of action, and the mechanism of resistance of Plasmodium Parasites. *J. Nat. Med.* **2016**, *70*, 318–334. [CrossRef]
209. Li, Q.; Weina, P. Artesunate: The best drug in the treatment of severe and complicated malaria. *Pharmaceuticals* **2010**, *3*, 2322–2332. [CrossRef]
210. Noubiap, J.J. Shifting from quinine to artesunate as first-line treatment of severe malaria in children and adults: Saving more lives. *J. Infect. Public Health.* **2014**, *7*, 407–412. [CrossRef]
211. Dondorp, A.M.; Fanello, C.I.; Hendriksen, I.C.E.; Gomes, E.; Seni, A.; Chhaganlal, K.D.; Bojang, K.; Olaosebikan, R.; Anunobi, N.; AQUAMAT Group; et al. Artesunate versus quinine in the treatment of severe falciparum malaria in African children (AQUAMAT): An open-label, randomised trial. *Lancet* **2010**, *376*, 1647–1657. [CrossRef]
212. Ferrari, G.F.; Ntuku, H.M.; Burri, C.; Tshefu, A.K.; Duparc, S.; Hugo, P.; Mitembo, D.K.; Rossi, A.; Ngwala, P.L.; Luwawu, J.N.; et al. An operational comparative study of quinine and artesunate for the treatment of severe malaria in hospitals and health centres in the Democratic Republic of Congo: The MATIAS study. *Malar. J.* **2015**, *14*, 226. [CrossRef]
213. Warsame, M.; Gyapong, M.; Mpeka, B.; Rodrigues, A.; Singlovic, J.; Babiker, A.; Mworozi, E.; Agyepong, I.; Ansah, E.; Azairwe, R.; et al. Pre-referral rectal artesunate treatment by community-based treatment providers in Ghana, Guinea-Bissau, Tanzania, and Uganda (Study 18): A cluster-randomized trial. *Clin. Infect. Dis.* **2016**, *63*, 312–321. [CrossRef]
214. Dobaño, C.; Nhabomba, A.J.; Manaca, M.N.; Berthoud, T.; Aguilar, R.; Quintó, L.; Barbosa, A.; Rodríguez, M.H.; Jiménez, A.; Groves, P.L.; et al. A Balanced Proinflammatory and Regulatory Cytokine Signature in Young African Children Is Associated With Lower Risk of Clinical Malaria. *Clin. Infect. Dis.* **2019**, *69*, 820–828. [CrossRef] [PubMed]
215. Das, S.; Manna, S.; Saha, B.; Hati, A.K.; Roy, S. Novel pfkelch13 gene polymorphism associates with artemisinin resistance in Eastern India. *Clin. Infect. Dis.* **2019**, *69*, 1144–1152. [CrossRef] [PubMed]
216. Kannan, D.; Yadav, N.; Ahmad, S.; Namdev, P.; Bhattacharjee, S.; Lochab, B.; Singh, A. Pre-clinical study of iron oxide nanoparticles fortified artesunate for efficient targeting of malarial parasite. *EBioMedicine* **2019**, *45*, 261–277. [CrossRef] [PubMed]
217. WHO. *Guidelines for the Treatment of Malaria*, 3rd ed.; World Health Organization: Geneva, Switzerland, 2015. Available online: https://www.who.int/docs/default-source/documents/publications/gmp/guidelines-for-the-treatment-of-malaria-eng.pdf (accessed on 26 October 2020).
218. Pull, L.; Lupoglazoff, J.M.; Beardmore, M.; Michel, J.F.; Buffet, P.; Bouchaud, O.; Siriez, J.Y. Artenimol–piperaquine in children with uncomplicated imported falciparum malaria: Experience from a prospective cohort. *Malar. J.* **2019**, *18*, 419. [CrossRef]
219. Leblanc, C.; Vasse, C.; Minodier, P.; Mornand, P.; Naudin, J.; Quinet, B.; Siriez, J.Y.; Sorged, F.; de Suremain, N.; Thellier, M.; et al. Management and prevention of imported malaria in children. Update of the French guidelines. *Med. Mal. Infect.* **2020**, *50*, 127–140. [CrossRef]
220. Lingani, M.; Bonkian, L.N.; Yerbanga, I.; Kazienga, A.; Valéa, I.; Sorgho, H.; Ouédraogo, J.B.; Mens, P.F.; Schallig, H.D.F.H.; Ravinetto, R.; et al. In vivo/ex vivo efficacy of artemether-lumefantrine and artesunate-amodiaquine as first-line treatment for uncomplicated falciparum malaria in children: An open label randomized controlled trial in Burkina Faso. *Malar. J.* **2020**, *19*, 8–13. [CrossRef]

221. Banda, C.G.; Chaponda, M.; Mukaka, M.; Mulenga, M.; Hachizovu, S.; Kabuya, J.B.; Mulenga, J.; Sikalima, J.; Kalilani-Phiri, L.; Terlouw, D.J.; et al. Efficacy and safety of artemether–lumefantrine as treatment for *Plasmodium falciparum* uncomplicated malaria in adult patients on efavirenz-based antiretroviral therapy in Zambia: An open label non-randomized interventional trial. *Malar. J.* **2019**, *18*, 180. [CrossRef]
222. Commons, R.J.; Simpson, J.A.; Thriemer, K.; Abreha, T.; Adam, I.; Anstey, N.M.; Assefa, A.; Awab, G.R.; Baird, K.J.; Barber, B.E.; et al. The efficacy of dihydroartemisinin-piperaquine and artemether-lumefantrine with and without primaquine on *Plasmodium vivax* recurrence: A systematic review and individual patient data meta-analysis. *PLoS Med.* **2019**, *16*, 1002928. [CrossRef]
223. Ballard, S.-B.; Salinger, A.; Arguin, P.M.; Desai, M.; Tan, K.R. Mphc Updated CDC Recommendations for Using Artemether-Lumefantrine for the Treatment of Uncomplicated Malaria in Pregnant Women in the United States. *Morb. Mortal. Wkly. Rep.* **2018**, *67*, 424–431. [CrossRef]
224. D'Alessandro, U.; Hill, J.; Tarning, J.; Pell, C.; Webster, J.; Gutman, J.; Sevene, E. Treatment of uncomplicated and severe malaria during pregnancy. *Lancet Infect. Dis.* **2018**, *18*, e133–e146. [CrossRef]
225. Ghantous, A.; Gali-Muhtasib, H.; Vuorela, N.; Saliba, A.; Darwiche, N. What made sesquiterpene lactones reach cancer clinical trials? *Drug Discov. Today* **2010**, *15*, 668–678. [CrossRef] [PubMed]
226. Zhang, Y.; Xu, G.; Zhang, S.; Wang, D.; Prabha, P.S.; Zuo, Z. Antitumor Research on Artemisinin and Its Bioactive Derivatives. *Nat. Prod. Bioprospect.* **2018**, *8*, 303–319. [CrossRef] [PubMed]
227. Slezakova, S.; Ruda-Kucerova, J. Anticancer activity of artemisinin and its derivatives. *Anticancer Res.* **2017**, *37*, 5995–6003. [CrossRef] [PubMed]
228. Dell'Eva, R.; Pfeffer, U.; Vene, R.; Anfosso, L.; Forlani, A.; Albini, A.; Efferth, T. Inhibition of angiogenesis in vivo and growth of Kaposi's sarcoma xenograft tumors by the anti-malarial artesunate. *Biochem. Pharmacol.* **2004**, *68*, 2359–2366. [CrossRef]
229. Crespo-Ortiz, M.; Wei, M. Antitumor activity of artemisinin and its derivatives: From a well-known antimalarial agent to a potential anticancer drug. *J. Biomed. Biotechnol.* **2012**, *2012*, 247597. [CrossRef]
230. Efferth, T. Artemisinin–Second career as anticancer drug? *World J. Tradit. Chin. Med.* **2015**, *1*, 2–25. [CrossRef]
231. Bhaw-Luximon, A.; Jhurry, D. Artemisinin and its derivatives in cancer therapy: Status of progress, mechanism of action, and future perspectives. *Cancer Chemother. Pharmacol.* **2017**, *79*, 451–466. [CrossRef]
232. Wong, Y.K.; Xu, C.; Kalesh, K.A.; He, Y.; Lin, Q.; Wong, W.S.F.; Shen, H.-M.; Wang, J. Artemisinin as an anticancer drug: Recent advances in target profiling and mechanisms of action. *Med. Res. Rev.* **2017**, *37*, 1492–1517. [CrossRef]
233. Von Hagens, C.; Walter-Sack, I.; Goeckenjan, M.; Osburg, J.; Storch-Hagenlocher, B.; Sertel, S.; Elsässer, M.; Remppis, B.A.; Edler, L.; Munzinger, J.; et al. Prospective open uncontrolled phase I study to define a well-tolerated dose of oral artesunate as add-on therapy in patients with metastatic breast cancer (ARTIC M33/2). *Breast Cancer Res. Treat.* **2017**, *164*, 359–369. [CrossRef]
234. Trimble, C.L.; Levinson, K.; Maldonado, L.; Donovan, M.J.; Clark, K.T.; Fu, J.; Shay, M.E.; Sauter, M.E.; Sanders, S.A.; Frantz, P.S.; et al. A first-in-human proof-of-concept trial of intravaginal artesunate to treat cervical intraepithelial neoplasia 2/3 (CIN2/3). *Gynecol. Oncol.* **2020**, *157*, 188–194. [CrossRef]
235. Burlec, A.F.; Cioancă, O.; Enache, L.C.; Hăncianu, M. Promising biological activities of sesquiterpene lactones. *Med. Surg. J.* **2017**, *121*, 645–652.
236. Krishna, S.; Ganapathi, S.; Ster, I.C.; Saeed, M.E.; Cowan, M.L.; Finlayson, C.; Kovacsevics, H.; Jansen, H.; Kremsner, P.G.; Efferth, T.; et al. A Randomised, Double Blind, Placebo-Controlled Pilot Study of Oral Artesunate Therapy for Colorectal Cancer. *EBioMedicine* **2015**, *2*, 82–90. [CrossRef] [PubMed]
237. Singh, N.P.; Panwar, V.K. Case report of a pituitary macroadenoma treated with artemether. *Integr. Cancer Ther.* **2006**, *5*, 391–394. [CrossRef] [PubMed]
238. Jansen, F.H.; Adoubi, I.; Comoe, K.; de Cnodder, T.; Jansen, N.; Tschulakow, A.; Efferth, T. First study of oral artenimol-R in advanced cervical cancer: Clinical benefit, tolerability and tumor markers. *Anticancer Res.* **2011**, *31*, 4417–4422.
239. Wang, S.J.; Gao, Y.; Chen, H.; Kong, R.; Jiang, H.C.; Pan, S.H.; Xue, D.-B.; Bai, X.-W.; Sun, B. Dihydroartemisinin inactivates NF-κB and potentiates the anti-tumor effect of gemcitabine on pancreatic cancer both in vitro and in vivo. *Cancer Lett.* **2010**, *293*, 99–108. [CrossRef] [PubMed]
240. Tilaoui, M.; Mouse, H.A.; Jaafari, A.; Zyad, A. Differential effect of artemisinin against cancer cell lines. *Nat. Prod. Bioprospect.* **2014**, *4*, 189–196. [CrossRef]
241. Zhang, Z.Y.; Yu, S.-P.; Miao, L.-Y.; Huanh, X.-Y.; Zhang, X.-P.; Zhu, Y.-P.; Xia, X.-H. Artesunate combined with vinorelbine plus cisplatin in treatment of advanced non-small cell lung cancer: A randomized controlled trial. *Chin. J. Integr. Med.* **2008**, *6*, 134–138. [CrossRef]
242. Liu, W.M.; Gravett, A.M.; Dalgleish, A.G. The antimalarial agent artesunate possesses anticancer properties that can be enhanced by combination strategies. *Int. J. Cancer* **2011**, *128*, 1471–1480. [CrossRef]
243. Beck, J.; Schwarzer, A.; Gläser, D.; Mügge, L.-O.; Uhlig, J.; Heyn, S.; Kragl, B.; Mohren, M.; Hoffmann, F.A.; Lange, T.; et al. Lenalidomide in combination with bendamustine and prednisolone in relapsed/refractory multiple myeloma: Results of a phase 2 clinical trial (OSHO-#077). *J. Cancer Res. Clin. Oncol.* **2017**, *143*, 2545–2553. [CrossRef]
244. Singh, N.P.; Verma, K.B. Case report of a laryngeal squamous cell carcinoma treated with artesunate. *Arch. Oncol.* **2002**, *10*, 279–280. [CrossRef]
245. Berger, T.G.; Dieckmann, D.; Efferth, T.; Schultz, E.S.; Funk, J.O.; Baur, A.; Schuler, G. Artesunate in the treatment of metastatic uveal melanoma–first experiences. *Oncol. Rep.* **2005**, *14*, 1599–1603. [CrossRef] [PubMed]

246. Liu, B.; Wang, C.; Chen, P.; Cheng, B.; Cheng, Y. RACK1 induces chemotherapy resistance in esophageal carcinoma by upregulating the PI3K/AKT pathway and Bcl-2 expression. *Oncol. Targets Ther.* **2018**, *11*, 211–220. [CrossRef] [PubMed]
247. Reungpatthanaphong, P.; Mankhetkorn, S. Modulation of multidrug resistance by artemisinin, artesunate and dihydroartemisinin in K562/adr and GLC4/adr resistant cell lines. *Biol. Pharm. Bull.* **2002**, *25*, 1555–1561. [CrossRef] [PubMed]
248. Kahler, M. Ueber einen neuen Stoff im Semen Cinae. *Arch. Pharm.* **2006**, *34*, 318–319. [CrossRef]
249. Sharma, S.; Anand, N. Natural Products. In *Pharmacochemistry Library Approaches to Design and Synthesis of Antiparasitic Drugs*; Sharma, S., Anand, N., Eds.; Elsevier: Amsterdam, The Netherlands, 1997; Volume 25, Chapter 3, pp. 71–123. [CrossRef]
250. Marshall, J.A.; Wuts, P.G.M. Stereocontrolled total synthesis of alpha- and beta-santonin. *J. Org. Chem.* **1978**, *43*, 1086–1089. [CrossRef]
251. Birladeanu, L. The stories of santonin and santonic acid. *Angew. Chem. Int. Ed.* **2003**, *42*, 1202–1208. [CrossRef]
252. Barton, D.H.R.; Moss, G.P.; Whittle, J.A. Investigations on the biosynthesis of steroids and terpenoids. Part I A preliminary study of the biosynthesis of santonin. *J. Chem. Soc. C* **1968**, 1813–1818. [CrossRef]
253. De Kraker, J.W.; Franssen, M.C.; Dalm, M.C.; de Groot, A.; Bouwmeester, H.J. Biosynthesis of germacrene A carboxylic acid in chicory roots. Demonstration of a cytochrome P450 (+)-germacrene a hydroxylase and NADP+-dependent sesquiterpenoid dehydrogenase(s) involved in sesquiterpene lactone biosynthesis. *Plant Physiol.* **2001**, *125*, 1930–1940. [CrossRef]
254. Wynn, S.G.; Fougère, B.J. Veterinary herbal medicine: A systems-based approach. In *Veterinary Herbal Medicine*; Wynn, S.G., Fougère, B.J., Eds.; Mosby: Saint Louis, MO, USA, 2007; Chapter 20, pp. 291–409, ISBN 978-0-323-02998-8.
255. Sakipova, Z.; Wong, N.S.H.; Bekezhanova, T.; Sadykova; Shukirbekova, A.; Boylan, F. Quantification of santonin in eight species of *Artemisia* from Kazakhstan by means of HPLC-UV: Method development and validation. *PLoS ONE* **2017**, *12*, 173714. [CrossRef]
256. Yang, D.-Z.; Du, L.-D.; Lu, Y. Santonin. In *Natural Small Molecule Drugs from Plants*; Du, G.-H., Ed.; PMPH Springer: Singapore, 2018; pp. 619–624. [CrossRef]
257. Zhang, H.; Liu, C.; Zheng, Q. Development and application of anthelminthic drugs in China. *Acta Trop.* **2019**, *200*, 105181. [CrossRef]
258. Xiao, S.-H. Progress in anthelmintic agent study since the founding of the People's Republic of China and current challenges. *Zhongguo Ji Sheng Chong Xue Yu Ji Sheng Chong Bing Za Zhi* **2009**, *27*, 383–389. [PubMed]
259. Yu, C.; Ai, D.; Lin, R.; Cheng, S. Effects of toxic β-glucosides on carbohydrate metabolism in cotton bollworm, *Helicoverpa armigera* (Hübner). *Arch. Insect Biochem. Physiol.* **2019**, *100*, e21526. [CrossRef] [PubMed]
260. Singh, B.; Kaur, A. Control of insect pests in crop plants and stored food grains using plant saponins: A review. *LWT* **2018**, *87*, 93–101. [CrossRef]
261. Wang, J.; Su, S.; Zhang, S.; Zhai, S.; Sheng, R.; Wu, W.; Guo, R. Structure-activity relationship and synthetic methodologies of α-santonin derivatives with diverse bioactivities: A mini-review. *Eur. J. Med. Chem.* **2019**, *175*, 215–233. [CrossRef] [PubMed]
262. Kim, S.H.; Song, J.H.; Choi, B.G.; Kim, H.-J.; Kim, T.S. Chemical modification of santonin into a diacetoxy acetal form confers the ability to induce differentiation of human promyelocytic leukemia cells via the down-regulation of NF-kappaB DNA binding activity. *J. Biol. Chem.* **2006**, *281*, 13117–13125. [CrossRef] [PubMed]
263. Khazir, J.; Singh, P.P.; Reddy, D.M.; Hyder, I.; Shafi, S.; Sawant, S.D.; Chashoo, G.; Mahajan, A.; Alam, M.S.; Saxena, A.K.; et al. Synthesis and anticancer activity of novel spiro-isoxazoline and spiro-isoxazolidine derivatives of α-santonin. *Eur. J. Med. Chem.* **2013**, *63*, 279–289. [CrossRef]
264. Domingo, L.R.; Ríos-Gutiérrez, M.; Acharjee, N. A Molecular electron density theory study of the chemoselectivity, regioselectivity, and diastereofacial selectivity in the synthesis of an anticancer spiroisoxazoline derived from α-santonin. *Molecules* **2019**, *24*, 832. [CrossRef]
265. Chen, H.; Yang, X.; Yu, Z.; Cheng, Z.; Yuan, H.; Zhao, Z.; Wu, G.; Xie, N.; Yuan, X.; Sun, Q.; et al. Synthesis and biological evaluation of α-santonin derivatives as anti-hepatoma agents. *Eur. J. Med. Chem.* **2018**, *149*, 90–97. [CrossRef]
266. Chinthakindi, P.K.; Singh, J.; Gupta, S.; Nargotra, A.; Mahajan, P.; Kaul, A.; Ahmed, Z.; Koul, S.; Sangwan, P.L. Synthesis of α-santonin derivatives for diminutive effect on T and B-cell proliferation and their structure activity relationships. *Eur. J. Med. Chem.* **2017**, *127*, 1047–1058. [CrossRef]
267. Quach, H.T.; Kondo, T.; Watanabe, M.; Tamura, R.; Yajima, Y.; Sayama, S.; Ando, M.; Kataoka, T. Eudesmane-type sesquiterpene lactones inhibit nuclear translocation of the nuclear factor κB subunit RelB in response to a lymphotoxin β stimulation. *Biol. Pharm. Bull.* **2017**, *40*, 1669–1677. [CrossRef]
268. Coricello, A.; El-Magboub, A.; Luna, M.; Ferrario, A.; Haworth, I.S.; Gomer, C.J.; Aiello, F.; Adams, J.D. Rational drug design and synthesis of new α-santonin derivatives as potential COX-2 inhibitors. *Bioorg. Med. Chem. Lett.* **2018**, *28*, 993–996. [CrossRef] [PubMed]
269. Filomena, P.; Luca, F.; Ian, H.; Matteo, B.; Asma, E.; Angela, F.; Charles, G.; Francesca, A.; David, A.J. Naturally occurring sesquiterpene lactones and their semi-synthetic derivatives modulate PGE2 levels by decreasing COX2 activity and expression. *Heliyon* **2019**, *5*, 1366. [CrossRef]
270. Chen, H.; Wu, F.; Gao, S.; Guo, R.; Zhao, Z.; Yuan, H.; Liu, S.; Wu, J.; Lu, X.; Yuan, X.; et al. Discovery of potent small-molecule inhibitors of ubiquitin-conjugating enzyme UbcH5c from α-santonin derivatives. *J. Med. Chem.* **2017**, *60*, 6828–6852. [CrossRef] [PubMed]
271. Issa, F.; Schiopu, A.; Wood, K.J. Role of T cells in graft rejection and transplantation tolerance. *Expert Rev. Clin. Immunol.* **2010**, *6*, 155–169. [CrossRef] [PubMed]

272. Dangroo, N.A.; Singh, J.; Gupta, N.; Singh, S.; Kaul, A.; Khuroo, M.A.; Sangwan, P.L. T- and B-cell immunosuppressive activity of novel α-santonin analogs with humoral and cellular immune response in Balb/c mice. *MedChemComm* **2017**, *8*, 211–219. [CrossRef]
273. White, E.H.; Winter, R.E.K. Natural products from *Achillea lanulosa*. *Tetrahedron Lett.* **1963**, *4*, 137–140. [CrossRef]
274. White, E.H.; Marx, J.N. The synthesis and stereochemistry of deacetoxymatricarin and achillin. *J. Am. Chem. Soc.* **1967**, *89*, 5511–5513. [CrossRef]
275. Kim, Y.S.; Bahn, K.N.; Hah, C.K.; Gang, H.I.; Ha, Y.L. Inhibition of 7,12-dimethylbenz[a]anthracene induced mouse skin carcinogenesis by *Artemisia capillaris*. *J. Food Sci.* **2008**, *73*, T16–T20. [CrossRef]
276. Zhang, R.; Wang, Y.; Hou, P.; Wen, G.; Gao, Y. Physiological responses to allelopathy of aquatic stem and leaf extract of *Artemisia frigida* in seedling of several pasture plants. *Acta Ecol. Sin.* **2010**, *30*, 2197–2204.
277. Kang, T.H.; Pae, H.O.; Jeong, S.J.; Yoo, J.C.; Choi, B.M.; Jun, C.D.; Chung, H.T.; Miyamoto, T.; Higuchi, R.; Kim, Y.C. Scopoletin: An inducible nitric oxide synthesis inhibitory active constituent from *Artemisia feddei*. *Planta Med.* **1999**, *65*, 400–403. [CrossRef]
278. Rivero-Cruz, I.; Anaya-Eugenio, G.; Pérez-Vásquez, A.; Martínez, A.L.; Mata, R. Quantitative analysis and pharmacological effects of *Artemisia ludoviciana* aqueous extract and compounds. *Nat. Prod. Comm.* **2017**, *12*, 1531–1534. [CrossRef]
279. Ho, C.; Choi, E.J.; Yoo, G.S.; Kim, K.-M.; Ryu, S.Y. Desacetylmatricarin, an anti-allergic component from *Taraxacum platycarpum*. *Planta Med.* **1998**, *64*, 577–578. [CrossRef] [PubMed]
280. Zaghloul, A.M.; Yusufoglu, H.S.; Salkini, M.A.A.; Alam, A. New cytotoxic sesquiterpene lactones from *Anthemis scrobicularis*. *J. Asian Nat. Prod. Res.* **2014**, *16*, 922–929. [CrossRef] [PubMed]
281. Banerjee, A.K.; Vera, W.J.; Gonzalez, N.C. Synthesis of terpenoid compounds from α-santonin. *Tetrahedron* **1993**, *49*, 4761–4788. [CrossRef]
282. Blust, M.H.; Hopkins, T.L. Gustatory responses of a specialist and a generalist grasshopper to terpenoids of *Artemisia ludoviciana*. *Entomol. Exp. Appl.* **1987**, *45*, 37–46. [CrossRef]
283. Sanchez-Carranza, J.N.; González-Maya, L.; Razo-Hernández, R.S.; Salas-Vidal, E.; Nolasco-Quintana, N.Y.; Clemente-Soto, A.F.; García-Arizmendi, L.; Sánchez-Ramos, M.; Marquina, S.; Alvarez, L. Achillin increases chemosensitivity to paclitaxel, overcoming resistance and enhancing apoptosis in human hepatocellular carcinoma cell line resistant to paclitaxel (Hep3B/PTX). *Pharmaceutics* **2019**, *11*, 512. [CrossRef]
284. Castro, V.; Murillo, R.; Klaas, C.A.; Meunier, C.; Mora, G.; Pahl, H.L.; Merfort, I. Inhibition of the transcription factor NF-κB by sesquiterpene lactones from *Podachaenium eminens* 1. *Planta Med.* **2000**, *66*, 591–595. [CrossRef]
285. Zapata-Martínez, J.; Sánchez-Toranzo, G.; Chaín, F.; Catalán, C.A.N.; Bühler, M.I. Effect of guaianolides in the meiosis reinitiation of amphibian oocytes. *Zygote* **2017**, *25*, 10–16. [CrossRef]
286. Li, Q.-Y.; Lou, J.; Yang, X.-G.; Lu, Y.-Q.; Lu, S.-S.; Lu, K.-H. Effect of the meiotic inhibitor cilostamide on resumption of meiosis and cytoskeletal distribution in buffalo oocytes. *Anim. Reprod. Sci.* **2016**, *174*, 37–44. [CrossRef]
287. Arias-Durán, L.; Estrada-Soto, S.; Hernández-Morales, M.; Chávez-Silva, F.; Navarrete-Vázquez, G.; León-Rivera, I.; Perea-Arango, I.; Villalobos-Molina, R.; Ibarra-Barajas, M. Tracheal relaxation through calcium channel blockade of *Achillea millefolium* hexanic extract and its main bioactive compounds. *J. Ethnopharmacol.* **2020**, *253*, 112643. [CrossRef]
288. Rustaiyan, A.; Sigari, H.; Jakupovic, J.; Grenz, M. A sesquiterpene lactone from *Artemisia diffusa*. *Phytochemistry* **1989**, *28*, 2723–2725. [CrossRef]
289. Rustaiyan, A.; Vahedi, M. Malaria parasites, traditional medicinal plants and artediffusin (tehranolide) as a new candidate of antimalaria agent. *J. Biological. Act. Prod. Nat.* **2012**, *2*, 200–217. [CrossRef]
290. Barrero, A.F.; Rosales, A.; Cuerva, J.M.; Oltra, J.E. Unified synthesis of eudesmanolides, combining biomimetic strategies with homogeneous catalysis and free-radical chemistry. *Org. Lett.* **2003**, *5*, 1935–1938. [CrossRef] [PubMed]
291. Patrushev, S.S.; Shakirov, M.M.; Shults, E.E. Synthetic transformations of sesquiterpene lactones 9. Synthesis of 13-(pyridinyl)eudesmanolides. *Chem. Heterocycl. Comp.* **2016**, *52*, 165–171. [CrossRef]
292. Rustaiyan, A.; Nahrevanian, H.; Kazemi, M. A new antimalarial agent; effect of extracts of *Artemisia diffusa* against *Plasmodium berghei*. *Pharmacogn. Mag.* **2009**, *5*, 1–7. [CrossRef]
293. Rustaiyan, A.; Nahrevanian, H.; Kazemi, M. Tehranolide, a sesquiterpene lactone with an endoperoxide group that probably has the same effect as the antimalarial agent artemisinin. *Planta Med.* **2009**, *75*, PD1. [CrossRef]
294. Rustaiyan, A.; Nahrevanian, H.; Kazemi, M. Isolation of artediffusin (tehranolide) as a new antimalarial agent. *Asian J. Chem.* **2011**, *23*, 4810–4814.
295. Wicht, K.J.; Mok, S.; Fidock, D.A. Molecular mechanisms of drug resistance in *Plasmodium falciparum* malaria. *Ann. Rev. Microbiol.* **2020**, *74*, 431–454. [CrossRef]
296. Rustaiyan, A.; Faridchehr, A.; Bakhtiyar, M. Sesquiterpene Lactones of Iranian Compositae Family (Astraceae); Their Chemical Constituents and Anti-plasmodial Properties of Tehranolide (A Review). *Orient. J. Chem.* **2017**, *33*, 2188–2197. [CrossRef]
297. Noori, S.; Taghikhani, M.; Hassan, Z.M.; Al-Lameh, A.; Mostafaei, A. Tehranolide could shift the immune response towards Th1 and modulate the intra-tumor infiltrated T regulatory cells. *Iran. J. Immunol.* **2009**, *6*, 216–224.
298. Noori, S.; Taghikhani, M.; Hassan, Z.M.; Allameha, A.; Mostafaei, A. Tehranolide molecule modulates the immune response, reduce regulatory T cell and inhibits tumor growth in vivo. *Mol. Immunol.* **2010**, *47*, 1579–1584. [CrossRef] [PubMed]
299. Sakaguchi, S. Naturally arising Foxp3-expressing CD25+ CD4+ regulatory T cells in immunological tolerance to self and non-self. *Nat. Immunol.* **2005**, *6*, 345–352. [CrossRef] [PubMed]

300. Noori, S.; Hassan, Z.M. Tehranolide inhibits proliferation of MCF-7 human breast cancer cells by inducing G0/G1 arrest and apoptosis. *Free Radic. Biol. Med.* **2012**, *52*, 1987–1999. [CrossRef] [PubMed]
301. Noori, S.; Hassan, Z.M. Tehranolide inhibits cell proliferation via calmodulin inhibition, PDE, and PKA activation. *Tumour Biol.* **2014**, *35*, 257–264. [CrossRef]
302. You, W.; Henneberg, M. Cancer incidence increasing globally: The role of relaxed natural selection. *Evol. Appl.* **2017**, *11*, 140–152. [CrossRef]
303. Sohrabi, C.; Alsa, Z.; O'Neill, N.; Khan, M.; Kerwan, A.; Al-Jabir, A.; Iosifidis, C.; Agha, R. World Health Organization declares global emergency: A review of the 2019 novel coronavirus (COVID-19). *Int. J. Surg.* **2020**, *76*, 71–76. [CrossRef]
304. Haq, F.U.; Roman, M.; Ahmad, K.; Rahman, S.U.; Shah, S.; Suleman, N.; Ullah, S.; Ahmad, I.; Ullah, W. *Artemisia annua*: Trials are needed for COVID-19. *Phytother. Res.* **2020**, *34*, 2423–2424. [CrossRef]
305. Zhuang, W.; Fan, Z.; Chu, Y.; Wang, H.; Yang, Y.; Wu, L.; Sun, N.; Sun, G.; Shen, Y.; Lin, X.; et al. Chinese patent medicines in the treatment of coronavirus disease 2019 (COVID-19) in China. *Front. Pharmacol.* **2020**, *11*, 1066. [CrossRef]
306. Zhao, Z.; Li, Y.; Zhou, L.; Zhou, X.; Xie, B.; Zhang, W.; Sun, J. Prevention and treatment of COVID-19 using Traditional Chinese Medicine: A review. *Phytomedicine* **2020**, in press. [CrossRef]
307. Efferth, T.; Romero, M.; Wolf, D.G.; Stamminger, T.; Marin, J.J.; Marschall, M. The antiviral activities of artemisinin and artesunate. *Clin. Infect. Dis.* **2008**, *47*, 804–811. [CrossRef]
308. Wang, C.; Xuan, X.; Yao, W.; Huang, G.; Jin, J. Anti-profibrotic effects of artesunate on bleomycin-induced pulmonary fibrosis in Sprague Dawley rats. *Mol. Med. Rep.* **2015**, *12*, 1291–1297. [CrossRef] [PubMed]
309. Li, S.-Y.; Chen, C.; Zhang, H.-Q.; Guo, H.-Y.; Wang, H.; Wang, L.; Zhang, X.; Hua, S.-N.; Yu, J.; Xiao, P.-G.; et al. Identification of natural compounds with antiviral activities against SARS-associated coronavirus. *Antivir. Res.* **2005**, *67*, 18–23. [CrossRef] [PubMed]
310. Islam, M.T.; Sarkar, C.; El-Kersh, D.M.; Jamaddar, S.; Uddin, S.J.; Shilpi, J.A.; Mubarak, M.S. Natural products and their derivatives against coronavirus: A review of the non-clinical and pre-clinical data. *Phytother. Res.* **2020**, *34*, 2471–2492. [CrossRef] [PubMed]
311. Lubbe, A.; Seibert, I.; Klimkait, T.; Van der Kooy, F. Ethnopharmacology in overdrive: The remarkable anti-HIV activity of *Artemisia annua*. *J. Ethnopharmacol.* **2012**, *141*, 854–859. [CrossRef] [PubMed]
312. Karamoddini, M.K.; Emami, S.A.; Ghannad, M.S.; Sani, E.A.; Sahebkar, A. Antiviral activities of aerial subsets of *Artemisia* species against herpes simplex virus type 1 (HSV1) in vitro. *Asian Biomed.* **2011**, *5*, 63–68. [CrossRef]
313. Rolta, R.; Salaria, D.; Kumar, V.; Sourirajan, A.; Dev, K. Phytocompounds of *Rheum emodi*, *Thymus serpyllum* and *Artemisia annua* inhibit COVID-19 binding to ACE2 receptor: In silico approach. *Res. Sq.* **2020**, in press. [CrossRef]
314. Kapepula, P.M.; Kabengele, J.K.; Kingombe, M.; Van Bambeke, F.; Tulkens, P.M.; Sadiki, A.; Decloedt, E.H.; Zumla, A.; Tiberi, S.; Suleman, F.; et al. *Artemisia* spp. derivatives for COVID-19 treatment: Anecdotal use, political hype, treatment potential, challenges, and road map to randomized clinical trials. *Am. J. Trop. Med. Hyg.* **2020**, *103*, 960–964. [CrossRef]

MDPI
St. Alban-Anlage 66
4052 Basel
Switzerland
Tel. +41 61 683 77 34
Fax +41 61 302 89 18
www.mdpi.com

Foods Editorial Office
E-mail: foods@mdpi.com
www.mdpi.com/journal/foods

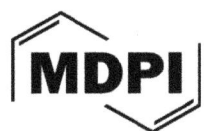

www.ingramcontent.com/pod-product-compliance
Lightning Source LLC
LaVergne TN
LVHW070504100526
838202LV00014B/1788